Principles of
Medicinal
Chemistry
Including **Proteomics**

A collection of theories and lecture notes for the students

Contributors

Amy De Nuan Huang Pharm D *(1.1.2.C)*
Thomas J. Long School of Pharmacy
University of the Pacific, Stockton
California 95211, US

Balaji Raghavan PhD *(2.4.4)*
Scientist, Laboratoire Roberval
UTC-CNRS (UMR6253)
Université de Technologie de Compiègne
Compiegne 60200, France

Betty De Suan Huang Pharm D *(1.1.2.D)*
Thomas J. Long School of Pharmacy
University of the Pacific, Stockton
California 95211, US

Janarthanan Krishnamoorthy PhD
(1.1.2.B; 2.3.2.C2.c; 1.5.11–Discussion 1.21)
Postdoctoral Fellow
Department of Chemistry and Biochemistry
Auburn University, Alabama 36830, US

J Sivaraman, PhD *(1.1.2.A)*
Associate Professor
Department of Biological Sciences
National University of Singapore
Singapore 117543

Contributed section numbers are given in parantheses with discussion numbers where applicable.

Principles of
Medicinal
Chemistry
Including **Proteomics**

A collection of theories and lecture notes for the students

Sushilee Ranganathan B Pharm MS
Resource Person, the Drug Design Workshop Series
Madras Medical College
Chennai TAMIL NADU INDIA

A Jerad Suresh MBA PhD
Principal, College of Pharmacy
Madras Medical College
Chennai TAMIL NADU INDIA

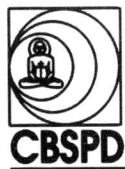

CBSPD

CBS Publishers & Distributors Pvt Ltd

New Delhi • Bengaluru • Chennai • Kochi • Kolkata • Lucknow • Mumbai
Hyderabad • Jharkhand • Nagpur • Patna • Pune • Uttarakhand

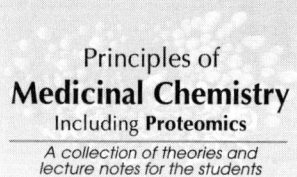

Principles of
Medicinal Chemistry
Including **Proteomics**
*A collection of theories and
lecture notes for the students*

ISBN: 978-81-239-1986-7

Copyright © Authors and Publishers

First Edition: 2011
Reprint: **2024**

Published by **Satish Kumar Jain** and produced by **Varun Jain** for

CBS Publishers & Distributors Pvt Ltd
4819/XI Prahlad Street, 24 Ansari Road, Daryaganj, New Delhi 110 002, India.
Ph: 011-23266838, 23289259   Website: www.cbspd.com
                                  e-mail: delhi@cbspd.com

Corporate Office: 204 FIE, Industrial Area, Patparganj, Delhi 110 092
Ph: 011-4934 4934   Fax: 011-4934 4935
                                e-mail: publishing@cbspd.com; publicity@cbspd.com

Branches

• **Bengaluru:** Seema House 2975, 17th Cross, KR Road, Banasankari 2nd Stage, Bengaluru 560 070, Karnataka, India
  Ph: +91-80-26771678/79   Fax: +91-80-26771680   e-mail: bangalore@cbspd.com
• **Chennai:** 7, Subbaraya Street, Shenoy Nagar, Chennai 600 030, Tamil Nadu, India
  Ph: +91-44-26680620, 26681266   Fax: +91-44-42032115   e-mail: chennai@cbspd.com
• **Kochi:** 42/1325, 1326, Power House Road, Opp KSEB, Power House, Ernakulam Kochi 682 018, Kerala, India
  Ph: +91-484-4059061-65,67   Fax: +91-484-4059065   e-mail: kochi@cbspd.com
• **Kolkata:** 147, Hind Ceramics Compound, 1st Floor, Nilgunj Road, Belghoria, Kolkata-700056, West Bengal, India
  Ph: +033-25633055, 033-25633056   e-mail: kolkata@cbspd.com
• **Lucknow:** Basement, Khushnuma Complex, 7 Meerabai Marg (Behind Jawahar Bhawan), Lucknow-226001, UP, India
  Ph: +0522-4000032   e-mail: tiwari.lucknow@cbspd.com
• **Mumbai:** PWD Shed, Gala no 25/26, Ramchandra Bhatt Marg, Next to JJ Hospital Gate no. 2, Opp. Union Bank of India,
  Noorbaug, Mumbai-400009, Maharashtra, India
  Ph: 022-66661880/89   e-mail: mumbai@cbspd.com

Representatives

| • Hyderabad | 0-9885175004 | • Jharkhand | 0-9811541605 | • Nagpur | 0-8692091830 |
| • Patna | 0-9334159340 | • Pune | 0-9664372571 | • Uttarakhand | 0-9716462459 |

Printed at Glorious Printers, Jhilmil Industrial Area, Delhi, India

Preface

The spectacular revolution in genomics and the extensive deployment of computing facilities around the world has paved the way for advanced proteomics and intelligent drug design. Today's research, job and academic scenario demands multidisciplinary knowledge and communication. We believe that research data *per se* is valueless to the student unless he/she is able to apply this information in a systematic and meaningful way. A gap analysis in these lines informs us that there is an unmet demand for texts that consolidate topics, projects and publications in medicinal chemistry and its various related fields. This book has been designed for students of life sciences doing their bachelors and masters as well as PhD having in mind the syllabi of the various universities across the country. This text does not present "everything one wanted to know about medicinal chemistry", but only a broad and multidisciplinary introduction to the field. For a book of this size, we present more than 300 original pedagogic illustrations, discussions, boxes and *did-you-know*s that informs the students of interesting principles and simultaneously preserves the flow of the main text.

Written in an informal style, the authors of this book intend that students be exposed to current computational techniques with an experimental background. Contributions in various fields such as nuclear magnetic resonance, X-ray crystallography, genetic algorithm, etc. from the invited contributors with sound experimental and theoretical knowledge greatly enrich the perspectives to medicinal chemistry contained in this book. The facets of drug designing have now been presented as a seamless fabric of interrelated principles. There are numerous reference works of exceptional depth and quality on proteins, therapeutics, computational chemistry, etc. There simultaneously exists a great disparity in the exposure received by the students in various fields of life sciences. The result: Students remain oblivious to current trends and freely accessible sources of information during the days of college education. This book intends to partly overcome this imbalance. It contains the research and opinions of scientists around the world that are aptly referenced. We have listed works of original authors, papers that contain methodology that might interest students, open access papers and latest exhaustive reviews. Last but not least, we are thankful to contributors who worked diligently to simplify and update their parts. We also appreciate the efforts of all those involved in proofreading the manuscript.

Sushilee Ranganathan is indebt to the committed mentoring of Dr. rer. nat. Elfi Kraka and Dr. rer. nat. Dieter Cremer during her MS degree in subject and otherwise, and wishes to dedicate this book to them.

Sushilee Ranganathan BPharm MS
Resource person, the Drug Design Workshop Series
Madras Medical College, Chennai, Tamil Nadu 600003, India

A Jerad Suresh MBA PhD
Principal, College of Pharmacy
Madras Medical College, Chennai, Tamil Nadu 600003, India

Contents

Plate 1

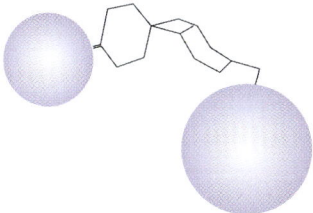

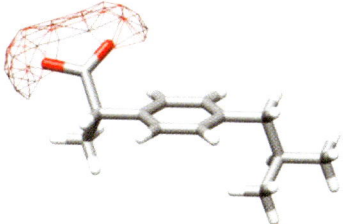

Some groups pose strong steric hindrance and can accommodate only very specific types and arrangements of proteins side chains around them.

Some moieties exert strong electrostatic influence and need to be complemented by residue side chains with contrasting properties.

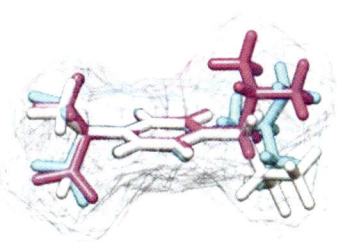

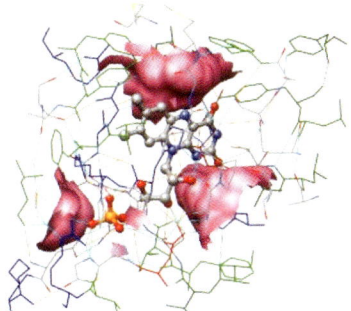

When 'circumscribing' the protein, a certain degree of flexibility must be allowed for the ligand to orient and flip around at the binding site.

The protein (receptor) is constructed around the ligand. The predicted structure of the protein in this area can be refined.

Fig. 1.42: Schematic representation of the role of receptor mapping in structure prediction; known ligands can be used to refine the structure of a protein of unknown structure

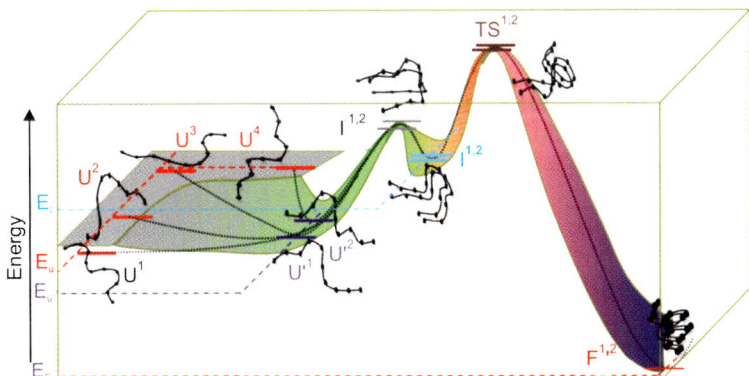

Fig. 1.50: The potential energy surface indicating the variations in conformations at selected points along the surface. Unfolded conformers (U^1–U^4) of approximately degenerate energy E_u form locally favored structures (U'^1, U'^2) of slightly lower energy ($E_{u'}$) at the start of folding. These latter conformations pass through a transition state (I'^1 or I'^2) and become stable intermediates of folding ($I^{1,2}$ of energy E_I). Next, the rate limiting transition to final folded conformer ($F^{1,2}$) of low energy (E_F) occurs by passing through the TS of folding ($TS^{1,2}$). At each stage from left to right, the variety of molecules (the diversity of the members of each ensemble) reduces, the unfolded molecule being most flexible and the folded, being most rigid, indicated by the spacing between horizontal lines that represent each conformer

Plate 2

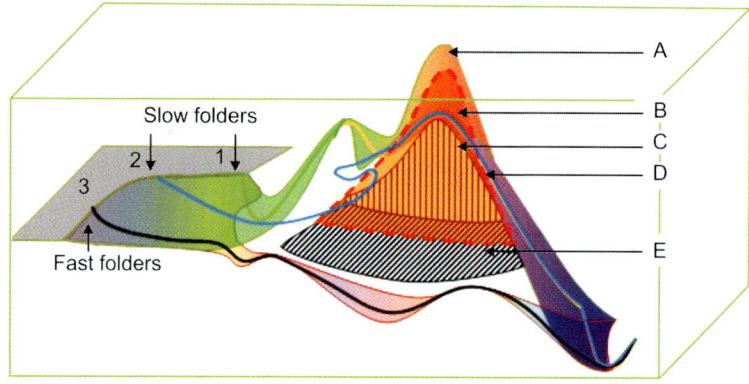

(A) "First Mountain", (B) Valley, (C) Cross section: Steep rise to a 2nd mountain,
(D) (red) Outline of 2nd mountain, (E) Base area of 2nd mountain

Fig. 1.53: The rate of folding depends on the path taken by the protein to reach the native state–a comparison among conformations 1–3

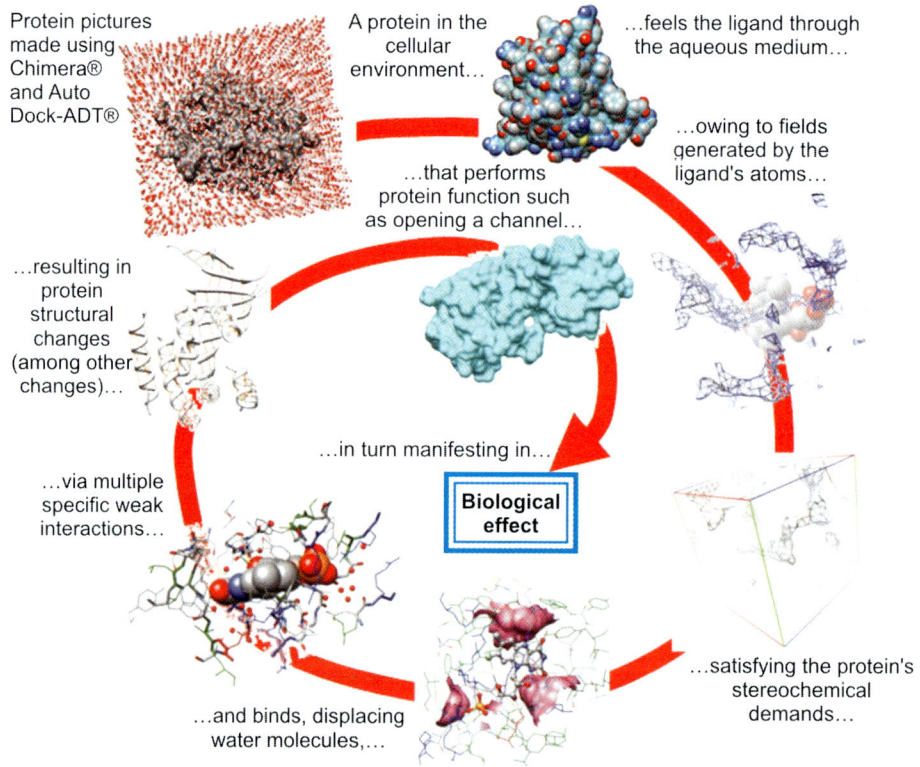

Scheme 2.3: An overview of protein–ligand interaction

Plate 3

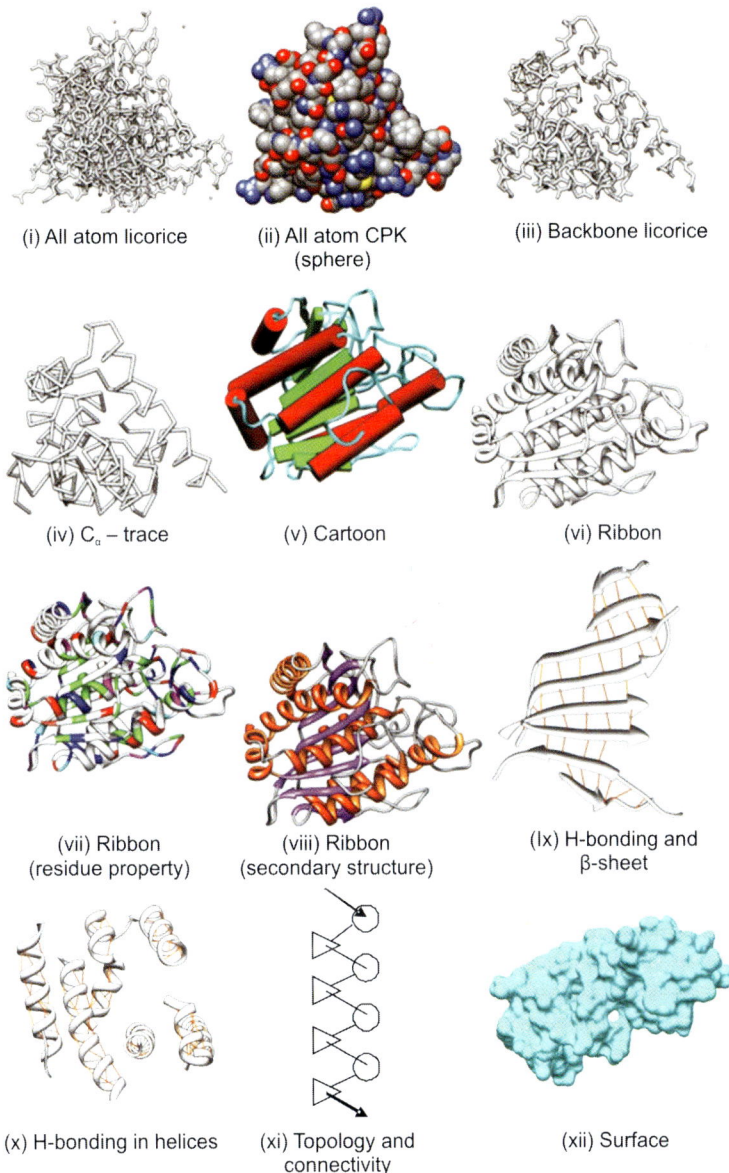

(i) All atom licorice

(ii) All atom CPK (sphere)

(iii) Backbone licorice

(iv) C_α – trace

(v) Cartoon

(vi) Ribbon

(vii) Ribbon (residue property)

(viii) Ribbon (secondary structure)

(lx) H-bonding and β-sheet

(x) H-bonding in helices

(xi) Topology and connectivity

(xii) Surface

Fig. 2.13: Representations of proteins

Plate 4

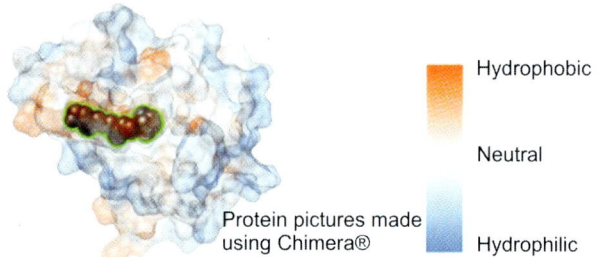

Hydrophobic

Neutral

Protein pictures made
using Chimera®

Hydrophilic

Discussion 2.17c: Hydrophobic retinol in the hydrophobic pocket of retinol binding protein is visualized by constructing an SES

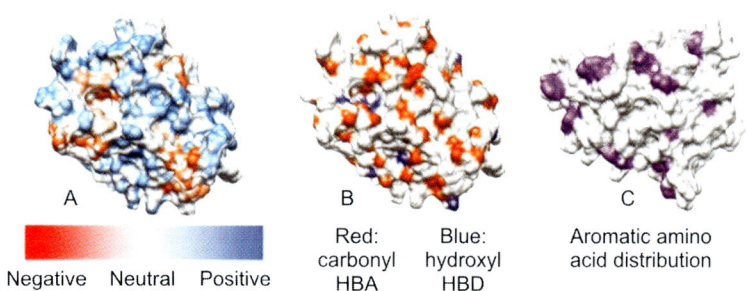

A

Negative   Neutral   Positive

B

Red: Blue:
carbonyl   hydroxyl
HBA   HBD

C

Aromatic amino
acid distribution

Fig. 2.14: Mapping properties on a surface

Part I
Receptors, Enzymes, Hormones, Carriers: The Proteins

Proteins are perhaps the most complex chemical entities in nature. No other class of molecule exhibits the variety and irregularity in shape, size, texture and mobility that can be found in proteins.

— Baxevanis, et al.

1.1 *Introduction*

The word *protein* is derived from the Greek word *prôtos*, meaning *of great importance*. It is also known to come from *Proteus*, a Greek sea god, who, being ever curious of what the land is like, and not being able to enter it in his original form lest he floods the cities, changed his form to that of a bird, beast or human. Even in early days, when scientist did not have a 600 MHz nuclear magnetic resonance spectrometer sitting in a lab right across the hallway, the variability of protein structure and versatility of its function has been suspected and appreciated—probably from studies on the "primordial soup" and the origin of life. Scientists from all fields, related in however remote a manner, embark upon this journey to determine protein structure, function and dynamics in a collective initiative to do what we would like to call "pinning proteus down". The first part of this book deals with the progress made in this incredible and adventurous quest wherein we follow the footsteps of time. The best chemist *nature* has taken over 3 million years to evolve its current biochemistry. Hopefully, with the help of computers, man does not need that long to catch up!

The study of proteins generously contributes to and greedily imbibes from numerous related and seemingly unrelated fields. Some of these fields are depicted in Scheme 1.1. This aspect makes the study of proteins interesting, informative, potent, prospective and speculative as to the scope of its applications and the impact of its findings on other fields.

Recent advances in technology in computers, chemistry and bioanalytical techniques, have allowed us to sequence the DNA, or genome, of a cell. Today, we have in various databases on the web, genomic sequence data for humans and many other species (insects, plants, simple multicellular organisms, microorganisms) and more are constantly being determined. This information, however, is useless unless we learn to read the genetic code meaningfully. The study of how one can relate this linear sequence of guanines, adenines, thymines and cytosines to cell function is called *functional genomics*. One of the most important genome products that deal with this function is the protein. They are also the most abundant–comprising of more than half the dry weight of a cell.

Details of its three-dimensional (3D) structure (dealt within chapter 1.2) are important to understand cell functioning and chemistry that sustain life, just as an understanding of DNA structure (the double helix it forms) led to the elucidation of the mechanisms that uphold the *central dogma* of biology - of how genetic information becomes functional and is passed on. Structure of proteins is not static like plastic models–there is no protein function without accounting for motion (chapter 1.3). However, in the form of pre-specified information, all the cell does is add together all ingredients of the protein recipe–the amino acids–in the order mentioned in the cookbook–the genetic code. Somehow, the protein is able to figure out what it must turn itself into, and how, without any hassle.

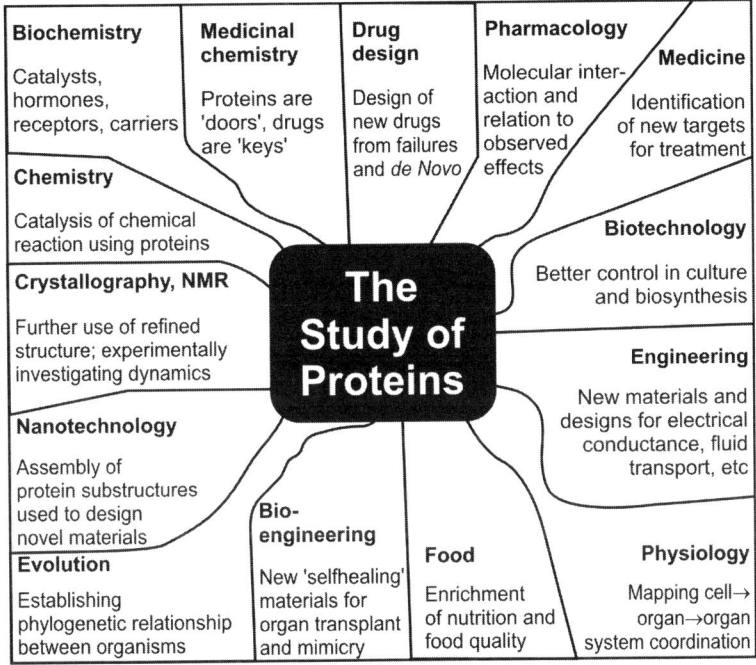

Scheme 1.1: The 'give-and-take' between the study of proteins and other fields of science

Investigations on how proteins know their final shape and how they attain it are presented in chapters 1.4 and 1.5 that deal with "protein structure prediction" and "protein folding" respectively. A simple understanding of isolated structure of protein alone does not suffice; the moral of biology is coordination and cooperation. Millions of cells in the body of any organism interact via messengers and keep each other constantly updates about current affairs in the cell. Proteins, being the "workhorses of the cell", interact and this is described in Part III.

Did You Know? 1
Important unsolved problems in science

Science magazine's description (2005) of the 125 most important unsolved problems in science states:

"Can we predict how proteins will fold? Out of a near infinitude of possible ways to fold, a protein picks one in just tens of microseconds. The same task takes 30 years of computer time."

Insight into protein functions and their mechanism allows, (1) Target discovery which is one of the stages of drug discovery wherein macromolecules in the body that regulate/carry out biochemistry are targeted to set right malfunctioning in a diseased state, and (2) Target selection (this is needed as there are many such macromolecules: proteins, DNA, RNA, etc.). The above information obtained in any way becomes useless

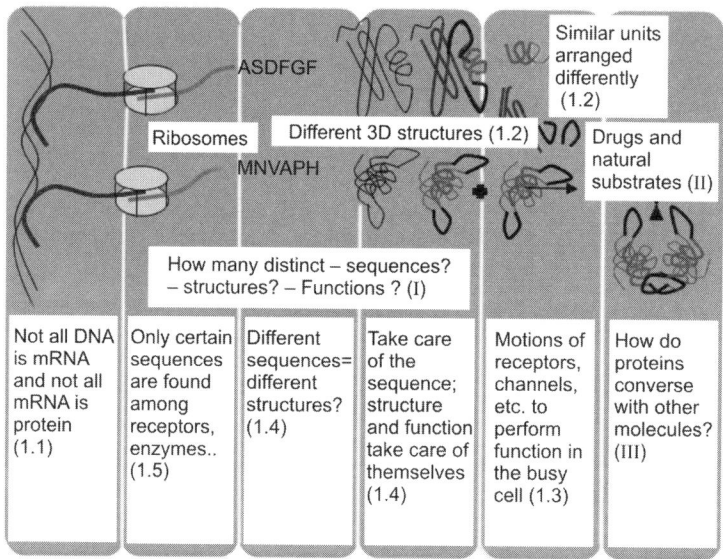

Scheme 1.2: Various aspects in the study of proteins

unless it is applied. With the availability of such a large number of protein structures and an even larger number of sequenced proteins, this information needs to be complemented with tissue distribution and pharmacological role in the body. Therefore, one needs an overall understanding of all protein-related processes experimentally and theoretically as the protein is identified, expressed, isolated, crystallized, purified, and its structure determined using nuclear magnetic resonance (NMR) spectroscopy/X-ray crystallography, refined for significant accuracy, deposited in a data bank in the form of coordinates making it available to researchers who wish to understand biology.

1.1.1 PROTEOMICS: THE STUDY OF PROTEINS

By analyzing the shape and size of a planet, NASA scientists are able to get an idea of its past-on how it was formed, as well as whether or not the planet is capable of supporting life. By simply looking at an airplane, even a layman can guess on the one hand, that it is built to fly and on the other hand, that it must be made of light-weight as well sturdy material. Similarly, analyzing protein structure gives us a tool to extrapolate in two different directions–on how amino acid sequences are organized to make up the protein, and, to perform what ultimate function the protein is enlisted in the genetic code. Transport proteins in the blood are globular in shape (in fact, a fraction of them are called globulins) because the sphere takes up the least surface area and volume, and this avoids interference with the million other activities taking part in the blood. Membrane proteins (that are either partly or completely buried in the plasma membrane) have a hydrophobic region so that they can remain in contact with the membrane lipids and function as the link between the intra- and extra-cellular environments. Similarly, spider silk fibroin is long and strong, spectrin C protecting erythrocytes is tough like luggage cases need to be across a trans-Atlantic flight, and titin, which is elastic, is integral to musculature. In addition, each sequence is unique– to match the protein's functioning.

The study of all these facets and more about proteins is collectively the field of proteomics. Proteomics is both deep and vast. Once interested and enthusiastic about this field, it is easy to loose oneself in its vast details and fascinating theories resulting from ongoing research. Although the first part of this book on medicinal chemistry attempts to put forth various aspects of the proteins (that medicinal chemists encounter as receptors, hormones, enzymes, etc.), it has been presented with information on how all this pure theory can be applied in drug design. *Proteomics roadmap to medicinal chemistry* is a chapter that is distributed in parts throughout the Part I and at the end of Part III of this book and is presented in the following way (Table 1.1):

Table 1.1: About the chapter "Proteomics roadmap to medicinal chemistry"	
Proteomics roadmap to medicinal chemistry 1	on protein structure
Proteomics roadmap to medicinal chemistry 2	on protein dynamics
Proteomics roadmap to medicinal chemistry 3	on structure prediction
Proteomics roadmap to medicinal chemistry 4	on protein folding
Proteomics roadmap to medicinal chemistry 5	on protein interactions

All these chapters put together serves to inform the reader of the medicinal chemistry goals that can be accomplished with this protein-knowledge. In addition, it also enumerates the ways in which theories and methods explained in this part can be used to take important decisions and interpret results effectively in all drug design projects that involve proteins. It helps to reinforce the theory based on which docking, rational drug design, 3D-QSAR and other computational procedures appearing in Part II and III are set up; and modern medicinal chemists need to deal with these procedures on a regular basis.

1.1.2 EXPERIMENTAL BACKGROUND

"The adventures first… explanations take such a dreadful time."
The Gryphon, in Alice's adventures in Wonderland by Lewis Carroll

Typically, in a molecular biology laboratory, the tissues of animals suffering from a particular disease condition are analyzed and compared with healthy tissues. A number of contemporary techniques (one of which is the DNA microarray) help to rapidly identify the differences in the cell constitution of the diseased and the healthy tissues. This might result in the identification of a few genes or genetic products such as proteins. Using another set of advanced recombinant techniques developed in similar labs, cell lines are constructed that contain the identified gene or express the identified protein (after the gene responsible for the protein has been found out and inserted). Even during the construction of the cell line, provisions are made to identify the protein and to favor its isolation, such as biosynthesizing them with fluorescent tags by tricking the genetic machinery of the cell (this is called a *gene reporter system*; *Ref.* textbooks on molecular biology such as (Elliott, 2009) for details). After isolation and cleavage of rthe artificially inserted tag, the protein is purified, crystallized, sequenced and subjected to X-ray analysis or the pure protein in a suitable solvent is subjected to NMR spectroscopy. A set of XYZ coordinates result, for every atom that can be detected by these techniques with the help of specialized software. Please *ref.* section 1.1.2 A. *Protein crystallography* and section 1.1.2 B. *Determining structure by nuclear* magnetic resonance spectroscopy for an outline of the principle involved in both these analytical processes.

In all the steps described above, there is chance for failure or error given the difficult, elaborate and time consuming nature of the tasks. The accessibility of the genomic product and the feasibility of setting up of bioassays that can screen for relevant active ligand compounds (at a high throughput, as done in industries) are the next major concerns. Research and technical advancements are constantly coming to the aid of these problems. An example is of how the large-scale production of proteins was made possible from recombinant DNA circumventing restrictions and regulations is presented in Discussion 1.1 progress in the above fields brings us closer to relating the sequence–structure–function of proteins. Computers are increasingly used to keep track of the knowledge gained in various fields via simulations. One cannot "look" at a molecule's conformation in the cell without *computations*. The closest one can get is to infer molecular structure from the patterns generated by a purified compound using X-ray or NMR information. The application of computers includes (as a small part) performing simulations. If the computer is able to mimic a system and give results comparable to those obtained in experiments, then we know, in terms of underlying theories, all we need to know about the system. This, of course, is easier said than done, but computational chemistry and computational biology are far from "unpromising". In many cases, computers are able to suggest structures that are more accurate than the experimentally determined ones–a repetition of experiment with great care and detail has showed how theoretical speculations of experimental errors in protein structures were correct (Sippl, et al. 1994).

Discussion 1.1: Breakthroughs are multifaceted

We are all familiar with recombinant DNA technology and the use of E Coli as a means of biosynthesizing proteins. However, not all proteins can be synthesized using bacterial cultures and during the time it was introduced, large scale synthesis of proteins using mammalian cells posed huge problems. In the 1980s, a breakthrough was achieved and the first large-scale process was developed by Genentech, Inc. (South San Francisco, California) for production of recombinant tissue plasminogen activator (tPA). This product is a fibrinolytic used in the treatment of heart attack and stroke. The following highlight the breakthroughs at the wake of marketing this drug:

1. Chinese hamster ovary (CHO) cell line was transformed, to replicate indefinitely so that cells will always be present to constantly produce tPA

2. It was required by FDA that cells used should be "normal" and these cells are not. Moreover, these cells are the precursors to cancer. Genetech convinced FDA for the first time that tPA injection does not contain carcinogens or carcinogenic substances

3. Till then, mammalian cell lines were only grown in rolling bottle cultures attached to the container's surface. This prevented large scale production because the bottles could not simply be made large-sized. Therefore, as a next step, Genentech introduced the suspension culture of the CHO cells in order to facilitate collection of protein

4. Serum-free medium was used (next large-scale breakthrough) to reduce complications in isolating and purifying the tPA protein. This greatly cut cost of production

5. The first ever large scale 'bioreactor' was constructed that involved detailed design of stirring and flow.
   a. The cells had to be stirred and required constant supply of oxygen and nutrients
   b. Special low shear filtration technology was needed to take care of removal of formed waste products
   c. Being extremely fragile, the stirring had to be done very carefully resulting in specially designed impellers with careful study of fluid flow. Engineers for this mission needed a recondite understanding of biology of cells in addition to their knowledge on fluid physics.

Such an enterprise brought together scientists and engineers from a wide variety of backgrounds. In addition, it also initiated several amendments to the existing regulations in drug manufacturing and marketing. (National research council, USA: Committee on challenges, 2003)

1.1.2A Protein Crystallography

J. Sivaraman

Introduction

The cell is the structural and functional unit of life. Cells contain organelles like mitochondria, supramolecular complexes like ribosomes, biological macromolecules and many simple molecules. Biological macromolecules are defined as large molecules made up of smaller organic molecules such as peptides, nucleotides and sugars. Three classes of macromolecules have been known to be present in cells namely carbohydrates, proteins and nucleic acids. Proteins are the most important biological macromolecules playing vital and integral roles in all living systems. The human body contains thousands of different proteins such as hemoglobin (oxygen carrier), ferritin (iron storage protein), immunoglobulins (immunoprotectants) and enzymes (biocatalysts), all playing essential roles in maintaining biological systems.

In general, a protein's structure determines the specific role it plays in the human body. The specificity of active sites and binding sites in proteins depend on the three dimensional structure of the protein. Inappropriate folding of proteins not only results in inactive proteins but sometimes also lead to pathological conditions. The case of prion proteins of the brain involved in the mad cow disease is one such example.[1] Several other diseases such as Alzheimer's, various cancers, and cystic fibrosis arise from defects in protein folding.[2] Currently, there is a lack of detailed knowledge about the structures of many proteins. Several techniques are employed to determine the three dimensional atomic resolution structures of proteins. Two major techniques that have been widely used to elucidate protein structure are single crystal X-ray diffraction and Nuclear Magnetic Resonance (NMR) spectroscopy. Structural studies of proteins using these techniques, in particular, will result in identifying the critical molecular determinants, which serve to inhibit and control the activities of these proteins. With an improved understanding of the molecular structures and interactions of proteins, new drug treatments could be developed to target specific human, animal, and plant diseases.

For proteins that form suitable crystals, X-ray crystallography represents a mature and rapid approach. It is a robust experimental technique, which enables determination of three-dimensional structures of proteins, and thus an understanding of their functional roles. As of February 2010, more than 85% of the structures deposited in the protein data bank [PDB] have been solved using X-ray crystallography (http://www.rcsb.org/pdb/home/home.do). In fact, the importance of structure determination by crystallography can be guaged by the awarding of several Nobel prizes in Chemistry and Medicine.[3] The history of X-ray crystallography dates back to the early 20th century. Bragg[4], et al. determined the first crystal structure, that of Sodium chloride [NaCl] in 1912. The first macromolecular structure for sperm whale myoglobin was solved in 1958 by John Kendrew, et al.[5] These discoveries won them Nobel prizes.

In general, X-ray crystallography works by determining the spatial arrangements of individual atoms in the crystal, by interpreting the scattering of the X-ray beam by electrons within a crystal. X-rays are reflected from evenly spaced planes of a crystal and this produces diffraction spots known as reflections on an image detector. Intensities of these diffraction images are measured as the crystal is rotated gradually in the X-ray beam. These diffraction images are subsequently analyzed mathematically and a three dimensional electron density map is calculated, which represents the atomic arrangement in the crystal.

The technique of protein crystallography can be summarized into three basic steps:

- In the first step, one starts with a single crystal of the protein grown to an adequate quality and size. The crystal should be regular in structure with no cracks, twinning or other deformities as observed in a macroscope (Fig. 1.1). This is often considered the rate limiting step in protein structure determination.
- The second step is the collection of diffraction data. It involves placing the crystal in the path of an intense X-ray beam of single wavelength. This produces a regular diffraction pattern of reflection with substantial number of diffraction spots of different intensities (Fig. 1.2). Multiple images are collected by rotating the crystal.

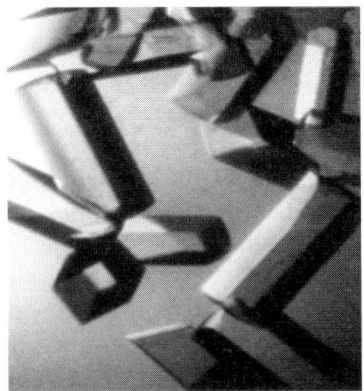

Fig. 1.1: Protein crystals: Crystals of a non-structural protein VP9 from White Spot Syndrome Virus[6]

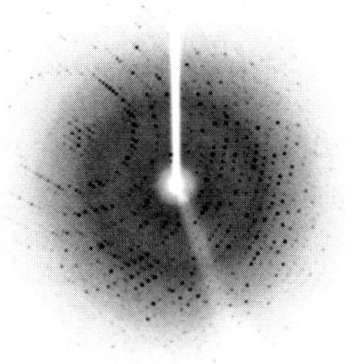

Fig. 1.2: Diffraction image: X-ray diffraction pattern of a protein crystal

- Finally, these data are computationally analyzed to produce an electron density map, which represents the arrangement of individual atoms in the crystal (Fig. 1.3). Based on the electron density map, a model of the protein molecule is built and refined using specialized computer programs.

The brief methodology for protein crystallography is discussed in the following paragraphs.

Protein Sample Preparation and Crystallization

Crystallization requires large quantities of highly concentrated pure protein which is often difficult to obtain from native source organism. Researchers thus resort to overexpression systems. The gene coding for the protein of interest is first cloned into a suitable vector and transformed into an appropriate host organism. The overexpressed protein is extracted from the cells of the host system by cell lysis and is then subjected to several purification steps. The purity and yield of the protein is monitored at each and every stage of purification by running Sodium Dodecyl Sulfate Polyacrylamide Gel Electrophoresis (SDS-PAGE), native PAGE, nonreducing PAGE, Western blot, and/or Mass Spectrometry to mention a few. The purified protein is then concentrated for crystallization experiments. The hydrodynamic homogeneity

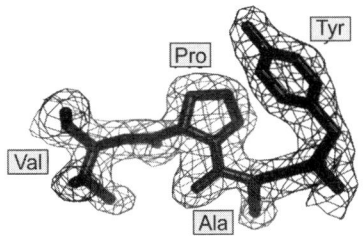

Fig. 1.3: Electron density map: Shows the electron density to model Tyrosine and Valine amino acids of the protein Sgm

of the protein sample significantly affects crystallization of the protein. Monodisperse protein samples have high chance of crystallization.[7] The hydrodynamic homogeneity is monitored using dynamic light scattering experiments. The obtained homogenous protein is subsequently subjected to crystallization trials which involve a search for an appropriate condition that will facilitate the protein to form the crystals.

Proteins stay in solution only up to certain concentration, once this concentration is reached, the solution will no longer be homogenous and will start forming a new phase depending on the crystallization buffer. The whole idea of crystallization trials is to identify a proper crystallization condition containing buffer, salt and precipitant that can slowly shift the highly concentrated homogeneous protein from a saturated state to a state of ordered aggregation (crystal formation). The identified initial condition from the screening experiments will further be optimized to obtain better quality crystals. There are different set-ups used for crystallization screening some of which are sitting drops, hanging drops, sandwich drops, free interface diffusion and microbatch under oil method. Protein crystals formed usually contain about 40–60% solvent by weight and are thus fragile and sensitive to drying out. Protein crystals diffract X-rays only when they are wet.

Amongst various parameters required for crystallization, the most important are the purity, homogeneity, solubility and stability of the proteins as well as their individual properties such as isoelectric focusing point and the balance between their hydrophilic and hydrophobic amino acids. Crystals can occasionally be grown from impure protein samples, but their size and quality improve only as the purity increases. If the protein contains significant amounts of contaminants, further purification is recommended. However, if the sample contains minor impurities and/or only a few milligrams of protein is available, it is worth trying screening conditions for crystallization. Further purification can be used to optimize the crystallization condition and thus to grow better quality crystals. Occasionally protein cleavage by proteolysis can be a reason for failure in crystallization or for crystals of a protein fragment to occur. If this is the case, a small percentage of cocktail protease inhibitors can be added with the purified protein sample. Sometimes, the presence of conformationally dynamic amino acid side chains on the surface of the protein may inhibit crystallization because of the entropic cost of immobilizing them in stable inter protein contacts. Surface entropy reduction by replacing the high entropy side chains of lysine, arginine, glutamate and glutamine residues to alanine can promote crystallization. These amino acids can be identified by using the Surface Entropy Reduction prediction (SERp) server.[8] Amino acids having a SERp value higher than the threshold value could be mutated to enhance crystallization.

Crystal and Symmetry

A crystal is a precisely ordered three dimensional array of molecules (Fig. 1.4), usually with some sort of internal symmetry. A unit cell, the smallest unit of the crystal, serves as the building block of the crystal. A unit cell is defined by 6 parameters; the lengths of the edges of the unit cell denoted by a, b, c and the angles between them namely α (between b and c axis), β (between a, c) and γ (between a, b) as shown in Fig. 1.5.

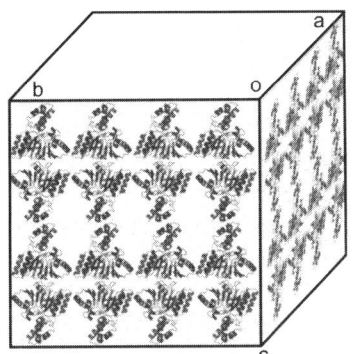

Fig. 1.4: Protein molecules in the crystal (Sgm molecules, pdb code 3lcu)

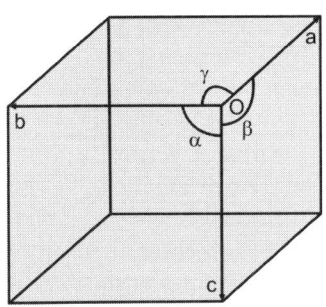

Fig. 1.5: Unit cell. The three axes x, y and z have unit dimensions of a, b and c respectively; α is the angle between b and c; β is the angle between a and c, and γ is the angle between a and b

The symmetrical arrangement of the molecules in the crystal can be described using various symmetry elements like rotation axis, reflection plane (mirror plane), translational elements (screw axis and glide plane) and an inversion point in the crystal. An object is said to have the symmetry, if, after applying a symmetry operation, the resulting object is identical to the original object. The complete details about the symmetry elements can be obtained from the International Tables for Crystallography, volume A (http://it.iucr.org).

There are seven three dimensional coordinate systems for describing the combination of symmetry elements in a crystal. Bravais discovered the combination of these seven crystal systems with lattice points at infinite repetition in 3D space give rise to 14 different lattice arrangements. Crystals could be described in terms of the group of symmetry operations relating their faces. Each of these groups is known as a point group. There are 32 such point groups possible among crystal systems. These 32 point groups combined with 14 *Bravais lattices* and translational elements result in 230 unique space groups which are the only ways in which identical objects may be arranged in an infinite lattice in the crystal. In protein crystals, individual protein molecules align themselves in a repeating series of unit cells by adopting a consistent orientation. The molecules in the crystal are mostly held together by the non-covalent interactions.[9] *Space groups* describe how a motif can be arranged in three dimensional spaces in a crystal. The presence of a chiral carbon in the amino acids except for glycine allows the possibility of L-amino acids and D-amino acids. However the exclusion of D-amino acids from proteins avoids mirror symmetry and this restricts the number of possible space groups to 65 in biological macromolecules.

X-ray Diffraction

X-rays are electromagnetic radiations with wavelength between 0.1 Å–100 Å. The wavelength of the X-ray used in the protein crystal diffraction is usually in the range of 1.5 Å, about the length of a carbon-carbon single bond, and the use of X-rays with this wavelength permits, in theory, resolution of individual atoms. Previously, for protein crystallography, X-rays were generated using conventional sealed X-ray tubes. At present, more powerful and advanced sources like rotating anode generators and synchrotron beam line facilities are being used.

The protein crystal is placed in the beam of monochromatic X-rays and a diffraction image is collected on an image plate or charge-coupled device (CCD). Crystal acts as a three-dimensional grating and scatters the incident beam of X-rays only in certain directions. The intensities of the diffracted X-rays from the single crystal together with some additional data (described below), allows one to determine the three dimensional structure of the protein present in the crystal.

A crystal can be imagined as consisting of various sets of parallel planes separated by a constant distance. Each set of planes is identified by three numbers, called the *Miller indices*. Miller indices are a symbolic vector representation for the orientation of an atomic plane in a crystal lattice and are defined as the reciprocals of the fractional intercepts which the plane makes with the crystallographic axes. These imaginary planes are brought in line with the X-ray beam by slowly rotating the crystal. The X-rays scattered from the set of planes may either interfere constructively or destructively depending on the distance between the planes and the angle made by the incident X-rays with the set of planes. This is explained by Bragg's law. When an X-ray beam falls on a set of planes oriented in a particular direction, they get diffracted and produce a spot on the diffraction image if Bragg's law is followed.

Bragg's Law

Consider two planes in a set of parallel planes as shown in the Fig. 1.6.
For constructive interference,
$AC + CB = n\lambda$ (n–is an integer)
$2AC = n\lambda$ (since $AC=CB$)
So $AC = n\lambda/2$
$Sin\theta = AC/d = n\lambda/2d$
Hence $2dSin\theta = n\lambda$

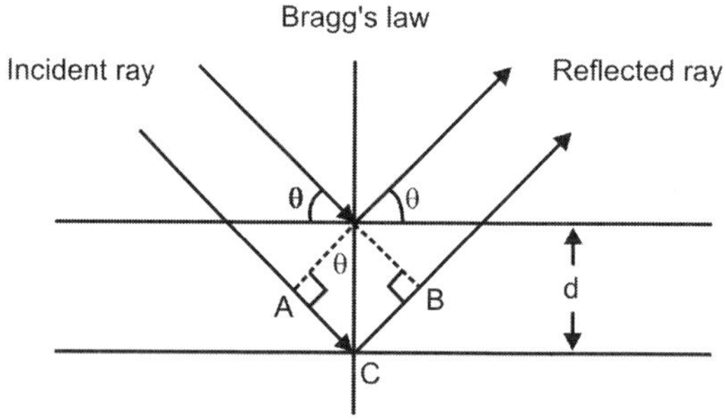

Fig. 1.6: Bragg's law

where d is the spacing between the lattice planes of a set within the unit cell, λ is the wavelength of the X-rays and θ is the angle of the incident and the reflected X-ray by the lattice plane.

Each set of parallel planes is brought in particular orientation by slowly rotating the crystal relative to the X-ray beam to satisfy the Bragg's law.

Structure Determination and Refinement

It can be shown that the amplitude of the X-rays diffracted by a crystal is the vector sum of the amplitudes of the X-rays scattered by the individual atoms in the unit cell (unit cell is the repeating unit of the crystal), each having an amplitude that is related to the number of electrons as well as a phase that is related to the special location of the atom within the unit cell. The sum of these individual contributions can be represented by a vector with an amplitude $|F_{hkl}|$ and a phase $|\alpha^1{}_{hkl}|$ where h, k, and l are the Miller indices that define the diffraction maxima. F(hkl), designated as the structure factor, can be expressed in terms of the f_j, the individual atomic scattering factor for the jth atom in the unit cell, and xj, yj, zj are the spatial coordinates of the jth atom in the unit cell

$$F_{hkl} = \sum_{j=1}^{n} f_j \, e^{2\pi i (hxj + kyj + lzj)}$$

where n is the number of atoms and j is an individual atom. Thus the structure factor can be defined as summation over the scattering factor of all the atoms in unit cell. The *Fourier synthesis* of the structure factor gives the electron density (ρ) Fourier transform distribution at any point in unit cell.

$$\rho(x,y,z) = \frac{1}{V} \sum_h \sum_k \sum_l |F_{hkl}| \, e^{-2\pi i (hx + ky + lz - \alpha'_{hkl})}$$

where V is the volume of the unit cell. From this expression it is clear that in order to calculate the positions of the various atoms in the crystal one needs the intensity of the diffracted X-rays and the phase angles. From the collected diffraction data the structure factor amplitude $|F_h|$ can be calculated. However, the phase information (α_h) in the structure factor equation is not experimentally measurable because the frequency of X-rays is ~10^{18} Hz per sec. This particular situation is termed as Phase Problem.

One of the three following methods is mainly used to calculate the phases. Two of these, i.e. Multiple Isomorphous Replacement (MIR)[10] and Multi wavelength or Single wavelength Anomalous Dispersion (MAD or SAD)[11] involve the presence of heavy atoms in the structure. The third procedure called Molecular Replacement (MR) is used when a homology model is available. When both the amplitudes and the phases of the scattered X-rays are known, they can be combined to produce an electron-density map of the atoms of the unit cell. The resolution of the electron density map generated depends on the angular extent to which the intensity data have been measured. After an electron density of good resolution is obtained, the polypeptide sequence of the protein is fitted to this map to generate the initial model of the protein. The initial model of the protein will contain significant errors due to the imperfect phasing of the experimental electron-density map. This model is then improved by a procedure called *refinement*. The aim of the refinement is to minimize differences between the calculated and experimental structure factors and at the same time, to optimize the stereochemistry.

A variety of software packages are available for refinement, such as CNS[12], Refmac[13] and others. The progress of the refinement can be indicated partly by the value of the R factor, given by this equation:

$$R\ factor = \frac{\sum \left\| F_{obs} \right| - \left| F_{calc} \right\|}{\sum \left| F_{obs} \right|}$$

where Fobs and Fcalc are the observed and calculated structure factors respectively. R factor can vary from 0.4 to 0.5 (or from 40% to 50%, if expressed as a percentage) for an essentially correct but unrefined structure.

For an exceptionally well-refined structure the R-factor can be as low as 0.12 (12%). Most well-refined structures produce R values <0.2 (20%).

After the initial structure of the protein is obtained, it is assessed for errors using the Ramachandran plot[14] to visualize dihedral angles ψ against ϕ of amino acid residues in protein structure (*ref.* chapter 1.2.2.1 method C). It will show the possible conformations of ψ and ϕ angles for a polypeptide. The Ramachandran plot is used by structural biologists to verify the stereochemistry of the determined structure. In addition, Brunger[15] has proposed a cross-validation procedure that involves omitting a certain percentage (approximately 10%) of the reflections in the refinement but using them only to calculate an R-factor known as Rfree, which will then provide an independent check of the validity of the structure. The difference between the value of R-free and R should be between 2 and 7%. If the difference is more than 7%, it indicates over-refinement. After having determined the structure of the proteins, some structure based functional studies that include site directed mutagenesis and biophysical interaction studies will help in understanding the function of these protein molecules.

Crystallography in Drug Design

Most enzymes are proteins and play a crucial role not only in maintaining the functional aspects biological systems but also in disease processes. The inhibition of enzyme activity serves as a major control mechanism in biological systems. Many drugs and toxic agents act by inhibiting the enzymes. Traditional drug designs rely on trial and error testing of chemical substances on cultured cells and animals, and matching the apparent effects to treatments. This method of drug design is time consuming and arbitrary.

A potential drug, in addition to being able to inhibit the target molecule, should have minimal structural requirements, high affinity, high selectivity and be cost effective. Current trend is towards rational drug design which makes use of the three dimensional structure of the target. Hence, the first step in rational drug design is to understand the mechanism of target action by determining the functional groups involved in enzyme activity. Crystal structures of enzyme-substrate/substrate-analog complex will help to map the functional groups crucial for enzyme activity. Once the key residues are identified, it enables the design of inhibitors that target residues specific to the active site thereby turning the enzyme inactive, and the development of substrate analogs.

Recent application of robotics to crystallographic studies as used in crystallization and data collection has enhanced the efficiency of drug discovery. Automated crystallization tools help in screening vast potential leads in short time, with minimal usage of the resources. Once the structure of the target molecule is known, a virtual screening is carried out to identify ligands that can inhibit the activity of the target protein. In the case of unsuccessful virtual screening, a combinatorial screening is carried out to identify the lead molecules that can potentially inhibit the target molecule.

References

1. Fei Wang, Xinhe Wang, Chong-Gang Yuan, and Jiyan Ma (26 February 2010) "Generating a Prion with Bacterially Expressed Recombinant Prion Protein" Science 327 (5969), 1132.

2. Philip J. Thomas, Bao-He Qu, and Peter L. Pedersen (1995) Defective Protein Folding as a Basis of Human Disease, TIBS, 20, 456–459.

3. Alexander Wlodawer1, Wladek Minor, Zbigniew Dauter and Mariusz Jaskolski (2008) "Protein crystallography for non-crystallographers, or how to get the best (but not more) from published macromolecular structures". FEBS Journal 275(1): 1–21.

4. W.L. Bragg, "The Diffraction of Short Electromagnetic Waves by a Crystal", Proceedings of the Cambridge Philosophical Society, 17 (1913), 43–57.

5. Kendrew, JC; Bodo; Dintzis; Parrish; Wyckoff; Phillips (Mar 1958). "A three-dimensional model of the myoglobin molecule obtained by x-ray analysis". Nature 181 (4610): 662–6.

6. Y. Liu, J. Sivaraman and C. L. Hew (2006). "Expression, purification and crystallization of a novel nonstructural protein VP9 from white spot syndrome virus". Acta Cryst. F62, 802–804

7. W Nicholson Price II et al. Understanding the physical properties that control protein crystallization by analysis of large scale crystallization data Nature Biotechnology (27): Number1 January 2009

8. Cooper, D.R. et al. Protein crystallization by surface entropy reduction: optimization of the SER strategy. Acta Crystallogr. D Biol. Crystallogr. 63, 636–645 (2007).

9. Lukasz Goldschmidt, David Cooper, Zygmunt Derewenda, David Eisenberg. (2007). Toward rational protein crystallization: A Web server for the design of crystallizable protein variants Protein Science. 16: 1569–1576 (2007 Aug).

10. Crick, F.H.C and Madgoff, B.S. (1956) The theory of the method of isomorphous replacement for protein crystals. Acta Cryst. 9, 901.

11. Hendrickson W, Ogata C (1997). "Phase determination from multiwavelength anomalous diffraction measurements". Meth Enzymol 276: 494–523.

12. Brunger AT, Adams PD, Clore GM, DeLano WL, Gros P, Grosse-Kunstleve RW, Jiang JS, Kuszewski J, Nilges M, Pannu NS, et al. Crystallography and NMR system: a new software suite for macromolecular structure determination. Acta Crystallogr. D Biol. Crystallogr (1998) 54(Pt 5): 905–921

13. Refinement of Macromolecular Structures by the Maximum-Likelihood Method" G.N. Murshudov, A.A.Vagin and E.J.Dodson, (1997) in Acta Cryst. D53, 240–255.

14. Ramachandran GN, Ramakrishnan C, Sasisekaran V (July 1963). "Stereochemistry of polypeptide chain configurations". J. Mol. Biol. 7: 95–9.

15. Brunger AT (January 1992). "Free R value: a novel statistical quantity for assessing the accuracy of crystal structures". Nature 355: 472–475.

1.1.2B Determining Structure by Nuclear Magnetic Resonance Spectroscopy

Janarthanan Krishnamoorthy

NMR spectroscopy has been instrumental in determining high resolution structure of molecules along side with X-ray crystallography. Conceptually, NMR differs from X-ray methods as it is an indirect method, which can only provide constraints, for calculating structure. For example, if three nuclei, i.e. A, B, C, are close to each other in space, through NMR experiments (NOESY) we can determine arbitrary distances between A–B, B–C, C–A (Fig. 1.7). Using these distance information as constraints (or conditions), we can compute structures which do not violate the given constraints. If

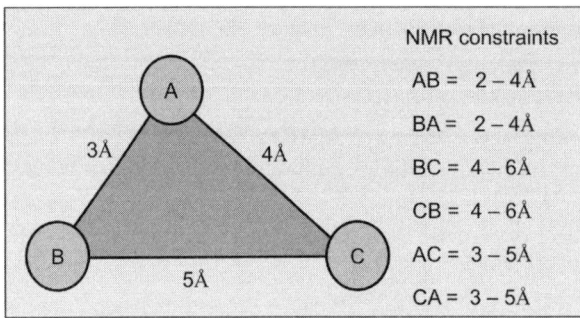

Fig. 1.7: Three nuclei A,B,C in space and the corresponding distance constraint

less number of constraints are used, large number of structures will result satisfying these constraints, many of which would probably not exist in reality. To confine the solutions to more accurate ones, more constraints are given in the form of angles (dihedral angles; the phi and psi angles), hydrogen bonds formation and orientation of bond vectors. Before getting into details of structure calculation, we will briefly explain the basic principles behind NMR experiments and how they are employed in obtaining constraints like the inter atomic distances (nuclear distances), bond angle between two bond vectors (dihedral angle) and orientation of bond vectors in space (Fig. 1.8).

Background Information

Since NMR deals with nuclei (subatomic particle), quantum mechanics is quintessential in understanding and interpreting the NMR experiments. Fortunately, physicists have developed two approaches to simplify this problem namely, product operator formalism and density matrix approach, which are similar in principle but differ in the representation. The product operator approach is simple and effective to analyze the NMR spectrum without much calculation. In

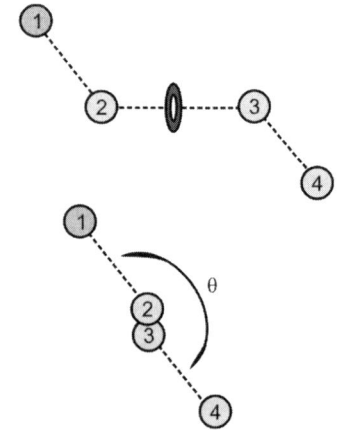

Fig. 1.8: Dihedral angle is determined by four atoms, i.e. the angle between two bond vectors connected via a single bond

contrast, complete experiments can be simulated using density matrix approach. (Keeler[1]).

Forgoing detailed theory in this chapter, we can state the objective of NMR experiments with structure determination in perspective, as to determine as many constraints as possible. In order to use these constraints effectively we need to relate the obtained NMR spectral parameters to the structural parameters (A. Bain[4]). For example, a peak in an NMR spectrum has four characteristics, namely, (Fig. 1.9)[3]

- Frequency at which it appears (Larmor frequency)
- Line width at half maximum
- Area of the peak
- Phase of the peak.

These are considered as the spectral parameters; on the other hand, there are the structural parameters that indicate the position of one nuclei with respect to the others in the three dimensional space.

In addition to the above spectral parameters, if a nucleus is chemically bonded to an adjacent one, the original peak would split in to multiple peaks (called *multiplets*). The number of split peaks depends on the number of adjacent nuclei attached to it. For example, for a methyl proton, all the CH_3 protons are magnetically equivalent, hence it should appear as a single peak with three times the magnitude of intensity, but when a CH_2 group is present nearby as in CH_3–CH_2–OH, then the two protons in CH_2 (n = 2) would split the single peak of CH_3 in to 3 (i.e. n+1 peaks). The magnitude of the distance between the split peaks is termed as the *coupling constant* (J) and is a measure of nature of the bond (i.e. single bond, double or triple bond, etc.) as well as the nuclei to which it is coupled or attached with. In fact, coupling effect is due to interaction of electrons surrounding one nuclei with its adjacent nuclei, hence it is an indirect effect, which contrast with direct effects like dipolar effect, where one nuclei interacts directly with its adjacent nuclei that is spatially close to it. If the coupling or scalar or bond effect is strong, then the magnitude of peak splitting would be large, on the other hand if coupling is weaker, the splitting effect would be smaller or negligible. In many cases, the relationship between the spectral parameters and the structural parameters are not straightforward, but will become clear with the explanation of some of the well known NMR experiments.

Fundamental Property of Nucleus

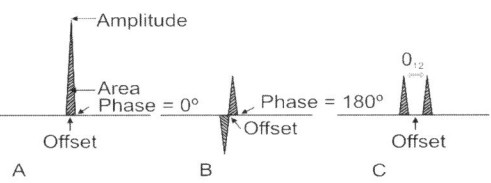

Fig. 1.9: The four basic characteristics of an NMR peak is highlighted in figure A and B; C shows how the J coupling splits the original peak into doublet

In NMR experiments the magnetic moment of nuclei are manipulated using radio frequency pulses in the presence of a strong magnetic field to obtain the desired information. In order to understand how a nucleus gives rise to a peak in the spectrum, we need to understand what magnetic moment/magnetization is, and how it is manipulated through experiments (Frank[3]). Let us consider a protein molecule, where amino acids are bonded together through peptide amide bonds. Each amino acid in turn has different nuclei such as H, N, C, S, O. Further down each element such as H, C, N can exist in many isotope forms, e.g. H can exist in H^1 (proton), H^2 (deuterium), H^3 (tritium) forms. In nature the ratio of $H^1:H^2:H^3$ is 99.89:0.085:<0.0001. Each isotope has its unique nuclear property called spin property, which is quantified in terms of spin quantum number. For example H^1 has ½ spin number, H^2 has an integral spin number 1. Nuclei with spin number greater than zero are said to be spin active.

Because of the presence of protons, nuclei inherently have some charge associated with it. In addition if that nucleus is spin active, as it spins along an axis, it generates a circular current with its associated magnetic field. Hence, when a spin active nucleus is placed in a strong magnetic field (B_0), it will behave like a tiny bar magnet and align itself along with the stronger magnetic field. The magnetic field of an individual nucleus is quantitatively defined as 'magnetic moment'(μ). As the nuclei's magnetic moment (μ) aligns along the main magnetic field, it will start precessing around the axis of the magnetic field (B_0) (Fig. 1.10). This phenomenon is similar to a top that is spinning and precessing around an axis under the influence of the gravitational field. The rate or the frequency in which nuclei precess is defined as the *larmor frequency*. Proton 'H' precesses at 400×10^6 times/sec or 400 MHz, N^{15} at 40.52 MHZ and C^{13} at 100.56 MHZ in 9.396 Tesla magnetic field.

Now when we consider all the protons ('H') nuclei present in different functional groups like NH_2, CH_3, CH_2, CH, C_6H_6 (aromatic) in a protein molecule, each proton has its own local environment defined by its functional group. In amino group, for example, NH_2, 'H' nuclei is adjacent to 'N' whereas in CH_3, 'H' nuclei is adjacent to 'C'. This results in protons experiencing different magnetic field from each another. Additionally, the protons may be well buried or exposed to the solvent in the structure. This also brings about the variation in the magnetic field experienced by the nuclei. The Larmor Frequency is directly proportional to the strength of the external magnetic field it experiences. For example, a proton nucleus (A) which is present on the surface, experiences stronger magnetic field compared to a proton nuclei (B) which is at the center of the molecule. Thus A will precess faster than B, because of the differences in shielding or screening effect caused by the adjacent nuclei in its surrounding. Indirectly we

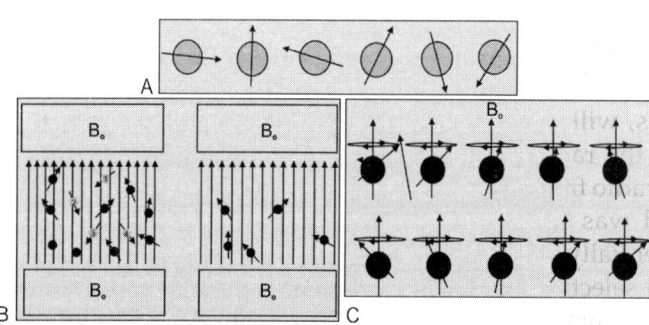

Fig. 1.10: To explain random orientation, aligning of magnetic moment, precession. A: The random orientation of nuclei present in a sample of molecules, B: The same nucleus, when placed in a strong magnetic field, the spin active nuclei will majorly align along the magnetic field and minorly against the field. The residual nuclei that actually contribute to the signal is the difference between these two sets of orientations. C: How a spin-active nucleus precesses with respect to magnetic field B_0 along 'z' axis

get the picture of the surrounding of each nucleus from its Lamor frequency. Chemical shift is the commonly used representation for lamor frequency, where the Lamor frequency of desired nuclei is expressed relative to a standard nuclei's Lamor frequency and finally written in parts per million. In real cases the frequency range of protons would be 500MHz ± 30 KHz at a 11.7 Tesla magnetic field. C^{13} and N^{15} nuclei also behaves like H^1, but its precession Larmor frequency would be around 125 and 50 MHZ respectively, note that naturally occurring C^{12} and N^{14}, are not spin active hence C, N are isotopically labeled through special means to enrich C^{13} and N^{15} nucleus in proteins.

Consider H^1 alone for the current discussion. If all the magnetic moments of the protons are aligned towards the magnetic field, they add up to give a 'bulk magnetization'. The magnetization by definition is the sum of all the individual magnetic moments (Fig. 1.11).

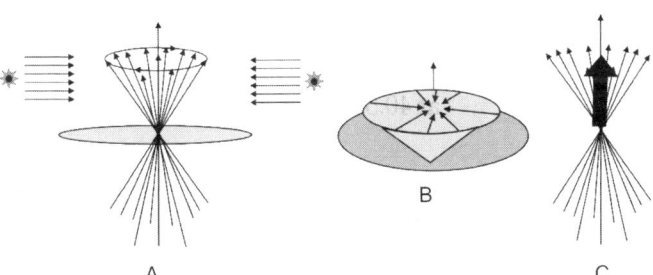

A   C

Fig. 1.11: Explaining longitudinal components. A: The magnetic moment of a set of nuclei precessing around 'z' axis is represented as red arrows. The direction of projecting these vectors onto 'z' axis is shown as grey arrows emanating from a light source. B: The top view of the projections, showing the maximum 'z' component. C: Shows the projected 'z' component as a vector also known as 'Bulk magnetization'

If we apply a stronger magnetic field in 'x' or 'y' direction, in contrast to the main magnetic field already present along the 'z' direction, the bulk magnetization will tend to align with the stronger field placed along x/y axis. In practice, this is effected by applying a strong *radio frequency field* instead of an alternate magnetic field. The Radio frequency waves being electro-magnetic in nature has both electric and magnetic component. The nuclei flip from 'z' to x/y axes, will happen only if its Larmor frequency matches exactly with the frequency of the radio frequency field. The degree of flip in turn depends on the strength of the radio frequency field. Decades earlier, continuous wave experiment or sweep method was routinely used where the frequency of radio frequency (rf) waves are sequentially and continuously varied from higher to lower field. As the field is swept, only selective nuclei take up the radio frequency and show up in spectrum. Nowadays, this method has been replaced with pulsed technique, where a short pulse of rf field generates all the required frequencies instantaneously along x/y axis. As a result all the nuclei with its Larmor frequency within the defined rf range absorbs and align along x/y axis. Immediately after the pulse, the magnetic moment vectors that are coherently aligned along 'x' or 'y' axis, start precessing in the x–y plane at the same time gradually moving away from x–y plane towards the initial equilibrium position along z axis. During this process, if a detector is placed perpendicular to the x–y plane, as the magnetization vector cuts across the coil, an induced current will be generated. This signal decays with time and is referred to as

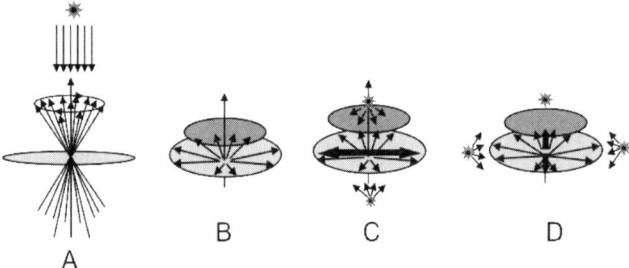

Fig. 1.12: Explaining, transverse components A, B Projection of the same vectors onto x-y plane, with the light source placed perpendicular to the x-y plane. C: Further projection of each vectors onto x axis by placing the light source perpendicular to 'x' axis. D: Similar projection of vectors on to 'y' axis

'*Free induction decay*' or the NMR time domain signal (Fig. 1.13).

Experiments are usually designed to manipulate the magnetic moments in diverse ways using multiple pulses at various intervals, before the final FID is recorded. By doing so, we transfer magnetization from one nucleus to another. One commonly used experiment called 'INEPT' (Indirect Nuclei Detection through Polarization Transfer) transfers the magnetic moment from a proton nuclei to its immediately attached C or N nuclei. Through this experiment, the Larmor frequencies of both the proton and its covalently attached C or N are obtained. Further, advanced experiments are available which are built on modulating the magnetization through 'pulses' and 'delays' in a specific way.

From all NMR experiments, we only get the time domain signal as shown in the following Figs. In order to interpret, the signal has to be transformed to frequency domain using *Fourier Transformation*. The characteristics of time domain signal are that it takes positive and negative values in an oscillating manner on progression with time. It also gets dampened or decayed during the process. The final 'FID' signal results not from a single nucleus but from all the available nuclei each precessing at different frequencies. The FT mathematically resolves the contribution of each individual nucleus from the FID signal. FT is worked out by multiplying, the time domain signal with a unique test frequency signal. If the FID signal has any of its component signal matching the test frequency then they will add up constructively. If the FID has no matching frequency then the summation would be destructive and result in zero value. Figure 1.14 explains this process in detail (Joseph[6]).

In the final Fourier transformed spectrum peaks will appear at positions corresponding to the Larmor frequency of the nucleus present in the sample. The intensity of the peak corresponds to the number of nuclei present at the same frequency.

In general, the Larmor frequency is referenced to a standard radio frequency wave, and expressed as offset value, i.e.

Offset frequency$^{(\Omega)}$ = Larmor frequency$_{(standard\ frequency)}$ – Larmor frequency$_{(nucleus\ of\ interest)}$

The above explained principles apply to H^1, C^{13}, N^{15} and other spin active nuclei alike. If an experiment considers and modulates only one type of nucleus, then such experiments are called one dimensional experiment. If additional nuclei type is also included, then it becomes multidimensional experiment. Practically, the dimension of an experiment is not based on the number or type of nuclei involved, but by the number of 'evolution periods' present in the pulse sequence. The evolution period, also referred to as 'Delays' is critical, as only during this period, the correlation between different

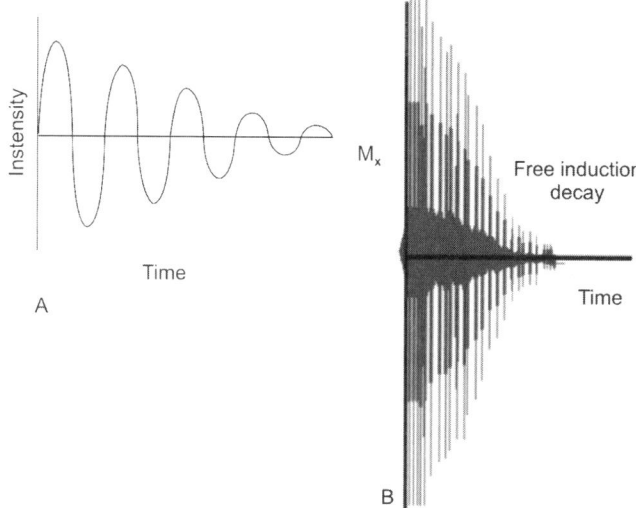

Fig. 1.13: Explaining, single frequency FID and original multiple frequency NMR signals; A: A dampened signal arising from a single nucleus. B: The free induction decay signal arising from a set of nuclei

nuclei are established. Each nuclei type is specifically modulated through one of the evolution periods present in the experiment. Hence the number of 'evolution periods' also corresponds to the number of nuclei type being manipulated.

An NMR experiment, with 2 evolution period is called two dimensional and the experiments with increasing number of evolution periods are accordingly called as three, four or higher dimensional experiments. It is not necessary that the dimension number matches with the different hetero-nuclear type present in the molecule. The hetero nucleus referred here can be any nucleus other than 'H' such as C, N, P, S, etc. Even 'H' present in different functional group, but within the same molecule can constitute the other dimensions. For example, in an amino acid, protons present in amide group, and protons attached to alpha or beta carbon can be considered as two different dimensions. Alternatively, amide proton of an amino acid and all the other protons present in its vicinity can also be considered as two different dimensions. In the former case the difference in the two types of protons is obvious as they are present in two different type of functional group. But in the latter case, the first dimension is straightforward as it is constituted by amide proton, but the second proton comes from all different functional groups including amide protons. Here, the second dimension is defined by the spatial proximity or vicinity rather than by according with functional group. Thus, the definition of the nucleus type corresponding to each dimension differs from experiment to experiment.

Based on the nuclear type that constitutes the dimensions, NMR experiments can be generally classified as homonuclear or hetero nuclear experiments. For example, In (H–H) COSY **(Correlation spectroscopy)** experiment, all protons present in the molecule constitute the first dimension, where as protons that are two or three bonds away with respect to the first dimension protons, constitute the second dimension. As both the dimensions are constituted by the same nuclear types, i.e. protons, this class of experiment is called homonuclear experiment. In ($N^{15}H$) HSQC experiment, proton forms the first dimension, where as the N^{15} hetero nuclei which are immediately attached to it through a covalent bond (i.e. a single bond away), constitute the second dimension. Since this type of experiment involves two different nuclei type, i.e. proton and nitrogen, it is classified as hetero nuclear experiment.

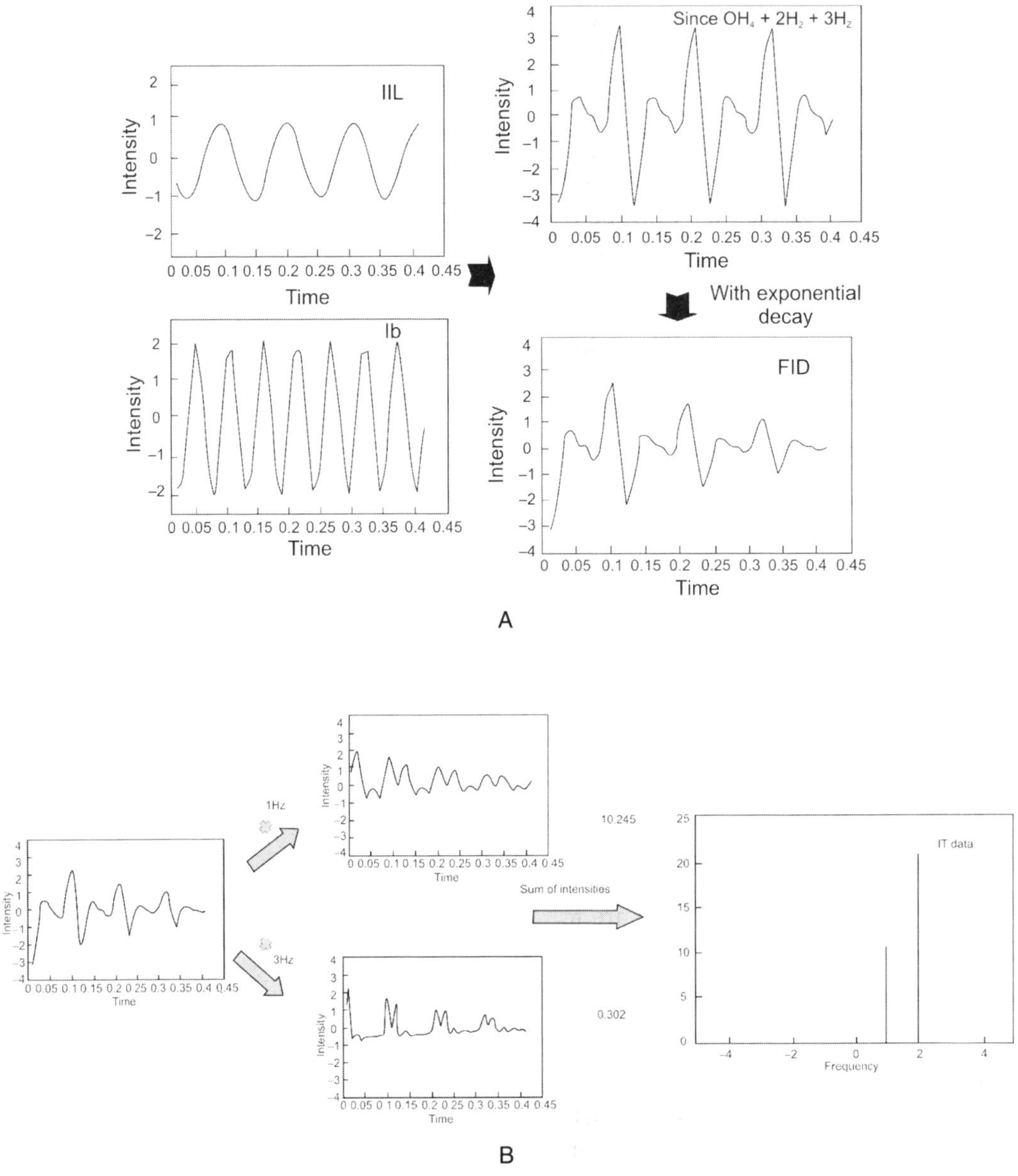

Fig. 1.14: A: Construction of FID using two frequencies 1,2 HZ. The resulting undampened signal. The same signal when multiplied with an exponential decay function (exp(- 3.5t)) gives the FID similar to NMR experimental data. B: Fourier transformation is employed to transform time domain to frequency domain signal. The FID is multiplied with 1Hz (test frequency), 3HZ (test frequency) and 2HZ (not shown). The resultant plot shows the intensity of 1HZ is positive (~10), where as 3HZ is negligible (0.33), as no such frequency is present in the FID. These intensities are plotted against the corresponding test frequencies; the intensity of 2 HZ is twice compared to 1HZ, as its amplitude in time domain signal is relatively doubled. This corresponds to two nuclei having the same resonant frequency, in an NMR spectrum

NMR experiments can also be classified based on the way the magnetization is transferred from one nucleus to other. For example, the magnetization can be transferred through the 'scalar or covalent bond' as in TOCSY experiments or 'through space' as in NOESY experiments. TOCSY experiments are designed to identify, all the nuclei that are adjacent to a nucleus of interest, and are attached to it through scalar bond. Whereas in NOESY, all nucleus adjacent to a nuclei of interest are identified, but the adjacent nuclei need not be covalently bonded to the nucleus of interest and must be spatially close to each other. To exemplify the difference, we can consider a protein molecule, in which each residue is connected through peptide bond. In NMR jargon each residue is considered as an individual system called 'spin system'. A proton from a specific residue, say 7th amino acid will be adjacent to protons from residue 6 and 8. But it will be far away from residues numbered say 20 or 35. But if the protein is folded in such a way that residue 100 is present adjacent to residue 7, then by sequence (covalent bonding ~ 93 peptide bonds) they are far apart, but by structure they are 'spatially' close. Hence in NOESY spectrum, we can see contribution of 100th residue to the 7th residue, and vice versa. The same effects cannot be seen in TOCSY spectrum as it is designed only to identify and correlate protons that are present within a single spin system or amino acid.

One Dimensional Experiment

Let us consider the following structure with two amino acids. Each amino acid is considered as an individual system or 'spin system'. It is possible to relate or correlate nuclei from one spin system to other nuclei within the same spin system (intra-correlation, e.g. TOCSY) or to other nuclei present in adjacent spin system (inter-correlation, e.g. NOESY). The correlation can be made either through scalar bond or spatial proximity/nearness. In a less complicated one dimensional experiment, one particular nuclei type is manipulated and observed without making any correlation with another nuclei type. If we are to record an NMR experiment for the above two amino acid peptide, we will get a spectrum as shown in Fig. 1.15 (Cavanagh[3]).

In the above 1D spectrum we see a pair of peaks corresponding to 'α' and 'β' protons from 1, 2 spin systems, i.e Alanine and lysine respectively and a single peak corresponding to each γ, δ, ε of 2nd spin system. The labeling in the figure has been done for convenience, but in practice, we don't know which peak belongs to which functional group and also from which spin system. The process by which each nucleus is designated to respective spin system is called "Assignment". 2D and 3D experiments are commonly used for the assignment purpose. Further, sophisticated 1D-experiments are available that are designed to observe nuclei in specific functional group. For example, experiments are designed to observe only the amide and amine protons, eliminating methyl, methylene, methyne and aromatic protons in the spectrum. The problem with one dimensional experiment is that, it suffers from poor resolution, with increase in number of protons in the molecule. For example, if only two protons are present in a molecule, it will probably appear as distinct, well resolved peaks. On the other hand if hundred such protons are present, then, the spectrum would be crowded with 100 peaks within the same spectral width or 'ppm' interval. To overcome

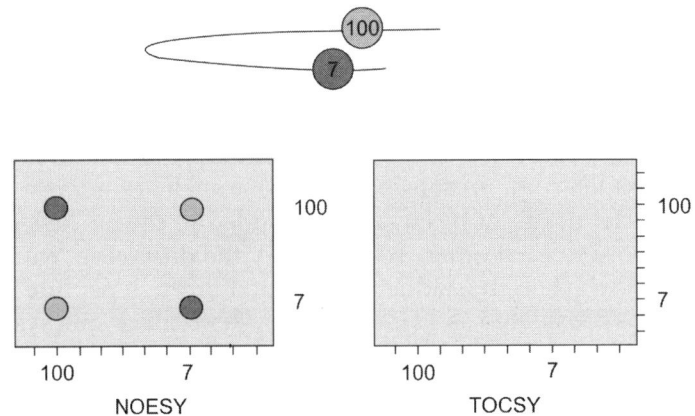

Fig. 1.15: A simplistic figure to differentiate TOCSY and NOESY. The pink peak corresponds to the NMR signal from 7th and 100th residue at an arbitrary chemical shift value, which is not mentioned here. TOCSY spectrum shows only peaks corresponding to residues 7 and 100. NOESY shows 'cross peaks' at symmetrical coordinates, shown in red, which is an evidence that 7 and 100 are correlated via spatial proximity. The figure is highly simplified to explain the difference between NOESY and TOCSY experiments. None of the x,y scale has meaning in practical sense

the resolution problem, higher dimensional experiments were developed, the concept behind extension of higher dimensional experiments from lower dimensional experiments are detailed in the figures.

Two Dimensional Experiments

For the same molecule, if we wish to identify the H_α and H_β that are directly correlated, we make use of 2D experiment called COSY (Correlation spectroscopy). In this experiment we get two characteristic peaks namely 'diagonal' and 'cross peaks'. Consider two nuclei that are covalently bonded together but two or three bonds seperate, and if we let '$\omega 1$' and '$\omega 2$' to be its chemical shift values (analogously, Larmor frequency). A diagonal peak will appear at ($\omega 1$, $\omega 1$) and ($\omega 2$, $\omega 2$) coordinates in a x–y axis system for first and second nuclei respectively. This does not contain any information, other than that two nuclei are present one at $\omega 1$ and other at $\omega 2$ position. Since the two nuclei are correlated through bond, two cross peaks will also appear at ($\omega 1$, $\omega 2$) and ($\omega 2$,

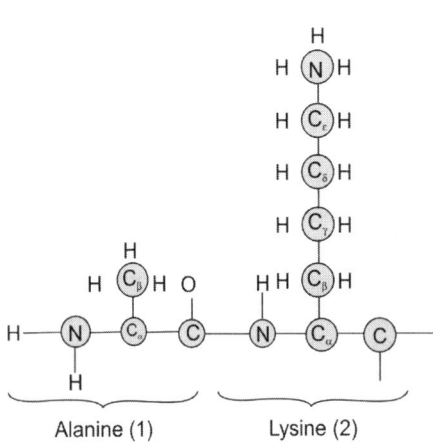

Fig. 1.16A: Structure of a dipeptide containing alanine and lysine

$\omega 1$) coordinates. This contains the structural information, that nuclei one is covalently attached to nucleus 2 and vice versa. In other words, cross peaks are peaks that are seen at the intersection of two different resonances, which are correlated, whereas,

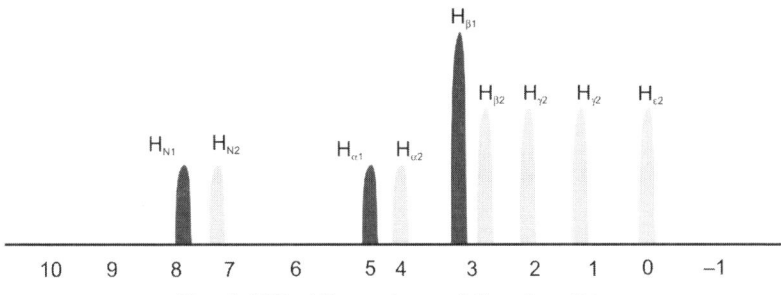

Fig. 1.16B: 1D spectrum of the dipeptide

diagonal peaks are the peaks that are seen at the intersection of same resonance. As each nucleus is related or correlated to itself, each nucleus will give rise to a single diagonal peak in the 2D spectrum. The number of covalent bond between the correlated nuclei can vary from 2 to 3, depending on which the intensity of the peak will decrease; the shorter the distance, the stronger the correlation and intensity.

In addition to correlating proton to proton type, there are experiments available that can correlate proton with heteronuclei like C^{13} or N^{15}. N^{15} HSQC (Heteronuclear single quantum coherence or correlation) experiment correlates amide proton with its respective amide nitrogen connected through a single scalar bond. TOCSY stands for *Total Correlation Spectroscopy*, it is a powerful experiment, which can correlate all the nuclei present within a single spin system to itself.

For example consider: NOESY (Nuclear OverhaussEur Spectroscopy) is another important experiment, which correlates all the nuclei that are adjacent to the nucleus of interest through space, not necessarily is connected to it through scalar bond. To compare TOCSY and NOESY, the former gives the details of all nuclei present within a spin system, but NOESY, information on all the nuclei that are present within a spin system as well as its adjacent spin systems but spatially proximal. This makes NOESY

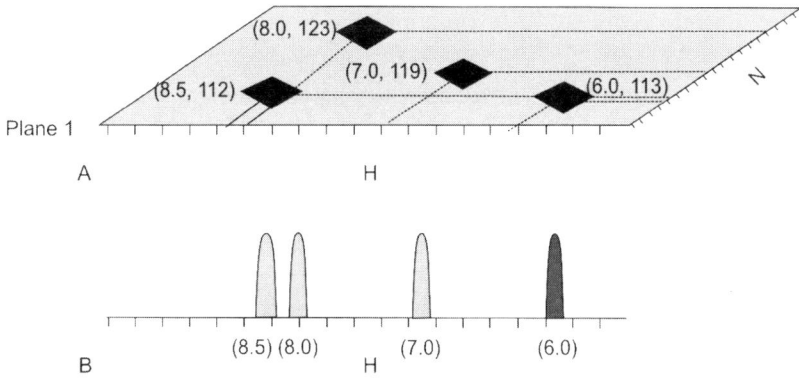

Fig. 1.17: Construction of 2D spectrum from 1D spectrum; A: One dimensional experiment showing four amide protons of a protein. B: The 2D experiment for the same amide protons, when a new dimension 'N' perpendicular to 'H' is introduced. In the 2D, the ppm of protons are identical as seen with 1D experiment, but have been spread out in the second dimension 'N', according to which it has been correlated

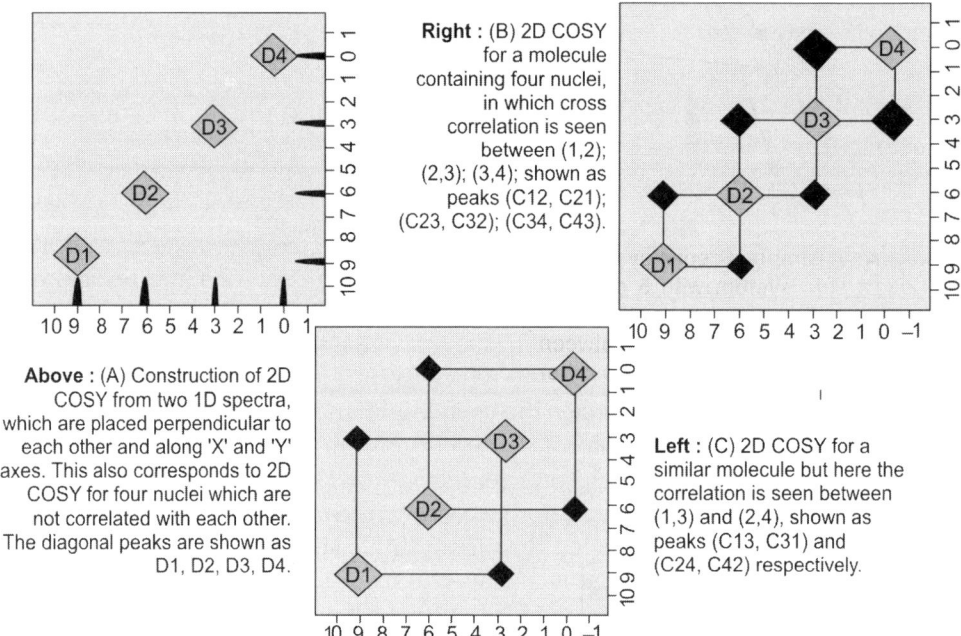

Right : (B) 2D COSY for a molecule containing four nuclei, in which cross correlation is seen between (1,2); (2,3); (3,4); shown as peaks (C12, C21); (C23, C32); (C34, C43).

Above : (A) Construction of 2D COSY from two 1D spectra, which are placed perpendicular to each other and along 'X' and 'Y' axes. This also corresponds to 2D COSY for four nuclei which are not correlated with each other. The diagonal peaks are shown as D1, D2, D3, D4.

Left : (C) 2D COSY for a similar molecule but here the correlation is seen between (1,3) and (2,4), shown as peaks (C13, C31) and (C24, C42) respectively.

Fig. 1.18: 2D spectrum of COSY, Uncorrelated spins, sequentially correlated spins, non-sequentially correlated spins

more useful in terms of the structural information it contains. The intensity of each cross peak in NOESY spectrum is related to the nuclear distance between the correlated nuclei. So the distance information on a pair of nuclei can be deciphered from the cross peak's intensity.

The determined intensity is used as a distance constraint in further structure calculation. In contrast to NOESY, correlation experiments like TOCSY, COSY are used to identify and assign peaks to its respective nuclei type.

Just as two dimensional experiment increases the resolution of peaks obtained in one dimensional experiment; three and four dimension experiments further extends the resolution of two dimensional experiments. The construction of higher dimensional experiments from two dimensional experiments is illustrated in the (Figs 1.17 to 1.21).

Structure Determination

The determination of protein structure is carried out in two steps,
• Assignment of each resonances or peaks in the spectrum
• Structure calculation using structural restraints obtained from the spectral parameters.

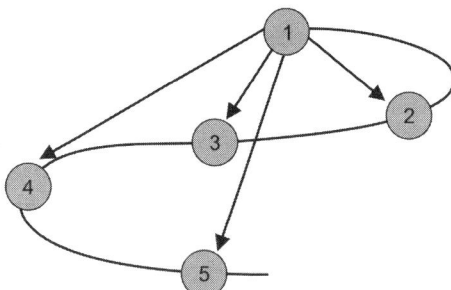

Fig. 1.19A: A simple 5 spin system. A hypothetical spin system with 5 different nuclei connected through bonds, shown as curves, the inter-nuclear distance between pair of nuclei is different from each other shown in arrows

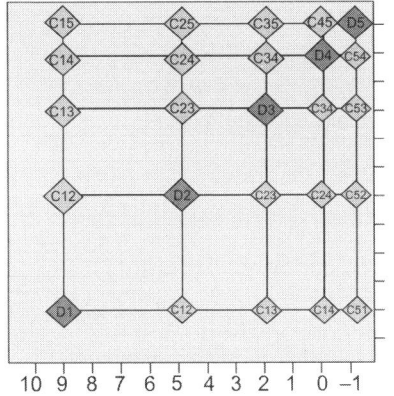

Fig. 1.19B: TOCSY spectrum of the same spin system (above). We see 5 diagonal peaks corresponding to 5 nuclei present in the spin system. As all the nuclei within a spin system are covalently correlated, despite the number of bonds separation, we see cross peaks for each bonded nuclei, e.g. nucleus 1 has a diagonal peak D1 and cross peaks (C12, C13, C14, C15 and its symmetrical counterpart C21, C31, C41, C51). Unlike COSY, in TOCSY, the correlation is not confined to one or two bond separation, it extends to even 5 or more bonds apart, but present within the same spin system

Assignment involves identifying all the chemical shifts of H, N, C, i.e. shifts of all the nuclei present in each spin system or residue.

Once we have the assignment, then we can identify and assign all the peaks in the NOESY spectrum and get information on inter-nuclear distance from the peak intensity. To emphasize, though different experiments are performed on the same sample resulting in different spectra, the chemical shift of each nucleus will be the same in all the spectra, i.e. an amide proton with a chemical shift 7.7 ppm will show up a peak identically at the same resonance in COSY, TOCSY, NOESY (Figs 1.18 and 1.19). Hence unique information concerning the same proton is obtained from each of these different experiments. The assignment step itself is carried out in two steps,

- Back bone assignment
- Side chain assignment

The backbone assignment involves assignment of protons like H(N), H(C$_\alpha$), and the hetero nuclei C and N which are bonded to it [i.e. (H)N, (H)C$_\alpha$, C'(O)]. In the above notation, the nucleus whose chemical shift is determined is outside the bracket, and the nucleus associated with it is placed within the bracket. A set of correlation based experiments that correlates a specific nuclei from one spin system (*i*th residue) to another specific nuclei in either its preceding (*i*th-1 residue) or its subsequent spin system (*i*th + 1 residue) is used for backbone assignment. CB–CA–(CO)–NH, HN–CA–CB, HN–CO and CO–(CA)–NH are some of the routinely used backbone assignment experiments.

In the side chain assignment protons like H(C$_\alpha$), H(C$_\beta$), H(C$_\gamma$), H(C$_\delta$), H(Cε) etc. and its associated heteronuclei such as (H)C$_\alpha$, (H)C$_\beta$, (H)C$_\gamma$, (H)C$_\delta$, (H)Cε are identified and assigned through TOCSY based correlation experiments. Now we can take a look at the details of how the backbone experiments are used for identification and assignment of peaks.

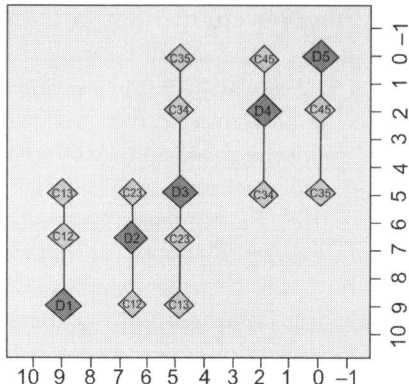

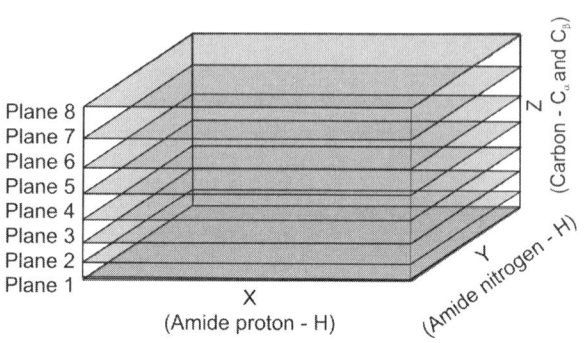

Fig. 1.19C: NOESY spectrum of a same spin system. Unlike TOCSY, the NOESY spectrum shows variation in intensity of cross peaks that correlates two nuclei. This intensity is related to the internuclear distance between them. Nucleus 1 has a diagonal peak at D1, and cross peaks at (C12, C13) and (C21, C31). Though nuclei 3, 4, 5 are covalently bonded to nucleus 1, since they are far apart (>5 Å) spatially, we do not see any cross peak for these nuclei. Please note that, though the pattern of appearance and disappearance of cross peaks varies among these experiments the coordinate or positions of both the diagonal and cross peaks are identical and do not change

Fig. 1.20: 3D experiments include one more dimension perpendicular to the two dimensions seen in conventional 2D experiments. The third dimension is shown as a series of planes along 'z' axis. Each dimension represents a nucleus type which is magnetically non equivalent

$CB_{(i-1)}$–$CA_{(i-1)}$–$(CO)_{(i-1)}$–$N_{(i)}H_{(i)}$ and $H_{(i)}N_{(i)}$–$CA_{(i)}$–$CB_{(i)}$ is a pair of experiments (Figs 1.22 and 1.23) used for correlating *i*th residue with its *i*th–1 residue. In $CB_{(i-1)}$–$CA_{(i-1)}$–$(CO)_{(i-1)}$–$N_{(i)}H_{(i)}$ experiment, the magnetization starts with amide proton $H_{(i)}$ of *i*th residue and transferred to its immediately attached amide $N_{(i)}$ of the same residue (i). From $N_{(i)}$ the magnetization is transferred to $C_{\alpha(i-1)}$ and then to $C_{\beta(i-1)}$ of the preceding residue (i–1), through the linking carbonyl group $[CO_{(i-1)}]$ of (i–1)th residue. During this process of magnetization transfer, the time domain signal is labelled with the larmor frequency of the amide proton ($H_{(i)}$), amide nitrogen ($N_{(i)}$) and finally with both $C_{\alpha(i-1)}$ and $C_{\beta(i-1)}$. Similarly, its complementary experiment, HN–CA–CB, transfers signal starting from $H_{(i)}$ to $N_{(i)}$, then to $CA_{(i)}/CB_{(i)}$ all within the same residue.

In both these experiments, three different nuclei are involved during magnetization transfer, hence when such a time domain signal is Fourier transformed, once for proton, once for nitrogen and finally for carbon dimension, the resulting frequency domain spectrum would result in a set of x–y planes stacked upon each other along the z direction. This is clearly illustrated in the Figs 1.20 and 1.21 how multidimensional experiments result from single dimensional experiments. For $CB_{(i-1)}$–$CA_{(i-1)}$–$(CO)_{(i-1)}$–$N_{(i)}H_{(i)}$ experiment the peaks will appear at the coordinate of ($H_{(i)}$, $N_{(i)}$, $C_{\alpha\,(i-1)}/C_{\beta\,(i-1)}$),

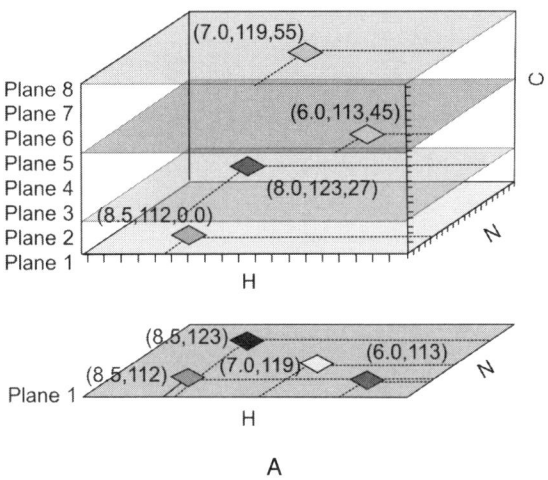

A

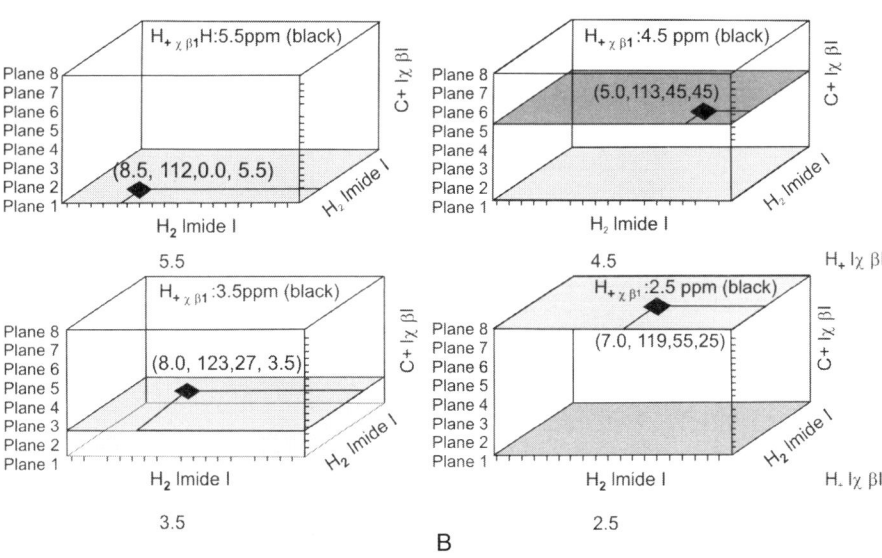

B

Fig. 1.21: Explaining the concept of 3D from 2D, and 4D from 3D. A: 3D spectrum with the third dimension represented by 'C'. The four peaks seen in the 2D is spread along the 'C' dimension into different planes, corresponding to which 'C', each amide proton and nitrogen are attached with. Each plane corresponds to one chemical shift value of 'C' dimension. B: 4D spectrum, where the 3D cubes are extended and resolved along one more dimension, 'H' (4th dimension). The fourth dimension is shown as linear axis below the cuboids represented at each ppm. Like each plane corresponds to one 'C' resonance value, each cuboid corresponds to one 'H' resonance value in 4D experiment

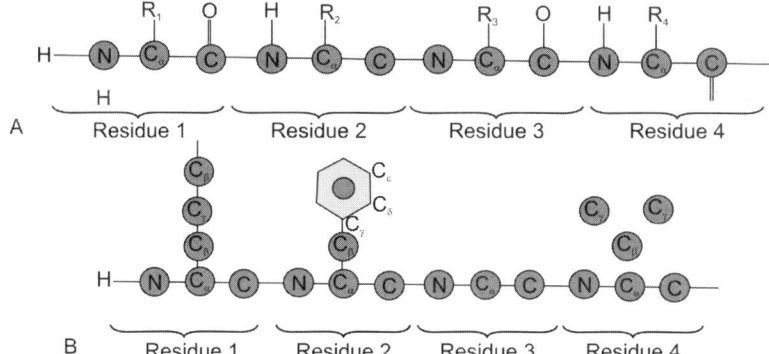

Fig. 1.22: A: Shows the back bone nuclei present in four consecutive residues assigned by backbone experiments. B: Shows the side chain nuclei present in four consecutive residues assigned by side chain experiments

but for HN–CA–CB, the peaks will appear at the coordinate of ($H_{(i)}, N_{(i)}, C_{\alpha (i)}/C_{\beta (i)}$). Sometimes we can also see the peaks of ($H_{(i)}, N_{(i)}, C_{\alpha (i-1)}/C_{\beta (i-1)}$) in HN-CA-CB, but its intensity will be much weaker than the ($H_{(i)}, N_{(i)}, C_{\alpha(i)}/C_{\beta(i)}$) peaks.

It is to be noted that the amide proton resonance in both of these experiments belong to the ith residue, i.e. hence the (x, y) coordinate corresponding to ($H_{(i)}, N_{(i)}$) chemical shift value would be identical in both these spectrums. The difference comes only in

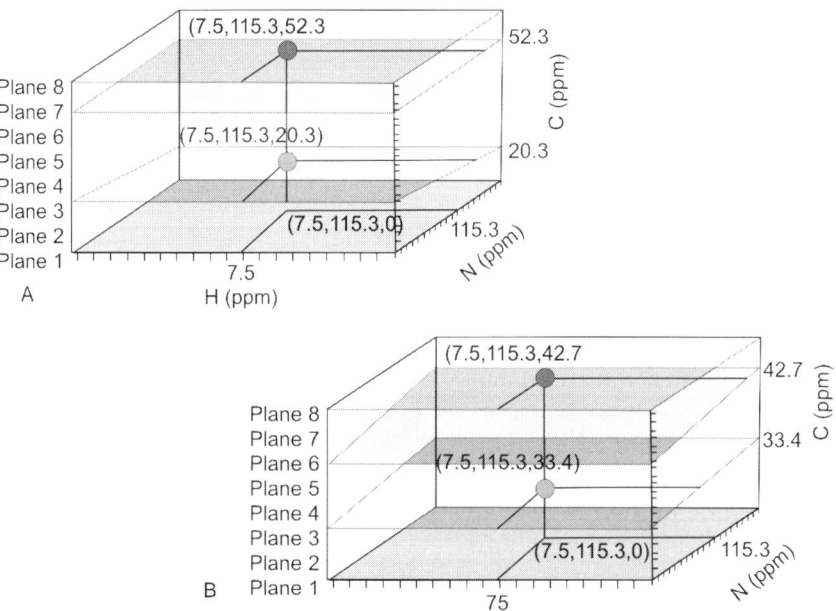

Fig. 1.23: A: Spectrum of CBCA(CO)NH experiment. The CA and CB of the (i–1)th residue appear at 52.3,20.3 and correlated with HN of ith residue at 7.5,115.3. B: Spectrum of HNCACB experiment. The CA and CB of the ith residue appear at 42.7,33.4 and correlated with HN of the same residue at 7.5,115.3

the carbon dimension, i.e the 'z' axis. In CB–CA–(CO)–NH, we can identify two peaks along carbon dimension (z) for the same $(H_{(i)}, N_{(i)})$ chemical shift value. These peaks correspond to the CA and CB of the preceeding residue (i-1). The HN–CA–CB, also shows two peaks along the carbon dimension, at the same $(H_{(i)}, N_{(i)})$ coordinates. These peaks correspond to CA and CB of the same (*i*th) residue. The amide proton of residue '*i*' helps us to correlate CA, CB of its own spin system and to its preceding spin system or residue. We can consider the following Table 1.2 where the peak pairs (CA, CB) identified from both experiments through its common amide proton resonance.

	HN-CA-CB				CB-CA-(CO)-NH			
Peak no.	$H_{(i)}$	$N_{(i)}$	$CA_{(i)}$	$CB_{(i)}$	$H_{(i)}$	$N_{(i)}$	$CA_{(i-1)}$	$CB_{(i-1)}$
1	7.5	115.3	**42.7**	**33.4**	7.5	115.3	45.7	-
2	6.8	107.3	**62.4**	**65.4**	6.8	107.3	**57.4**	**45.2**
3	8.3	121.5	53.4	20.3	8.3	121.5	**62.4**	**65.4**
4	7.1	119.8	**57.4**	**45.2**	7.1	119.8	**42.7**	**33.4**

Table 1.2

Here the peak numbers are arbitrary and do not correspond to the sequential number of the amino acid. We can see the CA/CB pairs sharing the chemical shift on both sides highlighted in different colors. On matching these values, as shown below we can identify which spin system or residue precedes it in terms of arbitrary number.

Table 1.3

Arbitrary no.	CA/CB of ith residue	CA/CB of (i–1)th residue
1	7.5, 115.3, **42.7, 33.4**	7.5, 115.3, 45.7, -
4	7.1,119.8, **57.4, 45.23**	7.1, 119.8, **42.7, 33.4**
2	6.8, 107.3, **62.45, 65.47**	6.8, 107.3, **57.4, 45.23**
3	8.3, 121.5, 53.4, 20.3	8.3, 121.5, **62.45, 65.47**

After connecting all the residues through their arbitrary number, we have to match it with its sequence by correlating with unique resonance pattern observed for residues like alanine, serine/threonine and glycine. Alanine has the lowest CB value compared to all the other amino acids and usually would not exceed 20 ppm. In the above table looking at the first column corresponding to *i*th arbitrary residue, the residue no. '3' would be alanine. Serine and threonine has its CB resonances higher than the CA value, contrasting all the other amino acids whose CA>CB. Also, CB of serine and threonine would be in the range 65 to 72 ppm. Analyzing the table again, residue '2' would be either serine or threonine. Glycine is unique among other amino acids in that it has only CA and no CB. The CA of glycine usually appear around 45 ppm. Hence we surmise the residue preceding '1' would be glycine.

If we represent the above matched residues with its guessed amino acid type, then the sequence is

Preceding residue$_{(Glycine)} - 1$ (not identifiable) $- 4$ (not identifiable) $- 2$ (S/T) $- 3$ (Alanine)

If we compare this pattern with the partial amino acid sequence of the protein,

TEEDLCSWQGFYSAHRGVLKGLP

we can identify that the section GFYSA, matches with the linked pattern of peaks, $N_G 1_x 4_x 2_S 3_A$.

By repeating this with all the available peaks, we can assign the CA, CB, N(H), H(N) of most of the amino acids in the sequence. The complete process starting from arbitrary alignment to final comparison with amino acid sequence and identifying the spin systems correctly is referred to as *backbone assignment*.

Side Chain Assignment

The side chain assignment is carried out using H(CC) (CO)NH and (H)CC(CO)NH–TOCSY based experiments. Both these experiments are similar to backbone experiments, except that the correlation is TOCSY based. As explained in earlier chapter, TOCSY gives the correlation between all the nuclei that are present within a spin system, and its implementation through experiment is unique. Instead of transfering magnetization sequentially from one nuclei to another, the magnetization gets mixed up by matching with 'Hartman Hann condition'. In a 3D H(CC) (CO)NH - TOCSY experiment, all the H(C) nuclei from different functional type (α, β, γ, δ, ε, etc.) transfers their magnetization to its immediately attached carbon and then to all carbons present within that spin system. After this 'mixing up' process, the magnetization is transferred to the amide nitrogen and then to the amide proton. The (H)CC(CO)NH–TOCSY is similar to the former TOCSY, except that carbon are detected rather than protons. In the former experiment, the first and second dimension would be H(N) and (H)N, and the third dimension would be proton that are attached to carbons, i.e. H(C) and in the latter experiment, the third dimension would be carbon that present in the side chain, i.e. (H)C.

Since we have already identified the chemical shifts of amide protons to its spin system, by going through the respective coordinate, we get the chemical shift of both carbon and protons of α, β, γ, δ, ε, etc. types present in the side chain. With the help of backbone assignment and side chain assignment, we can assign each peak present in the NOESY spectrum. Usually 3D or 4D NOESY experiments are used to avoid peak overlapping problem, though at the cost of losing some sensitivity. 3D H–HN–NOESY, starts with magnetization from all protons being transferred to its adjacent protons, through a 'mixing' delay, which is different from TOCSY's Hartman Hann mixing (where series of pulses are used). During the mixing time, through a process called 'relaxation', the magnetization from a nucleus starts leaking to its environment. If adjacent nuclei are present in close proximity to the relaxing nucleus, the magnetization transfer will take place. Unlike the conventional transfer through bonds, this process is space and distance dependent, hence the term 'through space' experiment. Following the proton to proton transfer, the magnetization is allowed to transfer to its attached amide nitrogen. During this process only the amide protons which have taken up the magnetization in previous step persists, whereas the rest of the protons will go undetected. On fourier transformation, we get both the first dimension and second dimesion to be proton types and the third dimension is (H)N.

Structure Calculation

Using chemical shifts of CA and HA alone, we can predict the secondary structure of the protein based on the fact that the CA/HA's chemical shifts for three different forms namely, the random coil, alpha helix and beta sheet are unique. But, for determining the tertiary structure, we need more structural constraints obtained through experiments.

- The distance constraint for each nucleus with respect to its neighbor nuclei are directly obtained from NOESY experiment. Another important constraint, the dihedral angle, is obtained indirectly using software called 'Talos' that uses two criteria to predict the phi and psi angles for each residue (Nmrpipe[5]). A standard database which has solved structure of proteins and highly accurate chemical shift values is used for this purpose. The test residue, whose dihedral angle has to be predicted from its chemical shift value, is BLASTED against this database, considering its flanking residues also (*ref.* section 1.4.3A, multiple sequence alignment). The resulting best sequences are taken and their structural aspects are obtained from another data base. The dihedral angle of the best search is then averaged and used as constraint for the residue in hand.

- The hydrogen bond constraints, is obtained by performing experiments such that those residues which form hydrogen bonds will retain their amide protons, while the others will exchange it with the solvent. In the spectrum, we can see prominent peaks for the residues forming H' bonds and slowly vanishing peaks for the rest. This valuable information is translated into distance information and used for structure calculation.

The structure calculation is more of an optimization problem, making use of *simulated annealing* or *genetic algorithms*. The objective is to get a globally energy minimized structure starting from random coordinates, satisfying all the provided experimental constraints. Both these algorithms, start with a set of random coordinates for all nuclei, and through a random operation, the nuclei are then moved slowly in a direction, which minimizes its overall energy. After each move, the potential energy of the molecule is calculated, along with a check on whether the experimental constrains are satisfied for the current state or structure, if so the current move will be highly favored and proceeds further. On the other hand, if either, the energy of the molecule increases or the constraints are violated, then penalty will be imposed for such moves. This process is repeated several times till a set of convergent structures are obtained.

Protein Expression for NMR Studies

In Protein NMR, it is quite routine to express/produce proteins in a highly controlled environment like recombinant bacteria, mammalian cells or in vitro systems. Which culturing such cells, the media will contain N^{15} ammonium chloride and C^{13} glucose as the sole nitrogen and carbon source. Thereby the proteins expressed/produced are labeled with NMR sensitive N^{15} and C^{13} nuclei. The expressed protein is purified and concentrated to 1mM or higher, in an appropriate buffer optimized for protein solubility and good spectrum. Usually 20 to 100 mM of phosphate buffer with sodium chloride or other salt (for solubility and stability reasons) and sodium azide (0.02%–anti fungal agent) is used. For small molecules (≤ 2 kDa) 1 dimensional or 2 dimensional experiments are good enough to get the required constraints. For medium sized molecules (>2 kDa to <25 kDa) 3 dimensional and higher experiments are necessary. For large proteins (>25 kDa), the protein is expressed in deuteriated medium rather than aqueous medium, while culturing the bacteria, this process is called *perdeuteriation*; as a result all the protons in the protein will be replaced with deuterium. This is to circumvent the signal relaxation problem, quite often faced in NMR experiments (relaxation rate is directly proportional to molecular weight of molecule). Special group of experiment called TROSY (Transverse Relaxation Optimized Spectroscopy) is used for structure determination.

References

1. Keeler J (2005) Understanding NMR spectroscopy, Wiley West Sussex. 459 p.
2. Frank. Van de van.(1995) .Multidimensional NMR In Liquids: Basic Principles And Experimental Methods
3. Cavanagh J (1996) Protein NMR spectroscopy: principles and practice, Academic Press. 885 p.
4. Bain AD (2003) Chemical exchange in NMR. *Prog Nucl Magn Reson Spectrosc* 43: 63–103.
5. NMRpipe 9. http://spin.niddk.nih.gov/NMRPipe.
6. http://www.cis.rit.edu/htbooks/nmr/
7. http://www-keeler.ch.cam.ac.uk/lectures/

1.1.2C Gene Expression

Amy De Nuan Huang

It is essential that the human body is able to produce normal proteins to maintain health. Proteins have a vast amount of important functions in the body such as catalysis of reactions, transportation of molecules and defending the body from infections. Serious problems may arise from the inability of the body to produce normal proteins due to genetic or environmental factors. For example, many people with diabetes cannot produce the protein insulin. This increases the risk of cardiovascular disease, blindness, and nerve and kidney damage. Therefore, pharmaceutical industries produce proteins, such as insulin, to be used as therapeutic drugs. In order to live normal lives, diabetic people must inject themselves daily with insulin. Pharmaceutical industries make insulin by the process of heterologous protein expression in bacteria and yeast.

Recombinant DNA technology allows scientists to produce proteins for both research and therapy. The most common bacteria used for gene cloning and expression of heterologous proteins is *Escherichia coli* because this organism has been extensively studied and is now the best understood bacteria. *E. coli* is a gram negative facultative anaerobe that is part of the normal flora in the human intestine. Some strains of *E. coli* can cause infections and diarrhea.

There are many advantages to using *E. coli* for the expression of proteins and cloning of genes. They are able to grow at high densities, they grow quickly, and they are relatively inexpensive to maintain. The cDNA of the gene of interest can be inserted into a plasmid vector, although a virus vector may be used as well. Scientists and researchers are able to create recombinant DNA plasmids to clone eukaryotic genes in bacteria such as *E. coli*. The ability to create recombinant DNA plasmids comes from the discovery of restriction enzymes. Restriction enzymes cut pieces of DNA at specific sites which allows scientists to cut out and fuse different pieces of DNA together to produce the plasmid they want. A cloning vector is a piece of plasmid that can carry foreign DNA into a cell. Cloning vectors can be extracted from the bacteria and then manipulated by inserting a gene into the vector (through the use of restriction enzymes) and then this recombinant plasmid can be reintroduced into the bacteria to be cloned.

Commercially available plasmids contain a selectable marker that most commonly confers antibiotic resistance. Therefore, growing *E. coli* cells on a medium with the antibiotic will isolate colonies that contain the plasmid and thus the gene of interest. Competent *E. coli* cells can uptake the plasmid vector through transformation. The competent *E. coli* cells may be heat shocked into uptaking the plasmid or electrically shocked. The *E. coli* cells can then be plated on medium that contains nutrients and an antibiotic. They will selectively grow and multiply resulting in millions of copies of the plasmid produced in a relatively short period. Usually, in 24 hours the colonies of *E. coli* formed are large enough to work with.

Challenges and modifications can arise when attempting to express a eukaryotic gene in a prokaryotic cell. For example, promoters and certain other regulatory sequences are different in bacteria when compared to a eukaryotic cell. The use of an expression vector has overcome the differences in promoters in prokaryotic and eukaryotic cells. An expression vector contains a highly active prokaryotic promoter just upstream of the site where the eukaryotic gene is inserted. This ensures that the bacteria will recognize the promoter and express the foreign gene. Another problem with expressing a eukaryotic gene in bacteria is the presence of introns in most eukaryotic gene. This is solved by using cDNA instead of the natural gene sequence itself. The cDNA of a gene lacks introns present in the original gene sequence.

Eukaryotic organisms are also used in protein expression and DNA cloning. Yeasts are common organisms to use because they have been well characterized and are able to perform post-translational modifications to proteins such as adding carbohydrate or lipid groups. In addition, yeasts offer a few advantages compared to other eukaryotic organisms. Yeasts are single celled organism and they are easy to grow like bacteria and they also have plasmids. Yeast artificial chromosomes (YACs) are chromosome vectors that can be used in cloning or expression of a protein in yeast. YACs contain essential DNA sequences including an origin for DNA replication, a centromere and two telomeres with foreign DNA. There are a few methods that scientists use to insert recombinant DNA into yeast. One method is electroporation in which an electrical impulse creates holes in the cell's plasma membrane which allows the foreign DNA to enter. Another method is the direct injection of DNA into the cell.

An example of yeast used as a system for heterologous protein expression is *Pichia pastoris*. This organism has been used to produce over 600 heterologous proteins including human insulin, cow rennin (used for cheese making), and certain drugs and vaccines. Many valuable human proteins have been produced in *P. pastoris* because it has many qualities that make it ideal for this application. For instance, the alcohol oxidase I gene (*AOXI*) can be inserted on the plasmid into *P. pastoris,* and when grown on methanol medium, this gene is induced. *AOXI* is the blueprint for the alcohol oxidase protein and it contains one of the strongest promoters known. There is almost a 1000 fold increase induction of transcription when cells are switched from glucose to methanol medium. In fact, about 30% of the total protein made is the alcohol oxidase protein when a *P. pastoris* cell is grown on methanol medium. Thus, from the alcohol oxidase gene, the *P. pastoris* cell is able to synthesize an amazing amount of alcohol oxidase protein. Therefore, when scientists are using *P. pastoris* to make their protein, they simply substitute the coding region of their protein (i.e. insulin) for that of alcohol oxidase. The plasmid with the desired gene can be cloned using *E. coli* and then purified so that it can be transformed into yeast. Once transformed, large amounts of *P. pastoris* can be grown in a liquid medium that contains methanol to induce transcription of the gene and therefore expression of the protein. The protein synthesized by the yeast is purified and used for further research, drug therapy or other purposes.

References

1. Campbell NA, Reece JB. Biology 7th edition. Pearson Education. 2005, 384–391
2. Lin Cereghino GP, Lin Cereghino JL, Ilgen C, Cregg JM. Production of recombinant proteins in fermenter cultures of the yeast *Pichia pastoris*. Elsevier Science. 2002, **13**:329–332.

1.1.2D Solid-Phase Peptide Synthesis

Betty De Suan Huang

Structures of enzymes and how it influences the function of the enzyme has been studied extensively. In the field of pharmacology, peptide drugs are being developed to treat many diseases, and even the older peptide drugs are still being studied, such as insulin and bacitracin.[1] Peptides also acting as an antimicrobial agent are being studied and are considered to have a very high potential for success as antibiotic resistance become more and more of a problem with conventional agents.[2] The field of peptide drugs today is growing enormously as the usefulness and interesting biological activities of these drugs are being discovered. However, before the development of peptide drugs, many natural enzymes in the body and its structure are analyzed to see how the enzyme works due to its shape. Usually, the globular form of the enzyme is broken down and looked at in its secondary form for simplicity, such as its beta sheets and alpha helices. In the lab, parts of the active site of an enzyme are reconstructed and analyzed using computational theoretical chemistry. By doing so, chemist can gain a better understanding of how the enzyme works relative to its shape.

Many labs also synthesize short peptide sequences and study the properties, gaining insight on how peptides work, and thus how enzymes in the human body work. Many times, the active site of an enzyme is recreated to help fully understand how that certain peptide sequence works in the human body. The approach to breaking down and studying a single component allows us to eventually understand how the whole component works. For example, the thioredoxin superfamily of enzymes (which play an important role in the reduction, oxidation, and isomerization of disulfide bonds) has been studied through reconstruction of its active site and has been analyzed for its properties that are evident in the human body.[3,4] In this specific example, the active site of the thioredoxin enzymes is a short peptide sequence containing the motif of CXXC, where X usually represents hydrophobic amino acids and the cysteine residues are responsible for the enzyme's main activity. It has been shown that the cysteine residues are unusually acidic.[5] In order to elucidate this phenomenon, a series of cysteine- polyglycine peptides were synthesized and its properties measured. As the articles have shown, it is very likely that the secondary structure-the alpha helix-of the peptide contributes to the overall acidity of the cysteine residues. With this understanding, it is clearly seen that it is not only the sequence of the enzyme, it is the overall conformation that can play a role in its mechanism. This allows us to appreciate and understand the importance of the shape of the peptide as a drug in medicinal chemistry.

There are many synthesis methods available to make peptides. There are biological techniques in which the gene of the sequence is isolated and inserted into a microorganism for synthesis. For those peptides that are difficult to express in bacteria, other techniques can be used. One of the most commonly used today is Solid-Phase Peptide Synthesis (SPPS). This was developed by Robert Bruce Merrifield in 1962, who won the Nobel prize for it in 1984. The ease of purification of synthesized peptide made this method become very widespread and popular. Merrifield used a peptide synthesis vessel, which consists of a frit that insoluble resins lie on and a valve that allows liquid solvents to drain out of the vessel. Solid phase peptide synthesis involves the initial coupling of the C-terminal residue of the amino acid to an insoluble solid support, deprotection of the labile protecting group on the N terminus of the amino acid, coupling with the next successive residue, and cleavage of the solid support after the peptide is completed. Since the peptide is attached to an insoluble resin, every step is washed with solvent and the peptide is easily purified.

Mass spectrometry is used to identify expected ionized fragments to confirm that the desired peptide has been synthesized. For every peptide sequence, the mass spectrometry is able to induce fragments unique to the sequence. Usually, a minute amount of the peptide is dissolved and used as the ion source. Through electrospray ionization and collision induced dissociation (CID), the ion source is sprayed into the mass analyzer and dissociates into ionized fragments. These fragments are measured by their mass to charge ratio and is unique to every peptide. Theoretical peaks of the fragments are matched with experimental peaks obtained. Usually with a confirmation of three or more matching peaks, it is concluded that the peptide was synthesized and that it was synthesized in the correct sequence. With this knowledge, the synthesized peptide can be further analyzed for its properties. The mass spectrometry is also used to compare the acidic and basic properties of the peptide using reference acids or bases. When the peptide is dissolved with an acid, a proton bound heterodimer is measured. Depending on the intensity of the peak, it is determined whether the peptide is more or less acidic than the reference acid.

In order to predict the conformation of a peptide, theoretical chemistry programs such as Gaussian are used and theoretical properties of the peptide are usually compared to the experimental. There are several methods mentioned in section 2.3.2.C3 available within the program to estimate and predict the properties of the peptide. Through comparing many short peptide sequences, the properties and effects of the peptide structure becomes more lucid.

Peptides are influenced quite dramatically by its structural conformation. By studying the effects of its structure, researchers can better understand the biological activity of peptide drugs and thus further develop the peptide drug research area.

References

1. Manosroi, A; Khanrin, P; Werner, R; Götz, F; Manosroi, W; Manosroi, J. Entrapment Enhancement of peptide drugs in niosomes. *Journal of Micoencapsulation.* 2010, 27, 272–280. Online at *http://informahealthcare.com/.*
2. Pan, C; Chow, T; Yu, C; Yu, C; Chen, J; Chen, J. Antimicrobial peptides of an anti-lipopolysaccharide factor, epinecidin-1, and hepcidin reduce the lethality of *Riemerella anatipestifer* sepsis in ducks. *Peptides.* 2010, 31, 806–815. Online at http://www.ncbi.nlm.nih.gov/pubmed/20138098.
3. Tan, J. P.; Ren, J. Determination of the Gas-Phase Acidities of Cysteine-Polyalanine Peptides Using the Extended Kinetic Method. *J. Am. Soc. Mass Spectrom.* 2007, *18*, 188–194.
4. Ren, J.; Tan, J. P.; Harper, R. T. Gas-Phase Acidities of Cysteine- Polyalanine Peptides I: A3,4CSH, and HSCA3,4. *J. Phys. Chem. A* 2009,113, 10903–10912.
5. http://www.pubmedcentral.nih.gov/articlerender.fcgi?artid=2286559.

1.1.3 PROTEINS ON THE WEB: THE RESULT OF EXPERIMENTS

Computational biology and chemistry serve to augment our knowledge in many ways, such as building and visualizing models, understanding catalytic reactions and their mechanism, rates and energetics, predicting 3D structure, estimating dynamic interaction of molecules and their functions, ultimately helping to fill up gaps in experimental data. Knowledge of structure of receptors and hormones can provide direct benefits to the improvement of medicines and disease prevention. The precise molecular structure and (lack of) symmetry of a protein gives it great selectivity in distinguishing among the various small molecules that circulate in the body evincing the search for the better drug. The historical hypothesis by Adrien Albert (see introduction passages to chapter 2.3) that acetylcholine (neurotransmitter) and D-tubocurarine (the compound in curare), both being quaternary ammonium compounds and yet having opposing biological action (the former contracts and the latter relaxes skeletal muscles), indeed acted on the same receptor and that the difference was in the latter blocking the action of the former at the receptor site owing to its larger size, proved to be the benchmark for such studies. As of March 2010, RefSeq (http://www.ncbi.nlm.nih.gov/refseq/)–the Swiss protein database that serves as a repository of protein sequences–reports 9,856,489 proteins. Several proteins in that database are relevant to the molecular pharmacological pathway of diseases, but till date having unknown structure, hinder pharmaceutical development.

The year 2000 marked two important incidents, one resulting from the other, of which drug designers must know. The first was the successful completion of the *human genome project* (for an overview of results and implications in medicine, *ref.* **Discussion 1.2**) as a result of which, the 21st century is constantly being referred to as the "post genomic era".

Discussion 1.2: The human genome project (HGP)

The ability to "tune" the molecular signaling that continually occurs in our bodies will eventually allow for more exquisite control of the cellular processes of life.

(National Research Council, USA: Committee on challenges, 2003)

As the highlight of the "biology century", the year 2003–the 50th anniversary of Watson and Crick's description of DNA structure–witnessed the completion of the human DNA sequencing. The mega project officially began in 1990 and ran for 13 years. The first draft of the human genome was produced in the year 2000.

"As of this writing, the HGP has produced finished sequence covering H"98% of the euchromatic human genome"

(Waterston, et al. 2003)

The project began in 1990 and was initially headed by James D. Watson at the US National Institutes of Health. A working draft of the genome was released in 2000 and a more complete version was published in 2003.

The primarily goal of the project was to chemically sequence the 3 billion base pairs of and to identify the 20,000–25,000 genes in the human genome. This intends to map the human genome in a physical as well as functional sense. The results of this project have immense scope for bioinformatics, and therefore setting up a storage and retrieval system was also one of the goals. A database of the sequence of the human genome is now available for public access and the link to it can be found in the website mentioned in the references to this discussion. During the project, major advancements in the sequencing and analyzing technology were made. The project also aimed to address the 'ethical, legal, and social issues' (acronym: ELSI) pertaining to this project. The project intensively involved both private and public agencies such as the US department of energy, the Wellcome trust from UK, numerous institutions of the academia, etc. from several countries such as US, UK, France, China, India, etc.

It is an undeniable fact that this grand project is an extraordinary accomplishment for biology, chemistry, pharmaceutical sciences, biotechnology, biochemistry, instrumentation and engineering, computer sciences, and other fields. Discoveries of the past 50 years were pooled together from polymerase chain reaction to short-gun sequencing. The contribution of the latter technique is noteworthy-short-gun sequencing enabled the sequencing of large segments of the genome in a few months. A 2,000 to 300,000 base pair long DNA fragment was fragmented to various sizes to generate a DNA "library". The library fragments are sequenced using an automated DNA sequencer. With the aid of a supercomputer, these fragments are pieced together to generate the complete original sequence.

The initial results of the project surprised researchers. Being at the highest level of organismal complexity, humans were expected to have more than 100,000 genes; however, the study showed that there were only 30,000 genes comparable to that of mice. These genes contained several key ones that are responsible for various diseases. The main areas of focus of the last 5-year plan of this project are Genetic Map, physical map, DNA Sequence (99% of gene-containing part of human sequence finished to 99.99% accuracy), Human Sequence Variation (3.7 million mapped human SNPs), Gene Identification (this included 15,000 full-length human cDNAs), the use of model organisms such as the fruit fly, functional analysis (such as scale-up for protein-protein interaction). Results from this enormous project are steady with the availability of genes that code for proteins and with the mapping of single nucleotide polymorphisms. The project has lead to the splicing and identification of 46,000 proteins, RNA classes have special functions, the presence of disease–genes located in the non coding regions (in contrast to what was believed), the possibility to investigate post-translational modification of proteins, etc.

*Selected references for this discussion: (Waterston, et al., 2002), (Waterston, et al., 2003), (Lander, et al., 2001), (Collins, et al., 2003), (McPherson, et al., 2001), (Venter, et al., 2001)

http://www.ornl.gov/sci/techresources/Human_Genome/project/about.shtml; http://www.ornl.gov/sci/techresources/Human_Genome/home.shtml;

The second milestone in this same year was the commencement of the **structural genomics initiative** to utilize the information about the coding regions (regions that code for proteins) in the DNA of humans resulting from the human genome project. The structural genomics initiative aims to solve the 3D structure of 10,000 proteins by the year 2010 (*ref.* **Discussion 1.3** for the mission statement). Achievement of such a goal requires combined efforts in the improvement of experimental and computational strategies to establish working sequence–structure–function relationships. This demands establishing sound correlations between sequence and structure, and further between structure and function such that the function can be directly predicted from the gene product–the sequence. This helps in structure prediction, folding pathway analysis and working towards "pinning proteus down".

Discussion 1.3: The structural genomics initiative

The launch and completion of a project as momentous as the human genome project produces considerable impact on the research community. Rising from its glowing embers is the Structural Genomics Initiative (http://www.structuralgenomics.org). This project aims to systematically elucidate the structure of all known proteins. The importance of this step to Medicinal Chemistry will become evident under chapter 2.1 in Part II of this book. Briefly, the availability of the 3D protein structure forms the basis of structure-based rational drug design. Though the sequences of several pharmacologically important proteins are known, their structure has not yet been characterized. The lack of 3D coordinates of target proteins forms the rate limiting step to rational drug design. The structural genomics project serves to aid medicinal chemists by prioritizing unsolved proteins for the experimental protein chemists and keeping track of solved ones for the computational protein chemists. This project that keeps track of the former process is called the protein structure Initiative. It

1. Is based on the high-throughput structure determination paradigm
2. Is set up to facilitate the tedious experimental process of determining protein structure by X-ray, NMR, and other techniques
3. Serves to improve the efficiency of protein synthesis and isolation techniques such as gene expression and cloning
4. Serves to prioritize targets in demand for structure elucidation as to save time for the drug discovery process
5. Extends advice to structure-based drug design, design of therapeutics for genetic diseases, etc.
6. Intends to serve as starign point for the investigation of protein folding, evolutionary relationships, structure prediction, and classification (these topics are dealt with in the chapters of Part I of this book).

The website http://kb.psi-structuralgenomics.org/KB/ keeps track of sequencing, structure determination and protein function.

The initiative also aims to automate all processes–from calculations and comparisons to decision-making and providing feedback.

The current database that acts as a repository of protein structures that have been determined experimentally is the protein data bank–PDB. It is the single most exhaustive database from which one can obtain protein *structure* – i.e. the coordinates of its atoms. Only when these coordinates are available, as mentioned in **Discussion 1.3**, structure-based drug design is possible, such as de Novo design, docking, etc. presented in chapters of part II. In addition to protein coordinates, the database also offers a host of other information as mentioned in **Discussion 1.4**.

Discussion 1.4: The protein data bank

The RCSB Protein Data Bank (hereafter, the PDB) is available at http://rcsb.org/pdb or newly at http://www.pdb.org/pdb/home/home.do. It was first established in 1971 at Brookhaven National Laboratory and was earlier called Brookhaven databank; then, it contained 7 structures. Now, it is managed by Rutgers (at the State University of New Jersey) and UCSD (University of California, San Diego) belonging to the RCSB (Research Collaboratory for Structural Bioinformatics) group.

The RCSB PDB is a member of the Worlwide PDB (wwPDB) along with PDBe (Europe), PDBj (Japan) and the BMRB (Biological Magnetic Resonance Data Bank; also from USA).The PDB has several mirror sites that archive and manage the huge amount of data contained in it to facilitate global access.

Growth of the database: The growth of the PDB is remarkable and some interesting numbers have been presented (compiled from http://www.pdb.org/pdb/static.do?p=general_information/pdb_statistics/):

	Protein	*Nuclei acid*	*All structures*
1976	13	0 (DNA)	13
1985	172	10 (DNA)	195
1995	3456	227 (DNA)	3,823
2000	12141	644 (DNA)	13604
2005	31,204	1,022 (DNA)	34,172
2010	59,711	1,262 (DNA)	64,500

Current Most populated X-ray resolution = 1.5–2 Å
Current most populated enzyme class = 3.2.1.17 (lysozyme)

Experimental method	*All structures*
NMR (2000)	2140
NMR (2005)	5133
NMR (2010)	8334
EM (2000)	13
EM (2005)	116
EM (2010)	284
Current: X-ray	55,731
Current: NMR	8,322

Some information present in the Database

For a particular protein, the database offers the following information:

- References–primary and other–that describe why the protein was studied and in what environment it was obtained.
- Name of the protein, organismal source, other molecules whose coordinates have been deposited along with those of the protein.
- Enzyme or protein classification code with a classification of its domains and a labeling of its secondary structural features by various methods.
- Sequence and structural similarities between the protein and other proteins in the database.
- Geometry, structure, Ramachandran map, multimer, monomer, biologically active form of the molecule.

- Coordinate files (see end of this discussion) for download.
- Links to a number of other databases of proteins, genome, etc. such as *PDBsum* (containing literature research and background connecting genomic and other information), *proteopedia*, comparison of surface topology, interatomic contacts, protein-ligand contacts, etc.

In general, it offers the following information
- Education tools and tutorials.
- Statistics on the growth of the database in various categories that reflect research trends.
- Information about proteins and their history in the form of "molecule of the month" and the Protein Structure Initiative–"featured molecule" bulletins.
- Built in Java based molecules viewer.
- News and publications, career, policies and others.

Searching for entries: Proteins and other entries can be searched by typing the key word(s) in the search box (when all related structures will be listed out) or by typing out the ID of the protein (such as 1GOX) if known. Advanced search help to simultaneously filter the dataset using several categories such as
- Experimental method of determination (X-ray, NMR, etc),
- The accuracy of the structure (X-ray: resolution),
- Protein classification (SCOP, CATH, etc… see later under chapter 1.2.2),
- Other molecules present (such as ligands),
- Unique sequences (the same protein might be repeatedly deposited in the PDB by the same group owing to different experimental conditions OR by different groups. This gives rise to redundancy. One can filter out similar sequences if one needs unique proteins), and
- Several other categories.

File for download: The experimentalists who determine protein structure use special software for refinement of the determined protein structure (*ref.* sections 1.1.2.A, B). The coordinates of atoms in the protein are then saved onto a text file and deposited into the PDB. This text file is given the extension '.pdb' such as '1GOX.pdb'. The contents of this file must follow a strict format called the PDB file format and this is discussed separately in **Discussion 31** under chapter 2.3.1.D in Part II. The PDB files are opened by most molecular modeling software. One or more files can be downloaded in various formats such as the PDB format, the MMCIF format, the Mol2 format for ligands, the FASTA file containing only the amino acid sequence of the protein, etc. Each format serves a specific purpose.

As of April, 2010, the databank contained 64,500 structures.

1.2 *Protein Structure Analysis*

There are some enterprises in which a careful disorderliness is the true method.

Hermann Melville

In 1950s, Linus Pauling predicted that the protein chain can exist in only two regularly repeating forms—the α-helix and the β-sheet and that the other forms of helices, though could be made, would be considerably strained. With the availability of X-ray crystallographic data on proteins, the first of which was determined by Sir John Cowdery Kendrew for which he was awarded the Nobel Prize in 1962, a complicated jumble of structures was observed. The earlier experiments of Anfinsen and coworkers (*ref.* chapter 1.5) that showed proteins as being capable of attaining their native folded forms perplexed researchers when they realized that this folded form was indeed so complicated.

The visualization and evaluation of protein structure is being increasingly done using computers because XYZ coordinates of each atom in a protein can be obtained from X-ray and NMR experiments. These Cartesian coordinates are stored in files along with other information such as the name of the proteins, the resolution in Å it was obtained at (for X-ray structures), the primary references for the way the protein was studied and to what purpose, etc. These files are stored in a worldwide databank called "the protein data bank" or in short, the PDB (*ref.* discussion 1.4). Each protein file is therefore referred to as a PDB file. Depending on the experiment, the proteins are sometimes studied along with ligand, cofactor, water molecules, peptide fragments, etc. and in turn, their coordinates also become available along with those of the protein. For a detailed discussion of the PDB file format, *ref.* **Discussion 31**. The Cambridge Crystallographic Data Centre (CCDC) at http://www.ccdc.cam.ac.uk/stores such structures for small organic and inorganic molecules.

Did You Know? 2

The Cambridge Crystallographic Data Centre recently reported the archiving of its 500,000th crystal structure—that of Lamotrigine! "However, the scientific community is hungry for the next 500,000..." writes Dr. Colin Groom, Executive Director of the CCDC. The structure of Lamotrigine was published by Balasubramanian Sridhar and Krishnan Ravikumar, Indian institute of Chemical Technology, Hyderabad (Sridhar, et al. 2009).

Figure 1.24 shows the levels of information that become available to researchers along the stages to determine protein structure and the role of computations. The XYZ coordinates, *per se*, are nothing but points in space. One can obtain meaningful structural information only using specialized software that combines the position of each point with the chemical information in the PDB. For example, the second atom in the protein of PDB ID 1A6I [deposited (Orth, et al. 1998)], which is a variant of tetracycline repressor protein class D, is located at coordinate (X, Y, Z = 11.854, 20.860, 6.211).

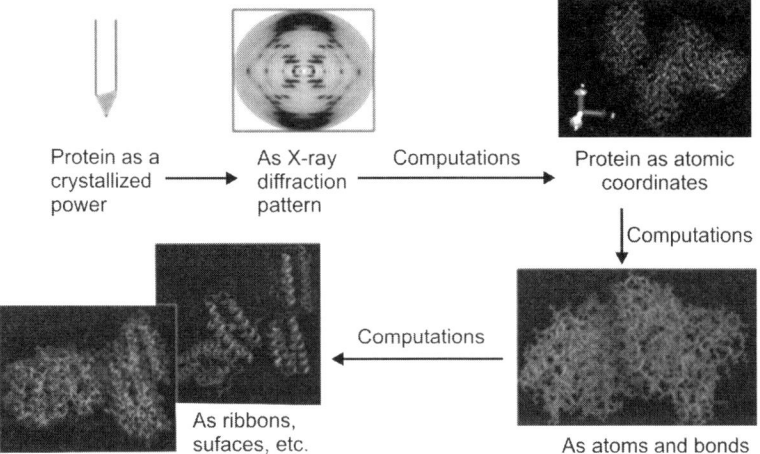

Fig. 1.24: Levels of information that become available to researchers along the stages to determine protein structure and the role of computations. Protein pictures made using VMD® and Molden®

The software combines this position with the fact that it is a C_α atom belonging to serine, the first residue of the protein (molecular visualization is outlined in Part II, section 2.3.2.D).

It is noteworthy that to just look at the shape of proteins in full color and represented by fancy ribbons is insufficient. "Protein structure analysis" always aims:

- To simplify structure by organizing it into various levels (as in chapter 1.2.1)
- To obtain a quantitative description of structure by geometry, conformation, periodicity, regularity and deviation from ideal, strain, energy content (chapter 1.2.2)
- To quantitatively compare structures and shapes in order to obtain an estimate of all the different patterns in nature (chapter 1.2.3) and consequently,
- To classify them in various ways (chapter 1.2.4) with the long-term goal to decipher protein function.

1.2.1 GENERAL OVERVIEW OF STRUCTURE

> *Alice had learnt several things of this sort in her lessons in the schoolroom, and though this was not a very good opportunity for showing off her knowledge, as there was no one to listen to her, still it was good practice to say it over.*
> *'Alice's Adventures in Wonderland', by Lewis Carroll.*

Proteins are the key to understanding biology. They are macromolecules; the polymers, or specifically, polypeptides made of amino acids linked via peptide/amide bonds. Protein structure is complex and so it is organized into primary, secondary, tertiary and quaternary structure. Figure 1.25A is a schematic representation of the various protein structure levels.

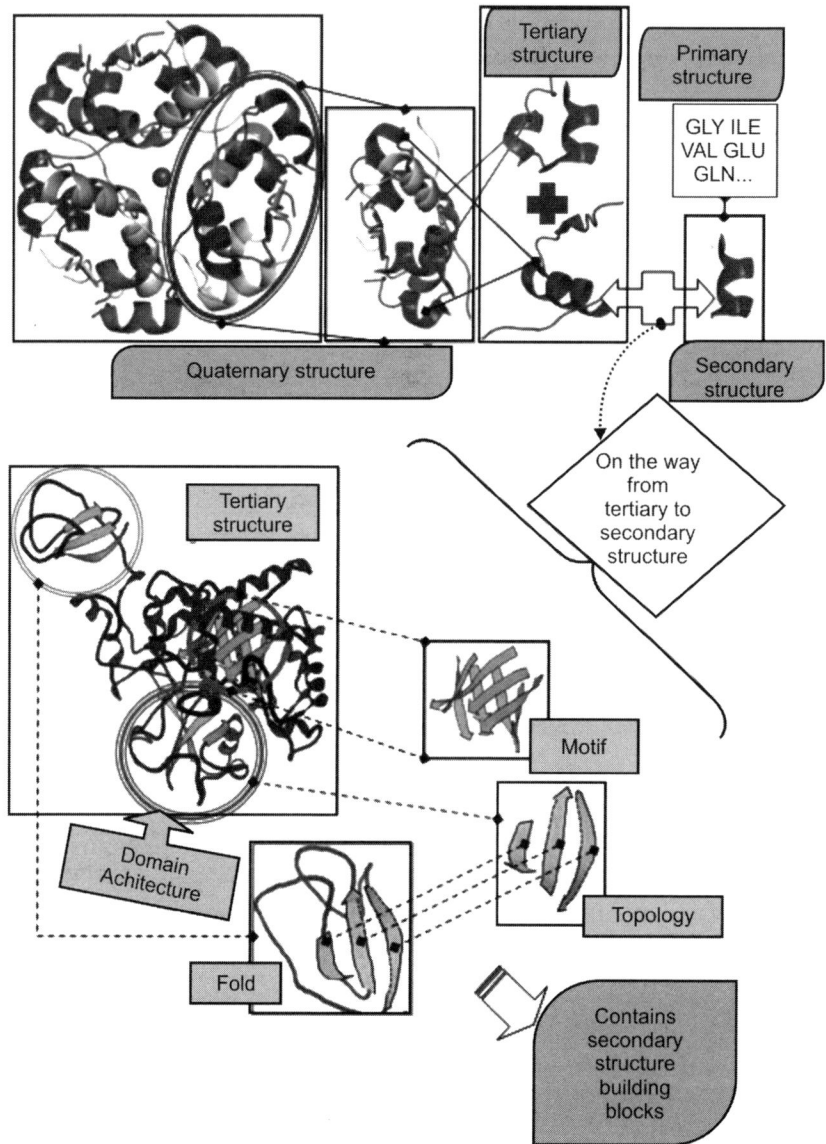

Fig. 1.25A: The hierarchy followed in organizing protein structure. Protein pictures made using Chimera®

1.2.1A Amino Acids: The Monomers

It is well known that although there are 300 different naturally occurring amino acids, the DNA cares to encode for only 20 of these and uses them in various combinations to make proteins. Amino acids combine to form the polypeptide chain via *covalent amide linkages*. The amide HNCO arrangement is planar due to anomeric effect–orbital interactions involving the lone pair on NH, the π-electron pair on the CO double bond, and antibonding π^* group-orbitals on Cα in the peptide linkage (Williams, et al. 1981). The arrangement is also almost always trans and is favored over cis arrangement by 10^3-fold.

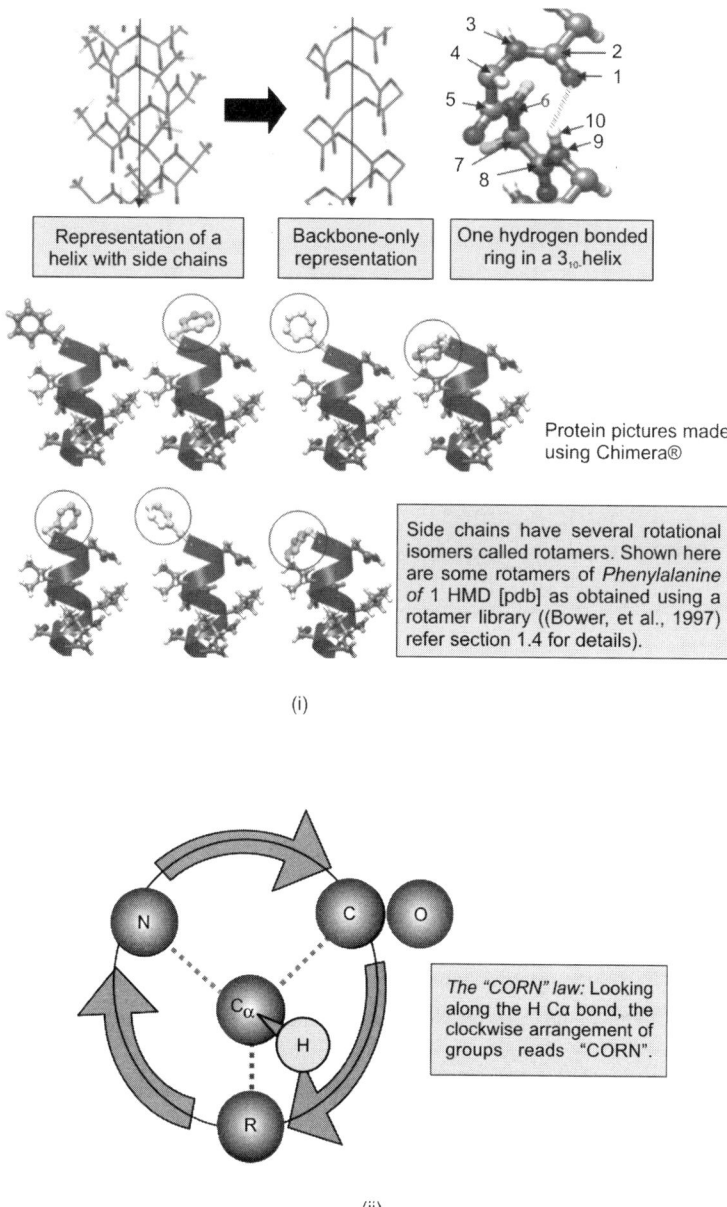

Representation of a helix with side chains

Backbone-only representation

One hydrogen bonded ring in a 3_{10} helix

Protein pictures made using Chimera®

Side chains have several rotational isomers called rotamers. Shown here are some rotamers of *Phenylalanine* of 1 HMD [pdb] as obtained using a rotamer library ((Bower, et al., 1997) refer section 1.4 for details).

(i)

The *"CORN" law:* Looking along the H Cα bond, the clockwise arrangement of groups reads "CORN".

(ii)

Fig. 1.25B (i) and (ii): Protein jargon: backbone, side chain, H-bonded rings and side chain-rotamers

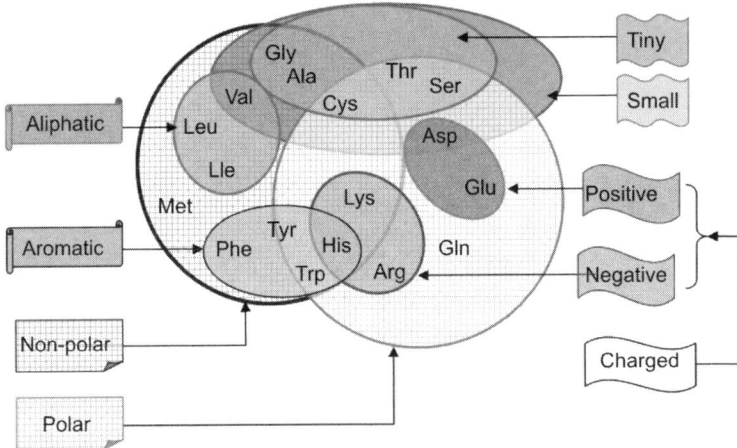

Fig. 1.25C: The amino acid monomers–stereochemistry and diversity

---

Question Box

Name the 20 amino acids in full, as their 3 letter- and single letter-codes. Construct a Venn diagram distributing all the 20 amino acids among as many properties (such as "acidic") as can be determined. What is the stereochemical property that is common to all amino acids (all are L)? Express all the 20 amino acids by their absolute configuration. Do you notice anything peculiar (all but cystein are R)? Can you identify the reason for the peculiarity?

1.2.1B The Primary Structure

The amino acids are the monomer units that make up the protein (*ref.* Table 1.4). We know that the sequence with which they occur in proteins is important; the amino acid sequence of a protein itself contributes to structure. This is easy to understand if one imagines the influence of very flexible amino acids such as glycine or very rigid structures such as proline occurring along the sequence. The amino acid sequence in a polypeptide chain is derived directly from the genetic code. The sequence of amino acids on insulin is for example, different from the sequence in G-protein. The protein is typical with respect to the number of residues in the chain, the number of chains in the protein, the presence of key residues bordering the binding pocket essential for the protein's functioning, the distribution of residues that maintain its structure by forming disulfide linkages/hydrogen bonds (etc). These are all features of a protein and due to their strong interrelationship with the protein sequence mentioned at the beginning, it has been increasingly appreciated that secondary and even tertiary structure of a protein is dictated by the amino acid sequence. Arriving at this conclusion is not surprising since all that a protein is "born" with is only its amino acid sequence (Fig. 1.26A). Determining the primary structure–protein shape correlation is done in protein structure prediction (*ref.* chapter 1.4). The Paracelsus challenge and its result (discussed under chapter 1.4), in addition to the work of Chou and Fasman (also

Table 1.4: A list of the 20 genetically recognized, post-translationally modified and synthetically used amino acids found in proteins

1. Coded for insertion into proteins			
19 α-amino acids $NH_2 - CH(R) - COOH$			
Glycine	$R = H$	Arginine	$R = CH_2-(CH_2)_2-NHC(NH)NH_2$
Alanine	$R = CH_3$	Lysine	$R = CH_2-(CH_2)_3-NH_2$
Valine	$R = CH_2(CH_3)_2$	Methionine	$R = CH_2CH_2-S-CH_3$
Leucine	$R = CH_2CH(CH_3)_2$	Serine	$R = CH_2OH$
Isoleucine	$R = CH(CH_3)CH_2CH_3$	Threonine	$R = CH(OH)CH_3$
Glutamate	$R = CH_2CH_2COOH$	Cysteine	$R = CH_2SH$
Aspartate	$R = CH_2COOH$	Phenylalanine	$R = CH_2C_6H_5$
Tyrosine	$R = CH_2C_6H_4OH$	Histidine	$R = CH_2C_3H_3N_2$
Tryptophan	$R = CH_2C_8H_5N$	Asparagine	$R = CH_2CONH_2$
		Glutamine	$R = CH_2CH_2CONH_2$
One imino acid			
Proline	$(C_4H_7NH)\,COOH$		
One rare amino acid			
Selenocysteine			
One amino acid in bacteria			
Pyrrolysine			
2. Produced post-translationally in proteins			
4-Hydroxyproline	Formyl methionine	Gamma carboxy glutamic acid	Hypusine
3. Other amino acids in the body			
Homocysteine	2-aminoisobutyric acid	Ornithine	Citrulline
Gamma-aminobutyric acid (GABA)	Lanthionine	3-aminopropanoic acid	
4. Biological β-amino acid			
β-alanine (3-aminopropanoic acid)			

detailed in chapter 1.4), are early proof for this hypothesis and highlight two complementary aspects of this relationship: that sequence dictates structure, and that a specific structure requires typical arrangement of only selective 'key' residues. Protein structure prediction has become a vast and growing field that has given new hopes to genetics, drug design, pharmacogenomics and disease research (*ref.* Part III).

1.2.1C Conformations of the Protein Backbone *vs* the Side Chain

An amino acid is so called because it contains a free amine and another free carboxylic acid group, both attached to the same carbon atom (the alpha-carbon, C_α). The free

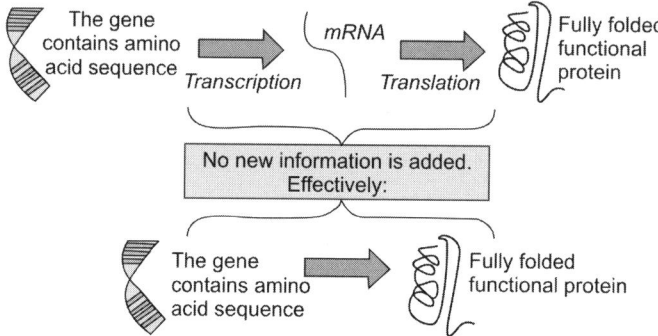

Fig. 1.26A: Gene → RNA → protein: only the amino acid sequence is available for a protein to survive

carboxyl group condenses with the free amino group to form an amide linkage and a dipeptide. This dipeptide has a free amino and carboxylic group too, but attached to two different residues (Fig. 1.26B). A protein of any length, in the same way, will have a free of amino group at one end and a free carboxylic group at the other end respectively called the N terminus and the C terminus (Fig. 1.26C). After the formation of the amide linkage, the N, C_α and $C_{carbonyl}$ atoms form a continuous chain repeating in that order. These atoms form the "backbone" of the protein (Fig. 1.26D) and the amino acid R-groups form the side chains. An essential feature of the backbone is that the amide unit is planar and folds on itself forming various shapes due to interaction between its various atoms. The side chain could be imagined as a "bunch of grapes" that hangs from the backbone with some freedom to rotate. These adjust to the folding of the backbone and also to the interactions of other side chains that may come closer to each other in space.

$NH_2 - CH(R_1) - \boxed{COOH + NH_2} - CH(R_2) - COOH$

A dipeptide has one peptide bond; there is still an amino and carboxyl group free

$NH_2 - CH(R_1) - CO - NH - CH(R_2) - COOH$

Fig. 1.26B: A dipeptide has a free amino and carboxyl group

$NH_2 - CH(R_1) - CO - NH - CH(R_2) - CO - NH - CH(R_3) - CO - NH - CH(R_4) - CO - NH - COOH$

A protein has a free amino group called amino terminus and a free carboxyl group called the carboxy terminus

Fig. 1.26C: An *N*-residue peptide also has a free amino and carboxyl group

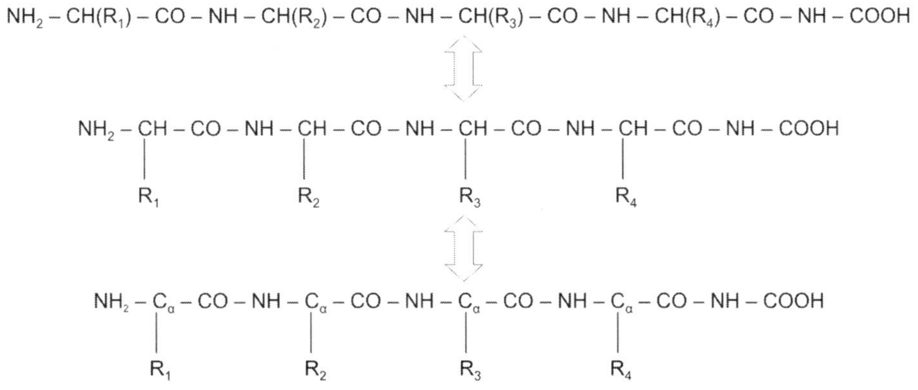

$$NH_2 - CH(R_1) - CO - NH - CH(R_2) - CO - NH - CH(R_3) - CO - NH - CH(R_4) - CO - NH - COOH$$

$$NH_2 - \underset{\underset{R_1}{|}}{CH} - CO - NH - \underset{\underset{R_2}{|}}{CH} - CO - NH - \underset{\underset{R_3}{|}}{CH} - CO - NH - \underset{\underset{R_4}{|}}{CH} - CO - NH - COOH$$

$$NH_2 - \underset{\underset{R_1}{|}}{C_\alpha} - CO - NH - \underset{\underset{R_2}{|}}{C_\alpha} - CO - NH - \underset{\underset{R_3}{|}}{C_\alpha} - CO - NH - \underset{\underset{R_4}{|}}{C_\alpha} - CO - NH - COOH$$

> After amino acid condensation, there is continuity in the protein via the $-N-C_\alpha-C-$ atoms. These are called backbone atoms as they form the "backbone" of the protein, the 'R' groups are imagined to be suspended from it.

Fig. 1.26D: Backbone and side chain

Protein structure analysts generally try to understand most structures by one of the following approaches:

a. Protein structure is mainly dependent on and evident from the backbone shape. The rotational and geometric conformation of the side chain (the rotational conformation of a side chain is called its *rotamer*, as indicated in Fig. 1.25B) is mostly influenced by the backbone's local conformation.

b. The side chains form the main bulk of the protein. The very fact that backbone atoms approach each other for interaction is due to the repulsion–attraction forces that operate among the various side chain atoms. So, it is the side chain that fixes protein shape (Dahl, et al. 2008).

The debate continues… one can never actually 'separate' the backbone and side chain; these are not two independent parts of a protein (as if one can exist without the other!). It must always be remembered that this debate is only conceptual, to decide where to start structure interpretation in proteins. In addition, it is only after polymerization of amino acids into proteins that one can *ref.* to 'backbone' and 'side chains'. It makes no sense to consider the free amino, the C_α, the free carboxyl groups of an uncombined amino acid as being a different entity from the R-group!

1.2.1D The Secondary Structure

The secondary structure is an independently folding localized unit of a protein with a distinct and well characterized shape. They are continuous regions of local structures along the polypeptide chain. They have been extensively studied in terms of conformations and hydrogen bonding. The secondary structures that have the regular and repeating conformation and hydrogen bonding pattern are **helices** and **beta-strands**. The conformation of the backbone is analyzed, for example, in terms of phi and psi values (*ref.* chapter 1.2.2 for Ramachandran angles and various other methods) to decide whether the given segment of protein is a helix, strand, etc. The 'hydrogen bonding pattern' often refers to the number of atoms in a *hydrogen bonded ring* (wherein the ring is "closed" by the hydrogen bond), in other words, the regularity of occurrence of donor and acceptors atom pairs along the protein backbone (as in Fig. 1.25B).

Helices are the portions of the polypeptide chain that have a well characterized hydrogen bonding pattern, and the backbone follows a helical path. These are the most common secondary structures found in proteins (only **3** architectures out of **40** are β-domains without large α-helices by the CATH classification scheme described later) and can be classified into three categories: the 3_{10}-helix (~0.01% standalone helices, i.e. uncombined with any other helix), the α-helix (~99% of the stand-alone helices are α-helices), and the π-helix [conflicting abundance: ~0.01 % of all helices; 1 π helix out of every 10 helices (Fodje, et al. 2002)]. Each helix has its distinct diameter, pitch and hydrogen bonding pattern (for a concise summary, *ref.* Fig.1.27A and Table 1.5).

The type of residues most commonly occurring in each type is also distinct, as is the function attributed to them. Some of the most important features of helices are as follows:

- There is a regular and repeating pattern of hydrogen bonding between the amide hydrogen and carbonyl oxygen (Fig. 1.27A)
- The side chains of helices are rotated and arranged in the most spatially efficient orientations, pointing away from the direction of polypeptide chain propagation (much like a tobacco mosaic virus protein coat, arranged as in Fig. 1.27A)
- If the polypeptide chain of a protein is uncoiled, its end-to-end length is 100 times greater than the diameter of the protein. Forming a helix is the most efficient way to roll up the polypeptide chain into a very compact structure. It is easy to imagine that the simplest way to store a garden hose is to roll it up: and that takes a helical path.
- From molecular dynamics calculations, it has been determined that *it takes approximately 10 nanoseconds for an α-helix to elongate by one residue* (*ref.* Discussion 1.15 under chapter 1.5 on protein folding).
- The helices (all three mentioned above) are right handed. Left handed helices occur for vey short stretches and are mostly composed of glycines because all other amino acids in proteins are of the L-configuration.

Question Box

Model a left handed helix made of L-amino acids and determine why this is not favored. Model the same using D-amino acids–what is your opinion about stability in this case? What about a right handed helix made of D-amino acids?

- An advanced and interesting property credited to helices is what is called the *helix macrodipole* (Fig. 1.27B). Each C=O bond has a small dipole with the partial positive located on the carbon and the partial negative located in the oxygen. As the polypeptide chain backbone of the helix winds, each C=O moiety is aligned in the direction of helix winding, and so are the partial positives and negatives.

Table 1.5: Some secondary structures in proteins

Structure	Helices						β-strand
	α	3_{10}	π	α_L	Polypro-line II[7]	Colla-gen[7]	
Formal name	3.6_{13}, (also 3.7_{13})	3_{10} (also 3.2_{10})	4.4_{16}	-	-	-	-
Popularity[1]	38%[1]	3%[1,2]	Rare[1,2,3]	Rare[1,2]			43%
φ, ψ angles ideal	−57, −47[4]	−74, −4	−57, −70	60, 60	−75, 145		−119, +113 (parallel)　−139, +135 (antiparallel)
φ, ψ angles common	−63.8, −41.1	−49, −26	−76, −41[5]	[6]			−121, 128 (group 1)　−66, +137 (group 2)
φ, ψ angles in r-coils	−50<φ <−120; −40 <φ <−30	-	-	[6]			−130 <φ < −105
H-bonding	i→i+4	i→i+3	i→i+5				
No. of res. per turn	+3.6	+3.0	+4.4	−3.6	−3.0		~2.2
Rise/residue (Å)	1.5	2.0	1.1		2.9	3.4	
Radius (Å)	2.3	1.9	2.8	1.6			
R-group arrangement (Fig. 1.27A)	Staggered into square	Staggered into a triangle	Staggered ~ circular				Alternately above and below the plane of the strand (see text)
Pitch (Å)	5.5	6.0	5.0				6.8
Preferred residues	Refer section 1.4.1.A						
Additional comments	All the CO groups point towards the C-terminus and the NH groups towards the N-terminus						Can exist alone or as sheets

[1]: Out of all residues in a protein

[2]: Less optimized h-bonds → less well-packed helix core → less stability of helix → less abundance

[3]: There are papers that claim these helices to occur in 1 out of almost every 10 helices (see text)

[4]: Several values are found in literature

[5]: (−71°, −18°) also found to be common

[6]: Left-handed α-helices are not common; left handed helices are found in turns

[7]: The polyproline II and collagen helices not part of globular proteins; these are left largely unfilled to avoid excessive detail

MAIN HELICES

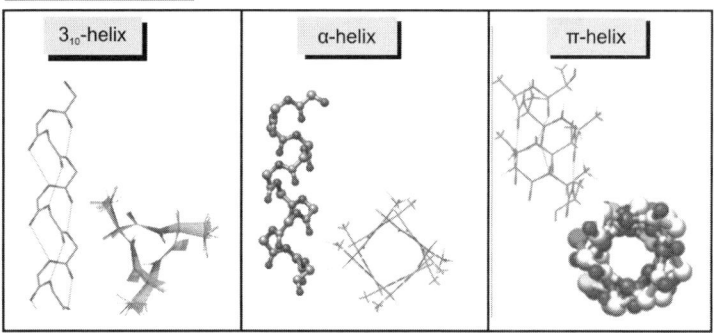

| 3₁₀-helix | α-helix | π-helix |

OTHER HELICES

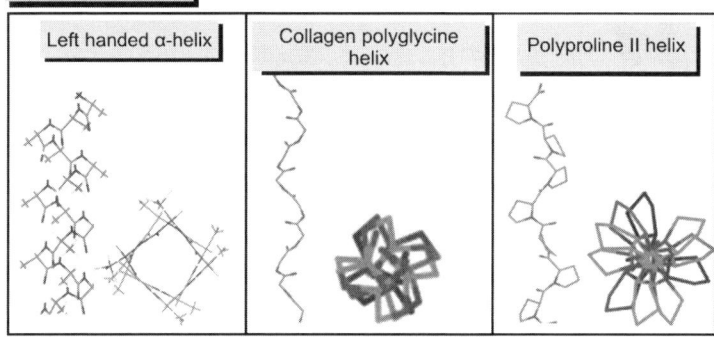

| Left handed α-helix | Collagen polyglycine helix | Polyproline II helix |

(i)

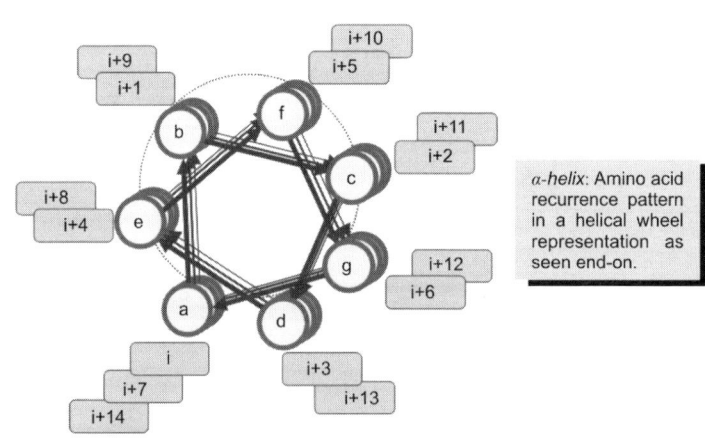

α-helix: Amino acid recurrence pattern in a helical wheel representation as seen end-on.

(ii)

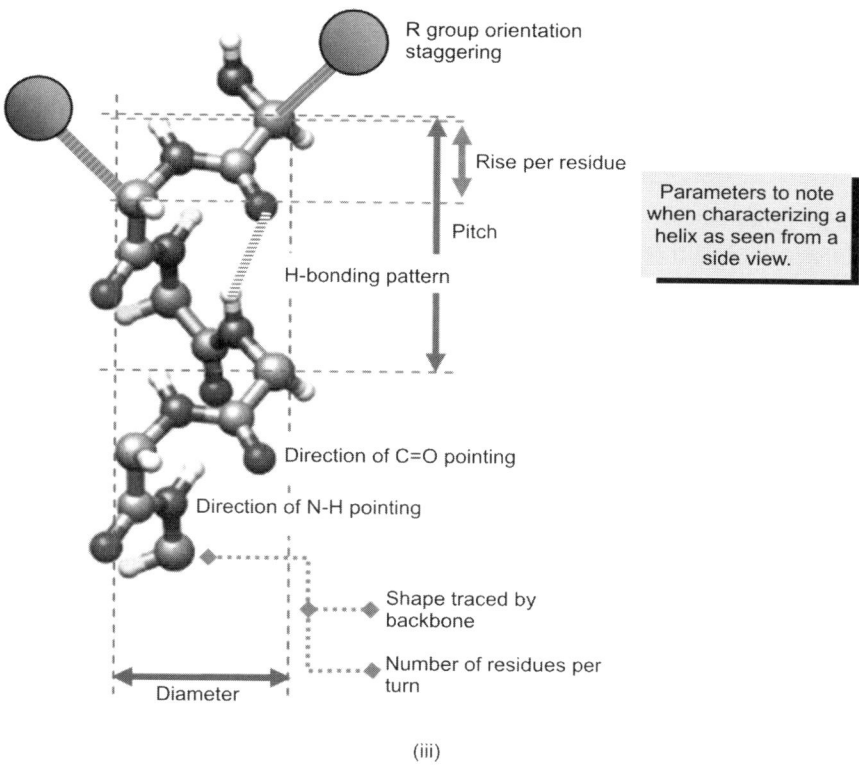

R group orientation staggering

Rise per residue

Pitch

H-bonding pattern

Parameters to note when characterizing a helix as seen from a side view.

Direction of C=O pointing

Direction of N-H pointing

Shape traced by backbone

Number of residues per turn

Diameter

(iii)

Fig. 1.27A (i) to (iii): The three main and the other helices in proteins; (iii) also general illustrations defining various parameters of helices. Protein pictures made using Chimera®

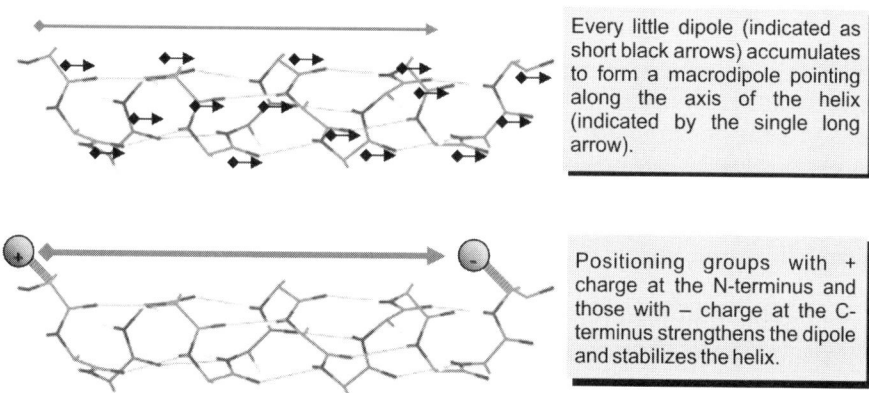

Every little dipole (indicated as short black arrows) accumulates to form a macrodipole pointing along the axis of the helix (indicated by the single long arrow).

Positioning groups with + charge at the N-terminus and those with − charge at the C-terminus strengthens the dipole and stabilizes the helix.

Fig. 1.27B: The helix macrodipole. Protein pictures made using Chimera®

Accumulation of the small dipoles of the C=O bond results in the entire helix acquiring a partial positive at the N-terminus and partial negative at the C-terminus, called the helix macrodipole. Accordingly presence of negatively charged residues at the N-terminus and positively charged residues at the C-terminus increase the stability of the helix because it strengthens the dipole. The vice versa arrangement decreases helix stability. This knowledge helps us in two ways: First, patterns have been identified in the amino acid distribution among natural proteins that amplify dipoles and stabilize helices. The helices of certain proteins are crucial for functionality-either by directly interacting with ligands (such as in the thioredoxin fold) or by contributing to the protein's conformation (as in *transmembrane proteins*). The backbone h-bonds of helices are readily attacked by water molecules. Secondly, this knowledge can be used while designing peptides and proteins for pharmaceutical purposes.

The other regular repeating secondary structure is the **beta-sheet**. We know that the helix is formed when one continuous segment of polypeptide chain rolls up, and stabilizes itself by forming h-bonds (Fig. 1.27A). The beta-sheet structure is slightly different: it is formed by bringing together several segments of the polypeptide chain, and fixing the different segments together by hydrogen bonds, resembling a railway line. These bonds form between the atoms of adjacent segments and not between those of consecutive residues as in a helix. They are also less susceptible to disturbance by water. The pair of h-bonded β-segment looks like a ladder (Fig. 1.28A); each such segment is called a beta-strand. When extended, these segments may be present one after the other in the polypeptide chain or may have come together from different parts of the protein (Fig. 1.29A). Depending on the relative orientations of β-strands, β-sheets can be parallel or antiparallel. The popularity of β-sheets in terms of the number of participating amino acids and other details are given in Table 1.5. One could argue that the sheet structure, when formed by strands that are not adjacent to each other can be classified "tertiary structure" rather than "secondary". This argument has indeed been put forth (Przytycka, et al. 1999) but that would mean sheets that contain adjacent strands should be treated separately as secondary structure. For simplicity and convenience, it is classified as secondary structure (Miles, et al. 2005).

Question

Model an ideal beta-strand: We know that an alpha helix has 3.6 residues per turn. How many residues "per turn" does a beta-strand have? *Ref.* Table 1.5 after you finish modeling, and compile your answer.

See Fig. 1.29 for an outline. Some important features attributed to beta-sheets are:

- The local conformation of the amino acids of the polypeptide chain backbone is different for the parallel and antiparallel beta-sheets. This difference can be numerically seen among the trends of phi and psi values as in Table 1.5. In Fig. 1.28A there is a difference in the shape of each hydrogen bonded ring along the beta ladder.
- The degree of compaction of the polypeptide chain that is achieved in a beta-sheet structure is much less than that achieved in a helix. Two consecutive C_α atoms of a β-strand span greater distance (6 Å) than 3.6 consecutive residues of an α-helix

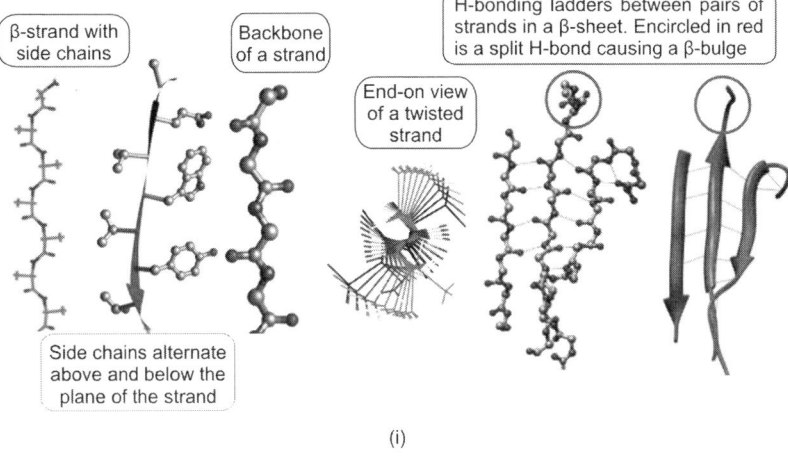

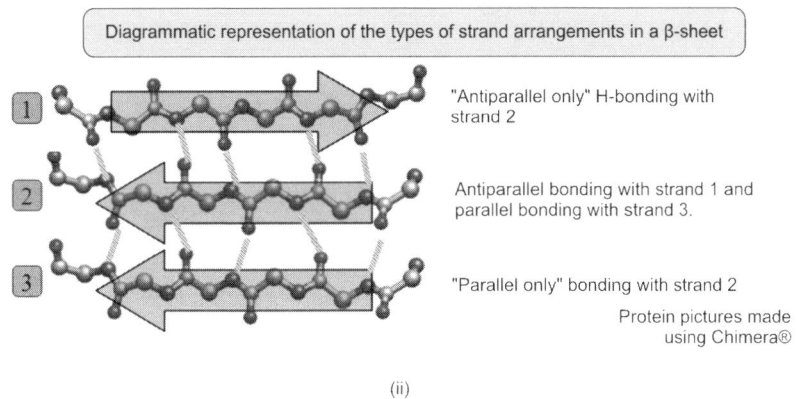

Fig. 1.28A (i) and (ii): The beta-sheet: Parallel and antiparallel types

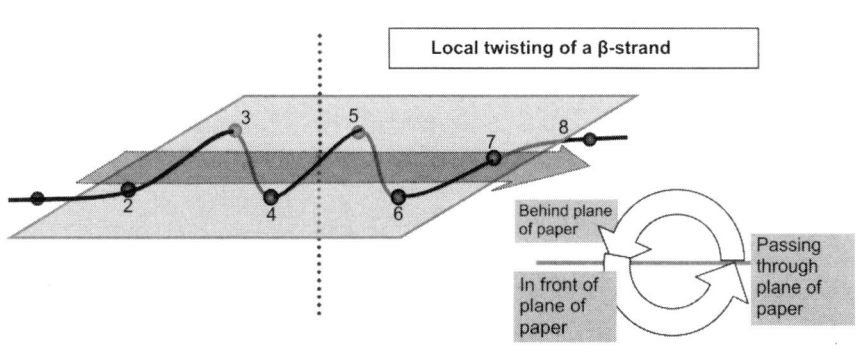

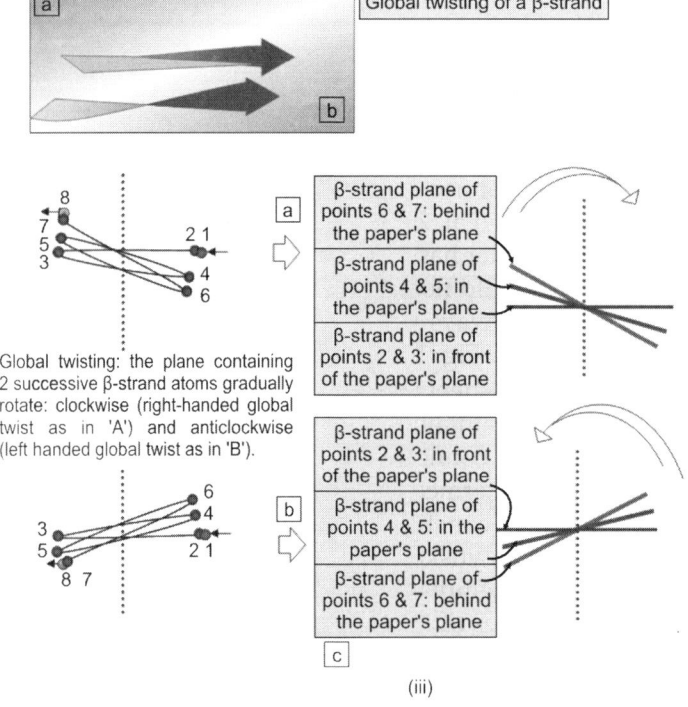

Right handed local twisting: right handed connection between points 3 & 4, 4 & 5, 5 & 6.

This shape can be traced out only by the right hand thumb.

(ii)

Global twisting of a β-strand

Global twisting: the plane containing 2 successive β-strand atoms gradually rotate: clockwise (right-handed global twist as in 'A') and anticlockwise (left handed global twist as in 'B').

β-strand plane of points 6 & 7: behind the paper's plane

β-strand plane of points 4 & 5: in the paper's plane

β-strand plane of points 2 & 3: in front of the paper's plane

β-strand plane of points 2 & 3: in front of the paper's plane

β-strand plane of points 4 & 5: in the paper's plane

β-strand plane of points 6 & 7: behind the paper's plane

(iii)

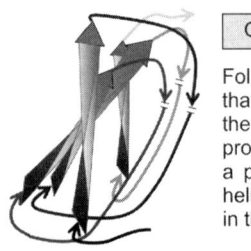

Global twisting of strands in a β-sheet

Following the protein chain (black lines that fade to grey & arrows indicating that the N-terminus lies towards the reader progressively layering backwards) traces a path that is curved along right-handed helix. The global arrangement of β-strands in this fold is thus a "right-handed twist".

(iv)

Fig. 1.28B (i) to (iv): Beta-sheet jargon: Local and global handedness of twisted strands, twisted sheets

(5.4 Å). The side chains in a beta-sheet structure point alternatively above and below the plane of the sheet (Fig. 1.28A); also *ref.* Table 1.5.

- These strands are known for their structural rigidity. Especially when sheets incorporate large number of strands, they form distinctive barrels that function as ion channels, etc. Depending on the amino acid composition, the sheets can act as an interface between aqueous and lipophilic environments (having polar residues on one side and non-polar ones on the other).

- *Beta-bulges:* There are a number of 'imperfections' found among the strands of a beta-sheet. One of them is called a β-bulge. It is a situation wherein two amide hydrogen atoms bond to one C=O group. Such hydrogen bonds are described as being *"bifurcated"*. The result is that one of the residues is pushed outward (away from the partner strand) forming a bulge, whereas the rest of the strand is relatively straight. Bulges are known to play a role in protein function (dihydrofolate reductase), resistance to mutation, and domain dimerization (Ig). β-strands are often kinked to varying degrees and have been classified (Ranganathan, et al. 2009).

- A beta-strand is also considered to be a helix that has rearranged its atoms slightly to attain a more stable conformation.

- Strands are often referred to as being "flat". This is only a simplified picture that arises when C_α atoms are connected. Some groups report that strands have left-handed twist (Ranganathan, et al. 2008–2), whereas earlier works mainly identified right handed ones. If the reader has indeed modeled the strand in light of the above question, this revelation should not come as a surprise! However, the way strands combine to form sheets is always in a right-handed fashion and is referred to as 'twist'. Is this confusing? *Ref.* Fig. 1.28B.

There are helices and beta-sheets scattered throughout the protein Fig. 1.29A performing various roles in maintaining structure and functionality of the protein. These secondary structures are connected by segments of the polypeptide chain that may be either relatively floppy, termed loops or relatively well defined and rigid called turns. The helices and sheets constitute only about 50–55% of the entire protein structure on an average (Leszczynski, et al. 1986). The remaining structure has been termed "random coil," and attempts to categorize these structures have resulted in the classification of several types of *turns* and loops.

As mentioned earlier, turns are short and well structured. They are defined as segments of the polypeptide chain consisting of consecutive residues such that the distance between the first and the last is less than 7–7.5 Å (Rose, et al. 1985) indicating strong change in polypeptide chain direction. Characterized "random coils" are longer than 4–5 residues and are termed *loops* (Leszczynski, et al. 1986). Compared to helices and β-strands, loops and turns are more difficult to classify owing to their lack of regular patterns. However, extensive study in terms of geometry, hydrogen bonding, amino acid distribution, and role in maintaining the structure and function of proteins gives us interesting insights (*ref.* **Discussion 1.5**) and show that "random coils" are not so 'random'.

"'Tut, tut, child!' said the Duchess. 'Everything's got a moral, if only you can find it.'"

in "Through the Looking Glass", by Lewis Carroll

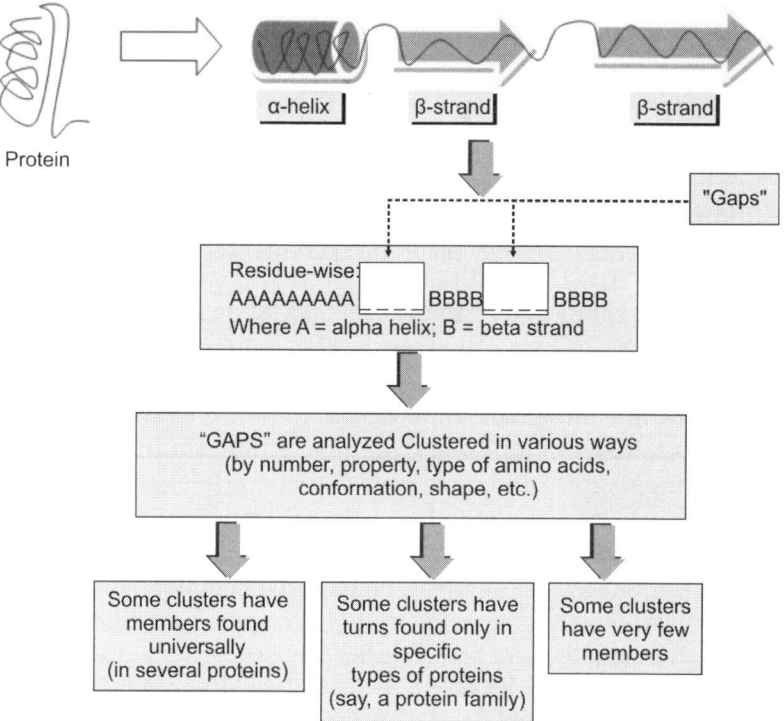

Fig. 1.29A: "Regular secondary structure" filtering and subsequent analyses

Discussion 1.5: Order in disorder

The above description on loops may give the readers the impression that these are "disordered", "random coils", or "un-interpretable segments". This discussion, however, wishes to clarify some related points. Literature records a certain degree of regularity in the occurrence of these disordered regions among proteins performing similar functions; hence the title. There is a certain order with which these ill-structured regions occur among proteins. For example,

- The topologically equivalent domains of 5 proteins–HIV–1 integrase, phage Mu A transposase, ASV integrase core, RNAse H domain of HIV–1 reverse transcriptase and the Ruv C Holliday junction resolving enzyme are known to contain a 5–residue loop located at structurally identical position (Veerapandian, 1997)
- Proteins with similar functions are known to have exposed loops with similar degree of flexibility. Binding surfaces that interact with ligands are known to be significantly more flexible than the regions of the protein that are expected to maintain its scaffold (Varley, et al. 1991)
- Domains are known to be connected by loose floppy segments of the protein chain. Sometimes this allows considerable domain motion in that these huge

structures "roll about". In other cases, these *linkers* of domains form the active site for ligand interaction (Tsou, 1995). In more specific cases, environment induced conformational changes in the linkers opens channels, etc. by domain motion (Yuan, et al. 2003).

- DNA binding proteins are known to be largely disordered until they bind to the target. Extensive studies in this regard resulted in the design, prediction and confirmation of binding sites within random segments (Longhi, et al. 2003).

- The correct binding of CYS2HIS2 zinc finger proteins to the DNA causes the flexible linker to perform its function.

"…fold, cap and thereby stabilize the preceding helix in the protein, and
to orientate the next zinc finger correctly for binding in the major groove of DNA"

Text quoted from (Dyson, et al. 2005)
On previous work (Laity, et al. 2000)

Inspite of all this importance of flexibility in binding, it has been established that increasing flexibility of "random coils" via site directed mutagenesis and other experimental techniques was found to abolish activity [shown for DNA binding proteins (Laity, et al. 2000)]. Thus there is a predetermined and calculated disorder introduced into these segments by the genetic code.

There are varying degrees of flexibility among proteins. Some segments have random structure. Any quantitative analysis of their structure shows no specificity or regularity of values. For reasons discussed in chapter 1.5 on protein folding, protein structure is considered never to be literally random; it is believed that there is always slight degree of order and preference for some conformations. Thus, although amino acid is not rigidly fixed into one or another conformation, the entire protein is globular and loosely packed (Uversky, 2002). This is referred to as the molten globule (*ref.* section 1.5.3.C). A higher level of order would be the linkers of domains mentioned above. The domains on either side of the linker have well defined structure within them. However, they "bounce about" in solution with the conformation of the linker becoming flexible to a large extent (called "modular" structure). As a next example, consider a protein with well characterized conformation A. After interaction with a certain ligand, it changes to another well-characterized conformation B. In this case, even though there is some degree of flexibility, it is very low–only allowing switch between conformations A and B. This portrays a higher degree of order. A rigid protein is one wherein being completely folded, the protein has all its internal interactions satisfied in the form of secondary structure and tertiary interactions. However, it is noteworthy that such a self-satisfied protein totally invisible to and ignorant of surroundings is hardly of any use in carrying out physiological and pharmacological roles!

There are two approaches in understanding the structural role and formation of turns. Firstly, they could be thought of as regions fixing and orienting helices and β-sheets within a protein. The second approach is that helices and beta-sheets arrange themselves by exerting an influence on each other and by experiencing the influence of the turn regions. Owing to their variety and complexity, a number of properties and features can be attributed to the turn regions: Scheme 1.3, Fig. 1.29B.

Theoretical methods use the coordinates of proteins obtained after experimental structure determination (X-ray, NMR, etc). The reason this is pointed out is because loops are naturally floppy and depending on experimental conditions, can crystallize (X-ray) or fold (NMR in solution) with slightly different local conformations (*ref.* protein dynamics in chapter 1.3). Static structure of protein studies each of the several closely related conformations of the native state called the ensemble. The various structure analysis methods use different approximations and principles. There is some degree of disparity in ascertaining structure (*ref.* section 1.2.2) that a leading review article (Chou, et al. 1977) published in the 1970s that was 50 pages of extensive insight into beta turns (see below) commented that *ambiguity is an "intrinsic property"* of the protein and that methods are therefore deemed to differ in assigning the extent of involvement of amino acids.

The ends of turns that connect two secondary structures often assume a conformation that resembles that of the respective secondary structure (Sun, et al. 1996), (Ranganathan, et al. 2008–2). Several structure determination methods therefore use *"effective turn lengths"*, i.e. they have a cut off characteristic based on which they include close-to-secondary structure conformations into the secondary structure itself. This is one technique that serves to reduce the length of turns thereby reducing its variability and dispersion while classifying and analyzing conformations. For the same reason of secondary structural influence, the local conformation of the ends of turns often influences the turn shape. Turn shape is assessed in several ways:

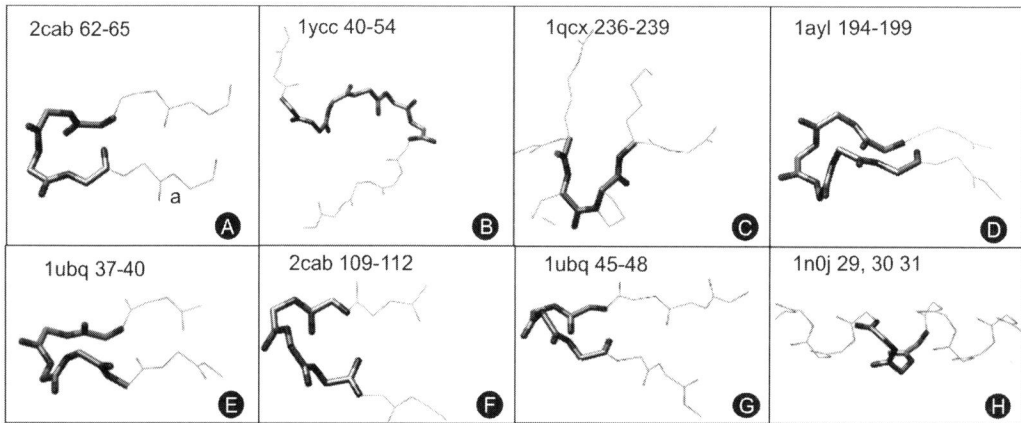

Fig. 1.29B: Stereochemical representations of turns. A: Reverse turn: 2cab 62–65 (Lewis, et al., 1973); B: Ω loop: 1 ycc residues 40–54 (Fetrow, 1995); C: CisPro touch turn: 1qcx 236–239; D: Alpha turn: 1ayl N 194–M199 (Dasgupta, et al., 2004); E: β-turn type I: 1 ubq 37–40; F: β-turn type II: 2cab 109–112; G: β-turn type III': 1 ubq 45–48; H: Pi turns: 1n0j 29, 3031 (Rajashankar, et al., 1996). See text for other references

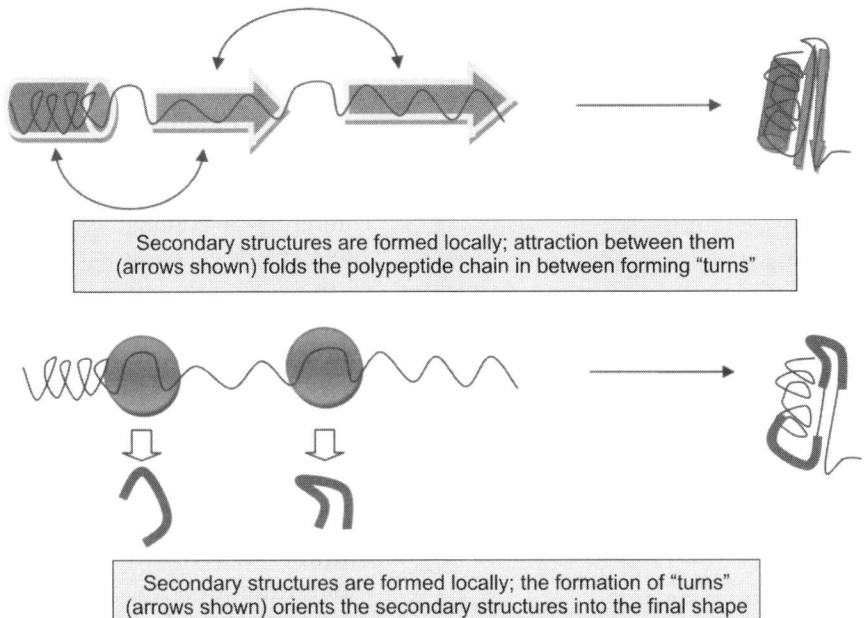

Scheme 1.3: Two approaches in formation of turns: "Helices and β-sheets create turns" approach shown above vs "turns orient helices and β-sheets" approach shown below

- *Cumulative turn property:* Linearity and planarity; distance cut-offs; hydrogen bonding pattern
- *Local conformation:* Backbone dihedral angles; virtual bond angles and dihedrals; distance matrices
- *Global perspective:* Orientation of turns determine 3D structure.

The presence and uniqueness of certain 'flexibility' in a loop segment is evolutionary and strongly depends on protein functions. There is an order in this sort of disorder (Discussion 1.5). In general, members of the same protein family perform the same function and are structurally similar. When proteins are classified into the same family, they are considered to possess structural similarities and are expected to be functionally similar also. Structural similarity is determined by quantitative structure comparison (*ref.* chapter 1.2.3 and 1.2.4) of entire 3D structure of proteins. However in some cases, differences in function have been observed among proteins classified in the same family. In those cases the basis of final difference was found to vary in structure of loops found on the surface (Fernandez-Fuentes, et al. 2006).

Only some conformations are accessible by a protein's amino acids. There is a natural tendency of protein structure to not vary too much from the native structure.

- *Physically:* Due to van der Waals (steric), electrostatic, exchange, hydrophobic, backbone, solvent, electronic, and long range interactions
- *Evolutionarily:* Due to the pressure of divergence (this results from a sequence-gene-protein structure relationship further detailed under chapter 1.5).

Polarity: The polarity of the disulphide group influences exposure to solvent and localization of turn in the protein side chain. The polarity of the turn as a whole results from the shape and amino acid composition of the turns. It is induced by the arrangement of the backbone/side chain atoms. This is similar to the macrodipole found in helices (Fig. 1.27B). These properties of turns are summarized in Scheme 1.4.

Nomenclature of turns: One of the widely used turn classification systems apply the following nomenclature:

- *α-turns*: These are 5 residue turns composed mainly of hydrophilic amino acids that can be categorized further into 9 classes having distinct arrangements of (φ, ψ) for each category. There is a hydrogen bond between the carbonyl group of residue 1 and the amino group of the residue 5 (Pavone, et al. 1996). Their presence and formation have been have been related to helix folding mechanisms.

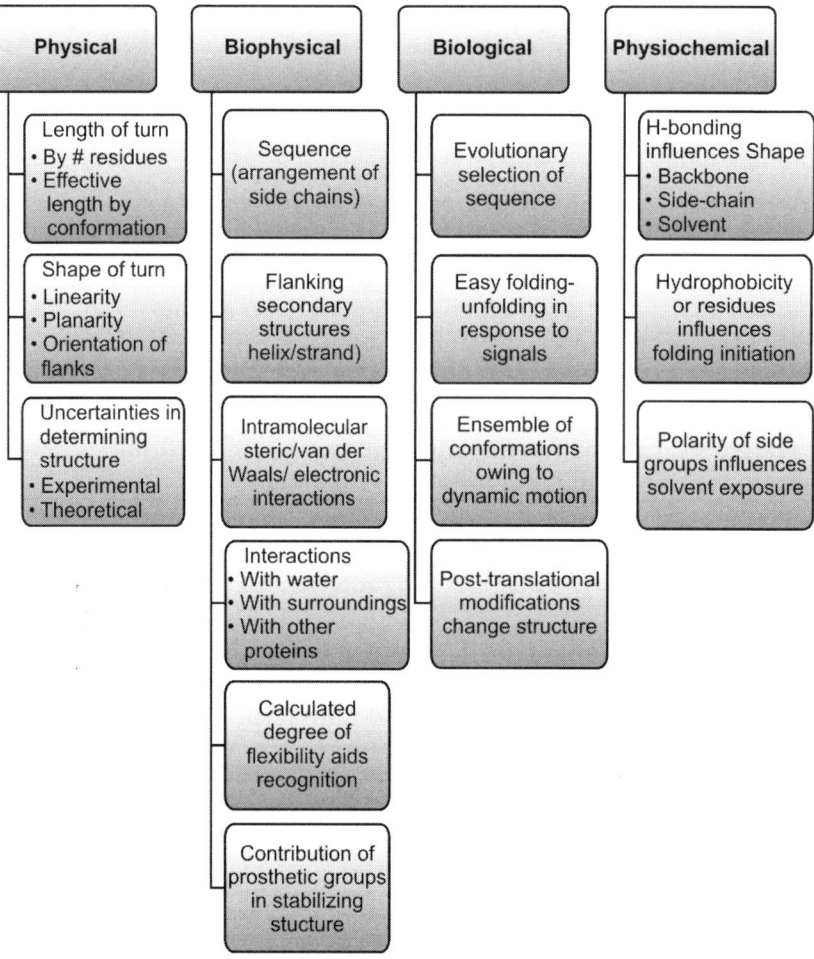

Scheme 1.4: Various aspects influencing turns/loops in proteins

- *β-turns*: These 4-residue turns connect the two strands of an antiparallel beta-sheet resulting in 180° reversal in chain direction and are found among 25 to 30% of residues in proteins (Wilmot, et al. 1988). An extensive treatise on beta turns was written early on (Chou, et al. 1977), (Rose, et al. 1985). Currently, 8 classes of beta turns are identified (types I, I', II, II', VIa1, VIa2, VIb and VIII; *ref.* overview under "Ramachandran angles" in section 1.2.2.C for an account of their evolution). These are mainly defined by the φ and ψ values of the two middle residues. One additional class (type IV) contains the β-turns that do not fit into the 8 classes.

- *γ-turns*: These are three residue turns and are further subdivided into classic and inverse, depending on the φ and ψ value of the middle of residue. These are found to occur in close association with beta turns and the inverse type is significant in protein folding (Milner-White, 1990).

- *π-turns:* These are also "tight turns" as the above, but are the largest, being 6 residues long. The first residue's CO is linked by a hydrogen bond to the 6th residues NH. Several classes have been identified (Rajashankar, et al. 1996). These are $\pi_{\alpha1}$, $\pi'_{\alpha R}$, π_β. The $\pi\alpha_L$ turn is a helix cap occurring at the α-helices' C–termini. The 'α_L' denotes the left-handed conformation (the α_L, region of the Ramachandran map) adopted by the fifth residue as it exits the α-helix. Similarly, 'β' and 'α_R' represent the β and right handed α-helix conformations of the residue at the same 5th position. The 'prime' represents a stereochemical mirror image of the base turn.

Analysis of regular yet long loops has also resulted in identifying typical linearity and planarity properties depending on whether they occur at the N- or the C-terminus of the protein (Ring, et al. 1992).

1.2.1D(i) Online

There are some *databases* that store just the loop segments: they recognize secondary structures, eliminate them and accumulate what is left, i.e. the loops and turns of the protein. The turn segments can be downloaded and studied by research groups who are interested in looking into all the types of turns that occur in proteins. These libraries also help in loop modeling during protein structure prediction. As discussed in chapter 1.4, a correlation can be found between sequence and structure. With sufficient analysis, regular amino acid-loop structure correlations can be unraveled (a partial list of these sites can be obtained in Table 1.6).

When analyzing a large number of turn segments from such libraries, some precautions need to be kept in mind as follows:

- One must know the method of analysis used to recognize and eliminate secondary structures and also know its strength and failures (results vary depending on the method: A turn identified using one approach might not be identified by the other).

- The conformations of the ends of turns are influenced by the adjoining secondary structures. In many cases, it might be meaningless to cut in the middle of a continuum of conformations that lead from turn to secondary structure or vice versa.

Table 1.6: Online resources for proteins

PDB	http://rcsb.org/pdb	Protein Data Bank
SCOP	http://scop.berkeley.edu/	Protein classification
CATH	www.cathdb.info/	Protein classification
Genetic sequence	http://www.ncbi.nlm.nih.gov/genbank/	
SWISS-PROT/TrEMBL	http://www.ebi.ac.uk/swissprot	European Molecular Biology Lab
ExPASy	http://www.expasy.ch/sprot	Main page that contains links to TrEMBL and SWISS-PROT
PROSITE	http://www.expasy.org/prosite/	Protein family, domain and functional site information
PIR	http://pir.georgetown.edu	Protein Information Resource – a protein sequence database
Entrez	http://www.ncbi.nlm.nih.gov/Entrez	Sequenced proteins
MIPS (Munich Information Centre for Protein Sequences)	http://www.helmholtz-muenchen.de/en/mips/services/index.html	Organism specific protein and genome information

1.2.1D(ii) Results of Extensive Analysis of Turns from 100s of Proteins

As above, some investigations concentrate on classifying and templating turn regions (Topham, et al. 1993) eventually aiming prediction rules. Others explore the significance of statistical clusters of turns (Brevern, et al. 2001), i.e. when the various structural clusters are obtained, it is believed that functional relation and relevance will become evident. From all these works and many more, it was found that the distinction between turns and coils is not clear as up to 13 amino acids have been analyzed and classified in various ways (Wojcik, et al. 1999; Fourier, et al. 2004; Li, et al. 1999; Michalsky, et al. 2003) and so gradually "loops" are becoming "turns". As such, turn classification has come a long way from the initial investigations of beta turns. After understanding what is meant by 'tight turns' (Richardson, 1981), 'alpha turns', 'gamma turns', 'pi turns', 'omega loops', 'closed loops' and 'paperclips' (*ref.* as discussed above), it is collecting these independent turn motifs and using them in harmony to describe the entire protein structure that is even more challenging. Instead, building the higher levels from a small number of averaged classes of sub-structures would yield better insights, especially when unified by applying a common approach. Attempts in this direction (Fourier, et al. 2004) (Sun, et al. 1996) (de Brevern, et al. 2001) suggest ideas that might result in a much smaller and tractable number of motifs. The need for unified approach is well documented at the tertiary level (Day, et al. 2003), (Taylor, 2002) where recognizing the boundaries of domains and classifying folds remain ambiguous. Some examples of what can result from such analyses in drug design (first, why should we expect some result? Only because we know that there exists sequence–structure correlation)–that drugs acting on more than one protein can have similar pharmacophores. That means the active site of these proteins are also similar – we expect similarities to exist in a general sense even if there are several specific differences. One cannot rule out the possibility that specific shapes and lengths of turns are needed among such proteins to directly react with the ligand or to arrange helices and beta sheets that line the active site. For example, one can search for all proteins into which a certain drug can fit. Finding proteins of different classes that will react to a particular pharmacophore might increase the potential uses the drug and can also be used to detect possible side effects of using the drug.

1.2.1E The Tertiary Structure

The arrangement of all secondary structures with respect to each other, basically, the global and overall structure of a protein and the 3D shape of a protein is referred to as its tertiary structure. In Figs 1.25A, 1.26A and 1.29A, etc. indicating a completely formed protein, helix 1 is ordered correctly with respect to β2 which in turn is ordered with respect to β3, etc. So the entire tertiary structure is in place. One can view it as the structure with the regular helices and β-sheets and non-regular secondary structures in their respective places. The 3D shape that a protein spontaneously assumes when allowed to fold is referred to as its "native" shape. In several situations, return of the protein to this structure (after deformation) is easy. The native tertiary structure is considered to be the stable form of the protein. In other words, denaturation/ disturbance from this form due to change in environment is generally not permanent (there are exceptions). The protein returns to native state when the external influence or change in environment is removed (i.e. returns to the preferred state). Investigating why proteins have this strong tendency to seek its native fold is a very deep and fast growing field with surprising influence on drug development, disease investigation, etc as described under chapter 1.5 (protein folding). Pertaining to this chapter, it is important to know that the native form is the most "stable" and mostly bioactive form of a protein.

The stability of a protein must not be compared to the stability of covalently bonded compounds such as ethane, or the amino acids of the protein itself. This is because the protein's native structure is maintained by numerous weak interactions such as hydrogen bonding, electrostatic, van der Waals exclusion, exchange repulsion, hydrophobic interactions, aromatic stacking interactions, dipoles, induced dipoles, and the strongest of them being the disulfide bridges (*ref.* part II and III of this book for an account of these interactions). The only covalent bonding is the chain of amino acids which does not change in both unfolded and folded states of the protein. A protein has a theoretically calculated internal energy of about 40 million kJ/mol (adding up the energy of every bond and interaction among all atoms of the protein) and the difference between its energetically stable (or folded or preferred) form and the unfolded (random) form is only about 20 to 65kJ/mol (discussed in detail under chapter 1.5 on protein folding; also *ref.* Fig. 1.30A). The difference is not high enough to prevent reversal of folding. In fact, proteins are very dynamic structures. Interaction with ligands, water, other proteins, plasma membrane, cofactors, etc constantly unfold or change the folded conformation of the protein. So, stability of the native structure of the protein in this context refers to the preference of the protein to adopt this form compared to other possible conformations such as the slight preference of ethane to

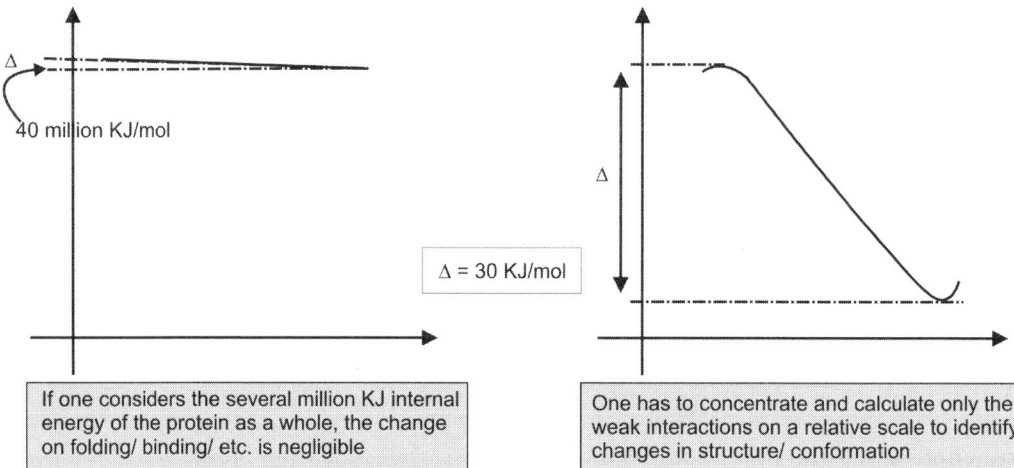

| If one considers the several million KJ internal energy of the protein as a whole, the change on folding/ binding/ etc. is negligible | One has to concentrate and calculate only the weak interactions on a relative scale to identify changes in structure/ conformation |

Fig. 1.30A: A change of 30 KJ/mol for a protein of 40 million KJ/mol energy is a drop in the ocean!

be in the staggered than in the eclipsed form. Such investigations of conformational flexibility study protein dynamics. This is also another vast field with applications in drug designing and computational chemistry, a brief introduction to which is presented in chapter 1.3.

The primary sequence of a protein is always a mixture of amino acids having various types of properties such as hydrophobicity, acidity, etc. Proteins are exposed to hydrophilic environment because the cell is predominantly aqueous (exceptions being those proteins integral within the plasma membrane). Thus amino acids that "like" water would face outward in the 3D or tertiary arrangement whereas hydrophobic residues would shun water getting buried in the interior region. In recent years the power of hydrophobic interactions (the force that drives hydrophobic groups away from water) is increasingly considered as the main contributor to initiating the formation of tertiary structure for proteins exposed to aqueous environment (*ref.* chapter 1.5). The protein tertiary structure therefore contains a hydrophobic interior that is often referred to as the "hydrophobic core" and the environment in the core is often compared to "the gas phase" because the strong influence that solvents are capable of exerting is very minimal (Fig. 1.30B). This is typical of the tertiary structure of globular proteins.

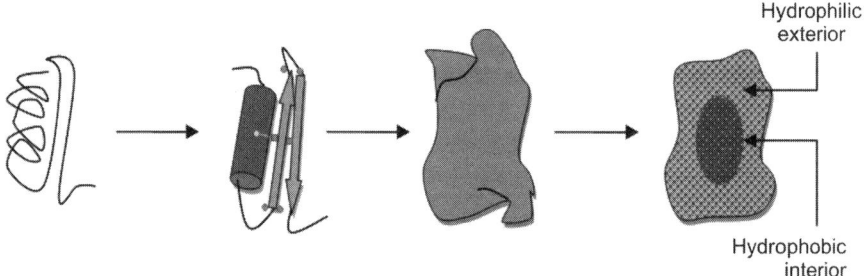

Fig. 1.30B: The hydrophobic core

A feature of the distribution of the physicochemical properties in 3D is affected by the arrangement of secondary structures with one edge submerged in the hydrophobic core and the other parts exposed to the solvent. Thus a helix would have a strip of hydrophobic residues that would face the interior core in the native state. This is indicated in Scheme 1.5 for a helix. Patterns in the distribution of hydrophobic residues have been observed. For example, if there are two helices connected by a turn, then typical distributions of hydrophobic residues resemble that shown in Scheme 1.6 (Efimov, 1993). Such discoveries of amino acid properties that distribute consistently among particular structures of particular family of proteins is valuable as this information is used for structure prediction (*ref.* chapter 1.4) and to infer the properties of the active site of the receptors. For example *Retinol Binding Protein* binds to retinol by hydrophobic interactions.

Hydrophobicity is one of several interactions that bring residues from just about anywhere along the polypeptide chain and at quite a distance from each other, close together in 3D space (*ref.* "the hydrophobic collapse theory" under chapter 1.5 on protein folding). Such interactions as hydrogen bonding and salt bridges are therefore

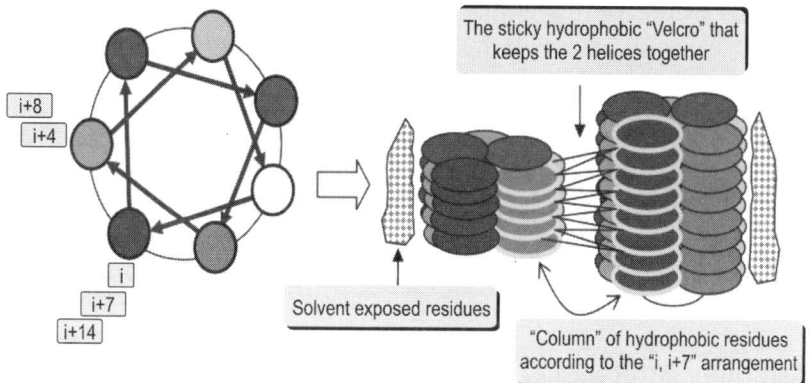

The sticky hydrophobic "Velcro" that keeps the 2 helices together

i+8
i+4

i

i+7

i+14

Solvent exposed residues

"Column" of hydrophobic residues according to the "i, i+7" arrangement

If *i* is hydrophobic, it is likely that any of *i+4, i+7, i+8, i+14*, etc. residues are also hydrophobic resulting in a "sticky strip" of residues that adhere and get buried into the protein.

Scheme 1.5: Hydrophobic strip of residues along a helix

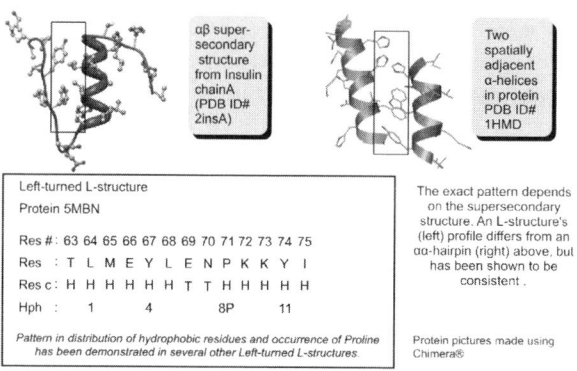

αβ super-secondary structure from Insulin chainA (PDB ID# 2insA)

Two spatially adjacent α-helices in protein PDB ID# 1HMD

Left-turned L-structure

Protein 5MBN

Res # :	63	64	65	66	67	68	69	70	71	72	73	74	75
Res :	T	L	M	E	Y	L	E	N	P	K	K	Y	I
Res c :	H	H	H	H	H	H	T	T	H	H	H	H	H
Hph :	1			4					8P			11	

Pattern in distribution of hydrophobic residues and occurrence of Proline has been demonstrated in several other Left-turned L-structures.

The exact pattern depends on the supersecondary structure. An L-structure's (left) profile differs from an αα-hairpin (right) above, but has been shown to be consistent .

Protein pictures made using Chimera®

Scheme 1.6: Hydrophobicity distribution in a helix-turn-helix structure

called "long range interactions". These initiate the formation of and maintain tertiary structure of proteins, as mentioned earlier. From the sequence, it is often a challenge to predict which residues will come into contact with each other by setting up "contact maps"–method is called "contact prediction"–by predicting the formation and arrangement of secondary structures.

Did You Know? 3
Convergent evolution and the catalytic triad

Subtilisin, a serine endopeptidase, is structurally unrelated to the chymotrypsin-family of serine proteases. However, both proteins possess the same arrangement of serine–aspartate–histidine in the active site – an arrangement called the "catalytic triad". This is a classic example of convergent evolution. Also ref. Scheme 13: convergence and divergence in protein evolution.

It is interesting to compare the different respiratory proteins present in various life forms (introduction to chapter 2.1). It easy to imagine that proteins with sequences differing for 1 out of every 10 residues (90% sequence similarity) are closely related whether they occur in a crow or in humans and their structures are known to be very similar. But in 1980s, it was discovered in the globin family of proteins that members with <15% sequence similarity actually have very similar 3D structures. Examples with even lower (8–9%) matching sequences have been shown to resemble in tertiary structure [(Rost, 1997), (Holm, et al. 1993), (Holm, et al. 1997), (Dokholyan, et al. 2001)]. This, of course, suggests strong evolutionary ties and has been attributed to similarities in the protein core. Such proteins have also been found to follow similar folding pathways (*ref.* chapter 1.5). The theory that tertiary structure of homologous (meaning "evolutionarily related") proteins is better conserved than the primary structure (in terms of sequence similarity) thus came about.

1.2.1F Quaternary Structure

The biologically active form of several proteins such as receptors, hormones, etc. is composed of more than one polypeptide chain. Either several copies of the same chain associate to form a multimer or the multimer may be composed of chains differing in structure, topology and amino acid composition. One reason for the formation of multimers of identical chains is avoiding excess information in an already long genetic code. Protein synthesis results in several chains all of which are independent (whether the chains are identical or different). The quaternary structure results from weak interactions and disulfide bridges bringing these various chains together just as the tertiary structure results from the assembly of secondary units. The quaternary structure is thus formed from dynamic interactions between the various independent monomer units. There is no covalent bonding between these chains and so they are described independently. This level directly relates to functionality of the protein-many proteins assume their biologically active conformation on association to multimers. The classical example about the arrangement and functioning of hemoglobin, which can be found in standard reference books (Nelson, et al. 2008), however, was recently shown to be a result of the pentanary structure rather than quaternary. Therefore, an outline of literature research on the *Leucine zipper motif* **(Discussion 1.6)** is presented as an example of quaternary structure. Of the two images for "quaternary structure" shown in Fig. 1.25A, the one on the left represents the insulin hexamer and that on the right, its biological subunit.

Discussion 1.6: The leucine zipper motif–relation between sequence, structure, and function

The DNA, various proteins and telephones (that have cords) are examples of systems in and around us that contain long helices that coil about each other. In protein terminology, they are considered a "motif", formed by secondary structures (i.e., helices) and are slightly higher in the structural hierarchy than secondary structures. It is known that α-helices follow a right-handed twist; the supercoiling is left-handed. One long helix from two identical domains each twists around and forms a stable dimer. The dimer, as in figure (1FOS), appears like a pair of tongs making it convenient for the protein to "hold" the DNA. The motif is known to be one of the 3 motifs *that mediate DNA binding*. The other two motifs are the Helix-Turn-Helix (one helix involved in DNA recognition, the other helix involved in stabilizing the first) and the Zinc Finger motifs (Zinc complex stabilizes the motif's 3D structure). This motif is a remarkable example of how structure and function go hand in hand. The Leucine Zipper motif (LeuZIPm) is found among the following classes of proteins:

- The CCAAT-box/enhancer binding proteins (in short C/EBPs) contain a basic amino acid–rich region followed by the leucine zipper motif, both occurring towards the C-terminus. Several isoforms of this protein are known all of which have ~90% residue similarity in this region. The C-termini of the protein are only about 20% similar in terms of amino acid composition. These belong to a family of transcription factors.
- Other transcription factors such as the members of Jun/AP1 family*
- The octamer-binding transcription factor 2 (Oct–2/OTF–2)*
- The cAMP Response Element (CRE) is a regulatory site in the DNA. Proteins that bind to this site of the DNA are known to form the Leucine Zipper Motif (CREB, CRE-BP1, ATFs).*
- The yeast general control protein GCN4.*
- The Fos oncogene, and Fos-related proteins (fra-1 and fos B).*
- The C-myc, L-myc and N-myc oncogenes.*
- Bactereophage Mu C–a member of the newly discovered family in which Helix–Turn–Helix motif and the Leucine Zipper motif are both present and interact cooperatively
- The viral envelope glycoproteins of many retroviruses such as the human immunodeficiency virus Type 1 (HIV–1) envelope glycoprotein called gp41. The latter protein is required for virus entry into host cells (Ramadevi, et al. 1998)
- Bluetongue virus minor protein VP4

*PROSITE documentation PDOC00029 @ www.expasy.ch/prosite/PS00029

Quaternary Structure:

It is evident from the figure that LeuZIPm is formed by two identical proteins. There are two aspects to dimerization in the LeuZIPm.

1. Dimerization is a prerequisite for protein function. LeuZIPm is the structural scaffold driving protein dimerization on which process the respective proteins are dependent to perform their functions. Some examples are:
    a. LeuZIPm is responsible for dimerization and the adjoining basic amino acid – rich region (also taking up α-helical secondary structure) is responsible for DNA binding and recognition in the C/EBP.
    b. Similarly dimerization of VP4 is essential for encapsidation by Core Like Particles formed by VP4.
    c. dimerization is necessary for the DNA binding of the entire GCN4 molecule.
2. The dimer is the more stable form.
    a. The residue composition and structure of this motif drives dimer formation. In fact, introduction of the Leu Zipper motif into a monomeric protein was found to oligomerize it.
    b. Owing to great similarity among most LeuZIPm containing proteins, certain heterodimers were found possible. This is known to increase the variety of recognition and regulation mediated by a limited number of these proteins
    c. Between the c-Fos and c-Jun proteins, heterodimerization was found to be favored as dimeric Fos was not stable
    d. Electrostatic properties of side chains influence whether the helices in register are packed in a parallel or antiparallel fashion

Mechanism of dimerization: The interplay between primary sequence, secondary structure, tertiary shape, quaternary arrangement and protein function can be beautifully seen in this example. Consider the primary sequence pattern: L XXXXXXL XXXXXXL XXXXXXL XXXXXXL (example: carboxy terminus of VP4 protein region 523 to 551). Leucines indicated occur at every 7th position (among other charged residues in VP4). The repetition of the above pattern one more time in a protein leads to the formation stable parallel helices that slightly coil around each other (LeuZIPm). Leucine is hydrophobic, and in 3D, after supercoiling, the Leucines end up facing each other. This symmetric interface arrangement (O'Shea, et al., 1989) makes the two helices stick to each other like Velcro. The hydrophobic side groups aggregate in space and zip into each other–hence the term "zipper" (Busch, et al. 1990). Although there is large overall similarity in the composition of LeuZIPm proteins, not all monomers can bind to each other (in other words, not all proteins can heterodimerize with each other). The presence of charged residues in between the Leucines incorporates selectivity in dimerization. In addition, the basic residues ensure that not just any of the formed dimmers bind to any of the susceptible DNA segments (i.e. the basic residues present in the region that comes in contact with the DNA is responsible for specific binding with certain palyndromic sequences in the genetic code). Such inferences regarding the role of amino acids in protein function is obtained by laborious and detailed experimental (such as site directed mutagenesis)/computational (such as molecular dynamics) investigations. Through these studies, the transition of conformation to the dimerized form was found to be cooperative (*ref.* chapter 1.5.4.B in protein folding). In addition, longer proteins were found to be more stable than shorter ones.

The above points show why the sequence, though apparently quite distant from higher levels of structural organization such as the tertiary and quaternary, drives their formation. Also, one could almost consider folding as a link between sequence and function.

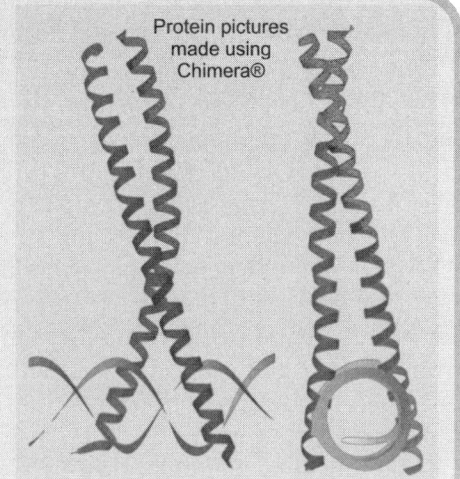

Fig. The inverted Y of Leucine Zipper motif bound to DNA: (left) a lateral-DNA view (right) head-on-DNA view

Consequent to all these studies, proteins have been designed. However, this is beyond the scope of this discussion that aims to convey the significance of quaternary structure in the light of primary structure and protein function (for an outline, *ref.* the chapters "proteomics roadmap to medicinal chemistry".

Selected references for this chapter: (Ramji, et al. 2002), (Skolnick, et al. 1999), (Agre et al.), (Chakraborty, et al. 2007), (Ramadevi, et al. 1998)

1.2.1G The Pentanary Structure

The pentanary protein structure is a concept that has just sprung up in the world of protein structure description. It is also called the fifth-order time-dependent or dynamic structure of a protein. Proteins are known to switch between states such as 'open ↔ closed' for channels, 'folded ↔ unfolded' in the intracellular environment, 'active ↔ inactive' for enzymes, etc. However, these changes are induced by molecular recognition. The description of the change of protein structure over time, generally without the influence of specific drugs or substrates, is attempted in this pentanary level. Detailed discussions of such changes are still not available; but the related study of protein dynamics is presented in chapter 1.3.

1.2.1H Other Intermediate Standard levels

Supersecondary, fold, domain, class: Although *"Primary → Secondary → Tertiary → Quaternary"* is the summary of protein structure organiza-tion, several intermediate structures are often analyzed. Similar to the case wherein carving a scene from one rock is more difficult than assembling separately carved smaller parts of the scene together the steep rise in complexity of structure from secondary to the tertiary level is broken up using what are called *"supersecondary structures"* and *"supersecondary motifs"*.

Why does moving from secondary to tertiary structure involve such a steep rise? Recognizing secondary structure involves identifying the conformation of residues and the localized shapes they build up to, such as helices, strands, and some turns. With just a list of secondary structures of a protein and the amino acids that form them (resulting from secondary structure recognition), it is a big step indeed to visualize the 3D arrangement of helices and strands with respect to each other and deduce the 3D shape of the protein. Supersecondary structures are pairs of secondary structures linked by the turn in between (Schemes 1.7 and 1.8). The focus of study at this level is the overall shape being formed (such as V-shape, L-shape, etc.) in addition to the arrangement/conformation of structures that form them, such as the φ-ψ value or hydrogen-bonding pattern of residues. Their study was first carried out by Rao and Rossman (Rao, et al. 1973). Even at this level, some structures are associated with specific functions–the helix-turn-helix with DNA binding, the perpendicular helices of the EF hand with calcium binding (Miles, et al. 2005). From a functional point of view the entire protein sometimes gets condensed to just its supersecondary structure. The rest of the protein serves to hold this structure in place allowing it to perform its function as in Discussion 1.6. To note is that there is no universal classification of

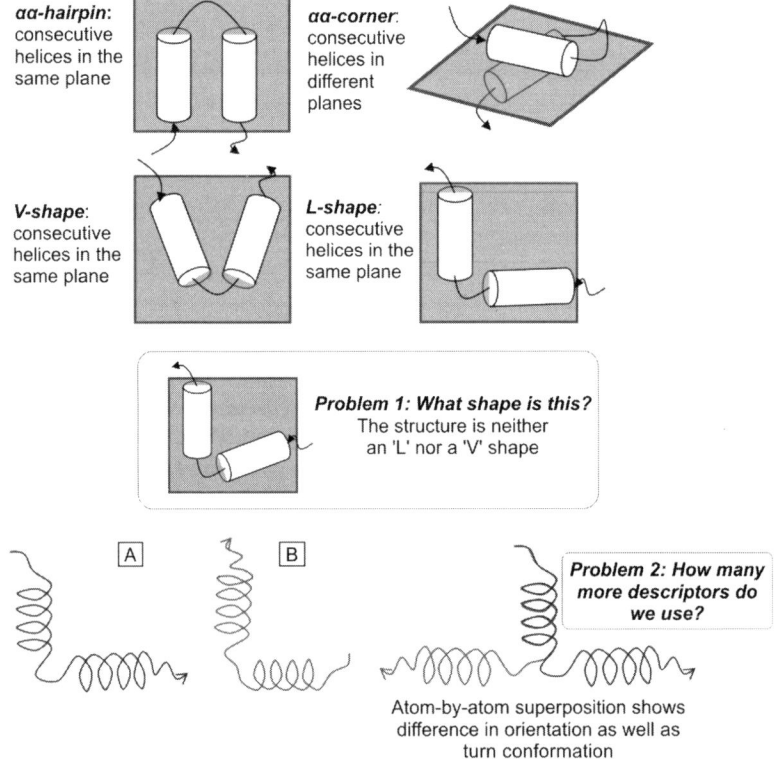

αα-hairpin: consecutive helices in the same plane

αα-corner: consecutive helices in different planes

V-shape: consecutive helices in the same plane

L-shape: consecutive helices in the same plane

Problem 1: What shape is this? The structure is neither an 'L' nor a 'V' shape

A   B

Problem 2: How many more descriptors do we use?

Atom-by-atom superposition shows difference in orientation as well as turn conformation

Scheme 1.7: List of supersecondary structures showing the loss of information when looking at the whole picture

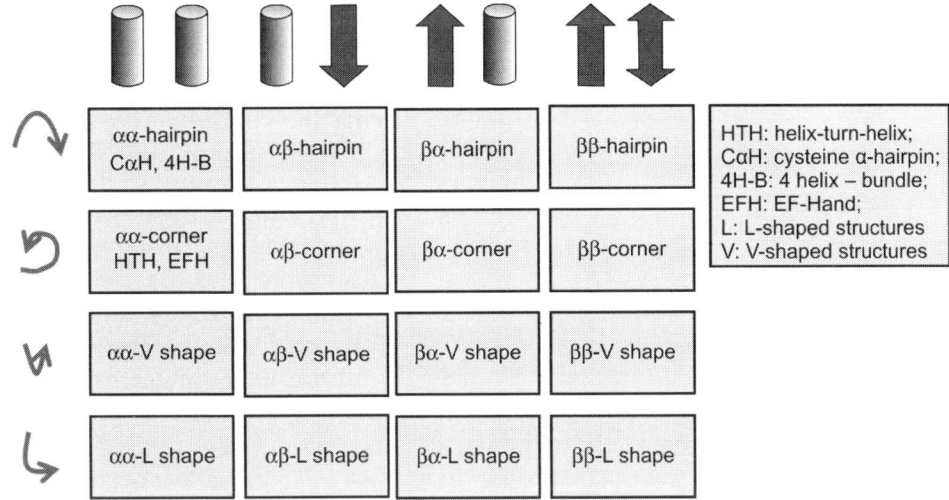

αα-hairpin CαH, 4H-B	αβ-hairpin	βα-hairpin	ββ-hairpin	HTH: helix-turn-helix; CαH: cysteine α-hairpin; 4H-B: 4 helix – bundle; EFH: EF-Hand; L: L-shaped structures V: V-shaped structures
αα-corner HTH, EFH	αβ-corner	βα-corner	ββ-corner	
αα-V shape	αβ-V shape	βα-V shape	ββ-V shape	
αα-L shape	αβ-L shape	βα-L shape	ββ-L shape	

Scheme 1.8: Supersecondary structures

these structures–the number of classes identified depends on the level of detail a particular method handles. In fact, even the word "supersecondary" is not generalized– it is sometimes hyphenated and sometimes not! A method that generalizes helices as "cylinders" by estimating only their direction in the form of a vector would not differentiate "L-shaped αα-structures" into 4 classes (with the second helix to the left, right, front and back respectively, as seen by the viewer, if the orientation of the first helix is fixed). This is because whether the second helix is right- or left-turned with respect to the first the vectors can always be rotated and superimposed making these classes indistinguishable (indicated in Schemes 1.7 to 1.9).

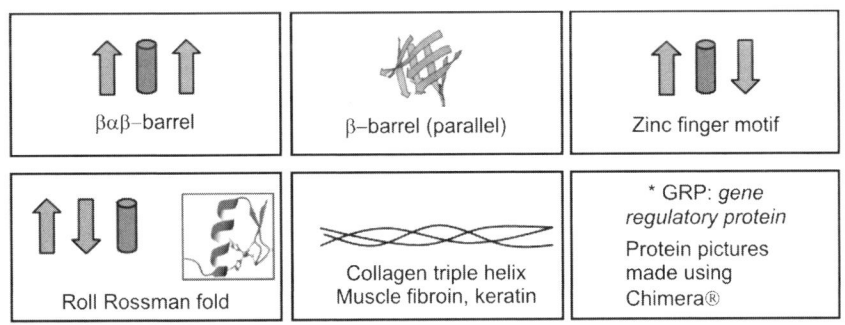

βαβ–barrel	β–barrel (parallel)	Zinc finger motif
Roll Rossman fold	Collagen triple helix Muscle fibroin, keratin	* GRP: *gene regulatory protein* Protein pictures made using Chimera®

Scheme 1.9: Higher order motifs

Supersecondary motifs are slightly larger in secondary structure composition than supersecondary structures (that is, motifs may contain more secondary structures). There are as many minus one supersecondary structure in a protein as there are secondary structures. If a protein has 3 helices and 2 β-strands, it has 4 supersecondary structures (Scheme 1.10). However, not all four of the latter may be functionally important. The protein may contain a functionally important pair of secondary

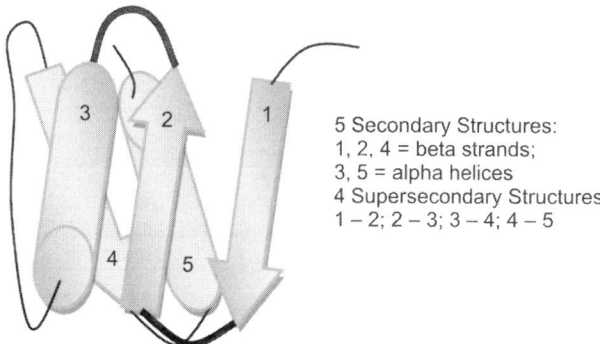

5 Secondary Structures:
1, 2, 4 = beta strands;
3, 5 = alpha helices
4 Supersecondary Structures:
1 − 2; 2 − 3; 3 − 4; 4 − 5

Scheme 1.10: Secondary and supersecondary structures

structures (a super secondary structure). When this arrangement is searched in other proteins, it might become evident that the supersecondary structure might be accompanied by a 3rd secondary structure in, say, 80% of proteins forming what is referred to as a supersecondary motif. The proteins studied might belong to the same family performing similar functions. In general both supersecondary structures (SSS) and motifs (SSM) are not energetically independent subunits of a protein in the sense that they are not attributed to form or exist independent of the rest of the protein in any way. Isolating that segment of the protein containing the SSS or SSM and allowing it to fold independently in a test tube does not result in a new protein segment having the same arrangement of secondary structures as in the original protein. The SSS and SSM are energetically stable combinations of secondary structures occurring within a protein, i.e., they lack steric strain (Miles, et al. 2005). It is useful to know that these terms sss and ssm are not as rigidly defined as primary, secondary, tertiary and quaternary structure are, and have even been used interchangeably in literature.

A domain is often considered, as summarized (Veretnik, et al. 2004), to be a structure
• Which retains a significant level of sequence homology.
• Which is the product of the smallest functional segment of a gene.
• Of a protein attributed a specific function.
• Similar to parts of other proteins.
• That is compact and visually identifiable a "lobe", "knob" of secondary structures.
• That is an independently folding part of a protein.

Proteins may or may not have more than one domain (*see* Scheme 1.11); each domain may have one or more *folds*. A fold is a structurally independent unit connecting distinct arrangement of secondary structures formed by a continuous segment of the polypeptide chain .A fold is a folding intermediate during domain formation (Scheme 1.11). It was mentioned that sss and ssm generally do not behave as an independent folding unit but, in contrast, folds do. Folds include typical composition, arrangements, and connectivity of secondary structures. In Scheme 1.11, structures 1 and 2 and in Scheme 1.12, structures 1−4 have the same composition and arrangement of secondary structures but different connectivity and hence have two different folds. A fold also has functional significance. It therefore can also be viewed as that part of a protein/ domain that performs a specific function or that supports a functionally significant part. An example is the immunoglobulin fold (this is found in the constant domain of IgG and other immunoglobulins). Table 1.7 gives a list of folds, domains, motifs and their functional relevance [reference: http://www.ebi.ac.uk/interpro/and (Day, et al. 2003)].

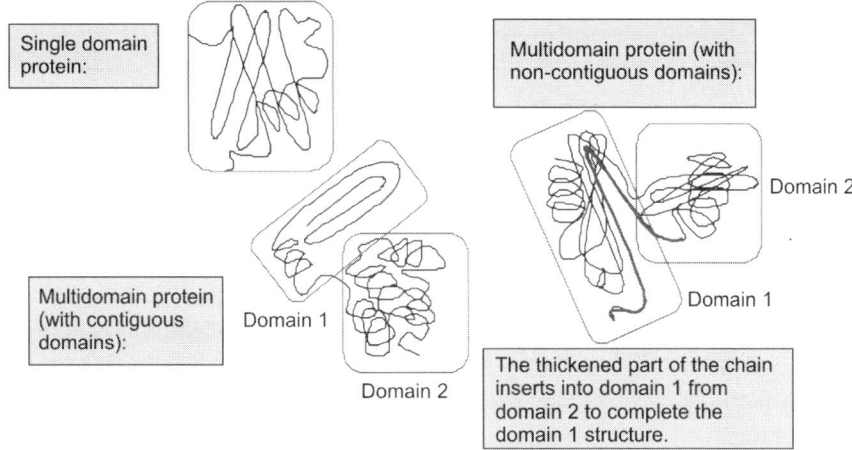

Scheme 1.11: Multi-domain and single domain

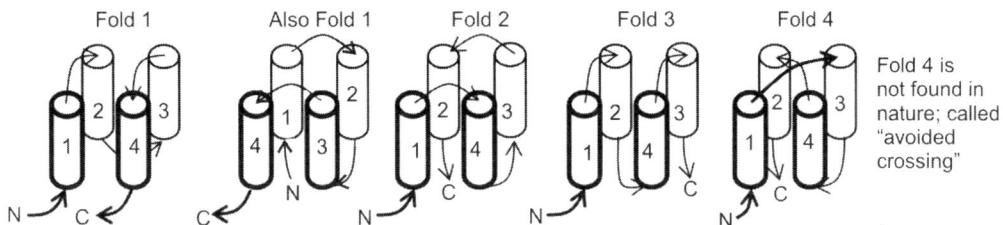

Scheme 1.12: Same topology, yet different folds

Architecture is yet another term describing tertiary structure. Domains/folds of the same topology need not have the same connectivity: structures 1 and 2 in Scheme 1.12 have the same topology. Only some architectures (out of all possible combinations of secondary structure) occurs among natural proteins. The architectures ensure extensive contacts between adjacent secondary structure elements (Reichmann, et al. 2007). For example, certain architectures facilitate the folding of protein into the hydrophobic interior and hydrophilic surface. A strict definition of what *architecture* is can be given only with respect to method used for analysis. Exact aspect in which families (of people) going on a vacation and a protein wish to gain an advantage is *packing*. By rolling-up or by folding-over, the aim is to reduce voids and optimize contact. As proteins (and unfortunately, not travel luggage!) self-pack independent of external help, it has been proposed that only certain architectures are preferred as they are advantageous during and after folding. Some domains are known to be very popular among proteins whereas others are hardly observed (Day, et al. 2003). A strict definition for each term, however, can be given only with respect to the method used for analysis.

- Some architectures are very popular among proteins. Example: α bundles. These are called *major architectures*.
- Some motifs are very popular. They are present in proteins as repeating units in folds and are ways of extending or expanding popular folds.

Table 1.7: List of domains, folds, motifs and their functional relevance ordered by abundance

Name	Function
1. Immunoglobulin-like	Defense
2. Rossman fold	Binds NAD cofactors
3. TIM barrel	Several enzymes
4. Jelly roll	*unknown*
5. DNA/RNA binding	~
6. 3-helix bundle	DNA binding
7. Globin	Carrier proteins in blood
8. Four-helix bundle	Among hormones
9. β-grasp (ubiquitin-like)	Protein folding
10. EF-hand	Calcium binding
11. Trypsin-like serine protease	Arrange amino acids for catalysis
12. Thioredoxin-like	Several enzymes
13. OB fold	Transcription, etc.
14. Cytochrome C	Electron transport
15. FAD/NAD(P) binding domain	~
16. Knottins	Regulatory protein
17. C-type lectin-like	Defense
18. Lipocalin	Fatty acid synthesis, etc.
19. Trefoil	In structural proteins, Defense
20. C_2H_2 & C_2H_4 Zinc finger	DNA binding and recognition

- Most folds and architectures are "layer based". These results in roughly globular shape and can undergo several mutations (substitution of/deletion of/formation of new secondary structures).

Structure is very much related to the evolutionary process. Scheme 1.13 explains how. A variety of proteins result from the diversification of one or more of the various levels. Inspite of this, some core motifs such as β hairpins or βαβ motifs are often identified to repeat in various ways. Genetically, gene segments are often repeated in various combinations to generate folds, domains and proteins and only those architectures that do not fall apart when shuffled are popular (Dokholyan, et al. 2002). The "layered architectures" and symmetry in arrangements of folds are considered to accommodate this way of working (Reichmann, et al. 2007).

Not all levels of the protein classification are based on structure. For instance, the *superfamily* (Gough, et al. 2001) is a sequence based and not a structure based stratum (Kim, et al. 2006). Sometimes, a superfamily often contains sequences that are less than 25% identical and hence it is often impossible to be sure that protein are divergently, rather than convergently, evolved on the basis of sequence alone (Scheme 1.13). Therefore superfamily has an alternative definition–that it consists of proteins that have similar structures and structurally equivalent functional groups (Wermuth, 2008).

1.2.2 METHODS AND MODELS FOR STRUCTURE ANALYSIS

"Everything should be as simple as possible, but not simpler."

Albert Einstein

How does one determine whether a segment of a protein is curled into a helix, pleated into beta-sheets or has sharp turns? How are well defined patterns identified in terms

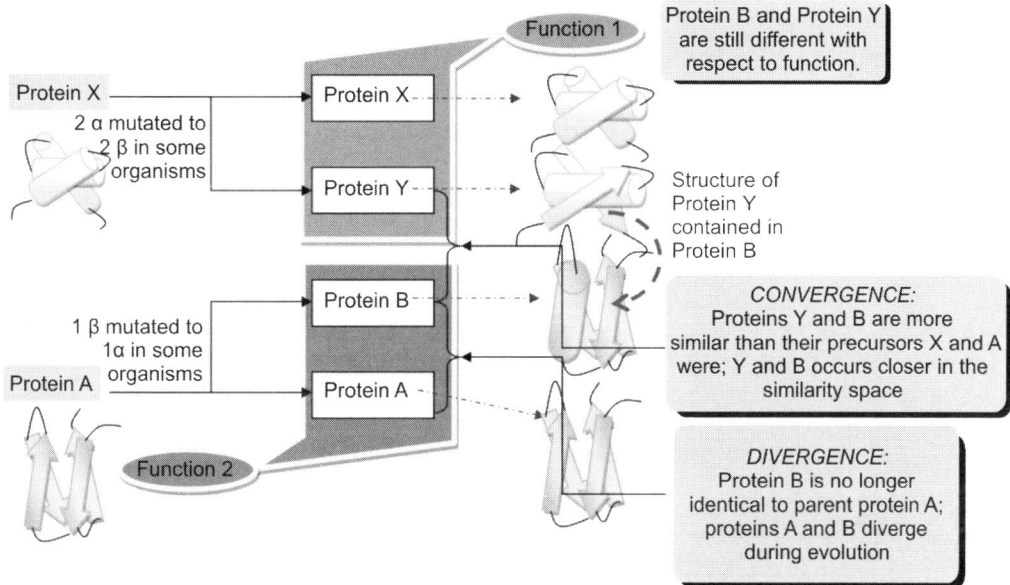

Scheme 1.13: Convergence and divergence in protein evolution

of geometry, conformation or hydrogen bonding? One can broadly classify some of the popular secondary structure assessment methods as in Scheme 1.14; the individual names of the methods are also given. Methods that appear under more than one category, use several approaches in combination for structure recognition. The approaches, terminologies, advantages and flaws of some of the popular methods are discussed in detail in this chapter. Related terminologies are first explained

Structure recognition: It is the (usually automated) recognition of structures using various computer algorithms. Focus is on determining what the type of structure is at secondary (whether α-helix, 3_{10}-helix, π-helix, parallel-, antiparallel-strands of β-sheets, specific types of turns, etc.), supersecondary (αα-V, αα-L, etc.), motif (DNA binding, calcium binding, β-barrel, etc.), etc. levels and the amino acids of a protein that are involved in each conformation. Assessment of structure applies one or more approaches described in Scheme 1.14. Thousands of structure assessment methods are available (for secondary and other levels including) and they generate slight differences in assignment; the choice of method depends on the goal of the study.

Fundamental unit: The term "fundamental unit" is used for that part of the secondary structure, either by H-bonding or by conformation, that repeats. Depending on the method of analysis, the assignment of fundamental units differs. Generally, the 4-membered loop is the fundamental unit of the α-helix and the β-bridge is that of β-sheets (*ref.* Fig. 1.27A for helices in section 1.2.1.D secondary structures).

Pseudo-atom: The term pseudo means 'false' or, here, 'a substitute'. Several methods that analyze protein structure do not take every atom on the protein. As mentioned

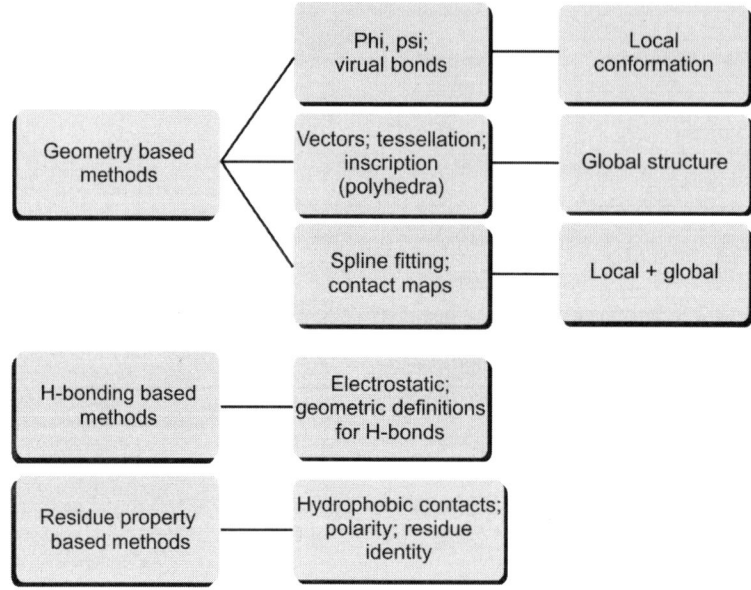

Scheme 1.14: Classifying protein structure analysis methods

earlier, many of them consider just the backbone, or further simplifying, just the C_α atoms. In the latter case, the C_α becomes the pseudo-atom, as it 'represents' or 'substitutes for' every amino acid in the protein (for example, *ref.* Scheme 1.15 on page 85 under Levitt and Greer's method–the C_α atoms are the only atoms retained for analysis along the protein backbone). The pseudo-atoms can also be a theoretically calculated point such as the mid-point of consecutive C_α atoms or the centre of mass of the side chains. It does not have to be a part of the chemical structure (here, the polypeptide chain). The justification for the popular use of the C_α atom to study enzymes, amino acids and other large protein system is that C_α atoms:

- Accurately reflect local conformation as they are flexible.
- Better reflect regularity in structure.
- Are estimated accurately even in low resolution.
- Are often used in protein folding analyses.

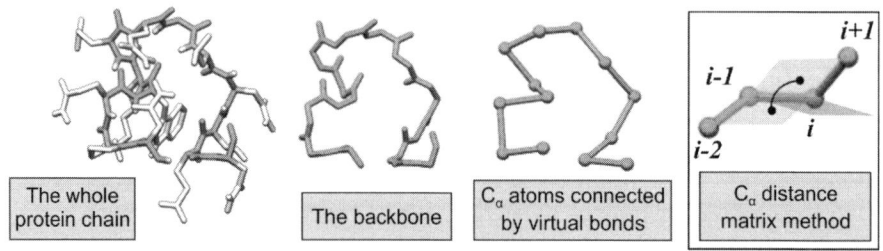

Scheme 1.15: Levels of simplification leading to C_α—distance matrices

Virtual bonds: These are 'lines' that connect simplified points or pseudo-atoms in proteins. For examples, instead of working with the "chemical bonds" in the backbone such as the N–C_α–C–N bonds, one could connect simply the C_α atoms of every residue with 'virtual bonds'. The less number of bonds, or atoms, the easier it is to determine protein structure, but there is some level of compromise on accuracy as explained in following paragraphs.

The local–global compromise: On an average, a "small drug receptor" contains about 500 amino acids; assuming each amino acid is made of 15 atoms on an average, one counts 7,500 atoms. One would imagine that the 'best' description is the most detailed, obtained by looking at the conformation of all these atoms. This however is a misconception. Looking at the bond–level structure of a protein, one might never get to tertiary or at times, even the secondary structure easily. In addition, one can never make comparisons between proteins. Letting go of some of the atoms and skipping over some bonds gives a clearer picture of higher level arrangement and more efficient use of computational resources. The degree of simplification is heavily dependent on the purpose of study. To analyze the way various secondary structures are oriented and connected (i.e. the fold), a helix could be simplified to a cylinder. But by doing this, one loses local distortions in the helix. If the purpose of the study is to view folds, this "coarse grained" approach is most appropriate. However, this does not help secondary structure assignment as one would expect distortions to be accounted for at that level. Thus there is almost always a compromise.

Discrete/continuous approach: These are two approaches used by geometric structure determination methods. For example Ramachandran's φ and ψ angles are calculated over a series of "broken lines" which are the backbone bonds; the value of φ is independent of the ψ value of neighboring amino acid, and not even influenced by the ψ value of the same amino acid. Such approaches are said to be discrete. Mostly in literature, one would not come across this as a special term–most of the protein structure analysis methods are discrete; an example of one of a very few continuous methods is Automated Protein Structure Analysis (APSA) [(Ranganathan, et al. 2009), a method that author was involved in developing]. It has been documented since early times (Levitt, et al. 1977) that φ, ψ angles are error prone as they directly reflect the error of the experimental method in each bond—this error would only add up when each individual bond is considered. A continuous method would include the contribution of nearby conformations and would asses local residue conformations with respect to those of nearby residues, thus reducing error.

Projection to low dimension: Protein structure is 3D. Using automated methods, one could project this 3D information into 2D or 1D. Let us consider φ and ψ angles–though these are mere numbers (2D) for every amino acid, they describe the 3D structure of the protein backbone. From a list of these values (a list of numbers is 1D information), one could obtain the 3D arrangement of atoms in proteins, however, not completely (*would you know the rotational conformation of, say, phenylalanine if the ø and ψ values are given?*). The projection to lower dimension, though useful and easy to handle, is always accompanied by loss of information (akin to the loss accompanying global assessment of structures in contrast to local conformations, i.e. the local-global compromise mentioned above).

Cut-offs: Most protein structure analysis methods use cut-offs for lengths, angles, energies, regions of the Ramachandran plot, etc. The value of the cut-off is chosen after the analysis of large number of protein conformation. The statistical results help to choose the best cut-offs. For example, for a segment of four residues to be labeled as a "turn" the distance between the first and the fourth residue was considered to be shorter than 6 Å. The disadvantage of this is however is that with increasing number of proteins being analyzed the value changed to 6.5 Å, 7 Å and 7.5 Å (references cited) depending on authors! Cut-offs are used in all methods. For example, two independent hydrogen-bonding based methods that used different cut-offs for calculating the H-bond produced contradictory results when used in determining the length of a β-strand–the presence/absence of one of the bonds influenced the classification of the following segment.

As noted earlier, though all methods aim to capture the same secondary structure that repeats over and over in every protein deposited in the protein databank, it is surprising as well as amusing that assignment differs considerably between these various approaches. This aspect has been extensively discussed in literature, and it is generally agreed that no one method is "the correct one" and that each method is correct only within its sphere of definition. Seeking the consensus of several methods has always been recommended. The choice of method also depends on the overall purpose of the investigation. For example, the study of overall shape of the binding pocket of a list of proteins to which a particular ligand is known to interact with, requires a protein structure analysis, method that well describes global shapes. In another instance, consider a study that looks into the influence of the presence/absence of the molecule on protein structure; one would look at local conformation as well as hydrogen bonding in the protein.

1.2.2.1 Automated Structure Assignment

A. *Complications*

- Certain aspects of the experimental structure determination phase and the following theoretical research phase contains errors that results in variations. The variations may exist in atomic positions, the innate behavior of proteins as biomacromolecule, the approach used by structure assignment algorithms or the cut-offs used to define the conformations. Some of these variations are inevitable; others include conflicts in structure assignments by methods utilizing different approaches.

- Error in structure determination using experiments and missing residues due to disorder in the chain, proteolytic cleavage, etc. During early days around the late 1970s when experimental resolution for determining protein structure was large (2–2.5 Å in general), errors were also large (Levitt, et al. 1977). Today, proteins are obtained at a resolution of 1.6 Å or less. At any rate, the C_α atoms are generally less likely to have error relative to the rest of the chain atoms as their position is cross-determined by the position of the side chain as well as other backbone atoms (Miles, et al. 2005).

- There are several ways of describing structure for a particular segment of the protein. It is most important to understand that ambiguity in structure is an inherent property of the protein, meaning, it is one of the basic properties of a protein to present a different structure each time a different approach is used to quantify it.

- The problem of *continuum of conformations* and the problem of boundaries of secondary structures: Richardson, et al. 1989 called the problem of defining the boundaries of secondary structures "trivial but difficult".
- The task of defining structural relationships is further complicated by the existence of multidomain proteins; more than 30% of non-identical structures in the current PDB contain two or more domains (Hadley, et al. 1999).

The first X-ray crystal structure dates back to early times. Since then, extensive work on crystallographic patterns of proteins and the assignment of secondary structures from the generated data has been performed by various groups around the world. Therefore, this is included as an approach and is presented first, followed by the groundbreaking work (Ramachandran, et al. 1968) that has resulted in the φ, ψ angles and the Ramachandran map appearing in every textbook of biochemistry. One of the first automated structure analysis by Levitt and Greer (Levitt, et al. 1977) that used a combination of H-bonding and geometric criteria is described next. What follows are descriptions of DSSP (Kabsch, et al. 1983), a very popular method, STRIDE (Frishman, et al. 1985), made to reflect crystallographic assignment applying H-bonding and φ–ψ criteria, and DEFINE (Richards, et al. 1988) that compares distance matrices of the structures of a protein and the ideal structures. The availability of so many methods is far from discouraging; it is noteworthy that each method has its strengths and weaknesses and the choice of method depends on the purpose of research. Therefore, a few "newer methods" are mentioned.

B. *Crystallographer's Definitions*

Crystallographer's secondary structure assignments are based on the following:
- (varying definitions of) Hydrogen bonding.
- Distance and angle of approach of donor-acceptor atoms.
- φ-ψ (backbone dihedral angles).
- Visual inspection. For further details, *ref.* chapter 1.1.2.A.

C. *Ramachandran Angles*

Has been referenced thousands of times since publication.

Original publication by: GN Ramachandran, C Ramakrishnan, V Sasisekharan (Ramachandran, et al. 1963), (Ramachandran, et al. 1968).

Synonyms: backbone dihedral angles, phi-psi (φ-ψ) angles, backbone torsion angles.

Principle: This is a geometry based method. It is one of the earliest and until today, most popular method used to mathematically analyze the conformation of amino acids in a protein. It is a discrete and bond-level description that analyzes the dihedral angle of the C–N–C$_\alpha$–C arrangement, called φ and N–C$_\alpha$–C–N arrangement, called ψ as shown in the familiar Fig. 1.31. These 2 values are specified for every residue along the backbone. The regularity of helices and beta strands is evident as repeating values (within a certain range provided to include slight distortions in nature) and patterns in values have also been observed among turn regions. The φ and ψ values for the 3

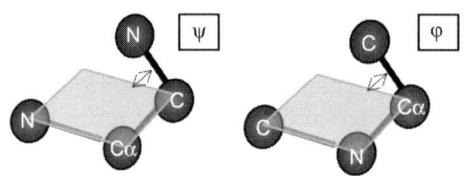

Fig. 1.31: Depiction of the dihedral angles φ and ψ

ideal helices and for β-strands have already been tabulated (Table 1.6, chapter 1.2.1). The authors further presented the 'Ramachandran plot' of φ values taken in the abscissa and ψ values in the ordinate. In such a plot, "islands" of frequently occurring (this statistical measure also corresponds to energetic preference) and theoretically possible conformations were located. The remaining regions were considered to be "disallowed" owing to steric hindrance.

Revisions of the Ramachandran map (*R*-map): With increasing number of proteins deposited (*ref.* chapter 1.1) in the PDB, the number of times the R-map has been revised (and is still being), the variety of applications it has been exploited for and the number of theories it has given rise to (and disproved) is enormous. Therefore, the following paragraphs are dedicated to the highlights of literature, ever since this work was published covering the aspects mentioned.

- *Allowed and disallowed regions of the map:* The map has been updated to keep in par with quantum chemical calculations (Miles, et al. 2005). In an α-helix, $\varphi = -\psi$ relationship was observed (Garnier, et al. 1990) that differed from the original description of helical conformations. The above relationship also demonstrated that the expected larger variability of φ (from −160 to −50°) compared to ψ (generally from −60 to −40°) as initially proposed by Ramachandran et al was not true (see reference (HovmoÈller, et al. 2002) that explains that even ψ varied to the same extent such that O–O and O–N distances were maintained around 3.5 Å).

- *Ideal secondary structures:* The latest survey of protein structures carried out on over 1,000 protein subunits in the PDB accounting for the backbone conformations of over 237,000 residues (HovmoÈller, et al. 2002). Although most α-helices were found to populate a very specific region on the plot (a reported 2% of the entire plot area around ε, ψ=−63.8°,−41.1°), β-sheets were found to segregate into two distinct regions on the plot with ε, ψ around −121, +128° and around −66, +137°. At the same time, no significant difference was observed between the parallel and the antiparallel sheets. Short (3-residue) stretches of left–handed α-helices were located around −60, −60°.

- *Turns:* In addition to the usage of φ and ψ angles to represent periodicity of secondary structures, the authors calculated hydrogen bonds between turns. They characterized β-turns of types I, II and III and their respective stereochemical mirror images I', II' and III' based on φ, ψ values and the presence of hydrogen bonds between the first and fourth turn residue. Additions and modification to this system were steadily made. In 1973, the need for defining turns based on the presence of hydrogen bonds was dropped as this was not the case for 25% of the β-turns (Lewis, et al. 1973). This was followed, in 1981, by the addition of 6 others and the removal of types III and III' that were none other than a four residues out of a 3_{10}–helix. [(Richardson, 1981), (Wilmot, et al. 1988), (Hutchinson, et al. 1994)]. These comprised of types I, I' II, II', VII, VIa1, VIa2, VIb and IV and is used upto date [implemented in PROMOTIF (Hutchinson, et al. 1994)].

• Numerous other investigations were carried out such as the identification of new secondary structures such as helix caps, protein structure prediction, verification of the accuracy of protein coordinates using R-maps, etc.

D. *H-bonding – C_α Distance matrix–α-Dihedral Angle Method*

Original publication by: Michael Levitt[1], Jonathan Greer[2,1]: Medical Research Council Laboratory of Molecular Biology, Cambridge, England, [2]: Columbia University, US

Purpose: In 1977, Michael Levitt and Jonathan Greer's H-bonding–cum–C_α distance matrix method became one of first methods automated for the determination of secondary structures using precise rules (and including H-bonds). It aimed to systematically label α-helices, β-sheets and reverse turns in a crystallographer-friendly manner.(In this paper, uniformity and agreement with crystallographers' assignments were not the case, the authors claim, when φ, ψ was used by individual protein crystallizing groups to assign structures).

Principles used: (*Ref.* Scheme 1.15) Only C_α atoms were used and connected by virtual bonds. The torsion angle formed by 4 consecutive C_α atoms (*i*–2, *i*–1, *i* and *i+1*) is called α_i angle (α angle of the amino acid residue *i*) and is most influenced by the *i*th C_α position. H-bond partners are calculated from the C_α positions itself and from that, strength and location of H-bonds are determined. Secondary structure is also obtained from C_α distances by forming a matrix that includes the distance between all the C_α atoms of a protein with respect to each other.

Methodology:

Geometric criteria: The α-angle:

Residues with the α-angle-value between 10° and 120° (and also those that have values between 120° and 140° provided the next α angle lies between 10° and 120°) form right-handed α-helices; those that have α angles between 120° and 270° define β-sheets and between –90° and 0° form left-handed α-helices. The combination of 4 or more consecutive residues having the same code forms a secondary structure, i.e four consecutive residues having α angle between 10° and 120° must occur to from an α helix.

Residues that have not been assigned as belonging to either an α-helix or a β-sheet are analyzed for the presence of reverse-turns. Thus residue *i* belongs to a right-handed turn category if it's α angle (α_i) 0° <α_i <90°, and to left-handed turn category if –90° <α_i <0° provided the following residue (*i+1*) is also assigned the same category.

Hydrogen bonding:

Hydrogen bonds form between CO and NH groups of the backbone. However, in this method, only C_α atoms are taken from the protein coordinates so the CO and NH information is unavailable from the protein coordinate file. From earlier studies (Levitt, 1976) it was shown that the peptide group can be approximated from the position of C_α atoms and the local conformation of the backbone.

Atom locations: A 'simplified peptide group' is generated for residue *i* with atoms N'_i, O'_i such that N'_i is midway between the C_α atoms of *i*–1th and *i*th residue and O'_i is 1 Å from N'_i and perpendicular to the plane defined by the C_α atoms of residues

$i-1$, i and $i+1$. Thus the relative positions of CO of residue $i-1$ and NH of residue i are both dependent on the conformation φ, ψ of residue i ($i-1$ conformation plays no part) corresponding to the fact that φ of residues in a protein is fairly unchanging compared to ψ (*vide supra*: means *ref.* above)

Presence: The following 'rules' were imposed: that at least 2 residues must separate the residues to which the donor and the acceptor belongs, that the distance of separation between their N' groups should be <6 Å and finally, that the 2 peptide dipoles (the dipole formed between O and N of one peptide group and the O and N of the other) must point in the same direction (or deviate by a maximum of 60°). The authors calculate that this arrangement of atoms must capture all H-bonds stronger than (or in other words, having lower energy value than) −2 kcal/mol. The ideal situation is when a distance of 4.2 Å between the 2 N' atoms and parallel arrangement (0° deviation) of dipoles results from the arrangement of the 2 interacting peptide groups resulting in an H-bonded interaction −5 kcal/mol in strength.

Pattern: α-helical regions are defined as the H-bonds formed by i and $i+1$ with j and j' if the difference between i and j, and that between $i+1$ and j' is 3 (wherein j' would be equal to $j+1$; although $|i-j|$ is 3, this again implies $i \rightarrow i+4$ H-bond in the traditional sense because according to this method, an H-bond at i involves bonding between $i-1$ and i). For values any other than 3, the segment is assigned an antiparallel β-strand. Parallel β-strands occur when the sum of j and i is equal to the sum of j' and $i+1$ (here, j' would be equal to $j-1$).

Geometric criteria: C_α distances

This criterion is used to detect secondary structures and also to present secondary and tertiary structure. The rule for identifying α-helices is that the distance between C^α_i and C^α_{i+3} should be less than 6 Å and that between C^α_i and C^α_{i+4} should be less than 6.5 Å (ideally these values are 5.1 Å and 6.1 Å respectively). If residues i to j have this pattern and if residue $j+1$ breaks it, then residues i to $j+1$ are labeled as α-helical. For short helices (5–7 residues), to avoid overlapping recognition with reverse turns, a least squares fitting procedure is undertaken with an ideally constructed helix such that the mean square difference between the two is less than 1Å (if this doesn't happen, the last residue of the helix is dropped out and the fitting is continued. If the helix is only 5 or 6 residues long to start with, a least square difference of 0.4Å or 0.5 Å are only accepted). With similar allowances operating among strands (the ideal distance of separation of the C_α atoms of antiparallel and parallel strands 5.6 Å and 5.5 Å respectively) the inter-strand C_α distance is set to be <6.5 Å for the parallel and antiparallel cases. Comparisons are again made to ideal β-sheets structures to obtain unambiguous results.

Combining both criteria for secondary structure assignment

A combination of 3 independent assessments is used to unambiguously identify and label secondary structures. It was reported that most β-sheets identified by H-bond were not recognized via the C_α distance matrix method. After the assignment of α-helices and β-strands, assignment of left-and right-handed turns is undertaken by the α-angle geometry method.

E. *Dictionary of Protein Secondary Structure: DSSP*

Original publication by: Wolfgang Kabsch, Christian Sander; Max Planck Institute of Medical Research, Germany (Kabsch, et al. 1983).

Purpose: To present an automated secondary structure recognition process that is simple, and at the same time capable of differentiating the many secondary structures. The authors aim at keeping the number of parameters that need to be adjusted to perform the recognition to a minimum (which, they opine is not possible while using $\varphi-\psi$ angles or C_α virtual bond methods that calculate distance, angle and dihedral). S-S bonds and solvent exposure is also calculated.

Principles used: The automated secondary structure recognition is achieved by programming the identification of the presence of specific backbone hydrogen-bond patterns and local geometric features from the X-ray coordinates of proteins. The elementary hydrogen-bonding patterns are the *turn* and the *bridge*. Repeating *turns* give rise to helices, and *bridges* to ladders; connected ladders are sheets. The presence of hydrogen bonds is calculated using energy cut-offs (details follow) and geometry is given by local curvature and torsion.

Methodology: (*Ref.* Fig. 1.32)

Hydrogen bonding

Presence: The presence of hydrogen bonds is decided by calculating electrostatic interaction energies between the H-bond donor N, the acceptor O, the hydrogen H and the carbonyl C. Partial charges are placed on C, O and H, N (+q1, −q1 and +q2, −q2 respectively) such that:

$$E = q1 * q2 \left(\frac{1}{r_{O-N}} + \frac{1}{r_{C-H}} - \frac{1}{r_{O-H}} - \frac{1}{r_{C-N}} \right) * f$$

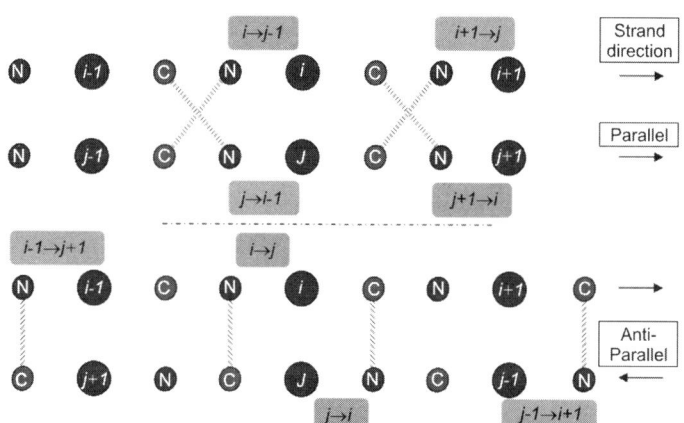

For β-strands, DSSP has a A parallel bridge pattern (that will build up to parallel β-ladders/sheet) is given by a zig-zag H- bonding between $i \rightarrow j-1$ and $j+1 \rightarrow i$ or $j \rightarrow i-1$ and $i+1 \rightarrow j$ and an antiparallel bridge (repeating to form antiparallel β-ladders/sheet), by a parallel $i \rightarrow j$ and $j \rightarrow i$ or $i-1 \rightarrow j+1$ and $j-1 \rightarrow i+1$.

Fig. 1.32: Hydrogen bonding in parallel (above) and antiparallel (below) β-sheet

Here, q1=0.42*e*, q2=0.20*e* (where *e* is the unit electron charge), *r* represents the distance between the subscripted pairs of atoms in Å and *f*, the dimensional factor equals 332. The *r* values are obtained from the XYZ coordinates of proteins. Energy is obtained in kcal/mol and has, ideally, −3 kcal/mol. As mentioned earlier, some structural distortions are coupled with weak and sometimes bifurcated bonds. To allow for such weakening, (given that 'weakening' results in less negative value than the ideal) a maximal cut-off of −0.5 kcal/mol is given allowing for N−O distance of up to 2.2 Å larger than the ideal and a 60° deviation from ideal alignment (compare with Levitt and Greer's values earlier).

Pattern: The pattern of H-bonding is expressed differently depending on whether the smallest unit is a *turn* or a *bridge*. For a *turn*, numbers are used to indicate between which 2 residues the H-bond exists. If the presence of an H-bond between the CO group of residue number 5 and the NH group 4 residues after has been confirmed for a *turn*, the *turn* is then called a 4-*turn*. In general, an *n*-*turn* has an H-bond between the CO of residue *i* and NH of residue *i*+*n*; it is well known that in an α-helix, the pattern of bonding is *i* → *i*+4−therefore by DSSP analysis, the smallest repeating unit of an α-helix will be the 4-*turn*. The shortest α-helix according to DSSP requires 2 consecutive 4-*turns*, which in the above example would occur at residue number 5 and 6. The α-helix would thus encompass residue numbers 6, 7, 8 and 9. Similarly repetition of two 3-*turns* forms 3_{10}−helices and that of two 5-*turns* forms π-helices.

Bridges are simply defined by the presence of H-bonds between residues that are not nearby in the primary sequence. The 2 residues *i* and *j* are considered to be a part of non-overlapping stretches of the polypeptide chain if *i*−1, *i*, or *i*+1 do not overlap with *j*−1, *j, or j*+1. A parallel bridge pattern (that will build up to parallel β-ladders/sheet) is given by a zig-zag H-bonding between *i*−1→*j* and *j*→*i*+1 or *j*−1 → *i* and *i* → *j*+1 and an antiparallel bridge (repeating to form antiparallel β-ladders/sheet), by a parallel *i* → *j* and *j* → *i* or *i*−1 → *j*+1 and *j*−1→*i*+1 H-bonding pattern as shown in Fig. 1.32. DSSP defines a 'ladder' to be "a set of 1 or more consecutive bridges of identical type" and a sheet to be "a set of one or more ladders connected by shared residues".

Geometric Criteria

Virtual bonds connecting 4 consecutive C_α atoms indicate whether these atoms are arranged along a right handed turn or one that is left. The torsional angle is positive or negative in value, respectively. Thus α-helices had positive torsion, and β-strands, when ideally twisted, were found to have negative torsion. Curved pieces are defined as "bends" and in the presence of certain H-bonded patterns, are called "hydrogen-bonded turns".

Bends are defined simultaneously by both H-bond patterns and angles; bends need the presence of H-bonds between residue *i*−2→*i* and *i*→*i*+2 with direction change of more than 70°. Chirality−the state of a segment of a protein being coiled left-handed or right-handed−is determined from the dihedral angle between four successive C_α atoms connected by virtual bonds.

Combining the two criteria for overall secondary structure assignment: The assessments of H-bonding and geometry are done independently for a protein. Structural overlaps are then sorted out such that residues are assigned as belonging to only one secondary structural element.

Other details: Solvent exposure is given as the number of water molecules in possible contact with a residue and *disulfide bridges* are also included in the calculations.

F. Secondary Structural Identification: STRIDE

Original publication by: Dmitrij Frishman, Patrick Argos; European Molecular Biology Laboratory, Germany (Frishman, et al. 1985).

Purpose: Automated secondary structure assignment made to reflect crystallographer's assignment strategy and results.

Principles used: (*Ref.* Fig. 1.33) This is a backbone analysis method. It combines the use of backbone hydrogen bond calculation and backbone dihedral angle information. The weighted contribution of both H-bonds and statistically derived φ–ψ values are taken to decide on the presence of a secondary structure (whether helix or strand). The identification is such that secondary structures are recognized by their fundamental unit (i.e. 4-membered "loops" for α-helices and "bridges" for β-strands as defined earlier in this chapter under terminologies. Thresholds are set up such that identification of helices and strands can take place even in the presence of irregularities in one of the two criteria. Expanding on the previous statement, the presence of strong hydrogen bonds can discount irregularities of the backbone (in terms of dihedral angle values) and the presence of statistically defined φ-ψ values can compensate weak hydrogen bonds.

Methodology

Hydrogen bonding:

The energy of the hydrogen bond is calculated such that $E_H = E_r \times E_t \times E_p$ where E_H is the energy of the calculated energy of the hydrogen bond, E_r is the energy term that depends on distance r in Fig. 1.33, given by:

$$E_r = \frac{-3E_m r_m^8}{r^8} + \frac{-4Emr_m^6}{r^6}$$

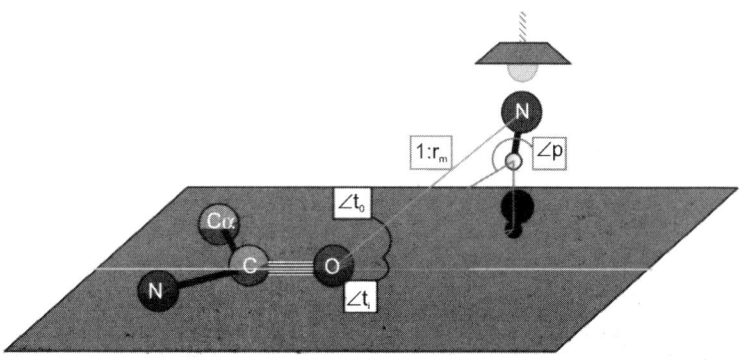

Fig. 1.33: A schematic depiction of how hydrogen bonds can be calculated just based on distances and angles

Ideally, hydrogen bond is defined with distance $r_m = 3.0$ Å and energy $E_m = -2.8$ kcal/mol. This equation actually resembles equations used in molecular modeling, with the distance term being expressed as an "8–6 function" as described in detail in Part II chapter 2.1. E_r becomes repulsive when bonding atoms get too close. This feature is needed only when modeling of atom behavior is undertaken. Here, as existing coordinates are being analyzed, if atoms get too close, i.e. if $r <$ the ideal distance r_m, E_r is considered to be equal to E_m.

E_t and E_p indicate the dependence of E_H on the angle of approach of the H-donor to the H-acceptor as calculated from the angle t_i, the angular deviation of the hydrogen atom from the bisector of the lone pair orbitals *within* the plane of the lone pair orbitals (this is the plane that is shown in Fig. 1.33), angle t_o, the same *from* the plane of the lone pair orbitals (i.e. t_o is the out-of-plane angle formed between H–O line and the plane in the figure), and angle p in the same Fig. 1.33. The reason these angles are considered is to account for the degree of interaction of the orbitals that are responsible for hydrogen bonding. The term $E_p = \cos^2 p$; the term E_t is defined depending on the positioning of the H atom with respect to the donor lone pair orbital in-plane angle (t_i). If t_i is greater than 110°, there is no bond formation ($E_t = 0$ and so $E_H = 0$ as $E_H = E_r \times E_t \times E_p$).

Dihedral Angles

The φ, ψ values of all residues of the dataset that have been described as α-helix or β-sheet (under "HELIX" or "SHEET" section of the PDF file header) in the PDB file submitted by the discoverers of the protein are determined (N_i^α, N_i^β respectively). Independently, the φ and ψ angles of all residues found in the dataset is obtained; the Ramachandran plot is then divided onto in 20°-by-20° regions (subscript *i* in the above notation) and all residues with φ, ψ values that fall within this region of the plot are counted (N_i^{total}). The probability that discoverers' assigned torsion angles for a secondary structure fall within the *i*th zone of the Ramachandran plot of the entire protein is determined, given by $P_i^\alpha = \dfrac{N_i^\alpha}{N_i^{total}}$ for helices and $P_i^\beta = \dfrac{N_i^\beta}{N_i^{total}}$ for β-strands. This allows STRIDE to assign α-helices and β-strands to match crystallographers' secondary structure definitions in φ–ψ terms as well as determine the extent of variation in φ and ψ values that occur amidst the latter.

Combining the Two Criteria

For α-helices, the presence of at least two consecutive H-bond between an atom k and the fifth atom down the line (k+4) in terms of energy E_H is combined with the probability that the conformation of the first and fifth residue is indeed helical. If this is true, all residues in between are assigned helical state, indicated by the letter H. The shortest helix is therefore 5 residues long. For β-sheet recognition, the shortest stretch is defined by the presence of two consecutive β-bridges. The quality of the β-sheet is calculated from firstly, the strength of both its H-bonds and secondly, from the P_i^β value of these two residues or those in between these two. The P_i^β value is not calculated for the two end residues of β-strands as the polypeptide chain drastically reverses at these points.

Results by the dataset/subsets: A dataset of 226 proteins (the size of datasets in the year 1995; today such analysis will include 1000s of proteins) was set up. After eliminating proteins that:

- Had only C_α atoms,
- Had no secondary structure assignments made by authors,
- Had incorrect assignments (wrong numbering, unrealistic coordinates etc),
- Had less than 70 residues,
- Resulted from modeling studies, the remaining were segregated into 3 non-redundant subsets (having proteins with sequence similarity no greater than 30%) and comments on the use of each subset are written within curling brackets:

a. X-ray structures of all resolutions + NMR structures (by STRIDE's automated secondary structure recognition, ~95% and ~93% of α-helical and β-strand residues, respectively, were identified correctly with respect to crystallographers results).

b. X-ray structures of resolution better than 2.5 Å (to determine STRIDE assignment when protein structure was "clear").

c. X-ray structures of resolution worse than 2.5 Å (to determine the difference between stride's performance with well-resolved and ambiguous structures. As the principle involved in strides depends on inter-atomic distances and angles, accurate resolution of structure becomes a necessity).

G. *Define (an overview)*

Original publication by: Frederic Richards, Craig Kundrot; Yale University, US (Richards, et al. 1988).

Principles used: Define establishes a distance matrix of the C_α atoms in a protein as a 2D display of 3D structure. This matrix is then compared to inter C_α distances of ideal structures and secondary structure is assigned if the two matrices agree within predetermined limits. In addition, the method is capable of a primitive supersecondary structure description. Both levels use just the C_α atoms as input. This algorithm is sensitive to the cumulative discrepancy between the ideal and observed distance matrix. The program assigns 90–95% of the residues in most proteins to at least one type of secondary element-helices, extended strands, sharp turns, or omega loops.

Methodology

- The program determines the initial and final residues in the various secondary structures assigned.
- The axial directions and locations are compiled from the input C_α coordinates; the helices and strands defined are thus idealized as straight segments. The secondary structure assignment is corrected by giving allowances for moderate curvature computed from the calculated axes.
- The geometric relations between each of these 'secondary structure line segments' are then calculated to yield first level supersecondary structure analysis.

- Even though a maximum of six parameters are required for a complete description of the relations between each pair of secondary structure, authors estimate that a less complete description will frequently suffice, for example just the separation and angle between two secondary structure axes.
- A matrix is used to represent the relative arrangement of C_α atoms in a secondary structure from which relative arrangement of the secondary structures itself can be obtained.
- Arbitrary motifs, substructures, higher levels of supersecondary structures and tertiary structures can also be searched among the domains of the PDB using this method.

Newer and Novel Approaches Continue to Develop

One would imagine that after all this work there is not much scope to develop new methods for secondary structure analysis and any such attempt is superfluous. This is not true. Some recent methods have given great insights into structure description and also suggestions to improve structure prediction and folding pathways. The first two methods involve the use of artificial neural networks (*ref.* chapter 2.4 on chemometrics). The unsupervised learning approach is presented as an example of how, forgetting all the discoveries of protein structure worked by thousands of groups all these years, the computer is able to "rediscover" history. In addition to using ANN method, they also represent proteins as "graphs" based on the graph theory of mathematics. For other representations on protein structure that involves graphs, *ref.* [(Xu, et al. 2001), (Brinda, et al. 2005)]. Very few quantitative continuous methods (in contrast to discrete methods) are available. A new method called APSA that uses spline fitted C_α atoms, developed to account for detailed local shapes a well as global orientations simultaneously, is presented.

H. Unsupervised Learning Approach

Original publication by: Barak Raveh, Ofer Rahat, Ronen Basri, Gideon Schreiber; Weizmann Institute of Science, Israel (Raveh, et al. 2007).

Purpose: To present an unsupervised *de-novo* "rediscovery" of secondary structures wherein the computer is used to find out regular patterns in conformation and bonding without supplying any sort of background information from literature (*ref.* chapter 2.4 under part II). Such an attempt is aimed capture conformations and non-conventional structures that might have been overlooked over the years.

Protein structure is mapped by the hydrogen bonded rings present; artificial neural networks are used to study the maps and decide the number of distinct patterns, their regularity and frequency of occurrence. Atoms in red and their linkages show hydrogen bonding (Fig. 1.34).

Method: The new method for unsupervised partitions undirected graphs, based on patterns of small recurring network motifs. The input was the network of all H-bonds and covalent interactions of protein backbones. The following were the involved steps:

Embedding protein structures in graphs: Protein structure was spread out (mapped) in the form of a "graph" shown in Fig. 1.34. This undirected graph G (V, E) has nodes/

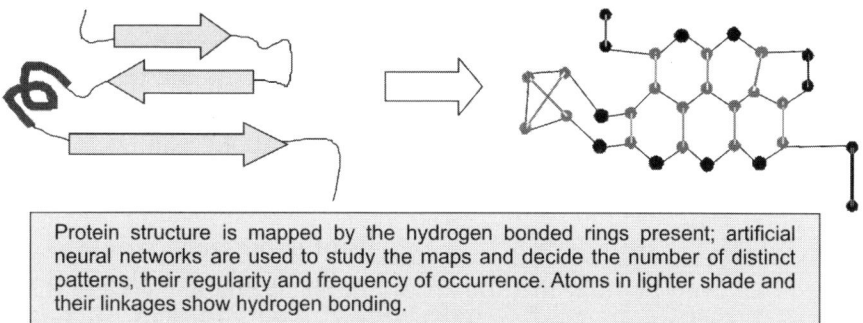

Protein structure is mapped by the hydrogen bonded rings present; artificial neural networks are used to study the maps and decide the number of distinct patterns, their regularity and frequency of occurrence. Atoms in lighter shade and their linkages show hydrogen bonding.

Fig. 1.34: Converting H-bonding patterns into graphs

vertices V and undirected edges E. Each node V represents a residue and each edge E is either a covalent bond or a hydrogen bond between two backbone residues atoms. The method included only covalent and backbone hydrogen interactions, since the study was mainly interested in a backbone description of folds.

Obtaining patterns: Having built a graphical representation of proteins, pattern of small network motifs were observed to appear frequently in the graphs (termed network motif vectors). For instance, hexagons were found to correspond to anti-parallel β-sheets, squares to parallel sheets, etc. Thus motifs represented the local environment of each node in the graph allowing the detection of recurrent patterns. A total of 1500 theoretically possible network motifs were elucidated; however in practice, only 180 motifs were observed.

Validation: To validate the efficiency and accuracy of pattern identification (of the network motif vectors), the method was applied to learn and predict the assignments of DSSP. About 90% success rate was found for all categories that DSSP is capable of labeling. Although the main purpose of the work is to rediscover secondary structures without assuming prior knowledge, the validation reassures that network motif vectors indeed 'work' to preserve the essential information needed for secondary structure classification.

Enrichment: The recognition of repeating adjacent motifs corresponding to secondary structures was "highlighted" in the algorithm by increasing weights of edges connecting similar patterns. This process was referred to as 'enrichment'. It is postulated that this process reinforces edges that form significant patterns, while reducing the weights of less significant edges that do not signify prevalent patterns.

Clustering: The obtained motifs and nodes were then clustered. Focus was laid on finding clusters of nodes with dense intraconnectivity owing to the presence of continuum of conformations.

Results: The conventional helices and sheets showed explicitly distinct patterns and were well recognized by the unsupervised learning. About 78% helices, 68% sheets and 86% loops of DSSP assignment were recognized. Some sheets in the unsupervised learning approach were reported to include neighboring DSSP-labeled loop regions as well. Eight families were recognized by this approach:

i. Types 1, 4, 5 and 6 all contained mostly loop areas

ii. Type 1 loop had a high content of sheets

iii. Type 5 loops contained helices that were mostly short

iv. Type 3, and to a lesser degree type 2, corresponds to DSSP sheets. Manual inspection revealed that type 3 is mostly assigned to anti-parallel sheets, whereas type 2 is assigned to parallel sheets

v. Types 7 and 8 are analogous to helices, but type 7 helices were shorter on average than type 8.

One helix of type 5 with less than one turn was classification by DSSP as a helix. This showed that even popular methods could be easily challenged and that caution must be exercised when utilizing results for further application. At any rate, this is a new method and needs further applications and investigations.

Advantages

- A method independent of current classification systems
- This method could also be used for other biological and non-biological networks.

I. *Another ANN Method: Structural Building Blocks (SBB)*

Original Publication by: Jacquelyn Fetrow, Michael Palumbo, George Berg; The University at Albany: State university of New York, US.

Principle: The method obtains a low dimensional representation of the backbone considering the conformation of not just one amino acid, but several (say, 'n'), such that an overlapping description of (almost) the entire chain is produced. Auto-associative ANN technique is used to discover distinct patterns and cluster the resulting n-residue segments. The clustering uses 'activation vectors' (these are vectors that represent members of a cluster as a group. To simplify understanding, compare this with the vectors used in the "unsupervised learning approach" described above) and each unique n-residue structure resulting from this approach is called *structural building block* (SBB).

Method: Only C_α atom positions are used. The 'n' above is set to 7, to parallel the fact that segments up to 6 residues long do not produce reliable matches during sequence similarity comparisons during knowledge–based structure prediction (*ref.* chapter 1.4). Thus, two successive SBBs in a protein chain overlap six of their seven residues. In other words, if one segment is from residue number 11 to 17, the next segment is from 12 to 18, reanalyzing the conformation of residues 12 to 17. Each 7 residue segment is analyzed using 43 parameters such as atomic distances, virtual bond angles, virtual dihedral angles, etc. referred to as units. This information is combined into an 'input vector' and each unit can take any value between 0 and 1.

The layers of the ANN are structured such that the hidden layer, which is sandwiched between the input and the output layers, searches for patterns and contains the weights that need to be optimized to give importance to those patterns that represent secondary structures. Except for this silent learning process that takes place, the 43 unit vector input is simply reproduced as a 43 unit vector output. The hidden layer is an 8 unit vector and trains by the standard back-propagation algorithm (chapter 2.4 on chemometrics). The training is considered complete when the input and output structures match (after optimization of weight and averaging structures in the clusters) by a root mean square error of less than 0.08. If this is achieved successfully, then the 7 residue segment, initially represented by 43 units, can now be represented by 8 units.

Results:

1. The regular secondary structures α-helix and β-strand were recognized in addition to other local structural features such as helix- and strand-caps. The network was also made to evaluate the preferences of amino acids to occupy specific SBB positions. "Random coil" regions were broken down into recognizable segments or "motifs" with suggested use for loop modeling and recognition during structure prediction.
2. Comparison with classical structure analysis methods:
   a. Except for the first 3 and last 3, the structure of all other residues are categorized in 7 SBBs. Compared to those methods that assign structure 'residue-wise' such as $\varphi-\psi$ method, this is proposed to reduce error.
   b. All residues along the chain belong to some SBB category and therefore residues are not left out.
   c. This is a geometry based method and therefore does not require the presence and calculation of H-bonds. Consequently, stretches of residues in the β-strand conformation that do not have a partner can be detected.

The authors note that the differences in the basic structures being identified by this method and several others (that use non-geometric criteria) prevent a quantitative equivalence being established between them.

J. *Automated Protein Structure Analysis: APSA*

Original publication by: Sushilee Ranganathan, Dmitry Izotov, Elfi Kraka, Dieter Cremer; University of the Pacific: Stockton campus, US (Ranganathan, et al. 2009).

Purpose: To develop a continuous geometry-based method that uses only one approach to accurately reflect the state of all parts of the protein's backbone (including detailed account of distortions) with the aim of simultaneously being able to access tertiary structure and orientation. When protein structure is analyzed by independent approaches (such as, combining independent geometry and H-bond assessments) a uniform description is not obtained for the entire protein. In addition, the failure of one parameter to recognize a certain regions as, say, being helical or not, gives us information on some disorder prevalent in that region compared to regions that are recognized. This information is overridden by the use of additional and independent criteria.

Method:

- The method uses only the C_α positions of the entire protein.
- These atoms are connected mathematically by a cubic spline resulting in a smooth 'backbone line'.
- The in-plane-curving and out-of-plane twisting of the line is obtained by differential geometry parameters of curvature κ and torsion τ respectively both as a function of

arc length s (See κ(s) and τ(s) in Fig. 1.35). The torsion here is not identical to the torsion angles that result from broken lines when $C_α$ atoms are connected by virtual bonds but is calculated for every point along the curved line.

- Torsion τ(s) is positive for a right-handed curve and negative for a left-handed one.
- A plot of curvature κ and of torsion τ, both against arc length s is generated. Arc length s is the length of the backbone line in Å. A piece of the spline between 2 successive $C_α$ atoms and is not necessarily equal to the distance between them–the line curves depending on the arrangement of atoms in space.
- The κ(s) and τ(s) of the backbone line also depend on the positioning of neighboring $C_α$ atoms. If, say, the $C_α$ atoms $i−1$, i and $i+1$ together form an α-helical shape, then

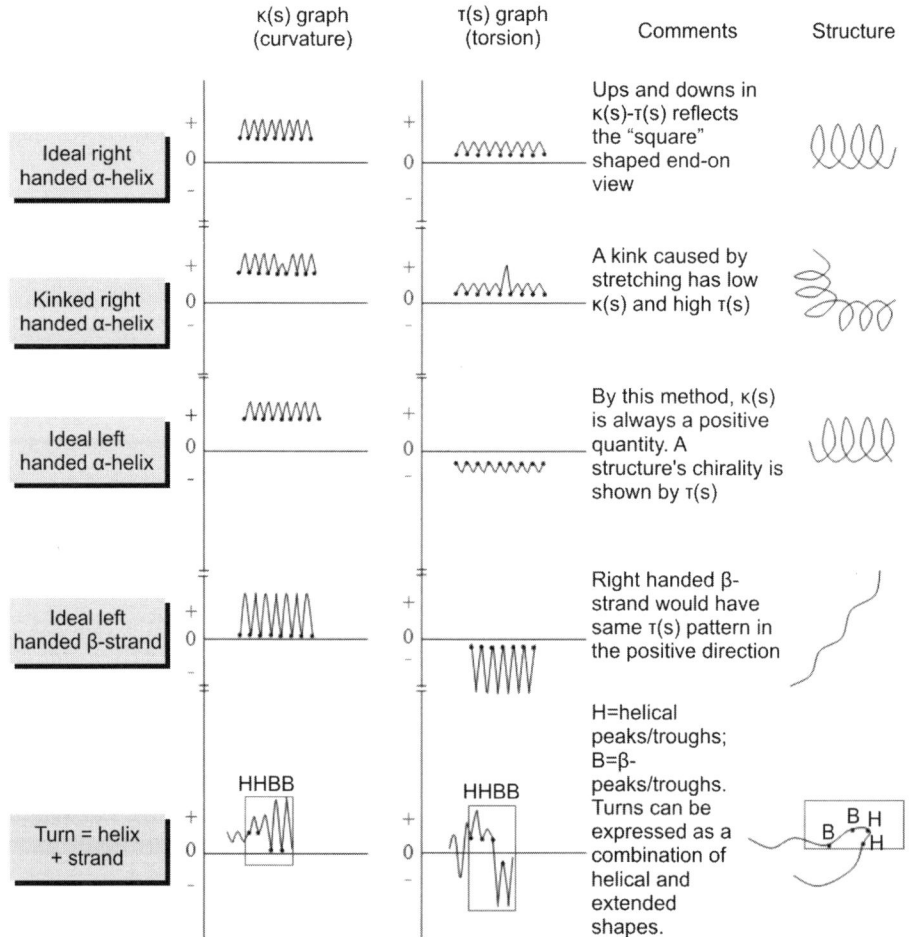

Note: Graphs not to scale; only a schematic representation; $C_α$ atoms are marked.
κ(s) & τ(s) graph x-axis: arc length s, κ(s) graph y-axis: curvature Å^{-1}, τ(s) graph y-axis: torsion Å^{-1}

Fig. 1.35: Continuous graphical interpretation of the protein backbone to detect local details as well as global directions

the backbone line curves assuming the α-helical outline (rather than the jagged set of lines obtained by virtual bonds). If $i+1$ ends the helix and is located at a position out of the helical path, the arc between i and $i+1$ also adjusts to this distortion with the κ(s) and τ(s) of i being influenced by the relative positioning of $i+1$. Thus, this non-local description of a local conformation defines the "conformational environment" of a residue.

Results:

i. The analysis of protein structure using a continuous method resulted in identifying backbone shape with great depth. The continuum of shapes formed (whatever be the local conformation each residue takes up) can be visualized clearly by the κ(s) and the τ(s) graphs and quantified on a scale ranging from strongly-helical to strongly-extended. Recognition of α– and 3_{10}-helices and of β-strands was automated.

ii. A classification scheme of all types of distortions found among secondary structures is suggested based on this method that included:

   a. Helix kinks (that change the direction of helix axis)

   b. Helix distortions (where the segment is still helical, but not α-helical)

   c. Helix termini, a subset of distorters, such as helical caps became evident

   d. Beta-strands kinked 'in-plane' (wherein the reference plane is the average plane containing the C_α atoms)

   e. Or 'out-of-plane' (the plane is as stated above).

iii. All turns and loops–basically the entire protein–is expressed as a quantitative variant of the extreme helical and extended conformations. Even an untrained eye can qualitatively glance at the plots and understand the 3D shapes of turns as being, say, right-handed helical in the first two residues followed by left-handed extended in conformation.

iv. The global changes in orientation (such as kinks and the direction of turns) are described just from the local conformation taken up by the backbone C_α atoms.

v. Evaluation of the assignment of helices and strands by this methods showed that strictly ideal structures were only ~63% of residues among α-helices and ~50% of residues among β-strands. This was pointed as the reason for disagreement between several secondary structure assignment methods in literature. Other methods also calculated disagreements to the same extents in terms of percentage residues (Arab, et al. 2007).

vi. The method has also been used for quantitative protein structure comparison and classification. Literature indicates the extension of the method to describe supersecondary-tertiary structures and protein folding (Ranganathan, et al. 2008–2), (Ranganathan, et al. 2008–3), (Ranganathan, et al. 2008–4).

1.2.2.2 Determination of Higher Levels of Structure

At the relatively higher levels of protein 3D structure such as the architecture of a domain, arrangement of secondary structures in the protein fold often has to be determined manually. The extensive variability at both local and global level makes automation difficult. Literature is often referred to for this purpose. There are plenty of examples where individual description of proteins done using contact maps, vectors, geometric shapes, is useful for identification of folds, architectures and domains often supplementing with energy calculations are presented. Two of them are:

   A. Inscribing a protein into shapes–the jellyroll topology being inscribed into a wedge (Chelvanayagam, et al. 1992)

   B. Globular helix packing (Barlow, et al. 1988).

  Attempt to automate tertiary level protein structure recognition is becoming more productive with increasing efforts. Some of these methods use recognition parameters for individual families of proteins as worked out by separate groups, whereas others aim to determine the entire range of a property (such as "connectivity") by developing methods capable of analyzing proteins in general for that one property. Examples are:

A. *Topology and Local Structure from GSSE*

Original publication by: Lukasz Jaroszewski, Adam Godzik; The Burnham Institute, US (Godzik, et al. 2000).

  Purpose: To simplify protein structure so that connectivity becomes evident in a way that global structure is based on the direction of the chain and local structure on the density of packing of the amino acids and the two perspectives are independent of each other, using a single method of analysis.

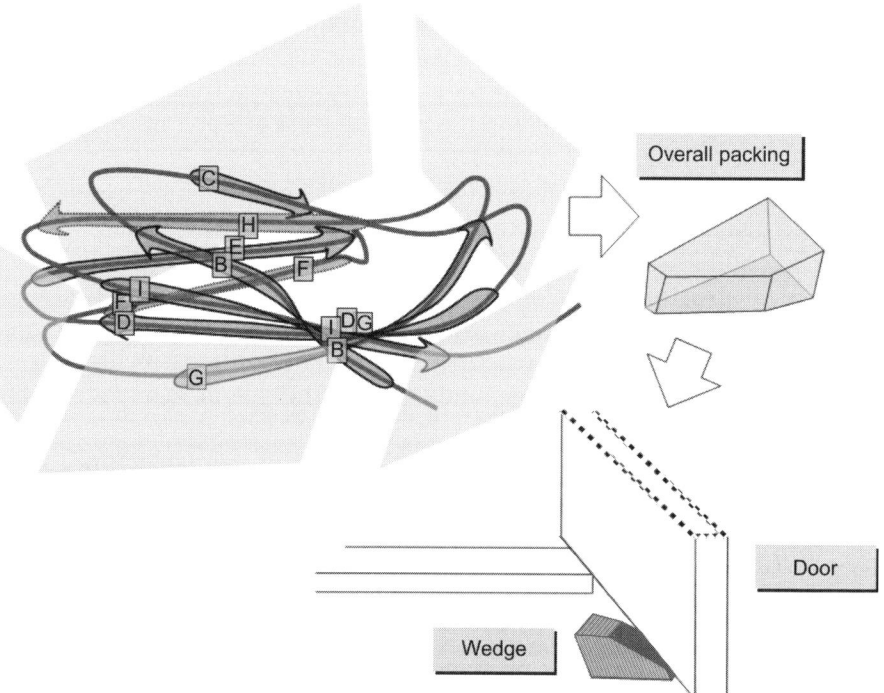

Fig. 1.36A: Packing of β-strands in the jellyroll topology: Viewed as a *wedge*

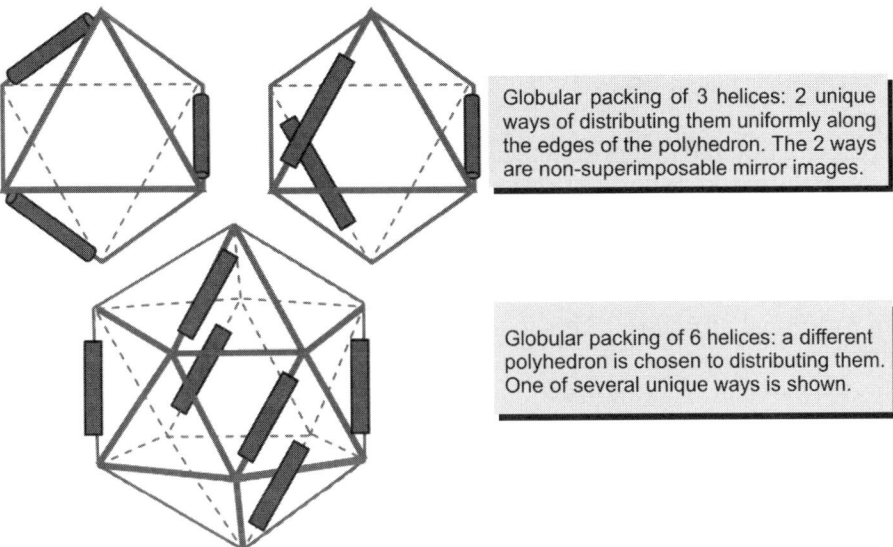

Globular packing of 3 helices: 2 unique ways of distributing them uniformly along the edges of the polyhedron. The 2 ways are non-superimposable mirror images.

Globular packing of 6 helices: a different polyhedron is chosen to distributing them. One of several unique ways is shown.

Fig. 1.36B: Packing of helices into geometric shapes identifies unique possible arrangements

Principle: Secondary structures of the backbone that do not significantly change in overall backbone direction are simplified to "rods" and are called Generalized Secondary Structure Elements (GSSE). These are then plotted on an adjacency matrix (similar to contact maps) to obtain which GSSEs are closer in space and which are farther away from a graph wherein the close GSSEs are placed at vertices and their interactions are edges. The method used to "smooth" the GSSE into rods produces a set of pseudo-C_α atoms along the chain such that its density is an indication of local structure.

Method:
- Averaging local characteristics: pseudo-C_α atoms are calculated by averaging 5 consecutive C_α residues resulting in a smoothed backbone.
- Definition of a secondary structure element: all relatively straight segments of the smoothed backbone. These could correspond to helices, β-strands, random coils, etc. structures defined in any way by other methods.
- Graphical representation—the angle between two vectors, each defined by consecutive pseudo-C_α points along the simplified backbone is obtained. A collection of these angles that define the relative orientation of all pseudo-C_α points are plotted to obtain an angular correlation matrix wherein angles close to 180° (representing parallel vectors and straight segments) are indicated by black areas, close to 90° by blue areas and close to 0° (indicating reversal of chain direction and antiparallel arrangement) by red areas.
- In addition to the angular correlation matrix above, an adjacency matrix is also presented that has '1's and '0's to show contact and no contact between secondary structures. It is using this matrix that new connections are made with existing positions of GSSEs or altogether new positions of GSSEs are evaluated.

Results:

Secondary structures are differentiated from the linear density of pseudo-C_α atoms along the chain. Helical segments have a high linear density of about 0.7 pseudo-C_α atom per angstrom (1.5 Å between pseudo-C_α atoms), segments with extended (β) local conformation have a local density of about 0.3 (i.e. 3Å between atoms). Several dense fragments were found not classified as helical by standard secondary structure classification programs.

In this method, the local and global structures are not the result of combination of independent approaches (such as the use of φ, ψ and hydrogen bonds for local, and vectors for global structure). This avoids assigning different numbers of secondary structures, their extent (i.e., the number of amino acids in them), etc. to proteins that are otherwise similar. This allows the method to be used to estimate number of possible topologies for a protein made of a certain number of secondary structure elements and also used to generate new topologies. In addition, the authors opine that the method can is easier to use in fold predictions.

Several promising applications in tertiary structure recognition and analysis have been shown to be feasible using this approach.

B. *Voronoï Tesselation Assignment Procedure: VoTAP*

Original publication by: Franck Dupuis[1], Jean-François Sadoc[2] and Jean-Paul Mornon[1]; [1]: Universités Paris 6 et 7, [2]: Université Paris 11, France (Dupuis, et al. 2004)

Purpose: To assign secondary structure by consensus of several established methods namely, DSSP, DEFINE, STRIDE and P-SEA and to couple this type of approach with the use of a geometrical tool based on 3D Voronoï tessellation. "Distance constraints between residue pairs lead to contact maps or contact matrices" that are mostly dependent on distance cut-offs that often become statistical and arbitrary. A new way to define contact maps is established that is independent of cut-off generally used in distance matrix methods that generate contact maps.

Principle: Imagine two points on a plane- the space between the two points can be partitioned by line. If these 2 points were in space, the partition can be done using two cubes such that the faces of the cubes touch (this would make sure that partitioning of space is complete with no space left out between the 2 points). If there were many points clustered in space, then space around each point can be "assigned" to polyhedrons (which are 3D) and the faces of each polyhedron can be made common to neighboring polyhedrons. Thus, with the existence of every point, a 'contact' is established via these polyhedral faces. The process of subdividing the space and associating each region with a polyhedron is called *Voronoï tessellation* or *decomposition*, and each polyhedron is called a Voronoï cell. Cells are made such that the intersection of contact planes (the faces) is built midway between the points. For a given set of points, the Voronoï decomposition is unique and absolute because there is no empty space between cells. This method considers the C_α positions to be the set of points around which polyhedra are to be built, wherein each cell is made to represent an amino acid.

Method:

- Decomposition of space and setting up of Voronoï cells is the first step. It involves a method called Delaunay tetrahedral decomposition. In this, tetrahedra are drawn such that the sphere around it contains only 1 C_α point such that it is placed at the vertex.
- As there are no points neighboring the C_α atoms of residues on the surface of proteins, these Voronoï cells cannot be closed. To prevent this, the protein is embedded in a random environment of spheres. Every step is taken to minimize errors as an artifact of the embedding process.
- Thus, the set of tetrahedra sharing a particular C_α as a vertex defines a residue's closest neighbor. In addition, properties such as the face area, the number of edges, the perimeter, the distance between the two C_α atoms, etc. can be characterized for the amino acids in contact.
- The contact between polygons less than 6 residues apart is categorized as being "strong" if the area was larger than the mean increase of 2 $Å^2$. Otherwise, it is considered "normal". The value of 2 $Å^2$ was chosen to obtain consensus agreement with DSSP, DEFINE, STRIDE and P-SEA.
- Based on this, contact maps are plotted. If a protein has 200 residues, a 200 × 200 contact map is drawn with normal contacts given by grey dots and strong ones, by black dots. The contact information of residues that are neighboring in the primary sequence (and hence is *within* a secondary structure) is obtained along the diagonal. An existing secondary structure assignment method is also marked outside the map region to ascertain contacts that are formed *between* secondary structures.

Results: Structure labeling

- i. Helices and β-strands have typical residues that come into contact with each other. Therefore, along the diagonal, patterns with respect to the thickness of obtained lines, the color, and the appearance of the dots (the "texture") indicate the secondary structure.
- ii. Depending on whether the dots are grey or black, one can assess whether the contact is favored or if it is enforced by the structure. For example, it was inferred that close contacts between i and i±2 in a helix is not favored, but is present due to helix geometry.
- iii. Antiparallel and parallel contacts between each of the secondary structures (whether 2 strands or 2 helices are parallel or antiparallel in respective alignment) can also be obtained. Thus alignment of secondary structures with respect to each other via contact maps will lead to the global structure of proteins.

1.2.2.3 Domain Assignment

Similar to the wide variety of definitions attributed to domains (mentioned under chapter 1.2.1 on protein structure), a wide variety of methods have been documented [(Veretnik, et al. 2004), (Day, et al. 2003)] to recognize conflicting segments of a protein to belong to a domain. Each classification system not only ascribes its own definition and name for its various levels in the hierarchy, the domains that result from each method are not comparable either. It becomes biased to results if we get to choose between the systems of classification depending on whichever suits our needs the best. The major reasons for this are:

- Some methods involve manual assignment done by experts whereas others are partly or fully automated.
- The basic approach to define the term "domain" is different and sometimes based on purpose (e.g. structure classification, versus folding database).
- Some structures have complex architectures, convoluted domain-domain interfaces, are very small and closely packed, or very large and diffuse.
- The difference in types and ranges (in terms of the participating amino acids) of secondary structures.

However, domain identification is important to us. This is because in those cases wherein multidomain proteins refuse to be isolated and crystallized, the protein can be expressed domain wise and then isolated. A well characterized domain is also known to be in a very narrow free energy minimum–i.e. a relatively large amount of energy is required to disturb its structure after formation. The following databases are mostly automated, except for final stage manual checking and in some cases reordering.

A. *3Dee DATABASE and the DOMAK (Domain Maker)*

(http://snail.biop.ox.ac.uk:8080/3Dee) The algorithm that assigns the domains present in the 3Dee database is called DOMAK (Siddiqui, et al. 1995). The database itself contains structures that separate the constituent folds (called subdomains) of multidomain proteins. As the domain appears as a lobe of the globular protein, it is easy to understand that it contains residues that form an independent unit (forming more internal contacts than external). This forms the basis of delineating domains according to this method. The maximum distance cut-off for residues to "be in contact" is fixed at 5 Å for heavy atoms. The algorithm was initially made to reproduce the domains of a small number of proteins with well established structures during which improvements were made to its parameters and secondary structure content is also included in its analysis. When the output is similar to what is present in the training set, it was tested on more proteins. Continuous domains (formed by one continuous segment of a polypeptide chain) as well discontinuous domains (those formed when different parts of the chain come together) can be identified. A ranking scheme is set up that identifies the definitions that are most likely to be correct. It can also provide hierarchical classification of domains in a protein.

B. *Others*

This is not intended to be an exhausted account of all methods. Two methods are mentioned as only a sample of how they vary by underlying principle (Islam, et al. 1995).

   i. DIAL (domain identification and alignment): DIAL is a domain recognition algorithm used (Sowdhaminini et al.) to construct a database of single domain families. The structural comparison procedure is called SEA.

ii. (Taylor, 1999) proposed domain identification based on the Ising model where the structural elements of the model change state as a function of the state of their neighbors. The method aimed to retain the integrity of β-sheets during domain separation and also to assign domains to tightly packed regions.

iii. *Numerous attempts are ongoing:* fully automated classification of domains accurate (about 80%) to the fold level detect new folds, reclustere existing databases, efficient structure comparison: existing protein classification methods have focused on classifying new domains into existing classification hierarchies, etc. In SCOP previously classified domains are often rearranged in subsequent releases, as new structures sometimes reveal more relationship amongst new and existing domains (Saini, et al. 2005). In addition, existing vs new domains are compared. For example, if a new domain provides evidence connecting previously unrelated domains, a cluster of these domains ensue. (Kim, et al. 2006).

iv. Detective (Swindells, 1995).

v. PUU (Holm, et al. 1993).

vi. CATH (Orengo, et al. 1997) considers domains for classification only after a consensus is achieved among the three independent domain assignment algorithms of DOMAK, DETECTIVE and PUU. It requires that there is at least 85% overlap in residues assigned to the domain between the 3 methods. After this consensus is achieved, DETECTIVE is used to chop the protein structure into its constituent domains. Where the algorithms disagree, the boundaries are examined by visual inspection and by reference to assignments in other databases, SCOP, 3DEE and literature.

1.2.3 STRUCTURE COMPARISON

When you analyze a large number of protein structures, one has to account for:

- How close/far the analyzed structures are compared to an ideal structure (for example, how much an α-helix or a β-strand differs from its ideal form)
- How structures are close to/far from each other (the distinct "families" of structures that you can create among existing proteins to determine diversity and uniqueness) (Sippl, et al. 2008)

The higher one climbs in proteins' structural hierarchy, the more difficult it gets to determine similarities owing to several reasons.

> *"There's a large mustard-mine near here.*
> *And the moral of that is – The more there is of mine, the less there is of yours..."*
> *– The Duchess in "Through the Looking Glass", by Lewis Carroll*

i. *The inclusion of loops that are long and variable:* Certain degrees of variation in loop regions occur even when the exact same protein is crystallized in slightly different environments.

ii. *Differing distribution:* The presence of isoforms in various environments (cytosolic, membrane inclusive, mitochondrial, nuclear, etc.) results in the same protein having slight differences in structure.

iii. *Evolution:* It has been shown that due to the effect of evolution resulting in sequence mutations (insertions and deletions) the 3D structure of proteins is conserved better than the sequence.

iv. *Compromise between detailed local conformations and overall global structure:* Some of the difficulty results from the various approaches used by structure assessment methods. Methods that aim to capture global structures tend to lose local information and the use of independent methods for the two levels may generate results that are not uniform, though this remains to be studied.

v. *Presence of multidomain proteins:* Among the many domains that belong to multidomain proteins, only a small proportion were found (Orengo, et al. 1997) to contain structures that matched those of single domain proteins or the domains of other multidomain proteins.

vi. *A large fold space resulting in a continuum of structures:* Even at the global level (presence of a continuum of conformations at the local level has been discussed above under APSA method) the presence of a continuum of structures has been observed for some architectures resulting in a spectrum of favored motifs. These motifs were found to occur in different combinations, with some being highly populated.

vii. *Presence of the Russian doll effect:* Structures within structure within structures makes it hard to find equivalence between folds of large domains and small domains, supersecondary motifs and folds, etc. as suggested by some references

viii. *Domain movement:* The assignment of domain boundaries is problematic because of "domain movement" and the dynamic nature of proteins–the popularity of certain motifs, folds and architectures indicates optimum conditions created by such arrangements in terms of contacts and long range interactions, as well as preferred folding pathways and the presence of nucleation sites that initiate folding. The symmetry of architectures has also been associated with its energy minima. These inferences remind us that protein structure is not as 'static' as the rigid set of coordinates that is used to view its structure.

ix. *Technical aspect:* Quantification. The deviation in atomic positions of 2 structures that have been superimposed on each other is expressed most often as an rms (root mean square) deviation. This is the statistical measure that averages differences between 2 peptide segments being compared by finding the mean of the squares of differences between the n pairs of C_α atoms of the two segments (in $Å^2$) and taking its nth root. This is the standard expression for quantifying differences and has the following features:

   a. A mathematical measure of deviation is therefore unbiased and uniform when the superpositioning of proteins is automated.

   b. The most widely used quantification of difference.

   c. Small change at one point that shifts C_α atoms by a few Å generates a huge difference numerically if it influences the arrangement of the rest domain (disadvantage).

   d. The overall measure does not give an idea about the *nature* and *location* of difference in structure (disadvantage).

The method is best used to compare similar structures; even very closely related 3D structures that differ in arrangement/orientation of, say, one helix cannot be compared using this parameter (and that is what comparison is all about; *ref.* the following discussion) .

At this point, in lieu of the concept touched upon in *point no. ix* above on quantification, one must understand the difference between *"classification"* and *"comparison"*. Stating (after analysis) that two proteins or their segments are "identical within a certain level of statistical significance" gives us an immediate understanding of protein structure with respect to each other (that they resemble). Contrary to this, if analysis establishes that the two proteins or their segments being compared are "not identical within the specified level of statistical significance" the same level of understanding as in the previous sentence is not achieved because after this, one has to identify what is different, why, and how it differs. Thus "protein structure comparison" mostly deals with solving a problem at hand in a quantitative manner to get a 'yes' or 'no' answer to the question, "Are the two structures different?", followed by "where is the difference located?", without going into their secondary structure composition, fold, class, etc. The following are broad situations where protein structure comparison is used:

- To establish the difference between ligand-bound protein and free protein after experimental (e.g. crystallization and X-ray analysis) or theoretical (e.g. docking studies, *ref.* Part III) techniques.
- To establish the evolutionary relationship between 2 proteins (3D structure is conserved better than amino acid sequence; *ref.* chapter 1.4).
- To evaluate the effectiveness of a predicted structure (see chapter 1.4) with the experimentally obtained structure.
- Comparing structure of unknown function with that of proteins whose structure and function are known.

Thus, accurate and powerful structure comparison methods are needed, better if they are tolerant to minor and biologically irrelevant deviations and able to grasp overall structure also. The current problem is not as much about computer capacity or resources, as it is about handling vast quantities of information. At any rate, the following are the limitations faced by various methods:

- Recognition of similarity in protein structure in the presence of large insertions and deletions, difference in loops lengths, etc.
- Recognition of similar topology when connectivity is different.
- A gradual continuum of conformations that lead from one structure/domain to the next limits assignments.
- Initial alignment cannot be automated.
- Massive CPU or memory resources are needed.

1.2.3.1 Methods

A. *Strategy 1*

As mentioned above, difference in structure is expressed as an rms deviation. For this, two structures have to be computationally placed on top of each other. In order to do this, the structures must first be oriented in the same way. Thus one could summarize the steps as:

i. *Alignment:* Position the N-terminus, C-terminus, the various equivalent secondary structures and the constituting atoms such that corresponding points in one protein are oriented the same way as the other protein.

ii. *Superposition:* To physically place the atoms on top of each other (for example, the CO group of residue 1 of protein 1 is made to coincides with the CO group of residue 1 of protein 2).

iii. *Quantification of differences:* After maximum coincidence and matching of atoms is achieved above, to calculate how far the rest of the atoms of one protein are from their counterparts in the other protein in Å and to calculate rms deviation.

Examples of this strategy can be found earliest in the work of Rao and Rossmann (Rao, et al. 1973) wherein this method was used to determine similarity among supersecondary structures via vectors. More recent methods are TOP developed in 2000 (Lu, 2000) and STON developed in 2009. TOP algorithm involves generating secondary structure elements and superimposing this to get an initial coarse alignment; the coarse superposition is followed by refining and is summarized in detail below. STON involves connecting 4 consecutive C_α atoms by virtual bonds, computing the three angles of each 4 C_α–structure and performing the rotations and translations on each substructure to get several suggestions for alignments (alternative alignments are discussed later in this chapter).

B. *Strategy 2*

An estimate of similarity can also be achieved by deriving structure information from the 2 proteins independently and comparing these derived profiles. If the profiles reflect the exact structure of the protein then their differences will also reflect difference in 3D. The level of being "exact" depends on the problem at hand that one is trying to solve; sometimes the question is "are the secondary structures of the 2 proteins connected in the same way" if one is trying to compare just the folds, or "is the binding pocket of the protein the same before and after ligand binding". Thus:

• Comparing profiles can be used to address a slightly broader range of questions than using *strategy 1*.

• The method used to derive the profile depends on the biological problem at hand, just as secondary structure assignment differs from one method to the next.

The profiles can be broadly classified into 2D and 1D and may involve inter-residue distances, properties such as solvent exposure, volume, etc. or conformations such as torsion angles and curvature.

B1: Three examples of similarity comparison using 2D profiles are:

2D fold fingerprints (Mezei, 2003): Fingerprints of folds are obtained from the angle between a virtual bond connecting C_α atoms and the C = O bond. It is shown that matches in the fingerprint matrices correspond to low r.m.s.d.

The method "CURVE" (Zhi, et al. 2006): the protein backbone is simplified to a highly smoothed 3D path by calculating the centre of gravity of a consecutive set of C_α atoms and using this calculated point as a pseudo-C_α atom. The 3D path is described by local curvature; alignment of proteins by their curvatures is then optimized by a "turning angle" deviation measure. Turning angles are the angles between virtual bonds that connect the pseudo-C_α atoms.

Differences between the distance matrices of pair of proteins (Holm, et al., 1993)

The method GRATH (Harrison, et al., 2003): A 2D graph of the secondary structure connections in a protein is generated such that the secondary structures are represented as straight vectors along their axes called the 'nodes' and interactions are the 'edges' of the graph (the graph of the type explained in Fig. 1.34). The α-helix and the β-strand are the two types of nodes that are identified. The *distance* and the *torsion angle* between the two vectors along the secondary structure axes are obtained. The fold of a new protein is then determined by searching the CATH database for a structure match.

B2: The 1D profile of proteins is obtained as a list of values or characters (mostly alphabets) that represent backbone structure such that each character represents a certain backbone conformation. Some examples are:

Coded regions of the Ramachandran plot – numerous modification and application of the plot exits, only 3 of which are presented here:

- *(Efimov, 1993):* After segregating the regions of the Ramachandran plot using greek letters that represent distinct residue conformations, Efimov compared strings of these conformations to identify standard structures for turns, loops, entries and exits of helices and β-strands, shape of supersecondary structures and also local conformations in folds. In addition, correlation between conformation and residue properties such as hydrophobicity, polarity, etc. were also established.

- The hybrid protein model (Brevern, et al. 2001) was generated from 16 identified protein blocks (PBs) 5 residues long. PBE (protein block expert) (Tyagi, et al., 2006) was developed into a web-based structure analysis method. Each of the 16 structures is given a letter and an alignment of these letters result in better 3D alignment than some of the popular structural databases and good comparison can e carried out simply by the alignment of the letters. The PBs are characterized by 8 φ, ψ angles of the 5 consecutive C_α atoms.

- Sun and Blundel (Sun, et al. 1995) used DSSP–definition of α-helices and β-strands (wherein residues were given labels H and E) and for other residues, Topham's (Topham, et al. 1993) sectioning of the Ramachandran plot into regions represented by letters a (approximate helix), b (approximate β-stand), g (glycine predominant), e, l, p (proline predominant), t (turn). They recognized 11 supersecondary structures that occurred more than 25 times among 240 proteins.

Coded faces of a polyhedron (Matsuda, et al., 1997): Protein backbone conformations are converted into character strings using an encoding scheme wherein each character represents the face of an octahedron towards which the following C_α atoms points. This encoding is followed by local alignment using Smith-Waterman algorithm to recognize similarity in structural motifs.

Coded values of torsion [τ(s)] curves [(Ranganathan, et al. 2009), unpublished work] The APSA method (*ref.* under *chapter 1.2.2.1 Automated structure assignment*) that generates curvature $\kappa(s)$ and torsion $\tau(s)$ plots of a smoothed backbone was simplified by considering just the torsion diagram and encoding the peaks and troughs using character strings. 16 types of ranges in $\tau(s)$ were specified to represent ideal helices (α- and 3_{10}-), β-strands, their frequently encountered distortions and several turn conformations. Comparison of the character code leads to identification of similar motifs.

Projecting the structure information into lower dimension thus not only serves structure assignment, but also aids in structure comparison saving 3D alignment and superposition problems. Comparing a series of letters or two graphs is much simpler than superimposing, aligning and comparing 3D structures. Projection, as mentioned earlier, is always accompanied by loss of some information. The aim is to not loose information that is important and thereby minimize (but not eliminate) errors that result.

C. *Strategy 1 using Strategy 2*

Most current methods based on strategy 1 (3D alignment) use the results of backbone representations and secondary structure assignments (used in strategy 2) as starting suggestions to speed up the *alignments and superposition* process. An example is TOP (Lu, 2000), a method developed in 2000. The latter was developed to search the large collection of structural information found in databases. A brief outline is presented in the following paragraphs. MatAlign (Aung, et al., 2006) is another method in which the tertiary structure of the pairs of proteins being compared is represented as a matrix of the distances between all its C_α atoms; the matrices are used to determine an initial suggestion for alignment of residue pairs in 3D and this coarse alignment is then refined iteratively using an objective scoring function:

TOP (*overview*)
Original authors: Guoguang Lu; Karolinska Institute, Sweden
   Purpose: To perform automatic structure comparison and similarity searches among a large number of proteins in the PDB. The method is implemented online with a web-server dedicated to process submitted job requests. A user friendly interface has also been implemented to facilitate browsing and access to information.
   Principle: The protein is considered to be a "rigid body" and the mathematical operations of rotation and translation are performed on it such that one out of n points on protein 2, say, corresponding to the C_α of protein/domain 2 is brought into close vicinity of one out of n points on protein 1 (say, the corresponding C_α to the point on protein/domain 1). The rotation is represented by R (an orthogonal matrix) and the translation, represented by **t** (a vector that represents translation vector t_x, t_y, t_z and the vectors of position coordinates $\mathbf{x}_{i,1}$ and $\mathbf{x}_{i,2}$ of points on proteins 1 and 2) according to the given equation.

$$x_{i,2} \sim R.x_{i,1} + t$$

   Here, $\mathbf{x}_{i,1} \in X_1 (\mathbf{x}_{1,1}, \mathbf{x}_{2,1}, \ldots \mathbf{x}_{n,1})$ and $\mathbf{x}_{i,2} \in X_2 (\mathbf{x}_{1,2}, \mathbf{x}_{2,2}, \ldots \mathbf{x}_{n,2})$. The degrees of rotational freedom are assessed using Euler angles θ_1, θ_2 and θ_3. This publication specifically and other standard works in general can supply more details. Next, TOP simplifies the number of points that have to be searched in X_1 and X_2 by considering secondary structure elements (SSEs), i.e. α-helices and β-strands. This is justified because, firstly, it simplifies computational effort by reducing the entire SSE to just 2 points (the start and the end) connected by a straight line. Secondly, matched SSEs give a better suggestion for alignment as they are spatially more conserved than, say, loop regions. Refining of this initial superposition is done by changing the variables in the above equation so that the root mean square deviations of the angles between the SSE axes are minimized. After this, atom level match ensues and the final necessary conditions before determination of a quantitative difference are

- At least 3 consecutive residues of one protein are aligned with the other
- The residues thus aligned above need to have <45° C_α–Cβ difference, and, to one of the C_αs, its counterpart C_α on the other protein should be the closest in space than any other atom in the region
- Inter C_α distance of the corresponding C_α atoms of the two aligned proteins must be <3.8 Å.

A structural diversity index is then calculated as follows:

$$\text{Structural diversity} = \frac{\text{rms deviation of distance between matched } C\alpha \text{ atoms}}{\left(\dfrac{\text{Number of matched } C\alpha \text{ atoms}}{N_0}\right)1.5}$$

If N_0 = total number of residues in protein 1 and 2/2, *mutual structure diversity* is obtained, that reflected "evolutionary distance" well. If N_0 = total number of residues in protein 1, the index is called *single structure diversity*, and is used in similarity searches for a new structure against a database. If N_0 = the number of residues in the smaller domain, a *minimum structure diversity* results, an index used when proteins of different sizes are being compared.

TOPS (Michalopoulos, et al. 2004) is a database (whereas TOP earlier is a method) of topologies of all proteins in the PDB in the form of arrangements in helices and beta strand as *TOPS cartoons* (triangles and circles) purpose: to search for a given fold and to view the kinds of folds available, multiple alignment and motif extraction. Extensive set of supersecondary structures (+pairwise relationships, H-bonding, special contacts of neighboring sec structure, chiralities of supersec structures); helices are described as straight, curved or kinked by the axis and then helix packing angle is calculated [significant deviation is for highly kinked/curved helices by HELANAL (Kumar, et al. 2000)].

Similarity comparisons must be performed when aiming to classify all protein structures in the PDB Databases. Example of such classification systems are CATH, SCOP, DALI, etc. that have been described in detail in the next chapter (*1.2.4 classification of proteins*). These methods must be able to perform rapid and simultaneously accurate analysis. The procedure used by **CATH** is listed stepwise below and shows the steps that involve structure analysis and comparison:

  i. Sequence alignment and clustering with the selection of cluster representatives
  ii. Selected representatives are examined for their secondary structure composition and placed into classes (all α, all β and α–β)

iii. Structures within each class are compared using the SSAP algorithm

    a. Secondary structures are represented by vectors.

    b. The vectors are aligned by a rapid version of SSAP.

    c. For good alignments (indicated by a score value) subsequent comparisons are perform that delve into their respective "structural environments".

    d. Similarity at this level is again scored, this time in a range of 1 to 100.

    e. Structure pairs having a high similarity score value ($\geq$75) in this fast but approximate comparison are sure to be similar.

    f. Structure pairs that are assigned a <75 score are selected and re-aligned using a slower version of SSAP, comparing just the structural environments.

    g. Pairs of structures with a high SSAP score of >70 and $\geq$60% of the larger domain structurally resembling the smaller (given that domains of different lengths need to be compared) are categorized into T (Topology) level of CATH (Class-Architecture-Topology-Homologous superfamily, *ref.* later in this chapter).

    h. The above pairs having a higher SSAP score (of >80) and simultaneously showing a functional similarity are further grouped into the same H–level.

Reference: Carugo, 2006

1.2.3.2 Averaging Fold Space

SCOP (Murzin, et al. 1995), CATH (Orengo, et al. 1997) and DALI (Holm, et al. 1996) are databases that classify protein structures and have been described elsewhere (chapter 1.2.4 classification of proteins) in detail. However, at this point, it is sufficient to know that the three databases use different criteria to recognize secondary structures, align them, compare them, compare sequences, and determine similarity and evolutionary relationship. These databases also have their own terminology for the various levels of hierarchy used in classifying protein structure that result from uniqueness in the aforementioned manipulations. This results in a disparity in the assigned ranges of 'domains' and 'folds' and makes comparison of the results from the different databases almost impossible. To solve this problem, just as mentioned earlier for secondary structures, a consensus protein-fold classification was determined (Day, et al. 2003) between the various methods. *Pairwise comparisons* of domains of the various systems were carried out to achieve consensus. Broad assignments were broken up and restrictive folds were combined. These resulted in metafolds, creating, in effect, an averaged view of fold space. Authors opine that such an averaging is useful to look for similar structures independent of the method used to compare proteins. From a non-redundant dataset generated from the PDB (the PDB contains several files of the exact same proteins under slightly different experimental conditions or as deposited by different authors. For all those investigations in which redundancy affects obtaining a neutral estimate of "averages", repeated proteins are removed by eliminating sequences that are similar) 30 metafolds were identified and these most populated folds were found to include about half of the investigated structures.

1.2.3.3 Multiple Protein Structure Alignment

Obtaining pairwise structure agreement by aligning the two protein structures being compared gives us an estimate of similarity between the two. But when a whole database of protein structures need to be compared and all proteins that are similar need to be segregated for manual confirmation, it is a cumbersome process to keep looking at only two structures at a time. If, say, there are 1000 structures that were considered similar and this needs checking, there are 3 ways to do this:

i. A pairwise comparison: this would require 1000 × 1000 comparisons.

ii. A representative structure is used out of the 1000 and the remaining 999 structures were compared to this representative: the analysis is complicated by the different types and extents of dissimilarities.

iii. About 10 structures are compared at once. This would require that only 110 sets of comparisons (i.e. 100 sets of 10 structures each; then 100 representatives, one of each set, compared with each other resulting in another 10 sets) be performed: multiple structures must be aligned at once.

As mentioned above, comparing multiple structures at once, much like multiple sequence alignment and comparison, reduces time and errors and is also more informative about the evolutionary distances and domain movement of all structures being simultaneously compared. However, in the above example, the 1000 structures belong to the same family. If one has to compare all proteins in the PDB, improved simplification techniques are a must. One possible simplification is to first segregate by similarity in sequence. However, risk lies in the presence of large insertions or deletions among proteins with low sequence similarity when the 'conserved core' becomes small.

Multiple protein alignment is a complex procedure requiring simultaneous rotations, translations and matching of a large number of points. A simpler method was devised wherein information of paired structure alignments was stored in a matrix and used for multiple alignment as lucidly outlined (Taylor, et al. 1994). However, the alignment of a protein with another of a distinct family 'A' differed from that with a protein of another distinct family 'B'. The same situation was encountered in multiple sequence alignments of sequences with differing similarity (*ref.* chapter 1.4) and, similar to the solution reached there wherein a consensus sequence was generated that contained the information of all matched sequences, a consensus of structure environments of all residues in all the proteins being aligned has been attempted by combining SSAP and MULTAL algorithms (Taylor, et al. 1994). Thus the solution used to align multiple sequences was adopted for multiple structure alignment, with an additional advantage of being able to generate sequence–structure correlation.

1.2.3.4 Alternative Alignments

It is easy to imagine, from the above discussion and methods that the idea of structure comparison is based on increasing the number of main chain atoms that match and decreasing the r.m.s deviation of the matched structures. However, a little reflection upon the matter will tell us that these are 2 procedures that yield conflicting results –

which is the better fit if, for a particular alignment, a large number of C_α atoms can be matched with high r.m.s deviation and, in the other situation, by matching a fewer C_α positions, one can achieve a low r.m.s deviation? This dilemma is becomes pronounced the larger the diversity of the structures being compared—and one cannot avoid comparing remotely resembling structures. These alignment suggestions are called "alternative alignments" and it has been recognized that there can be more than one alternative alignment for a pair of structures. Depending on the decision of the alignment, the results of sequence-structure correlation, assignment of homologous family, model building by homology, refining fold recognition, designing novel proteins, drug design, etc. are affected. It is of utmost importance to recognize the fact that there can be more than one solution and evaluate all the possible alignments before taking decisions. For a detailed comparison *ref.* [(Zu-Kang, et al., 1996) and other works published later]

1.2.4 CLASSIFICATION OF PROTEINS

Anything in biology makes sense only in the light of evolution

Dobzhansky

One of the most important goals of protein structure analysis and classification is to establish something akin to "structure–activity relationship" for proteins. Classifying, and determining functionality, correlate. A classification system needs to do more than just find out how many different classes of proteins there are in nature based on certain criterion (such as structure). One step further down this road would be to derive these classes in such a way that it interconnects structure, evolution, genome, function, etc. For example, a system could try to establish new structural classes that include members performing a similar function in the cellular pathway such as the Leucine zipper, 3-helix bundle, 4-helix-bundle, calcium binding domains and many more, some of which have been discussed earlier. Fully automated methods are yet to be developed: manual intervention is often required to complete the classification at higher levels such as domains. Expert analysis is somewhat subjective and integrates various discoveries reported in literature such as for sandwich, barrel and propeller structures. This is especially applicable for new structures and those that do not have sufficient number of representatives currently. Presented here are the most commonly used databases for receptor study: SCOP, CATH and Dali. Other databases also exist (The ENTREZ database of (Hogue, et al.), (Kim, et al. 2006) that are of great use depending on the research topic at hand.

A. The Structural Classification of Proteins (SCOP) Database

Original Authors

Origin: To arrange structures by their occurrence among plant, animal and microorganisms; to determined their similarities and differences during evolution. This was aimed to be accomplished by establishing a database of sequence-structure relationships.

Purpose

   i. To facilitate the understanding of and expedite access to all the proteins in the protein data bank

  ii. Gives a detailed description of structural and evolutionary relationships of these proteins

 iii. It includes all proteins in the current version of the PDB (from NMR, X-Ray and theoretical sources) and proteins for which structures have been published but whose co-ordinates are not available from the PDB.

TAXA: (Box 1) According to SCOP, the various taxa for structural classification are, from the bottom (i.e. from the most specific to the most general).

Family: This criterion is based on common evolutionary origin. Proteins belong to the same family if:

- They have 30% or more of their primary structure in common
- They perform similar functions and have similar structures. These proteins may have a lower sequence similarity than 30% (for example, globins with sequence identities of 15%).

Box 1: Snapshot of the SCOP webpage showing classification of heme-binding proteins

Family: Globins

Heme-binding protein

Lineage:

1. Root: scop
2. Class: All alpha proteins [46456]
3. Fold: Globin-like [46457]
   core: 6 helices; folded leaf, partly opened
4. Superfamily: Globin-like [46458]
5. Family: Globins [46463]
   Heme-binding protein

Protein Domains:

1. Hemoglobin I [46464]
   1. Ark clam (Scapharca inaequivalvis) [TaxId: 6561] [46465] (19)
   2. Clam (Lucina pectinata) [TaxId: 29163] [46466] (4)
2. Trematode hemoglobin/myoglobin [63438]
   1. Paramphistomum epiclitum [TaxId: 54403] [63439] (2)
3. Glycera globin [46467]
   1. Marine bloodworm (Glycera dibranchiata) [TaxId: 6350] [46468] (8)
4. Myoglobin [46469]
   1. Sperm whale (Physeter catodon) [TaxId: 9755] [46470] (174)
   2. Sea hare (Aplysia limacina) [TaxId: 6502] [46471] (7)
   3. Common seal (Phoca vitulina) [TaxId: 9720] [46472] (1)
   4. Pig (Sus scrofa) [TaxId: 9823] [46473] (17)
   5. Horse (Equus caballus) [TaxId: 9796] [46474] (32)
   6. Human (Homo sapiens) [TaxId: 9606] [46475] (1)

Superfamily: A superfamily may contain families of proteins, even though of low sequence identities, suggesting common evolutionary origins owing to
- Similar structures
- Also functional features

For example, actin, the ATPase domain of the heat-shock protein and hexokinase (Flaherty, et al., 1991).

Commonfold: This taxon is based on topological features of a domain:
- Arrangement and
- Connectivity of secondary structures

These families and superfamilies are said to have a common fold. A descriptive name highlighting its important structural (or sometimes functional) feature is often given for these folds. An understanding of "fold" is important. Among these are proteins that resemble each other to various extents, those that, for example, are similar to ubiquitin in arrangement of helices and β-strands with respect to each other and in the ways the strands are connected, even though the proteins as a whole may differ in size (there may be more amino acids in the helix making it longer for one protein or some extra "tails" may not present in the other). In extreme cases, up to one half of each structure may differ. It is noteworthy that the cause for structural resemblance could be physical constraints or chemical interactions that may favor specific arrangements of the secondary structures termed "secondary structure packing" ultimately resulting in topological similarities. It is believed that the various superfamilies of a fold share a common evolutionary origin even if this is not evident with sequence composition and that the identification of new superfamilies will bring out intermediate sequences within the same fold that bridge these various groups of vastly difference sequence compositions.

Class: The secondary structures, namely helices and β-sheets, combine at various ratios and with differing connectivity to form folds. It is therefore convenient to group folds that are similar in secondary structure composition. This forms the topmost taxon of the classification system–the class.
  i. All alpha (for proteins that are predominantly made of α-helices),
  ii. All beta (for those proteins essentially composed of β-sheets),
  iii. Alpha *and* beta (wherein there are both α-helices and β-strands, and these are interconnected: a β-strand may be followed by a helix which is in-turn connected to another β-strand from the N-terminus to the C-terminus),
  iv. Alpha *plus* beta (wherein the α-helices and β-strands occur separately such that the helices are connected in a series in one part of the protein, followed by a bunch of β-strand forming a sheet structure),
  v. Multi-domain (equivalent to a collection of "miscellaneous class" of protein folds that have no known homologues), and
  vi. Others (including proteins with their structures predicted by homology modeling, unusual proteins, peptides fragments, nucleic acids and carbohydrates).

Species: In addition to the above, the lowest structural taxon (the family) is further subdivided. To distinguish between structures deposited in the protein data bank with insignificant differences in which similarity of protein structure is 'obvious' (they are essentially the exact same protein) such as:

  i. Differences in the environment of structure determination (differing solvents in NMR, differing solutions as source of crystallization),
 ii. Difference in binding state and the ligand it is bound to,
iii. Variations caused by mutations introduced during the course of the experiment and structures of the same protein from different organisms (wherein the difference in source is significant and therefore the similarity between such proteins is also a significant occurrence and not 'obvious'), proteins listed within a family are sub-classified by species.

Method

  i. Comparison is primarily done by visual inspection and computational techniques are used only as tools that aid the human eye.
 ii. Protein domains are classified for small and single domain proteins: The whole protein is considered as one domain. In large proteins, domain boundaries are delineated manually and each domain is classified independently.
iii. Each taxon from the bottom to the top includes members that are increasingly different by sequence, structure (in addition to sequence), and ultimately function (including the other two criteria) and a hierarchy is established.
 iv. Similar sequences have similar structure, whereas the vice versa is not necessarily true. Therefore, an initial grouping based on sequence similarity is followed by manual identification of distant structural relations.

One glance at the SCOP website (database is accessible at http://scop.mrc-lmb.cam.ac.uk/scop/) would show that throughout, α– and β– are replaced by a and b for convenience.

Question Box

Choose 2 proteins, say 1ABC and 2DEF from the PDB. What are your comments on the features you can identify for each protein independently comparing its various parts/components (answer: whether they have one or more domains). Now compare the 2 proteins with each other (a) without using additional information than the PDB file and (b) using only molecular viewing software? (c) predict their relationship by SCOP. (d) Now, *ref.* SCOP. Where does this classification system place them from each other?

SCOP statistics: Among the 38221 PDB entries as of June 2009, SCOP (1.75 release) has classified 110,800 domains.

Advantages

  i. The database has links to a number of other useful sites. (*Go through SCOP and list them*).
 ii. It is easy to navigate through and access various points of this classification system appropriate both for researchers and students.

iii. Gives a generalized understanding of the proteins that have been analyzed, the species that have been most studied, the environments and conditions used in experiments, purpose of study and ligands bound as deposited in the PDB.

iv. Distribution among the various classes give us an idea of diversity of protein structures.

v. The lower the level, the more narrowed down the structures within a group become and greater the similarity. Individual structures can also be easily compared to their evolutionarily and structurally related counterparts that occur between groups.

vi. Powerful search tools and easy access to data and images.

vii. SCOP was proposed as a "general-purpose interface to the PDB".

viii. It is maintained up to date with the structures in the PDB. New structure in PDB is taken up simultaneously by SCOP for classification and analysis.

Disadvantages

i. The method is not automated and requires extensive manual comparisons. There is always the risk of human errors and introduction of bias even if software is used to complement human observations and decisions

ii. The SCOP database is updated twice a year only. One would have to wait for this biannual update to ascertain the classification of a newly deposited structure in the PDB.

iii. With the appearance of new protein structures, new folds and families are found to constantly emerge to accommodate these structures. This gives rise to doubts whether the classification is robust or subjective to what is being identified as 'extremes'.

iv. Uses information from literature to support the manual classification.

B. Class, Architecture, Topology, Homologous Superfamily: CATH

Original authors: C.A. Orengo, A.D. Michie, S Jones, D.T. Jones, M.B. Swindells, J.M. Thornton (University College London, UK)

Purpose: From the very first paragraph of the abstract of CATH's primary reference (Orengo, et al., 1997) as follows:

Background: "Protein evolution gives rise to families of structurally related proteins, within which sequence identities can be extremely low. As a result, structure-based classifications can be effective at identifying unanticipated relationships in known structures and in optimal cases function can also be assigned. The ever increasing number of known protein structures is too large to classify all proteins manually, therefore, automatic methods are needed for fast evaluation of protein structures."

It is clear why some works [(Day, et al. 2003), (Hadley, et al. 1999), (Miles, et al. 2005)] consider CATH protein classification system to be a "competitor" to the SCOP system. Whereas sequence similarity and evolutionary relationship form the basis of SCOP, they are considered more as "derived" information by the CATH system. The purpose:

i. To determine the diversity of protein structure and the relative population of each type of structure.

ii. To generate classification system that is based only on structure.

iii. To bring out similarity in sequence and derive evolutionary relationship from the classification of proteins by their structure.

As in SCOP, numbers are assigned for each member at every taxon. The advantage of CATH numbering as claimed by the authors is that although the four classes (C level) are numbered in increments of 1 (1 to 4), the numbers assigned for A, T and H levels are in increments of 10 to accommodate new structures easily.

Project: Interrelate the topics: evolution (*hint: convergence and divergence*), genomic variations (*hint: what is best is retained*), sequence similarity (*hint: some mutations in genes does not affect sequence but affects only transcription-translation mechanism, so sequence similarity is not necessarily genomic variability*) and protein structure (*hint: this is basically SCOP vs CATH*). How well can classification based on each of these principles be used to predict functionality? Divide the class into 4 groups, assign a topic to each group and hold a debate in class...

CATH distribution: CATH (version 3.3) has classified 97,625 PDB chains into 14,473 domains. The paper published in the year 1995 observed that among the then known 5000 or so protein structures deposited in the PDB, CATH classification resulted in only about 500 different folds. Of the non-homologous single domain structures among these 5000 proteins, approximately 43% were found to favor ten T-level folds or families. These families are called 'superfolds' to indicate their unusually high popularity and the existence within them of many protein pairs with no significant sequence similarity or functional similarity. Within these superfold families, sequences and functions could differ quite considerably. At least three different functions could usually be discerned for a given superfold family (e.g. the OB folds that was recently added). For the majority of folds outside these superfold families, however, protein function was typical of the proteins within the family. The underlying reason for such popularity is, however, unclear. The abundance doesn't stop with fold. Majority of the superfolds occurring under architectures were also found to be highly populated and could perhaps be referred to as 'superarchitectures' or major architectures.

TAXA: The hierarchical classification results in a classification tree. From the top, one encounters the following taxa:

Class (C-level): Secondary structure composition determines the class; three major classes are recognized: mainly-alpha, mainly-beta and alpha-beta. A fourth class contains protein domains that have low secondary structure content.

Architecture (A-level): This describes the overall shape of the domain structure as determined by the orientations of the secondary structures but ignores the connectivity between the secondary structures. It is currently assigned manually with reference made to the literature for well-known architectures (e.g. the beta-propellor or alpha four helix bundle). A simple and descriptive name is assigned for each architecture, such as 'barrel', '3-layer sandwich', etc.

Topology (Fold family: T-level): Structures are grouped into fold groups at this level depending on both the overall shape and connectivity of the secondary structures. Structure comparison algorithm SSAP and CATHEDRAL are used. Parameters for

Box 2: Screenshot of the top part of the CATH page showing hierarchy of taxa for heme-binding proteins

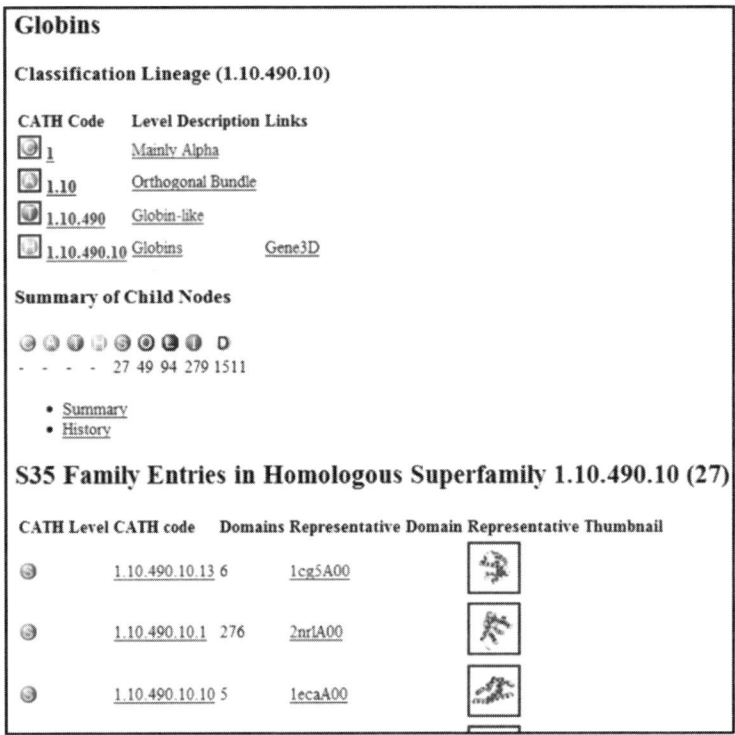

clustering domains into the same fold family have been determined by empirical trials throughout the databank. Structures where at least 60% of the larger protein matches the smaller protein are assigned to the same T level or fold group. Some fold groups are very highly populated.

Homologous superfamily (H-level): This level groups together protein domains which are thought to share a common ancestor and can therefore be described as homologous. They have high structural similarity and perform similar functions with resemblances in core packing or active sites. Similarities are identified either by high sequence identity or structure comparison using SSAP. Structures are clustered into the same homologous superfamily if they satisfy one of the following criteria:

i. Sequence identity ≥35%, overlap ≥60% of the larger structure equivalent to the smaller.

ii. SSAP score ≥80.0, sequence identity ≥20%, 60% of the larger structure equivalent to the smaller.

iii. SSAP score ≥70.0, 60% of the larger structure equivalent to the smaller, and domains which have related functions, which is informed by the literature and Pfam protein family database.

Sequence family levels: (S, O, L, I, D) Domains within each H-level are sub-clustered into sequence families having 80 % overlap using multi-linkage clustering, onto levels

S, O, L, and I such that the proteins within each level have sequence identities of 35%, 60%, 95% and 100% respectively. The mentioned percentages are calculated as follows:

$$\text{Percentage sequence identity} = \frac{\text{Number of identical residues}}{\text{Length of the shortest sequence}} * 100$$

$$\text{Percentage overlap} = \frac{\text{Number of aligned residues}}{\text{Length of the longest sequence}} * 100$$

The D-level acts as level that counts the number of proteins within each S100 family and is appended to the classification hierarchy to ensure that every domain in CATH has a unique CATHSOLID classification. The sequence identity and overlap used for clustering are obtained from an implementation of the Needleman-Wunsch algorithm using a gap penalty of 3 (*ref.* sequence alignment algorithms under chapter 1.4).

Method: The following steps are involved:

i. *Selection of structures for CATH database:* Only well-resolved crystal structures (3.0 Å resolution or better) and NMR structures are considered from the PDB. Structures were automatically labeled according to the method of determination and whether or not they are native structures: 1, native (X-ray); 2, mutant (X-ray); 3, native (NMR); 4 mutant (NMR); 5, C_α only; 6 model and 7, design protein are removed. As of September 1st, 1996, out of 8260 entries 5993 were selected for classifying within CATH.

ii. *Creation of homologous families:* Structures from the PDB are first compared by their sequences and clustered.

iii. Assignment of domain boundaries.

iv. Creation of structural (or fold) families: SSAP (a structure comparison algorithm), further groups the above clusters.

v. Automatic construction a database of single-domain fold families from the above
   a. Proteins with single domains are classified as such
   b. Multidomain proteins are broken automatically into their constituent domains and deposited into the database.
   c. Further clustering by sequence and structure,
   d. Recognition of some familiar families are done if detailed description in literature is available
   e. Also grouped according to similarity in protein class (i.e. secondary structure composition and contacts).

vi. The architecture of each protein fold is assigned manually.

Advantages

i. The method is semi-automated–most of the structure comparison is done by computational algorithms.

ii. The website has links to a number of other useful sites such as the gene bank, the PDB, etc.

iii. The user can scan through the hierarchy of protein structures, with graphical representations depicting the shape of the fold at each level.

iv. Derived data such as structural alignments and protein family templates are also stored.

v. The CATH server will allow the user to scan a new protein structure against the CATH database of unique folds.

vi. The 10 highly populated 'superfolds' revealed in the analysis serve as important tools for structure prediction.

Disadvantages

i. Recognition and classification of architecture is still manually done with the decisions possibly becoming subjective.

ii. References to literature are constantly made; there is possibility that the level of description of each structure, being done differently in literature, is also reflected here.

C. Distance Alignment (DALI) Domain Dictionary and FSSP (*overview*)

FSSP stands for Families of Structurally Similar Proteins; it is also known by the expansion 'Fold classification based on Structure-Structure alignment of Proteins'.

Original Authors: Liisa Holm, Chris Sander; European Molecular Biology Laboratory, Germany [(Holm, et al., 1994), (Holm, et al. 1996)]

Features: Two protein's secondary structures are compared pair-wise. A structural similarity value termed the S-score is assigned based on the extent of agreement between the pairs of structures being compared. For a collection of proteins, the S-scores for all pairs of proteins are obtained and are converted to Z-scores such that proteins with similar folds are assigned comparable Z-score values. FSSP is accessible at http://www.bioinfo.biocenter.helsinki.fi:8080/dali/index.html.

TAXA: There are no taxa! Proteins are simply clustered by their Z-scores. The structure comparison algorithm DALI is used to recognize structural neighbors. There is no formal ordering of proteins in the PDB into families. (Holm, et al. 1994)

FSSP application in structure alignment: (Holm, et al. 1992)
All proteins in the "twilight zone" of sequence similarity (below 30% similarity; *ref.* chapter 1.4 on structure prediction for significance) in the PDB are first obtained and considered to be the representatives of other proteins with which they share a greater (30 to 70) percentage of sequence. Thus each "dataset" of proteins contains structures that are similar. Comparison can be performed either in totally rigid way, or including interdomain motions and geometrical distortions, or in a sequential way (wherein one structure is compared followed by the next), or paying attention to connectivities among secondary structures depending on the needs of the user. Authors suggest that this method can expand current knowledge on protein folding and can be applied in protein design.

The alignment of remotely related proteins by sequence is an important aspect as it is done by structure, as mentioned under "multiple structure alignment" earlier. Through this, similarities in architecture are also clearly displayed.

1.2.5 PROTEOMICS ROADMAP TO MEDICINAL CHEMISTRY–1

References for this chapter: (Chothia, et al., 1987), (Foye, et al., 2008), (National Research Council, USA: Committee on challenges, 2003), etc.

This first chapter of proteomics dealt with protein structure in some detail. Knowing the structure and identifying their exact function deepens our understanding of human disease processes and helps in the development of therapeutic drugs. The availability of the concrete and relevant information, such as the amino acid sequence, binding ligands, clinical and experimental results, pharmacological pathway, etc brings the steps needed for the determination of optimal drug moieties for treatment of disease conditions into a well-defined protocol for a computational biologist to follow (*ref.* chapter 1.4 "receptor mapping" and also part II chapter 2.3.2 on 'techniques for lead design'). Drug discovery is no longer a "random search for plant products"-kind-of-field and the simultaneous research in all aspects of drug design is the reason behind this change.

1.2.5A Proteomics and Disease

- Immunity response is always based on structure and conformation of interacting molecules – the protein antibody and the smaller antigen. It is very specific and powerful, if one arrives at the right complementarity of structures. The following examples indicate this point:

  a. *Haptens* are small molecules whose chemical structure can be recognized by certain types of antibodies. Well designed haptens can be used to boost immunity (as prevention to certain infections), to diagnose the presence of certain antibodies that act as disease markers, and to control their levels. All of this is possible only with complete knowledge of antibody structure.

  b. An *epitope* is a specific chemical moiety that occurs as a part of a large organic molecule that are recognized by antibodies. Monoclonal antibody techniques allow the design of antibodies that target this epitope. For this, a thorough understanding of the structures of the antibody and the pathogen is required.

  c. Immunoglobulin G (Ig G) has a well conserved structural motif called the *Ig Fold* in its constant domain whereas the variable domains associate to form antigen binding sites that are not only different for each variation, but are also quite flexible for an induced fit (in contrast to the lock and key hypothesis). The study of hypervariable regions of immunoglobulins led to the proposal of a set of canonical structures.

  d. The information in (c) above was later applied to understand evolution, protein function and also for therapeutic and analytical design. *For example:* Antibodies are therapeutically administered to enhance immunity but are known to cause strong reactions of incompatibility as they are generally synthesized from non-human sources such as mouse. One can replace the hypervariable loops of these antibodies with those found in humans and this is called "humanization". However, after substitution, the loops must precisely resemble the loops found in human antibodies (not even 1.0 Å deviation) as otherwise, antigen–antibody binding will not take place and the humanization will also fail.

- Pathogenic proteins (prions) were reported in the year 1986. They cause fatal diseases like the 'mad cow' disease (Bovine Spongiform Encephalopathy) and in humans, the Cruetzfelt-Jacob syndrome. Study of their structure, folding propagation and pathology mechanisms will lead to the prevention and cure of such disease. These have been detailed further under chapter 1.5 along with the protein misfolding problems encountered in the Alzheimer's and Parkinson's diseases.

- Drug design using conformationally constrained peptides: a peptide is artificially synthesized such that it resembles a small part (usually, the active site) of a protein's structure and adopts this structure rigidly (because its conformation has been artificially constrained). Study of the binding affinities of various drug candidates in this peptide that mimics the receptor's active site can be performed in a cost effective way (for an example, *ref.* the work on *Bradykinin receptor antagonists* in the following: [(Kyle, et al. 1991), (Kyle, et al. 1993)].

- *Peptidomimetics:* In order to make proteins resistant to cleavage by peptidases present all through the Gastro-intestinal tract, peptides of therapeutic importance are sometimes synthesized with compounds that are not one of the 20 α-amino acids. These compounds are often called *peptoids* and may contain monomers other than the genetically transcribed amino acids (*ref.* Table 1.1 at the beginning of part I); they are designed often for the purpose of increasing bioavailability. Cleverly designed peptoids, as well as peptides with a proline or a D-amino acid substitution, cannot be cleaved by peptidases (simultaneously, it must be ensured that biological activity is not disturbed by the substitution). Sometimes, the pharmaceutical peptide is also hidden in a larger protein and folded into its interior. Metabolism of residues in the interior of the protein is not as high as at the surface and the after a series of superficial cleavages, the desired intact peptide is released for absorption.

- A long list of anticancer drugs discovered using computational modeling of proteins and their binding affinities can be provided (though owing to an equally long list of side effects, drug delivery and formulation problems, these were not successfully released in the market). Some examples are the design of purine nucleoside phosphorylase inhibitors (Montgomery, et al.), enedyine antibiotics (Tuttle, et al. 2005), etc.

- The functional proteins of the human immunodeficiency virus (HIV-1) are obtained after the cleavage of one continuous polypeptide chain by the proteolytic enzyme aspartyl protease. With the availability of the X-ray crystal structure of this enzyme, inhibitors were designed that were potent as well as selective in their action with the help of computational techniques (*ref.* part II).

1.2.5B Proteomics and Computer Aided Drug Design Strategies

- Knowledge of protein structure helps us study, understand, use and edit the PDB files and apply them in docking, simulations, etc. ...(part III)
- The study of protein structure gives us an idea of the error with which protein structure can be determined by experimental methods. This can help us estimate the error propagated to the calculation of binding affinity (*ref.* part III). Some errors

are *explicit* such as the absence of some residues from the protein chain. ...(part III chapter 3.2)

- The availability of sufficient literature on the concerned protein can help us reconstruct this missing segment.
- The placement of side chains in their correct rotamers is necessary in docking, especially if the protein structure is kept rigid (see *rigid docking* under types of docking in Part III) ....(chapter 3.2).
- The study of structure-function correlation helps fill up several gaps in our knowledge of either aspects of biological proteins.
- Study of conformational changes in the protein on ligand binding using structure comparison techniques provides insights on protein effector pathway signaling and ideas for novel drug design (chapter 2.3.2).

1.3 *Modeling Protein Dynamics*

Nothing is permanent except change.
From Lives of the Philosophers, By Diogenes Laertius

The aim of molecular dynamics simulations is to model systems that cannot be seen with naked eye. It acts as a bridge between pure theory and pure experiment. Such simulations are often used as a black box. A force field is tentatively set up that contains terms that are very fundamental and very likely to mimic forces between atoms in a molecule. These terms are repeatedly modified until the simulation reproduces experimentally observed phenomena. During this modification, not all changes are soundly based on the principles of physics. Some terms are simply added so that the results obtained are convincing. Evidently, one can only construct atomic behavior based on observations; the better when the latter is obtained from diverse aspects. Simulations that successfully capture molecular behavior then use this information to answer fundamental microscopic questions at the interfaces of biology, chemistry, and physics. Advancement in experimental techniques as well as increase in computational power increases the desire to answer complex natural phenomena using computations. Theoretical research has reached a point where calculated results match with experimental values in many investigations.

1.3.1 DYNAMICS...WHY?

The underlying cause for most reactions in chemistry is motion (*see* Fig. 1.37 for some fundamental vibrations in molecules). It is motion that brings atoms of various molecules together in various probabilities of arrangement resulting in a chemical reaction once the right arrangement is struck. Atoms are never "frozen" even at 0 K according to the Heisenberg uncertainty principle. It is therefore a totally unrealistic picture (a major approximation) that atoms of a protein exert steric and electrostatic influence in the intramolecular environment or on other molecules such as ligands, from static (fixed) positions in space. Stable interactions between chains are responsible for fibrous protein functioning as structural elements of the cell. Similarly, weak yet numerous interactions occur between globular proteins and other molecules. These interactions are significant but transient, allowing the proteins to respond rapidly to environmental changes and metabolic needs. Dynamics is being increasingly calculated

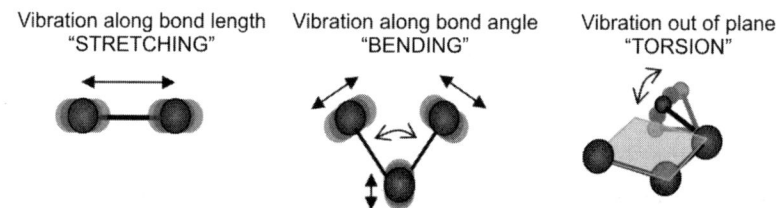

Vibration along bond length
"STRETCHING"

Vibration along bond angle
"BENDING"

Vibration out of plane
"TORSION"

Fig. 1.37: Conformational strain in molecules can be summarized relative to stretching, bending and torsion

for understanding all aspects of proteins, RNA and DNA such as structure, stability, folding, conformational changes, photosynthesis, molecular recognition and interaction, enzyme catalysis, ion transport, ATP synthesis, etc. The contribution of water molecules to protein structure is significant in some catalysis and here, dynamic water molecules need to be modeled to obtain the right mechanism with the right thermochemistry. Thus molecular motions can be classified as follows based on the number of involved moieties, amplitude of motion and time-scale (Yuan, et al. 2003):

Table 1.8: Types of motions found in proteins		
Type	Amplitude and frequency	Parts of the molecule
Local motions	.01–.5 Å, 10^{-15}–10^{-12}s	Atomic fluctuations, side-chain motions, loop motions
Rigid body motions	1–10 Å, 10^{-9}–10^{-6}s	Helix motions, domain motions, subunit motions (of covalently linked moieties)
Large scale motions	>5 Å, 10^{-7}–10^{4}s	helix-coil transitions, folding and unfolding, dissociation and association

Reference: http://www.ch.embnet.org/MD_tutorial/pages/MD.Part1.html

Dynamics simulations aim to capture this motion. However, an important question remains–are these modes of motion just an inherent property of atoms in a molecule, forming a "background response" to solvent, etc.? Or are they purposeful, contributing to protein functionality? This question has been addressed since early times[(Chothia, et al. 1983); (Gerstein, et al. 1991); etc.] with the characterization of specific conformational changes that lead to protein functioning such as allosteric effects, motor protein conformational changes, immunoglobulin flexibility, enzyme induced fit, etc. So what about the general atomic vibrations and "breathing" of the protein about an average geometry? This is still not clear since 1985 when this was first addressed (Fersht, 1985). The conformation induced in a protein by the approach and recognition of a ligand remains as long as the ligand is present (unchanged).

Atomic motion in proteins is often related to the atomic temperature factor or the *B-factor*. This quantity is obtained during X-ray determination of protein structure (*ref.* chapter 1.1.2.A on X-ray analysis of protein structure) when electron density distribution is relatively spread out owing to thermal motion of atoms. Analysis of this B–factor in regions suspected to aid protein function has been carried out extensively (Parthasarathy, et al. 2000) but are found to be contradictory [(Artymiuk, et al. 1979) vs (Zhang, et al. 1999)]. X-ray diffraction studies have confirmed that conformations of the bound and unbound protein are different; this same experiment however cannot determine the series of events that are responsible for the change such as hydrogen bond formation or electrostatic interactions. It is shown (Yuan, et al. 2003) that the segment of protein chain to which ligand binds does not have to be initially flexible to undergo the conformational change.

Explained in detail at the beginning of part II, quantum mechanical solution that constructs atomic behavior starting from the motion of electrons is accurate but extremely expensive in terms of computational resources and time. Therefore molecular mechanics methods are employed that uses *Newton's classical equations*. This becomes a major simplification and takes its toll on results that are calculated such as energy, enthalpy, binding interactions, etc. In order to bring calculated results in par with experimental ones, sometimes quantum mechanical or experimentally obtained values are brought into the force field. This empirical substitution might sometimes appear to be meaningless but nevertheless greatly improves results obtained at the end of theoretical modeling.

In order to make the computer to simulate molecular behavior, we must specify for every atom in the molecule its position, momentum, charge, arrangement with respect to other atoms, connectivity (chemically, what we call covalent bonding), etc. The force field of the molecular modeling software takes in all this information to calculate energy, vibration, structure, dynamics etc. Motion is calculated as atomic acceleration which is obtained from force, given that the mass of each atom is known once the atom type is specified (from the "$F_i = m_i a_i$" equation). The force is obtained from the potential energy function as its gradient ($F_i = \nabla_i V$ and so acceleration is determined as in box 4 later in this chapter. All atoms influence each other, the intensity of which is specified in the force-field as bonded (covalent) and non-bonded (Van der Waal's, electrostatic, etc.) components.

In a hypothetical situation, a single molecule isolated in a box tends to bounce around as a whole. This bouncing can be differentiated into rotational and translational components. But each atom within the molecule possesses a certain motion with respect to the other atoms. These are classified as stretching (along a bond), bending (of two bonds about their central atom) and torsion (or rotation about the bond axis). All these motions are mimicked in a dynamics simulation. A protein molecule modeled in this way accounting for all the various motions gives a far more realistic estimate of energy than a static single point calculation. For further details on how chemistry is condensed to physics which is in-turn described by mathematics (a language that computers can understand), ref. part II chapter 2.2, especially discussion 2.4: From observations to simulation' and discussion 2.5: Single, double and triple bonds'.

1.3.2 Terminology

Having this vague outline of how modeling protein dynamics is approached, it is useful to understand some of the terminology involved:

- *Phase space:* The conformational space, described in Scheme 1.16 and Fig. 1.38.

- *Ensemble*: a group of (conformationally and state-wise) different molecules of the same compound that share the same thermodynamic state. *Ref.* Discussion 1.7.

- *Trajectory:* This (*see* Fig. 1.38) is the 6N-dimensional phase space (3N positions and 3N momenta; *ref.* Discussion 2.15: Degree of freedom of molecules under part II, chapter 2.3.2.C1)

- *States:* States are the microscopic states that molecules occupy such as the ground state and excited states. The Aufbau principle, Hund's rule, and other electron filling rules describe arrangement of electrons in molecular orbitals in the ground state (*see* Discussion 2.19: A Molecule's states in Part II chapter 2.3.2.E).

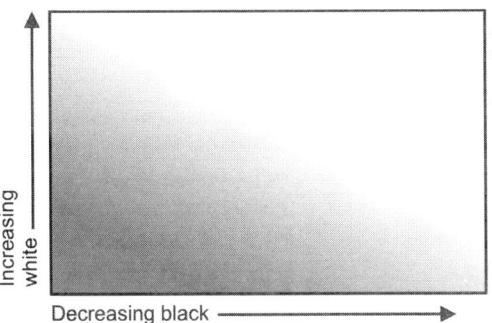

Just as grey can exist in several shades all of which can be represented in 2D format (one dimension = black; other dimension = white), a molecule can assume several conformations, all of which make up the "phase space". This space is multidimensional; moving along one dimension produces a change in a specific geometric criterion such as "c–c bond length".

Scheme 1.16: Comparing phase space to a shaded box and conformational sampling to color-picking. (*see* text)

- *Physical properties:* These are macroscopic properties of molecules that can be measured in laboratory. The microscopic or atomic arrangement and behavior is what leads to the macroscopic properties of molecules. *Ref.* Fig. 3.1 in Part III chapter 3.1.1.

- *Approaches in protein dynamics* (*ref.* Scheme 1.16): Consider yourself operating a color generating software (as in digital paint mixing centers) that works computationally. You have a certain color in print and want to generate the same using the software. The color is a certain grey: Now we know that grey is a combination of black and white and all its shades can be specified in the form of the 2D area in the Scheme. Every spot in this area has a unique ratio of black and white. There are 2 computational strategies to pick the optimum shade of grey–either black: white ratios are randomly changed looking through the various shades of the enclosed area until the right shade is hit upon (which is a *stochastic approach*), or the black: white ratio is systematically changed till the right shade is arrived at (which is a *deterministic approach*).

1.3.3 CALCULATION OF THE MACROSCOPIC PROPERTIES

Selective references: (Allen, et al. 1989), (Frenkel, et al. 2001), (Schlick, 2002), (Leach, 1997), (Tobias, et al. 1993), (Carignano, 2002).

Protein dynamics considers all atoms of the protein to move about and for each resulting snapshot of geometry, the energy and forces operating in the molecule are calculated. The aim of this modeling is to produce an estimate of macroscopic properties as derived from a microscopic environment. The effect of changes in volume, pressure, temperature, number of molecules, etc on macroscopic properties such as density, binding energy, entropy, internal energy, strain energy, etc. (this field that related probabilities of finding molecules in various states and conformations under certain conditions is called statistical mechanics) is understandable.

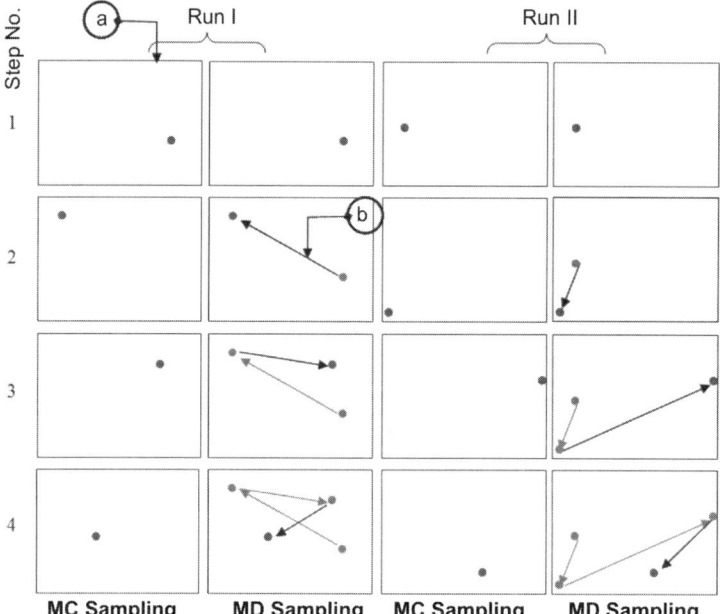

MC Sampling: 4 independent conformations obtained by sampling 4 points in the conformational space; each conformation is obtained by randomly changing the bond length, angle, dihedral.

MD Sampling: 4 conformations obtained by arriving at 4 points in the conformational space; each conformation is obtained by applying a force and moving the atoms about.

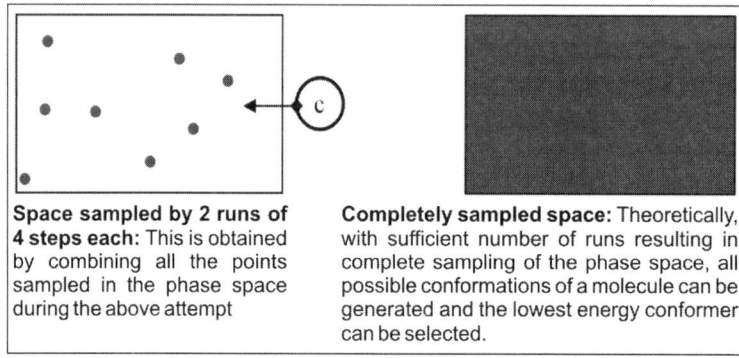

Space sampled by 2 runs of 4 steps each: This is obtained by combining all the points sampled in the phase space during the above attempt

Completely sampled space: Theoretically, with sufficient number of runs resulting in complete sampling of the phase space, all possible conformations of a molecule can be generated and the lowest energy conformer can be selected.

a: phase space; **b**: trajectory and **c**: the ergodic hypothesis that whether using MC or MD for conformational sampling, (for specific examples) with sufficient number of steps called iterations, the entire phase space of a molecule can be covered, or in other words, the macroscopic property being calculated will be the same and close to the true value.

Fig. 1.38: Sampling of phase space: The MC way *vs* using MDS

Discussion 1.7: The ensemble

It can never be overstresses that a medicinal chemist should understand what is being done in simulations. The main aim of simulations is to calculate equations relating to molecular structure in such a way that macroscopic lab-measured properties can be obtained by calculating microscopic environments within molecules. So far, in most chapters detailing the principles of modern medicinal chemistry, we have encountered the description of one molecule; in part I, the molecule is a protein, in part II, it is a ligand, and in part III, it is the protein-ligand complex. In all 3 cases, except in this chapter 1.3 of molecular dynamics and except in those situations that *ref.* to techniques used in this chapter, the subject of study is a single molecule all by itself, in the gas phase or in solvent. This is a major approximation (chapter 2.1). Macroscopic properties are not obtained from a single molecule. There are millions of molecules in a tiny drop of a substance. The conformation and state of all the molecules are also not identical. There is a distribution of a whole range of conformations (ethane gas at room temperature is a mixture of the eclipsed form, the staggered form and all the forms in between) and various states (elements absorb light of a certain frequency and their atoms reach an excited state; when the excited atoms re-attain the ground state they emit waves having distinct patterns in the electromagnetic spectrum by which the element can be identified in spectroscopy). Thus we talk about an ENSEMBLE (pronounced "on-some-bl") which we can understand as a group of similar yet not necessarily identical molecules of a compound subjected to the same environmental conditions. The probability of an ensemble of molecules to have a certain value for a physical property can be calculated as per the expression:

$$P[\Gamma_i] = \frac{e^{-\beta E_i}}{\sum\limits_i e^{-\beta E_i}}$$

Where Γ_i, the phase space, $= (r_1, r_2, ..., r_N, p_1, p_2, ..., p_N)$. β in the above expression expresses probabilities, the Boltzmann way (*ref.* chapter 2.3.2.E).

Various ensembles have been defined; three such are the *canonical*, the *microcanonical* and the *grand canonical ensembles*. In a microcanonical ensemble, macroscopic properties of a compound are calculated by placing the group of molecules of the compound at constant energy (or heat). This is denoted as an NVE ensemble indicating the number of molecules N, the volume occupied by the N molecules V and the total energy of the N molecules E are a constant. In a canonical ensemble, the group of molecules is allowed to exchange their energy with the surrounding environment–the molecules are allowed to either absorb or release heat to the surroundings; the 'surroundings' is a heat bath. It is represented as an 'NVT' ensemble (T standing for temperature). In the grand canonical ensemble– way of calculating macroscopic properties, the number of particles are allowed to vary (by undergoing diffusion, etc.), as well as energy is allowed to be exchanged with the surroundings.

An ensemble is comprised of different molecules of the compound. The macroscopic properties calculated for each of these different molecules are then averaged out. The ensemble average <Q> is considered a far more realistic estimate of the property Q than the estimate produced from a single molecule. How are different molecules obtained? By following a trajectory that explores the conformational space!

Similar to ensemble averages, one also obtains *time* averages. Applications of study of dynamics spread to structure analysis, protein folding, drug design (molecular binding, affinity, recognition, specificity), receptor modeling and functioning (ion channel behavior), etc. often times involve time averages. When all these movements are recorded over a period of time or over a number of simulations, the resulting estimates of physical properties are considered closer to the real picture. A simplified overview of some features underlying molecular simulations is attempted:

- A molecule with atomic coordinates $r = (r_1, r_2, ..., r_N)$ has potential energy $V(r)$.
- A molecule with momenta $p = (p_1, p_2, ..., p_N)$ has kinetic energy $K(p) = p_i^2 / 2m_i$ summed over all values of i.
- The molecule has energy $E(r, p) = K + V$ where K stands for the Kinetic energy and V stands for potential energy.
- Any macroscopic property can be compared to experimentally obtained values only if it is taken as an ensemble average (Discussion 1.7) (a *time average* performed over sufficient time, it is believed, will yield the same results as an ensemble average; *ref.* 1.3.4.E on the ergodic hypothesis).
- One must *weight* the properties of all members of the ensemble because although all conformations in all possible (closely spaced) states are considered, those states that are strongly preferred by the molecule must be allowed higher contribution to the macroscopic property being calculated
- The preference of some states over others (the weighting) is done using the Boltzmann distribution (*ref.* 2.3.2.E)
- For example, energy E, pressure P, entropy S, etc. are some of the macroscopic properties calculated. Internal energy of a molecule, instead of being calculated only for a single conformer or state, can now be calculated for (say) ethane gas at *room temperature and pressure* over all its eclipsed-staggered-gauche conformations in ground as well as excited state; this calculated value approaches the value that this gas would possess in nature under those conditions specified. The pressure is related to the macroscopic work done by the system as a result of the change in energy and other parameters can be calculated from these.

The number of states that become available to a molecule is high at *higher temperature* and therefore the probability that the molecule will occupy a particular state becomes small (*ref.* chapter 2.3.2.E wherein the Boltzmann distribution is discussed a little further).

Box 3: The probability that one would do something depends on how many others he wants to do of equal priority

If one likes all the dishes set before them equally well, then there is a big confusion as to what to taste first, and eventually, what all to taste. The next point to consider is "how much of each"- given the limited capacity of our stomach, and that we can taste only one dish at a time, we would spend very little stomach space on each item. This is similar to molecules occupying various states that become available to them, however, under equilibrium conditions. There is equal probability that a certain molecule will occupy any of the states that become available to it. If the temperature is raised, the number of accessible states is increased and if it is reduced, this total number drops. Probability of occupation is therefore influenced only by the total number of states available. This holds at equilibrium conditions only, where the molecule *per se* does not prefer a particular state. The above equation in the text needs modification if the molecule is not under equilibrium and if, independent of other conditions, the molecule itself is predisposed to occupy only certain states when others are available. The "non-equilibrium situation" is similar to determining the probability that a person will sample all dishes given that *that* person likes a few strongly, but we do not know which!

Computational modeling of molecular dynamics therefore boils down to setting up the right probability distribution, and generating enough conformations to sample a significant region of the phase-space.

1.3.4 TECHNIQUES

The details (in the form of equations) that go into the setting up of a simulation always depend on the purpose of the study – whether it aims to simply differentiate between good and bad theories (in which case very basic and most important aspects of the simulation is sufficient) or it aims to construct theory that cannot be obtained experimentally (in which case meaningful modeling of every atom and every force becomes relevant). Either way, snapshots of the way atoms are moved about are taken and each set of motion samples a certain part of the phase space. The variations in momentum and position are brought about in order to generate various conformations. The sampling and analysis could be

- Statistical or 'stochastic' (which takes snapshots of the system in independent randomly generated conformations) or
- Deterministic (which takes snapshots of the system as it evolves in a systematic time-dependent manner).

In the stochastic methods, such as Monte Carlo simulations (MCS), a conformation is randomly picked and calculated, and this is done a number of times. In the deterministic methods, such as Molecular Dynamics Simulation (MDS), a certain time-traced path is followed along which all the atoms are moved about. MCS and MDS are the two main families of simulation techniques used in molecular modeling. There are other simulation techniques that combine MCS and MDS in several ways. *Brownian Dynamics* method is a variation of MDS wherein major approximations allow calculation over long time scales (*ref.* MDS technique below for an explanation). In *Normal Mode Analysis* method, all atomic motions are treated as simple harmonic vibrations about a local energy minimum considering the natural vibrational frequency of molecules. Sometimes dynamics is guided or "steered" so that the simulation takes a short cut to reach the end. Thus, the driving force for dynamics simulation is the desire to relate motion to mechanism (Benkovic, et al. 2006).

A. Treatment of Solvent

How can one not consider the water molecules when *Proteus* is the God of the Sea? As clarified under chapter 2.1, there are a number of approximations operating in molecular modeling–some of these have a large effect on the result of calculations whereas some are insignificant. Ignoring the effect of water and modeling the behavior of proteins is a major approximation. The resulting properties that are calculated (whether it is binding energy (chapter 3.2), structure (chapter 1.1), dynamics (chapter 1.3), folding (chapter 1.5), etc.) actually correspond to the property of the protein in the "gas phase"! Water is dubbed the 21st amino acid (Wand, 2006) for a reason and this chapter deals with modeling solvent, especially water. Water influences physicochemical properties of biomolecules–small and large–and this can be considered in two ways:

- *An effect as a medium:* The effect of water "as a solvent medium" is on charges calculated by water's dielectric constant. The surface charges on proteins need recalculation in the presence of water than in vacuum. The main reason why polar amino acids are stabilized on the surface and hydrophobic residues are located in the interior of soluble proteins is because of the presence of water. This stability must be brought out in calculation. *When corrections are present in the force field so as to mimic the effects of water on the system, the modeling is called "implicit solvation".*

- **As** *a group of molecules:* The steric effect of H_2O molecules needs to be accounted for because water molecules occupy some space. In addition, they interact directly with the superficial protein atoms forming hydrogen bonds and stabilizing protein structure. There is also the non-bonded water–water and water–protein interactions to be considered. The computational time required to calculated non-bonded interactions is proportional to the square of the number of atoms in the system. In the natural situation, water molecules are hydrogen bonded, disordered, undergo proton exchange and give a number of other dynamic performances that contribute to enthalpies and entropies of various systems in it. *When hundreds of H–O–H molecules are added around the biomolecule and the entire system (1 biomolecule + hundreds of water molecules) is subjected to the calculations of the force fields, there is chemical as well as steric account of water. This type of solvent modeling is called "explicit solvation".*

The calculation of protein properties in the second situation is very close to an aqueous solution of the protein, but is computationally very expensive. One has to account for the presence and interactions (among themselves and with protein atoms) of *hundreds* of water molecules (*ref.* Fig. 1.39A). For example, TRP cage is a 20 residue protein whose folding simulation was carried out in an environment of 2000 water molecules.

Tightly–bound water molecules have numerous implications in protein simulations and drug design (*ref.* chapter 3.2 docking and 3.3 protein-protein interaction). Extensive analyses correlate these water-binding sites with numerous pharmacologically important regions in the protein (Marrone, et al. 1997).

B. Periodic Boundary Conditions

Now that we have understood this far, lets us take another look at the solvent box in Fig. 1.39A. If this set of molecules were to be subjected to the force field, it would appear as if there is a frozen cube of water with a protein the middle surrounded by vacuum. The force field would calculate a vacuum-water interface on the molecules that lie along the 6 faces of the cube. The number of molecules on which it would apply this type of conditions is also not insignificant. Consider $10 \times 10 \times 10$ molecules arrangement of water. One face of the cube would contain $10 \times 10 = 100$ molecules. When all 6 faces are included, we understand that nearly half of the molecules are treated with this interface–an interface that does not exist, is not supposed to exist

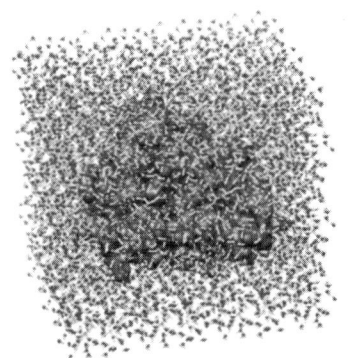

and is only an artifact of bad modeling. The properties that are calculated from this system will not be reliable. One would conclude that for the resources spent on this modeling, the gas phase simulation of this system is far better. One needs to improve the situation without making it significantly computationally taxing by include more molecules. How is this done? By creating an "image" of the presence water beyond the box as if by placing a mirror. Instead of having a boundary the way it is shown in Fig. 1.39A, one repeats the same environment that is found within the boundary in the space beyond it. This process is referred to as introducing *periodic boundary conditions* depicted in Fig. 1.39B.

Fig. 1.39A: Solvation box around a protein showing water molecules

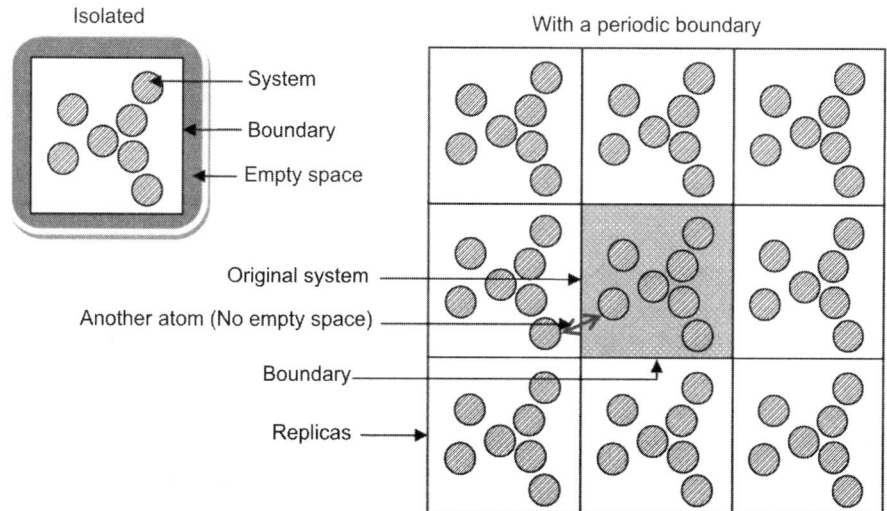

Fig. 1.39B: Periodic boundary conditions: Diagrammatic

The principle is that atoms (in one box) interact with its neighboring atoms which may be from the same box or from the neighboring boxes and there are no more empty spaces. The square-type arrangement of replicas shown in Fig. 1.39B is only one of the several methods that handle boundary conditions. There are several shapes of water boxes such as truncated octahedral, orthorhombic, etc.

Recommended references: (Smit, et al., 2001), (Leach, 1997)

Detailed references: (Allen, et al., 1989), (Allen, 2004), (B. R. Brooks, et al. 1983), (Jorgensen, et al. 1996), (S.J.Weiner, et al. 1984)

Interesting materials: Water transport through a protein channel; simulation by E. Tajkhorshid, K. Schulten, Y. Wang, J. Yu, F. Zhu, and M. Jensen at movie from http://www.ks.uiuc.edu/Gallery/Movies/

C. Molecular Dynamics Simulations (MDS)

> *"I am convinced that He (God) does not play dice."* Albert Einstein

Molecular dynamics simulation is very widely used theoretical tools for studying molecular behavior of fluids and solids. In MDS, at a given temperature atoms and molecules are made to interact and the evolution of the system over time is observed. The MDS approach is not probabilistic as that of MCS. The motion of atoms are mimicked such that an atom in 'conformation 1' obtained at a particular instant of time *moves to* its corresponding position *with a certain momentum* in 'conformation 2' at the next instant of time. The phase-space is spanned in this way. Even from this superficial description, it is evident that successive conformations are related and sequential (in contrast to MCS). It appears as if one MDS run generates a bunch of conformations that are not drastically different from each other and several totally independent runs might be required each starting with a different geometry to cover the phase-space. The same happens in an experimental solution when a physical property is measured [Q (r, p)] is obtained as an average over a certain time period Δt).

Box 4: Newton's equation and its application in MDS

Acceleration is rate of change of velocity and velocity is rate of change in distance. Therefore, Newton's equation of motion is written as:

$$F_i = m_i a_i = m_i \, (d^2 r_i / dt^2)$$

In another way, $$\text{Momentum } p_i = m_i v_i = m_i \, (dr_i / dt)$$
$$\text{Force } F_i = (dp_i / dt)$$

Expressing *force* this way is advantageous because it can be obtained as a gradient of potential V_i. Does potential *V* seem familiar? Yes, this is built into the force field (force times distance = potential)

$$F_i = - \, (dV_i / dr_i)$$

Now, the *aim* of MDS is to obtain the trajectory using these simple Newton's equations. This is done using:

Initial atom positions obtained from the PDB file such as the coordinates of a protein as determined by X-ray, NMR or model building methods.

Initial velocities for the atoms which depend on the temperature of the environment in which we wish place the macromolecule

Acceleration which can be calculated from *force* which in turn is a derivative of the potential energy (above).

Acceleration is related to time. At a certain instant of time t, with initial coordinates $r(t)$, the potential $V(r)$ of the molecule (applying the force field) is known. Consequently, the force 'F' and from that acceleration 'a' can be calculated [using $a_i(t) = -(1/m)\{dV(r)/d\,r_i(t)\}$]. Initial positions of various atoms are obtained from protein coordinate files such as the PDB files that contain X-ray, NMR or theoretically derived protein structure. If coordinates at time t is known, then the coordinates at time $t+\Delta t$ can be deduced because acceleration 'a' has been calculated (and so velocity $v(t)$ and $v(t+\Delta t)$ are known). Coordinates $r(t)$ has now become $r(t+\Delta t)$ and so a new potential $V(t+\Delta t)$ and acceleration $a(t+\Delta t)$ are freshly obtained. As the simulation proceeds, we follow the huge protein as it develops along the entire path of the simulation–i.e. along t, $t + 2\Delta t$, $t + 3\Delta t$, etc. and this is called the trajectory of the simulation. The simulation is generally carried out at a particular temperature that determines initial velocity v_0

and then kinetic energy $K = \left(\dfrac{3}{2}\right)NkT = \sum_i \dfrac{1}{2}m_i v_i^2$. In a general case of constant 'a', $v(t)$

$= at + v_0$ and the instantaneous velocity is obtained by "adding the effect of acceleration" $a = - (1/m)\, dV/dr$" to initial velocity v_0. Integrated with respect to initial coordinates (r_0) and v_0, the following equation is used:

$$r_i(t) - r_0 = v_0.t + \tfrac{1}{2}\,a\,t^2 \text{ (resembling "S = ut + ½ at}^2\text{")}$$
$$r_i(t) = r_0 + v_0.t + \tfrac{1}{2}\,a\,t^2$$

Coordinates (position of atoms) at time t represented as $r(t)$ is obtained from velocity $v_i(t)$ according to $v_i(t) = d\,r_i(t)/dt$

Summarizing the above treatment, one starts with an initial set of coordinates $r(t)$ at time t, whose $V(r)$ is calculated as implemented by the force field. Then with the acceleration (that changes for every time step) resulting from force calculations carried out on $V(r)$ at every time step, the trajectory along which atoms are to be moved from coordinates $r(t)$ to the coordinates $r(t+\Delta t)$ after time Δt is obtained, as velocity and acceleration are known.

Thus if we know coordinates (and velocity) at time t, we can find out what the same will be after time Δt using the above expansion. There are several algorithms that carry out this integration to move atoms along a trajectory. In order to cover the phase space of a system with little computational expenditure, large time steps need to be taken. However, the smaller the Δt, the more accurate the integration. Also, the more the steps taken around the phase space, the greater the spread of conformations and states, the more uniform the ensemble generated and the more representative the ensemble averages become of experimental values. It has been documented (in all of the books in the reference chapter) that the force calculation is the most elaborate and resource-consuming of all steps and that integration algorithms are therefore targeted to reduce the number of steps, with one force calculation per step. Calculation of *non-bonded interactions* using the *Lennard-Jones potential* and *coulomb interactions* have to be carried out over all pairs of atoms. Thus, *if there are N atoms, N² calculations need to be carried out*. A protein is nowhere close to a tiny

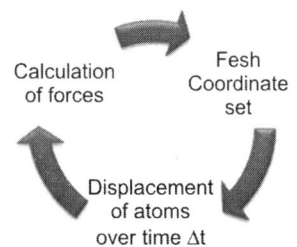

Calculation
of forces

Fesh
Coordinate
set

Displacement
of atoms
over time Δt

Scheme 1.17: Steps in MDS cycle

system and so standard integration algorithms need to be tailored to suite computational demands, resulting in the birth of *Verlet, Velocity Verlet, LeapFrog*, etc. Considering that this book is application oriented, we wish to skip detailing further on the technical aspects of this topic.

Advantages of MDS

Tremendous advancement in hardware and software resulting in enhancement of available computer capacities has enabled the handling of complex simulation problems. The study of protein structure MDS combined with such advancements has enabled extensive database storage and retrieval, structure prediction, study of protein folding mechanism, prediction of kinetics of folding, study of protein interaction, study of signaling pathway in the cell, modeling of disease progression, design of new proteins that are meant to catalyze synthetic reactions or mimic real proteins for better disease management, etc.

The significance of the MDS method lies in the fact that in addition to representing the time-dependent evolution of a system, it mimics the process by which experimental data is obtained via measurement. As microscopic physical forces are made to decide macroscopic physical properties, the system studied in an MDS (if not limited by computational resources and approximations) will be thermodynamically meaningful and can be used to extract all sorts of values that current experimentation cannot yield. Computational simulations can accomplish two aspects that industries are looking for–novelty (because of patentability) and low cost study (the connections with thermodynamics and kinetics can be used to predict feasibility of reactions and optimum reaction conditions avoiding expensive trial and error experimentation).

It was mentioned that calculation of the trajectory is the aim of the simulation. Thus, from the trajectory, we can obtain:

* Average energy of a molecule
* RMS between two structures at two points along the trajectory
* Fluctuations of atomic positions and Temperature Factors
* Radius of gyration

Calculation of these parameters is responsible for most of the applications of MDS in drug design as mentioned towards the end of this chapter.

Selective references for this chapter: (Allen, 2004), (BR Brooks, et al. 1983), (Frenkel, et al. 2001), (Leach, 1997), (Tobias, et al. 1993), (Rapaport, 2004), (Jorgensen, et al. 1996), *www.ch.embnet.org/MD_tutorial*, Course notes *"Molecular modeling"* by Dr. Elfi Kraka at University of the Pacific (USA).

D. Monte Carlo Simulations (MCS)

> *"The more he looked inside the more Piglet wasn't there."*
>
> By Winnie the Pooh in *"The House at Pooh Corner"*, by Milne

Monte Carlo is a city in Monaco where gambling and other games of chance were popular in the 1940s. The term "Monte Carlo method" was coined then (1949) by

Ulam and Metropolis, and referred to the technique that uses random numbers to solve problems. An MC simulation is one wherein the computer is made to generate random numbers within the simulation (and a different number is generated for different simulations as well) in order to evaluate the performance of a deterministic system (this is one that gives the same result for a particular input, repeatedly). It is noteworthy that a computer itself is a deterministic system–it uses logic and algorithms to function. Therefore to even generate random numbers, it requires extensive programming and rigorous testing of the randomness of results! That is why computer generated random numbers are called "pseudo-random"–the closest it gets to randomness is that the numbers are *unrelated*. A seed number is required as a starting value which the random number generator uses to generate output. The seed could be the date on the calendar, time on a clock, etc.

When a random number generator is used to change from one conformation to the next, successive conformations "appear out of nowhere" and are independent of each other. In fact, there is equal probability that the same conformation results again because the conformations being generated are not stored and tracked in any way. Thus the conformational space aims to be covered by random sampling at various points all over it. Thus in a MCS, there is no "evolution over time", no "mechanism" and no *momentum* (p_i). **Macroscopic properties** estimated are averages of independent values that result from seemingly unrelated conformations that belong to the ensemble. These properties are only dependent on the coordinates of atoms.

So how can a random number generator solve a problem? The technique is called a *"hit and miss"* integration method. The area of a circle (or the value of π) can be determined by inscribing the circle within a square (*ref.* text-books cited at the end of this chapter). A uniform sampling of the area of the square results in some n points lying within the area of the circle (called *hits*) and others outside it (*misses*). The area of the circle can be calculated from the ratio of the number of *hits* 'n' to the total number of points covering the square's area 'N' (*hits* + *misses*). The larger the total number of points, the more completely the area of the square is covered and therefore greater the accuracy of the area of the circle. Area of circle A = area of square A' ($\lim_{N \to \infty} n/N$) where error in calculating the area is inversely proportional to N. The uniform coverage of the area of the square needs a random number generator to get points all over the surface. Each random number being generated is used as a coordinate to position the sampling points somewhere within the square.

A MCS of protein dynamics is done in a similar fashion, governed by the *Boltzmann sampling of states* and determining the partition function Z (=$dr^- e^{-V(r)/kT}$). A molecule has 3N dimensional phase-space (if N is the number of atoms contained in it; *ref.* Scheme 1.16 above and also texts of Part II chapter 2.3.2.F for more). A molecule with just 10 atoms therefore has a phase-space of 30 dimensions. In other words, one random number places one atom (out of the N) at one point along 1 dimension (out of 3 dimensions available for that atom) and this is done for all of the N atoms.

From above, 30 random numbers describe various positions of the 10 atoms within a molecule resulting in 3^{10} conformations (10 atoms and 3 possible directions of movement for each along the X, Y or Z axes); and a small protein has 1500 atoms. For each conformation generated in the ensemble, V(r) and the Boltzmann factor are calculated, and macroscopic properties are derived as an ensemble average. If a little chemical meaning is brought into such a conformational sampling, it is easy to understand that only those conformations with low energy are important to us – and such a sampling is called *importance sampling* in which the probability of generation of a random conformation is biased towards a region of the phase space where the function f(x) for each conformation contributes the most to the macroscopic function <f> being investigated. Focusing over a particular region 'R' that is important to us is done as follows: <f> = $\int_R$ f(x) ρ(x) dx/ $\int_R$ ρ(x) d(x). If the same bias is carried out towards ρ(x) also in addition to f(x), this is called the *umbrella sampling technique*. In other words, one can concentrate on that region of the phase space that is chemically relevant such as the happening of a reaction and generate a population of conformations densely located around that area.

A further treatment that avoids astronomical V(r) calculations is called the *metropolis monte carlo technique*. In accordance with Boltzmann distribution, for all newly generated conformations, the change in potential $\Delta V(r)$ with respect to the previous is accepted if the new random number is < $e^{-\Delta V(r)/kBT}$. This is made clear in Fig. 1.40 which depicts a Monte Carlo integration to find the area of a circle (shown is that for a quadrant of the circle). The *ovals* are misses and *boxes* are hits. The area of the circle can be obtained from a large number of tries in which some will fall within and some outside of the quadrant. Figure 1.40B shows the more advanced sampling method called the Metropolis Monte Carlo technique. It is used to select low energy conformations of a molecule. The low energy conformations of $\Delta V < 0$ are always accepted (hatched region).

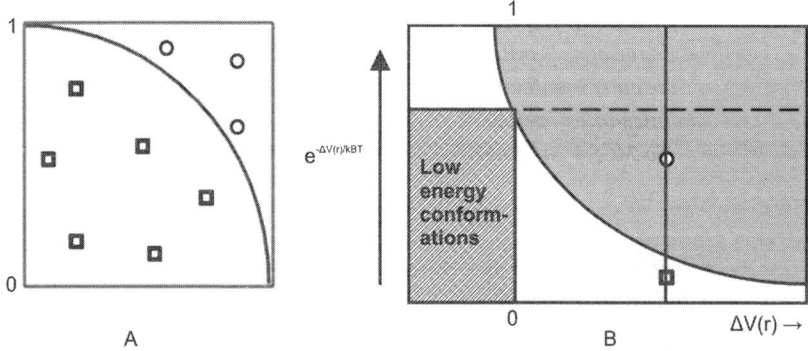

Fig. 1.40: MC and metropolis MC used in a simple example

Among high energy ones, if the conformation generated using a random number (between 0 and 1) results in the colored region, it is rejected (the oval) and if it falls in the area below the Boltzmann distribution curve (the box), it is accepted for a particular change in potential energy with respect to the previous conformation [$\Delta V(r)$].

MC Techniques become Invaluable

i. When simulating a complex multidimensional system such as protein folding where using a MDS, folding never goes to completion.

ii. As, experimental chemistry always follows the rules of statistical mechanics (the Boltzmann distribution).

iii. As there is never a single geometry for a protein–a large ensemble of unfolded protein conformations converges into a small ensemble of folded conformations.

iv. As MDS can get "caught in kinetic traps"–in MCS, all conformations are independent and equally probable of being generated (the system is said to be *ergodic*; *ref.* chapter 1.3.4.E) whereas in MDS, as one conformation is derived from the previous, structures can sometimes not overcome the barrier following a local minimum (*ref.* Discussion 2.16 for details).

v. When a lattice modeling of a polymer is undertaken, because there are well established ways to derive thermodynamic relations.

vi. When large time steps and large number of time steps are equally a problem when using MDS techniques.

Limitations of MC Simulations

i. A distribution function (at equilibrium, of course; non-equilibrium functions are difficult to set up as discussed earlier) needs to be available.

ii. Extensive sampling of the configuration-space is needed.

iii. $<Q(\Gamma_i)> = <Q(r_i)>$. In other words, MCS obtains ensemble averages $<Q>$ for parameter Q only pertaining to atomic positions (r_i) and leaves out momenta (p_i) from the phase space (Γ_i) therefore information on kinetics of the system cannot be obtained. *It is said that simulating molecules as being made of rigid bonds is not the same as simulating it as being made of very strong springs:*

> *Even if, physically, the difference is very subtle,*
> *it is crucial as it influences the distribution function for*
> *the other coordinates. In the case of "tight springs",*
> *an integration over all momenta ($p1,...,pN$) is non-zero.*
> *So MCS is not preferred for several investigations*
>
> *Allen, 2004*

Box 5: One of the longest simulations of protein folding

A time step implemented in practical MDS spans 1 to 2 fs (one femtosecond = 10^{-15} s). Now imagine a protein folding simulation that aims to mimic natural folding. The fastest ever known folding of a protein in nature takes about 100 nanoseconds ($100 \times 10^{-9} = 10^{-7}$ seconds). Simulating

10^{-7} seconds of folding using time steps that take 10^{-15} seconds each will require 10^8 (i.e., 100,000,000) MDS steps to be carried out. That means 10^8 changed sets of coordinates (r), 10^8 V(r) calculations, 10^8 force calculations, etc. A "tiny" protein has about 100 residues and 1500 atoms (1500^2 atom pairs) not including solvent water molecules needed for folding. The pioneering work carried out by Kollman and coworkers was one of the longest simulations of their time–the folding of the villin protein for 1μs by. Although the folding did not complete, important inferences were made. Physiological proteins generally do not fold in 100 ns. They take seconds, or even minutes (*ref.* chapter 1.5.11 on kinetics). Therefore MCS methods are often used. (Duan, et al., 1998)

Note: Selective references for this chapter: (Frenkel, et al. 2001), (Grant, et al. 2003), (Leach, 1997), (Schlick, 2002) (Tobias, et al. 1993), Course notes *"Molecular modeling"* by Elfi Kraka at University of the Pacific (USA).

E. MDS *vs* MCS and the Ergodic Hypothesis

In an MDS, $\bar{Q} = <Q>_{NVE}$ wherein Q *(with a bar on top)* represents an average over very long time t. However, the experimentally comparable situation is obtaining an *ensemble* average because a measurement is taken over an ensemble of millions of molecules in various states distributed by the Boltzmann rule. To explain this, the ergodic hypothesis was set up. It states that the same quantity above is equal to the statistical averaging over an NVE microcanonical ensemble (if the time average in the MDS method does not depend on initial conditions). This equivalence between an MDS and an MCS derived parameter is thus demonstrated; however, this equivalence is not universal (Leach, 1997). A potential energy function is said to be *ergodic* if it is continuous, allowing access from any conformation/state in the phase-space to any other. Although under specific conditions equivalence exists between the two simulation methods, one is often preferred over the other depending on the purpose of investigation (*ref.* any of the mentioned text-books for details). MDS can simulate coordinated molecular motions; on the other hand, MCS does not get trapped in wells and therefore generates greater variety of conformations. Whereas MCS can handle simulations that involve varying particle numbers (due to generation or destruction of particles), MDS is a must when calculating time-dependent bulk properties such as viscosity and also when simulating solvent interactions. The emergence of hybrid techniques aims to gain from both methods (Hashem, et al., 2009).

1.3.5 PROTEOMICS ROADMAP TO MEDICINAL CHEMISTRY–2

It is clear from this chapter that molecular simulations need study and practice for any researcher to be able to understand and apply them, in any field. Thus, it is natural that any student of pharmacy would be curious to know how these procedures can be applied to drug design. We hope that this list of points would convince them on this point and would also serve as a summary of this chapter:

Macroscopic properties of molecules that can be measured in a laboratory are due to phenomena taking place at the atomic level of the molecule (*ref.* Fig. 3.1 in part III chapter 3.1.1).

Thus the following can be ascertained by MDS/ MCS calculations:

- Proteins structure stability, protein folding (in the following chapter),
- Molecular recognition and its mechanism (*ref.* part III) between various classes of biomolecules (carbohydrates, lipids, nucleic acids, proteins, etc.)
- Enzyme activity by conformational change in the protein and the induction of the same in the ligand facilitating the ligand to reach the TS (*ref.* 2.3.2.F *analysis of reactions*)
- Rational drug design is improved by allowing a list of drug candidates to evolve in the presence of the protein. Although such an investigation is time consuming, the binding affinity and other parameters obtained would be from an average of an *ensemble of conformations* rather than a value from *one single conformation* in rigid docking procedure (*ref.* part III).
- Investigating the interrelation between (small and large-scale) conformational changes and molecular properties (such as charge distribution, etc) and their combined influence on biological function such as ion transport, receptor functioning, DNA activation, protein translation by RNA, etc.

Thus, *biological activity is the result of time dependent interactions between molecules.* MDS determines the trajectory which molecules follow as they become influenced by various forces over time. The exchange of forces take place at the surface, more accurately, at the *interface* of molecular pairs such as protein-protein, protein-nucleic acid, protein-ligand and protein-solvent, nucleic acid-ligand, nucleic acid-solvent, etc.

Dynamics techniques are the most important of the computational armamentarium of drug designing and molecular pharmacology strategies that aid us to understand phenomena that are impossible to visualize experimentally. Some specific examples:

- MDS calculations of acetylcholinesterase by McCammon and coworkers lead to the identification of secondary channels for acetylcholine. These secondary channels were found to open transiently and allowed the ligands to reach the active site. (Shen, et al. 2002), (Tai, et al. 2001).
- It is known that certain beta-Peptides have *antibacterial and antifungal* properties [(Koyack, et al. 2006), (Karlsson, et al. 2006)]. MDS showed that amphiphilic helical peptides composed of 2/3 hydrophobic groups were found to be surface active, and to adopt an orientation parallel to the air-water interface. The orientation of molecules at the air water interface is a macroscopic property. MDS helped to derive this from microscopic environment (the property and placement of side groups) and molecular conformation (the helicity of the molecule). The discovery helps in formulating these peptides for drug delivery (Miller, et al. 2009).
- Determining the start and end of a protein's domain has been discussed as being important for deriving evolutionary relationships all the way from bacteria. A dynamics-based solution to the problem was recently discussed (Navizet, et al. 2004).
- Mutation of the Histidine 44 → Alanine on the nucleocapsid protein of the HIV resulted in less strong nucleic acid-binding of the protein. An additional property of the protein to bind to zinc was induced in the mutant protein that remained unanswered, experimentally. MDS evolution of the molecule showed that a

reorientation of main-chain carbonyl oxygen atoms stabilized the ion zinc. Research is in progress on utilizing this difference in properties for drug design [(Stote, et al., 2004), (Osapay, et al. 1991)].

Note: Other selective references: Introduction to Molecular Dynamics Simulations; Roland H. Stote; Institut de Chimie LC3-UMR 7177; Université Louis Pasteur, Strasbourg, France [*the author wishes to thank R. H. Stote for his greatly simplified presentation on the web*]

Materials

• Molecular Dynamics Simulation programs and their tutrorial guides and websites: AMBER, CHARMM (http://www.ch.embnet.org/MD_tutorial/), NAMD, POLY-MD, http://www.pharmacy.umaryland.edu/faculty/amackere/research.html, etc.

1.4 *Protein Structure Prediction*

Take care of the sense, and the sounds will take care of themselves.
The Duchess, in Alice's adventures in Wonderland by Lewis Carroll.

So far, our understanding of protein structure can be summarized as in Fig. 1.41. The primary to the quaternary levels of organization is hierarchically arranged with one level leading to the next and with progressively increasing complexity. The above figure can be explained further. Structure analysis involves the study of protein's structure with the help of X-ray or NMR methods once the entire protein has been isolated. When the protein is isolated, its function becomes known. Often either the quaternary or tertiary structure is obtained experimentally. Structure and function complement our understanding of protein relationship and diversity. An alpha helix is marked in all those regions of a protein's known structure that fit the definition of certain parameters. So, secondary structure delineation is a theoretical process and is obtained by study of tertiary structure. The justification for why the primary structure (the amino acid sequence) is so composed explains the relationship between structure and function. Structure prediction, on the other hand, is totally based just on the primary sequence. All higher levels of structure are predicted just from the primary level. The information about protein structure and its relation to sequence (along the black lines in Fig. 1.41) accrued during protein structure analysis is applied now on the sequence to predict structure (the grey lines). Protein function and evolutionary inter-relationship are estimated from the structure predicted as well as from the sequence.

Tertiary and quaternary structures are directly associated with protein functionality making target discovery and lead optimization possible with the availability of protein structure coordinates (*ref.* part II Discussion 2.10: Target identification and chapter 2.3.2.B. *Lead optimization*). The primary structure arises from the genetic code in the DNA giving us a way to map the genome by knowing the sequence of proteins, even

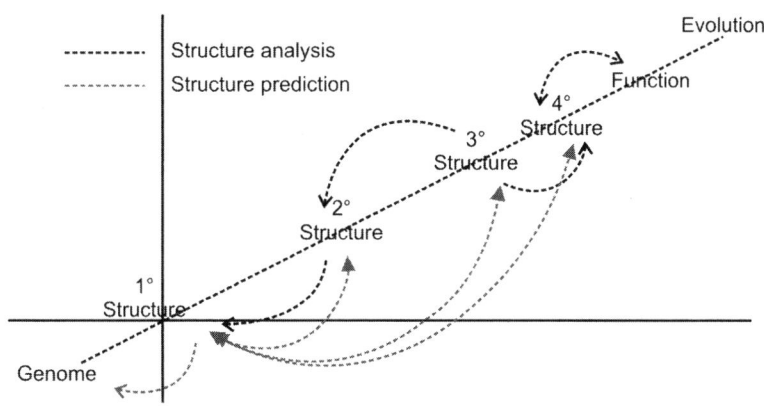

Fig. 1.41: Our understanding of proteomics

though not a significant fraction (23,000 protein-coding genes is only about 1.5% of the genome) code for proteins. However, with extensive research, it is being established to a large extent that the primary structure of the protein is responsible for the secondary and tertiary structures. An example is the successful fulfillment of the *Paracelsus challenge* (Discussion 1.8). Being able to predict the three-dimensional structure of a protein from its amino acid sequence is called protein structure prediction. Thus, central to all aspects of structural biology, literally at the origin, lies the primary structure, connecting function to information in the genetic code.

As mentioned so far, and so forth, sequences with low similarity are found to take up the same 3D structure. This has been theoretically understood from folding models (*ref.* under chapter 1.5 on protein folding). The same fold can also perform different functions (Todd, et al. 2001). The relationship between the composition of the genome, the sequence and the fold is complicated. In some cases, a particular sequence is found (Teichmann, et al. 1999) only in a particular fold, and this fold is significantly different from all others ("orphan folds"). In other cases, the same fold is present in functionally different proteins (Teichmann, et al., 1999) with its corresponding genome segments found everywhere. Although a sequence folding into a fold is generally independent of any other process once it has been synthesized (chapter 1.5), the relationship between genomic representation and function and all that in between is still a mystery.

So, what form is Proteus going to assume next? It is well known that the complete and intact 3D structure of a protein (whether tertiary or quaternary) is required for biologically activity. Proteins are the "workhorses of the cell". Yet, all that is available in the form of pre-specified information to a cell to generate these horses and get them to work is the 1D amino acid sequence information in the genome. Even after isolation from the cell, most proteins can spontaneously fold and refold after denaturation and only to one specific structure. One can break this phenomenon into two parts: first, that there is correlation between 3D structure taken up and the amino acid sequence of a protein. Consequentially, this should allow *protein structure prediction* (dealt with in this chapter). Second, that proteins are macromolecules, and when several millions of conformations are possible, the same 3D structure is taken up each time the sequence is allowed to fold. This results in the conclusion that *protein folding* must be an energetically favored process. So, how different is one protein from the other in terms of there sequence? In other words, can we change one protein's sequence to make it into another? And by how much?

Discussion 1.8: The paracelsus challenge

In 1994, George Rose and Trevor Creamer posed the Paracelsus challenge, named after the 16th century alchemist: that a protein with one structure should be transformed into another entirely different 3D global folding pattern by changing not more than 50 % of its sequence – the reward was $1,000. That amino acid sequence determines tertiary protein structure is a known concept; the challenge, however, aimed to ascertain the relative importance of individual amino acids in specifying folds. The challenge was met in 1997 by Dalal, Balasubramanian and

Regan (Dalal, et al. 1997), from the Department of Molecular Biophysics and Biochemistry at Yale University, US although the challenge required that there should be only a change in tertiary structure, the approach used by the successful group was reported as being more "guided" (Rose, 1997) as they started with protein G (the B1 domain of Streptococcal IgG-binding protein consisting of a helix and beta sheets) and proceeded to convert it into a four helix bundle. The newly transformed protein was called 'Janus' and the transformation was accomplished by replacing residues that support β-sheet-formation with those that supported the formation and stabilization of helices (the residue composition and long range interactions found in the four-helix-bundle of Rop–Repressor of Primer–was used as reference). Energy minimization procedures and secondary-structure prediction techniques were used to optimize and verify the resulting structure. It is amusing to read the advice of Rose and Creamer-that future proposers of challenges should offer Tee-shirts as prizes rather than cash, as their challenges would most probably be met!

The state of the art in structure prediction is assessed every two years by competitions called CASP (Critical Assessment of methods of protein Structure Prediction), and CAFASP (Critical Assessment of Fully Automated methods of if protein Structure Prediction). *Ref.* Discussion 1.9.

Discussion 1.9: CASP–an outline

Started in the year 1994 by John Moult, CASP 1 released 24 target sequences and 35 groups had participated. Ten years later, in CASP 6, over 200 groups from 24 countries participate to predict the structures of over 64 target sequences generating 30,000 predictions in total. CASP 8 (in 2008) received more than 80,000 submissions (Kryshtafovych, et al., 2009). In these competitions, a list of recently sequenced proteins whose structure has not been released so far is made available and in 3 to 5 weeks' time for methods that involve human interventions, and 48 hours' time for automated server prediction, the 3D models for the various sequences have to be submitted. Up to 5 models are allowed to be submitted per research group per sequence with one structure as their best. The best prediction of various groups are compared with the experimentally determined structure and match is determined over several criteria using standard structure comparison methods such as root mean square deviations. A GDT-TS score is assigned to each model and used for ranking. This comparison and assessment is independent. A "CASP meeting" is held in Asilomar, California when the reviewers are done with assessments and the best predicted structures, progress in various methods and shortcoming that need to be focused on are discussed. The original CASP organizing committee included John Moult, Kryzstof Fidelis and Adam Zemla. The two CASP websites are the Protein Structure Prediction Center at predictioncenter.llnl.gov and CASP discussion forum at www.forcasp.org.

Results–Selective Points

1. Both physics and bioinformatics based methods participated; the best modeling was in helix, strand and hydrophobic core
2. Bioinformatics methods have benefited from the growth in size of the PDB
3. Web servers and software packages often predict the native structure of small, single domain proteins to within about 2–6 Å of their experimental structures
4. Limitations were found in prediction accuracy serve to be the main bottleneck. In one of the earlier CASPS, the prion protein's predicted native structure was actually its misfolded conformation (Baxevanis, et al. 2005)
5. Problems were found in predicting loops especially on the protein surface and also among membrane proteins
6. Predictors aim to reduce errors to routinely better than 3Å, particularly for large multidomain proteins or those with huge β-sheets.

Applications of Protein Structure Prediction

i. A non-active form is obtained when proteins such as estrogen receptor and G-protein that need a lipophilic environment to maintain tertiary structure are crystallized. Their bioactive conformation needs to be predicted from the amino acid sequence.

ii. Predict the target structure of drugs with unkown mechanism of action

iii. Predicted models that are quick and cheap to test drug action on

iv. Helps in designing new proteins.

Most commonly used approaches for prediction can be classified as follows (Rost, et al., 2003):

Prediction in 1D:

• Secondary structure
• Solvent accessibility
• Transmembrane helices.

Prediction in 2D:

• Inter–residue/strand contacts.

Prediction in 3D:

• Homology modeling
• Fold recognition and threading
• *Ab initio* prediction (e.g. via molecular dynamics)
• Methods that use a combination of the above strategies
• Receptor mapping – a drug design based approach to structure prediction (*ref.* Part II also).

Selected titles from this list are presented here.

1.4.1 PREDICTION IN 1D

A. Secondary Structure Prediction

Protein structure prediction dates back to the 1960s. Groundbreaking research of Peter Y. Chou and Gerald D. Fasman demonstrated that certain residues formed helices readily and with this information, devised prediction rules for helices and coils (Chou, et al. 1974). These rules were extended to β-strands and in a dataset of 19 proteins, a success rate of prediction of 80% helical and 86% β-sheet. The following statement quoted from the 1974 *Biochemistry* article by the two authors mentioned (Chou, et al. 1974) shows the strategy:

> **Did You Know? 5**
> **The beginning of protein structure prediction**
>
> *"Briefly stated: When four helix formers out of six residues or three β formers out of five residues are found clustered together in any native protein segment, the nucleation of these secondary structures begins and propagates in both directions until terminated by a sequence of tetrapeptides, designated as breakers."*
>
> *Peter Y Chou & Gerald D Fasman (Chou, et al. 1974)*

Probability of occurrence of residues among helices and β-strands were calculated that lead to the classification into (with the charges mentioned in parenthesis):

- Among helical segments,
  a. H_α strong α former: Glu(-), Ala, Leu
  b. h_α, a former: His(+), Met, Gln, Trp, Val, Phe
  c. I_α weak α former: Lys(+), Ile
  d. i_α, α indifferent: Asp(-), Thr, Ser, Arg(+), Cys
  e. b_α, a breaker: Asn, Tyr
  f. B_α, strong α breaker: Pro, Gly
  g. Pro and Asp near the N-terminal helix and Arg near the C-terminal helix are assigned I_α.

- β-sheet assignments,
  a. H_β, strong β former: Met, Val, Ile
  b. h_β, β former: Cys, Tyr, Phe, Gln, Leu, Thr, Trp
  c. I_β, weak βformer: Ala
  d. i_β, β indifferent: Arg(+), Gly, Asp(-)
  e. b_β, β breaker: Lys(+), Ser, His(+), Asn, Pro
  f. B_β, strong β breaker: Glu(-)
  g. Trp near the C-terminal β region is assigned b_β.

The helix–β sheet–coil categories of conformations are often referred to as the 3-state assignment.

Box 6: Rules are steadily added to improve prediction

There are additional rules (from just occurrence of the above residues) that govern prediction (Rost, et al. 1994). For example, "*i, i+3, i+4, i+7*" pattern is conserved among helices whereas among β-strands, residues having same side chain properties are found along one face of the strand. Conserved glycine and proline residues are found to be strongly distributed in loops.

When pairs of secondary structures are compared between 2 proteins, a very high degree of similarity can be obtained even if sequence matches <20% (Klepeis, et al. 2003). Therefore secondary structure prediction itself can expose any structural similarities among distantly related sequences. The success of secondary structure predictions have always been strongly fluctuating. Today, a number of these methods are available via online servers such as PSIPRED (Jones, 1999). Several use various techniques to derive secondary structure prediction "rules" such as matrices that note the occurrence of residues at specific structural positions from the entire PDB database. Structure–sequence information has been represented as strings (Koretke, et al. 1999); yet other use techniques such as neural networks (Rost, et al. 1994) to train recognition of patterns among secondary structures. As always, some methods predict structures by obtaining a consensus of several existing methods (Cuff, et al. 1998). Composite secondary structure prediction attempts to simultaneously predict the presence of all secondary structures of a protein (An, et al. 2002) though literature discusses several complications in this matter (Honig, et al. 1995).

The various fields of research related to proteins are structure analysis, dynamics, prediction, folding and interaction, as conveniently described in this book. Results obtained from extensive work on protein structure analysis are neatly used as a start for protein structure prediction. For example, (Doig, 2008) extensively accounted helix – coil transitions described the formation of helices as resulting from local interactions and some methods such as the helix prediction part of Astro-fold (the complete program described under 3D *ab initio* prediction) analyze 5 – residue fragments throughout the protein (that will include a 3-residue nucleus). The study of 3_{10}-helices (Benedetti E, 1991) lead to typical residue preferences that could be used for prediction. Extensive analysis of β-turns in proteins, their occurrence, structure, amino acid preference, solvent exposure, hydrophobicity of residues, etc. (Rose, et al. 1985) have successfully contributed to their prediction. More recently in 2004, α-turns were predicted (Kaur, et al. 2004) using artificial neural networks to analyze earlier detailed structural characterizations.

B. Solvent Exposure Prediction

As discussed in early chapters, the folded protein has an "interior" and a "surface". As cellular environments are majorly aqueous, cytoplasmic and blood proteins have surface residues are generally polar. Hydrophobic residues at the core contribute to maintaining the folded shape of the protein whereas surface residues are involved in interaction and recognition needed to carry out protein function. Therefore a strong correlation can be expected between protein function and conserved surface residues. "Solvent accessibility" is a physical parameter that specifies the area (in $Å^2$) that is exposed to water molecules (also *ref.* part II chapter 2.3.2.A and 2.3.2.E) for a particular residue. The value could range from 0 (entirely buried) to 300 (on surface) and these values cannot directly be compared between residues because one has to consider the total area that a residue *can possibly* expose to the solvent. Small side chains like glycine ('side chain' is just hydrogen) have inherently very low surface area compared to say, phenylalanine. Therefore values are normalized by expressing solvent accessibility as the percentage out of maximal exposable area that is being exposed to solvent.

Exposure to solvent can often be predicted simultaneously to secondary structure prediction. For example, among α-helices, alternating hydrophobic residues in a "i, $i+3$, $i+4$, $i+7$" pattern and among β-strands, hydrophobic "i, $i+2$, $i+4$" pattern indicate that the respective secondary structure are at the surface. Interior β-strands are generally made of stretches of *conserved* hydrophobic residues. Similarly among loops, those located in the interior have hydrophobic regions that are well conserved, not containing insertions or deletions. Comparison with solvent accessibility trends among known proteins structures in the PDB show (Rost, et al., 1994) that values in the hydrophobic range (<10%) are conserved among the residues of homologous proteins, more than solvent exposed residues are. But even with the availability of such theories, predictive capacity is not sufficient just from sequence (correlation coefficient between predicted and measured accessibility to solvent is much less than 1, i.e. close to 0.5).

1.4.2 PREDICTION IN 2D: CONTACT PREDICTION

In this chapter, we wish to simply present the meaning of the term "contact prediction". Propensities of residues to come into contact with each other over long distance are counted from known structures in the PDB. Such a counting gives rise to tables and charts that show the probability those 2 residues i and j along a given blind sequence will come in contact with each other, given a certain environment in a certain type of protein. These derived values are called "contact potentials" and are used in threading methods (*ref.* under prediction in 3D) as a part of the force field that guides prediction.

1.4.3 PREDICTION IN 3D

Prediction in 3D can be divided into homology modeling, fold recognition and *ab-initio* methods, as described above. However, literature also suggests alternative ways of classifying these methods, namely:

- Methods that refine a crude template (these methods can only handle a protein that has been neatly pieced together by various strategies, as happens for sequences with >30% similarity as explained under homology modeling)

- Methods that can make templates (by aligning appropriately selected sequences and/or structures and building the template when sufficient sequence matches are not readily available in the database)

- Methods that can simply whip-up an appropriate structure when sequence matches with other proteins in the database cannot even be made with difficulty – this is called "free modeling".

As further explained below when introducing *ab initio* prediction methods, the distinction between various methods by the traditional classification become blurred. This can be resolved and understood better when considering methods in the light of "what they do" as detailed above.

A. Homology Modeling for 3D Structure Prediction

There is no structural data for most pharmacologically relevant target proteins (Wermuth, 2008). In this scenario, if one wishes to use rational drug design strategies to develop novel drugs for a certain target, with the availability of the target sequence and no more information, the only solution is to construct the target protein computationally from other proteins of known structure and similarity in sequence. This is called *homology modeling*, also called *comparative modeling* or *knowledge-based prediction* or, colloquially, *model building*. It is one of the most successful structure prediction methods to date. In the CASP competitions, 9 out of 20 models were predicted well by homology modeling methods (Tress, et al. 2005). The method is based on the principle that an agreement in sequence between two proteins or their parts [even if just ~40% (Schlick, 2002)] often shows similarity in 3D structure. Comparative modeling techniques are not yet perfect. But these are already helping to answer questions related to biology such as identification of possible binding sites. The method is also cost effect compared to determining protein structure experimentally. The following points outline the fundamentals of comparative modeling (*ref.* Scheme 1.18) in terms of its steps, attributes and precautions.

Steps in Homology Modeling

   i. *Collecting information in a database:* Information stored in databases and classified for easy access are invaluable reference. They bring together data generated by research groups all over the world. Examples: PDB, Swissprot, RefSeq , GenBank, Cambridge Crystallographic Database, etc.

   ii. *Finding basis structures*: "Known" structures (called *"basis"*) that are used to construct the structure of a blind sequence (the sequence whose structure is to be determined is termed 'blind'). Search for basis structures is done either by matching amino acid sequence or by matching the fit of a sequence to a fold (using threading methods-this is explained under "fold recognition" in this chapter). It has been reported that the larger the basis structure set, the more accurate the modeling (Chakravarthy, et al. 2008), because:

      a. One can be aware of all possible alignments and matches so that one can choose the best out of them

      b. One can be aware of the variety of tertiary structures that have been generated by sequence matching.

      c. In the above case, one can use local segments alone from the various tertiary structures to model the blind sequence

      d. Errors are reduced and model building becomes more robust.

   iii. *Alignment of sequence:* It is said that modeling is straightforward if a basis structure is obtained whose sequence has >30% similarity with the blind sequence. Sequences

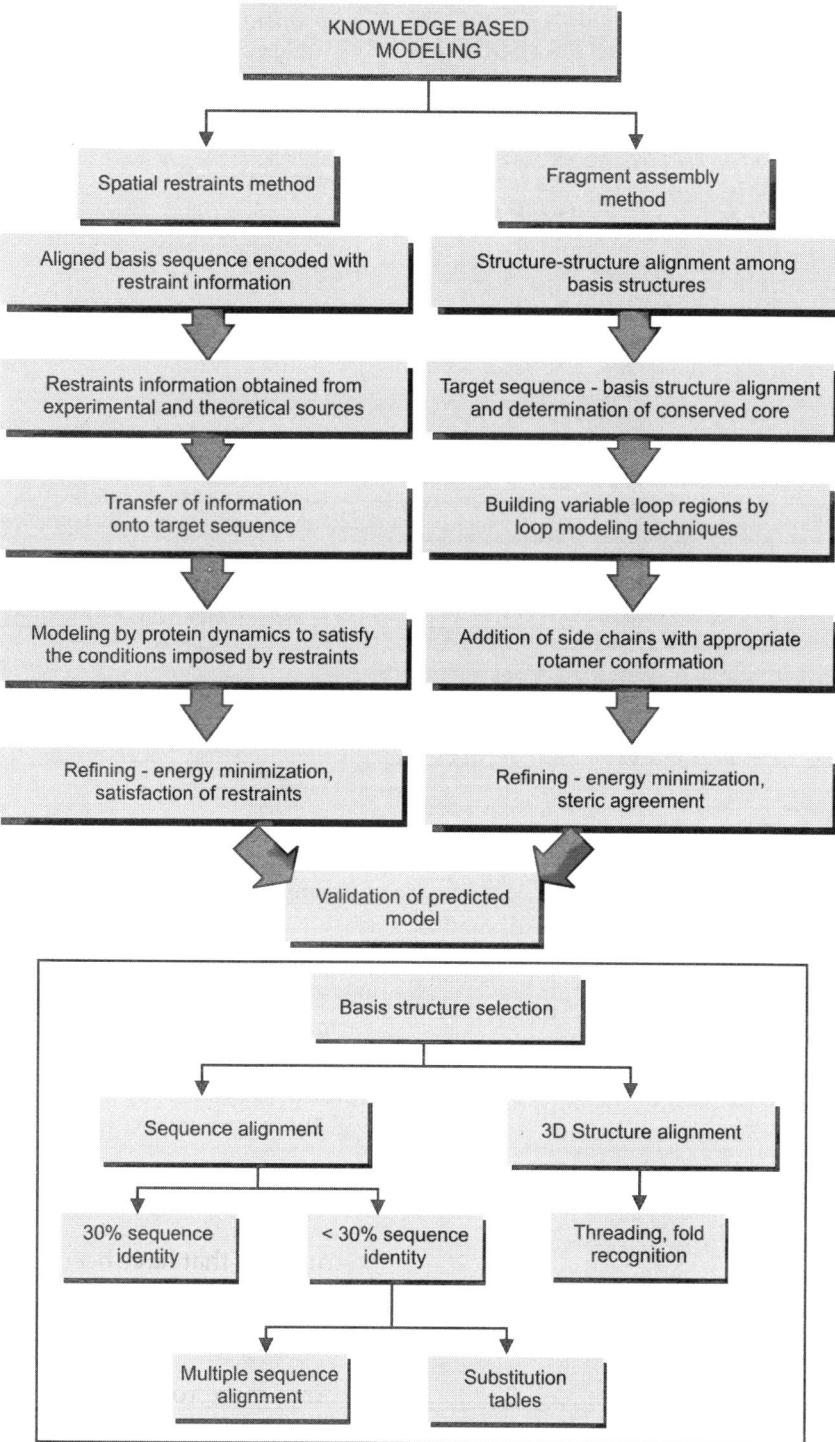

Scheme 1.18: On comparative modeling and fold recognition

for which such bases cannot be obtained are said to lie in the "twilight zone" of sequence similarity. The 3D structure may be conserved with little similarity in residues. In such cases, sequence similarities can only be obtained for portions of the blind sequence and the modeling must be done piecewise. At any rate, efficient alignment is a must, and also meaningful techniques to identify and quantify similarities are performed using scoring functions–the aligned amino acids are categorized as being "identical", "having similar properties", "not a match" (like the principle used in multiple choice examinations with negative marking that give +4 for a right answer, 0 for no answer and –1 for a wrong answer).

There are three ways to model matches between the target (or blind) sequence and the basis sequence:

Think Box 1: On homology modeling

Homology modeling is like trying to take a decision on an issue. The more people we get to voice opinions, the more likely that we take a good decision. When holding discussions on an issue, it might not be too surprising if people who come from similar environments have a common opinion. Therefore, one aims to include people who are experts, exposed to different scenarios and yet are relevant to the topic being discussed. If a consensus opinion can be obtained from such a group, we believe that a sound decision is achieved. Statistically, for the same level of significance, proving or disproving a hypothesis is stronger (given by the 'α value') if the dataset is heterogeneous than if its members belong to one tight group. Similarly, the larger and more diverse the size of the basis set, the more 'robust' the model obtained.

Pairwise sequence alignment (performed by FASTA (Pearson, et al. 1988), SSEARCH that aligns, scores for every pair of residue aligned against each other, shifts the alignment by one residue, recalculates alignment scores and the process continues till a maximum score is achieved.

Multiple sequence alignment (BLAST (**B**asic **L**ocal **A**lignment **S**earch **T**ool (Altschul, et al., 1990)), PSI-BLAST, HMM, Intermediate Sequence Search) that aligns several sequences against each other simultaneously by:

• Either accumulating pair-wise scores or
• By creating consensus sequences wherein the properties of several residues are added

By comparing with more methods, a consensus check of the effectiveness of the alignment can be obtained (Notredame, et al. 2000), (Thompson, et al. 1994).

Discussion 1.10: Sequence alignment

Consider the following sequence: "123456789". If this sequence of numbers is to be aligned against a database of number combinations, and if the following basis sequence is present in the database: "92348512345678935447541945927540" then the following alignment:

```
Basis: 9 2 3 4 8 5 1 2 3 4 5 6 7 8 9 3 5 4 4 7 5 4 1 9 4 5 9 2 7 5 4
Match: ` ` ` ` ` : : : : : : : : : ` ` ` ` ` ` ` ` ` ` ` ` ` ` ` `
Blind:           1 2 3 4 5 6 7 8 9
```

If the sequence in the basis is interrupted by an insertion, then a gap is produced:

```
Basis:9 2 3 4 8 5 1 2 3 4 5 9 8 7 6 5 4 3 2 6 7 8 9 3 5 4 4 7 5 4 1 9 4 5 9 2 7 5 4
Match:` ` ` ` ` : : : : : ` ` ` ` ` ` :: : : ` ` ` ` ` ` ` ` ` ` ` `
Blind:         1 2 3 4 5 x x x x x x x 6 7 8 9
```

The 8 character insertion generates a gap in the alignment. If one gives a "gap penalty" of 8 when matching protein sequences (meaning 8 other residues can come in between) then the algorithm will look for a match across 8 residues.

Sequence alignment is reported in CASP competitions (reports available at http://predictioncenter.org) to be the limiting step because:

- The shorter the stretch of residues that have been successfully aligned, the higher the level of similarity required between the residues to produce structural significance
- The presence of mutations such as deletions and insertions makes alignment difficult because there will be a gap.
- Even barring all these technical difficulties, a perfect sequence match itself does not guarantee that the structure taken up by the blind sequence will resemble the one built by tackling gaps and substitutions. In addition, one must expect a certain degree of flexibility in the loops or at the ends of domains or slight changes in domain orientations.

Famous algorithms for alignment are the Smith-Waterman alignment (Smith, et al. 1981) and the Needleman –Wunsch alignment (Needleman, et al. 1970).

Setting up of substitution tables [such as BLOSUM – *BLOcks of Amino Acid SUbstitution Matrix* (Henikoff, et al. 1992), PAM - **P**oint **A**ccepted **M**utation matrix (Dayhoff, 1978)] derived from the PDB that provides allowances for certain residue pairs after alignment by looking up a table. The highest score indicates the best alignment. The scoring function, as mentioned above, could be simply based on the identity of the residues (called identity scoring) or there could be other criteria, such as chemical properties, or genetic sequence.

iv. *Fragment assembly method:* This is a two-step process. First, the basis structures are matched among themselves and their structures are aligned so that their core regions (or if they are different proteins, the regions that they have been chosen for) are brought in place to form a "scaffold structure". In the second step, the residues in the blind sequence are made to march up the scaffold (like a line of marksmen on a fort) and take their positions such that their residues are aligned against matching basis residues. The structural information such as "helix", etc. is then transferred from the reference basis set onto the target sequence. It has been observed that the regions of the scaffold at this stage are mostly from the secondary structures. The rest are loops and are modeled in two ways (the process is termed "loop modeling"):

a. A knowledge based approach that identifies several basis structures and calculates statistical frequency of occurrence in similar environments or

b. An *ab inito* approach that starts with the flanking secondary structures, their respective orientations, the distance of separation, the sequence, etc. information and with conformational search, arrives at the most probable loop structure.

   As with any such empirical method, this method also involves simplifications (in that mostly only C_α atoms are considered) and lacks physical and chemical justification.

v. *Adding side chains:* So far, the $C\alpha$ atoms, and at the most, the atoms of the backbone alone are treated. Even though strong correlation is established between backbone's local conformation and the side chain rotamer (Bower, et al., 1997), constructing protein side-chains is a tricky process. In a structure modeled in the above way, each segmented of the chain would have been copy-pasted from various members of the basis set. Standard methods are available though with conflicting efficiency and are discussed later in this chapter that put the side chains in order.

vi. *Spatial restraints method:* In contrast to assembling the model from fragments, one can keep an account of various types of information in the primary code itself. That is, all proteins in the databank can be represented by characters that simultaneously combine sequence with other information. A serine in a helix conformation that is exposed to solvent can be represented as, say, a bold 'S' character underlined wherein the bold could indicate helical backbone conformation and the underlining could represent solvent exposure. Other representations can be used to indicate other properties in a category such as, say, italics for β-strand conformation and no formatting for loops. Once the entire database of proteins is "encoded" in this way incorporating secondary structure, solvent accessibility, backbone-backbone and backbone-side chain H-bonding, disulfide bonding, φ–ψ values, cis-trans (stereochemical) configuration (all these parameters are incorporated in a single method (Matsuda, et al. 1997)). Sequence alignment of the target with the database will lead to a bunch of basis structures that can first be compared among themselves with respect to the environments of the focused stretches of sequences. When this comparison leads to a consensus (i.e., when majority of aligned residues agree such as, say, "solvent exposed helices at positions 1–5, followed by buried loops at 6–8") as obtained from the encoding, this consensus is applied on the blind sequence. The atoms of the target sequence are made to take up conformations in space as dictated by the consensus characters, and they become "constraints" that limit the number of conformations that can theoretically be taken up.

Question

Compare and contrast fragment assembly with spatial restraints method (*hints*)
- Flexibility: The representation of protein structure is used for comparison as well as modeling purposes
- Several sources are available: One can get supporting information from theoretical as well as experimental studies

- A fine-grained description of secondary structure packing, hydrophobic patch distribution, correlated mutations, etc can be used to generate a detailed prediction model
- Comparative modeling can be improved in par with experimental data generated from NMR, genetic engineering, etc.

vii. *Refining:* The structure that is obtained by progressively modeling segments of the protein backbone acts as only a placeholder for backbone, and to some extent side chain, atoms. It has been shown that serious steric clashes arise (Lovell, et al. 2000) when rotamer libraries are used to determine side chain conformation. Whatever the source of modeling, at this step of refinement, energy is minimized (removing strain due to unnatural conformations) and Van der Waals clashes are checked. If the modeling was performed by spatial restraints method, then refining would involve minimizing violations of all restraints.

viii. *Validation:* Predicted models can be analyzed for its quality by calculating energy using energy minimization and molecular dynamics methods, by determining normality indices between the model and the real structures (*ref.* prediction assessment methods used in the CASP competitions on their website http://predictioncenter.org), by analyzing the distribution of φ and ψ of the proteins residues on a Ramachandran plot, etc. Standard software is available such as PROCHECK (Laskowski, et al. 1993) and PROCHECK-NMR (Laskowski, et al., 1996) [available for free download at http://www.ebi.ac.uk/thornton-srv/software/PROCHECK/].

Although knowledge based methods are known to be very successful (extolled further in the highlights of CASP competition results in this chapter) the same "knowledge" tells us that there are many chameleon sequences in proteins. These sequences are known to take up helical as well as β-strand conformations depending on the overall tertiary structure they occur in (Mezei, 1998).

B. Fold Recognition Methods for 3D Structure Prediction

Knowledge-based methods are statistical, yielding discrete sets of data that establish correlation between local protein structure and amino acid distribution. The underlying assumption is as follows: the reason why a certain feature (such as a conformation, a secondary structure, an amino acid at a certain position, a fold shape, etc.) is popular is because it is supported by evolution, conformational energy, atomic interactions, etc. Thus, physical rules that govern folding and structure stability are implicit in these results. However, it is impossible to calculate the 3D structure of a protein from discrete structural information of the amino acids of the polypeptide chain such as by adding "alpha-helix", "beta strand", "random coil", etc.

> "*A success rate of 100% in secondary structure prediction would therefore be insufficient to predict the native fold of a protein*" (Sippl, 1995).

Statistical methods are also influenced by the size and the variety of examples that are available for study. For example, the sectioning of the Ramachandran plot into regions changed with increasing number of examples (*ref.* "methods" under chapter 1.2). The fundamentals of the fold recognition approach are based on physical principles that ultimately aim to connect thermodynamics and statistical mechanics. They are in line with the efforts taken to solve the protein folding problem (see chapter 1.5). The native fold conformation is assumed to be the energetically most stable and favored one among all conformations that are possible. Therefore, the aim would be to artificially keep changing the conformations of the fold until the minimum energy one is hit and then to evaluate if this is the native state that one is looking for. In this approach, however, there are several difficulties:

- From the Levinthal's paradox (under chapter 1.5.1) it is clear that even using computers, it is an impossible task to sample all possible conformations.
- If one obtains a conformation that seems to have the lowest energy among a bunch of generated ones, how can one be sure that this is not one of the local minima, but is the global minimum?
- How can one be sure that the global minimum calculated corresponds to the native fold conformation? In other words, how does one know the complete set of parameters that determine the fold's energy?

One has to start somewhere, and the following points form the basis of fold recognition methods:

- The energy of the fold is considered to result from the interactions of all pairs atoms in it. The interactions that have to be accounted for can be categorized into covalent and non-bonded.
- Almost all interactions of atoms such as dipole and ion pair interactions, hyperconjugation, aromaticity, hydrogen bonding etc have been described as basic principles of quantum and classical mechanics. These descriptions are used to set up what are called "potentials". Potentials may use parameters previously determined (experimentally or theoretically). The energy of an interaction between two atoms in a protein molecule can thus be calculated with the help of *force fields* that result from the potentials and the parameters. For a detailed description, *ref.* protein dynamics (chapter 1.3) for applications and part II (section 2.2.10) for technical aspects.
- Pair-wise atom contact and solvation terms [example: (Jones, et al. 2003)] are used and the former values are often derived statistically from the protein database.

It is important to recognize that in order to determine the correlation between the global minimum and the native state, generation of all possible conformations of a sequence, even after eliminating ones that are chemically meaningless (such as those that have van der Waals clashes) is not the aim of simulations. Working in these lines requires that all possible conformations be generated and analyzed. Even if the structure corresponding to the global minimum is hit early in this search, there is no way to realize that this has happened until the search is complete because only then one can safely call it the global minimum eliminating other minima of lower energy (i.e. one can label a structure as global minimum only if the sampling of all the possible conformations is complete). Physical methods, as opposed to statistical ones, are conceptually sound and correlate strongly with the protein folding problem. Computationally, however, the problem boils down to finding the global minimum amidst some 10^{100} possible conformations, a large number of which could be local minima (*ref.* Part II chapter 2.3 for details on techniques).

It is thus clear that a lot depends on identifying the correct energy function that can be used to set up the force field. One cannot use the above laborious process to just verify the validity of a force field. For this latter purpose methods simply try to determine a conformation that is lower in energy than the native state. The presence of even one other such structure shows that the achieved state is not the global minimum when energy is calculated using that particular force field or method. The situation at hand can therefore be tackled using a two stage approach–first, to obtain the right energy function that stations the native state at the global minimum, and second, to find a method that, given the sequence, can locate the global minimum conformation. The reader is advised to *ref.* to the principles of protein folding under chapter 1.5 that were derived from the observations obtained from experiments that analyze protein structures in various environments. These observations indicate the various interactions that operate in a protein that make a protein finally look the way it does.

Although the term global minimum is used to *ref.* to a single conformation, we know that this sense is not literal. Even among proteins crystallized from the same environment, small localized changes in conformation can be seen in their crystal structure. Thus, we are looking at an ensemble (means collection) of conformations that represents the global minimum and is close to equilibrium point. Physical methods do not necessarily mean the absence of the statistical approach as envisaged by the Boltzmann distribution that establishes the relationship between energy and likelihood of occupation of a molecular state (for a short description, *ref.* chapter 2.3.2.E in part II). This ensemble of conformations can be obtained from the deposited crystal structures of proteins in the protein data bank for the same protein or for different proteins. A study of their conformation and structure (i.e, at a local and global level respectively) should tell us (1) why a particular sequence prefers a narrow range of conformations amidst a large theoretical number and similarly, (2) why only some folds are prevalent among proteins when various combinations of the secondary structures can theoretically form infinite folds.

Fold recognition deals with both the above aspects, however at the moment we concentrate on the former. The energy functions that guide a blind sequence to fold computationally must be able to capture the interactions that exist between all atoms in the amino acid sequence when it is at or close to equilibrium. An example of how the energy functions are described is presented below as implemented by the "knowledge-based mean fields" approach. After the setting up of optimum potentials that is capable of placing the native fold in the global minimum, one is able to predict this native fold for the given blind sequence. This is often checked by a "*jackknife test*"- a protein from the database is selected to act as the test sequence and is removed from the database before the mean field is compiled. The capacity of the force field to correctly identify the native fold of this protein given its sequence is tested.

Structure prediction encompasses the entire protein, wherein each domain may contain more than one fold, and the protein, more than one domain. Therefore, all possible folds in the blind sequence must be identified and then, the homologous members of families that contain the folds. Further complications in identifying the native arise when the fold is stabilized by cofactors, prosthetic groups and post-translational modification. Fold recognition and identification of homologous proteins are steps that proceed without the above complications. The technique used to determine how well the target sequence arranges itself on a particular fold is called 'threading'. Thus, with the availability of many fold structures in the Protein Data Bank (PDB), the target sequence can be made to dress and pose as the various folds and its resulting energy is compared with the energy of the fold in its native sequence (as pulled out from the PDB).

Inverse folding: Inverse folding is literally the inverse of folding and fold recognition. Whereas the latter strategies aim to identify the best fold for a given sequence, this technique fits all known sequences to a given fold to determine all those that fit best. An overview if this method is as follows:

- Structure is described using a series of characters/strings attributed to every amino acid position and the proteins of the PDB are expressed in terms of this 1D string.
- The structural encoding of proteins are compared with the respective amino acid sequences and "profiles" are generated wherein the tendency of residues (also encoded, by name or by property) to occupy specific structural positions (surface/interior, strand/helix/turn, etc) are determined.
- The structure of a fold with which other sequences are to be matched is encoded into the 1D string and all sequences other than the one native to the fold are aligned along the structure encoded string. After alignment, if the match between encoded structure and encoded sequence reflect the propensities derived from the database, the sequence is a good candidate for fitting the fold's structure.

Mutations and homology: Low sequence conservation among structurally homologous proteins has affected all spheres of computational protein analysis, such as structure classification, determination and comparison, prediction and folding. Mutations in the form of deletions and insertions have forced researchers to look for techniques flexible enough to tolerate gaps (although substitutions are also a form of mutation, they do not generate gaps). The same applies to fold recognition as well as inverse folding methods. As with sequences, there is also a continuum of structures (at a local as well as global level) that makes it difficult to segregate folds into structurally distinct groups. Any method that is sufficiently generalized to handle proteins in the PDB independent of their classification must take both structural as well as sequential variability into account. Fold recognition and inverse folding investigations are therefore applied to sequences that are not too similar and are made to handle the identification of discrete stretches of similarity (in sequence/structure) dispersed throughout the protein.

Discoveries reported in literature often help out tremendously–for example, it is known that closely related structures can have mutations in solvent exposed loops and that 3_{10} helices and α-helices can freely interconvert due to allowed Ramachandran angles during the conformational transition. However, it is also known that small changes at key residues are often responsible for one fold to completely fall apart and another to start forming (as shown by the outcome of the Paracelsus challenge, earlier in this chapter in Discussion 1.8). Even if changes in sequence to fit structure alignment are performed, how sure can one be that the original sequence will assume the same structure as the changed one? The problem is more fundamental than just being an artifact of computational methods of analysis and sequence alignment must be used only as a starting tool rather than as a foundation for the solution.

Threading: Fold recognition is simply compiling strongly conserved sequence features among proteins that contain the same fold and trying to locate these conserved features among the residues of the blind sequence. As such an approach fails to locate structural similarities when the sequences differ beyond recognition (remember: in a database of thousands of proteins, comparing sequence is easier than comparing 3D structure), sequence-structure alignment is done as described above by "threading". The term threading is therefore an extension of traditional fold recognition methods and performs the positioning of target sequence on the structures of folds in a database. The alignment is done by the *Needleman–Wunsch dynamic programming algorithm* (*ref.* Discussion 1.10). It was originally created for sequence–sequence alignments. A fold is selected from the database of structure complete with its native sequence in place, and residues of the blind sequence are substituted one by one into this fold with the rest of the sequence remaining undisturbed. An energy measure is used to ascertain the effect of substitution. The Needleman–Wunsch algorithm is used in this context to score the energy against residues of the blind sequence by constructing a matrix. A "thread" of low energy arrangement of residues on the fold can be seen.

Discussion 1.11: Knowledge-based mean fields

The methodology behind the construction and use of "knowledge-based force fields" is presented here for an educational purpose because it unifies several concepts discussed under part I including protein dynamics, structure, prediction, folding and even under part II such as the Boltzmann distribution, force fields, etc. The details and work presented have been referenced.

Authors: Manfred J Sippl, Institute for Chemistry and Biochemistry, University of Salzburg, Austria (Sippl, 1995)

Principle: To derive a force field based on the principles of statistical physics wherein the probability of occurrence of two atoms at a certain distance in space belonging to two amino acids is related to the preferred conformation and hence has favorable energy. By obtaining distances, the authors implicitly include all forces such as electrostatic, steric, etc avoiding the need to *ref.* to each term separately, hence the term "mean fields".

Method

Background–setting up of force field

  i. The Boltzmann distribution is written as:

$$P_{i,j,k...} = e^{-E_{i,j,k...}/kT}/Z$$

where Z represents the Boltzmann sum:

$$Z = \sum_{i,j,k...} e^{-E_{i,j,k...}/kT}$$

Here i, j, k… represent the various conformational states of the polypeptide chain and the probability $P_{i,j,k...}$ evaluates the tendency of the polypeptide chain to occupy the conformations represented by these states. Z is used for normalization as explained under chapter 2.3.2.E so that the probability of occupation of states $P_{i,j,k,...}$ obtained above is no longer written in a relative sense. In other words,

$$S_{i,j,k}...P_{i,j,k}... = 1.$$

ii. The probabilities are obtained as mentioned under 'Principle' in this discussion: The protein databank is scanned for the occurrence of two atoms c and d at a certain distance r from each other in space belonging to two amino acids a and b separated by a certain distance k in the primary structure. The distance r in space is specified in Å is a continuous variable and is converted into a discrete variable by setting up ranges–atoms c and d separated by say 5.5 to 6.5 Å belong to a specific category. The frequency of this particular arrangement of particular atoms is then represented as "f_r^{abcdk}". The Boltzmann rule states that lower energy states are more frequently occupied resulting in the following expression:

$$E_r^{abcdk} = -kT \ln f_r^{abcdk}$$

iii. It is ensured that values are not counted twice (redundancy is eliminated by subtraction of relevant quantities)

iv. The resulting expression gives the potential and for each value of k and r and depending on the atoms c, d and residues a, b, various interactions, whether hydrogen bonding or electrostatic, can be accounted for at once. Thus, scanning the database and filling up frequencies based on the above variables, give us (as the authors put it) a tool kit of mean force potentials

v. The conformation all energies of amino acid sequence is calculated as a summation over all sequence positions i and j and all atoms c and d.

vi. A small protein is about 500 residues long. Assuming a minimal average of 15 atoms per residue, the small protein will contain about 7500 atoms. To construct a force field for each of these atom pairs might be a waste of time and effort if reasonable results can be achieved by taking significantly fewer atoms and presenting a reduced description of protein structure. The mean field is constructed only of C^b atoms to start with (i.e. c and d are the C^b atoms of the respective residues) as this avoids construction of the entire side chain.

Verification of the Force Field –The use of a Polyprotein

i. The first part of this approach, as listed earlier, aims to test whether there are any other conformations lower in energy than the native. For this, the force field is applied to recognize the lowest energy conformation among a large number

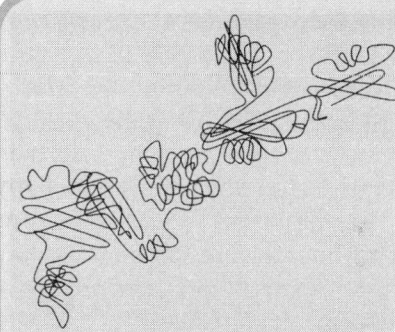

Fig. Schematic of a polyprotein

of artificially generated structures. If the identified conformation is indeed the native state, one can be certain that the derived energy function is indeed the right one.

ii. In order to make the test rigid, the native structure is hidden among several that look similar – i.e. they are made to vary only in side-chain rotamer conformation and hence in the positioning of atoms (c and d).

iii. As mentioned earlier under fold recognition, the fold is a part of a domain and recognition methods must be able to catch the right fold and place it in its native (or at least lowest energy) conformation in the presence of "miscellaneous residues" before and after it. The authors therefore hide the native fold within a structure called the "polyprotein" which is artificially constructed such that segments of its residues correspond to some meaningful conformation or the other, when compared with the structures present in the protein data bank. By this process, the native fold cannot be detected by a simple sequence comparison.

iv. The force field is made to work with the huge polyprotein starting from its N-terminus. The test sequence (whose native structure is known), which is say 200 residues long, made to assume the conformation represented by the first 200 residues of the N-terminus of the polyprotein. The energy of the resulting structure is calculated and recorded.

v. The force field is then applied on the next 200 residue fragment of the polyprotien starting from the second N- terminal residue and the new fold taken up by the test sequence is recorded along with its respective energy.

vi. This sequence shifting, structure recognition and energy calculation is successively performed until the force field hits the polyprotein's C-terminus and runs out of 200-residue-segments.

vii. All the recognized folds are next sorted by energy. If the 'lowest' energy structure recognized by the test sequence indeed corresponds to its native structure (as mentioned earlier, this is a test sequence, and hence its structure is known) the potential thus derived for the force field is correct. As the folds contained in the polyprotein are close to each other in overall structure and the native can be recognized among them only by very sensitive and well tuned methods.

Fold recognition by Threading

Fold recognition is basically matching how well a sequence of residues can take up various fold conformations. Given the several difficulties outlined above encountered by fold recognition methods, authors used *knowledge based mean fields* to simply generate the best possible alignment and minimize wrong alignments, as one can never be sure if the mutated sequence indeed represents the original in all aspects. The sequence-structure alignment is done by the Needleman–Wunsch algorithm. The level of comfort of a residue (of the blind sequence) substituting an already existing residue in the fold is judged using mean field energy generated by the fold's sequence. The matrix is set up as with the sequence on one side is matched against the calculated mean field energy for each residue of the sequence on the other side. All residues not paired with structure are removed and the final model is generated. The normalized score used by the authors when comparing proteins of different lengths is used here to determine low energy arrangements.

Starting point for ab inito predictions: So, is the global minimum the native state when energy of the fold is calculated by this method?

That is, when a random conformation of the sequence is given, can the force field guide the folding of a sequence to its native structure? Given that the mean fields approach has only included C^{β} atoms so far, it is easily conceived that the force field is incomplete. As a start to this investigation, mean field energy was first plotted against amino acid position. Although on a residue-level zoom energies were found to oscillate considerably between positive and negative values, averaging the values over 10 residue window showed some regions of strain that were being compensated by other stabilized regions. An even larger window consisting of 50 residues was able to distinguish between purposely misfolded structures (these are sequences of one protein made to assume the shape of another that is totally unrelated) and native structures as the former had positive values for energy whereas in the latter case, it was negative. Authors highlight that the method was capable of recognizing models of intentionally misfolded proteins as well as unrefined structures of proteins as having high energy, compared to the native state. Hence, the high energy unfolded conformations accessible to a sequence during early stages of folding were considered to be capable of being eliminated using this mean fields approach. The problem was therefore considered to be technical on how to sample and determine the global minimum.

One of the strategies used by authors is to generate multiple conformations for all possible 6-residue segments in the sequence and to assemble overlapping regions to generate a comple model. The stable and variable segments were marked and latter segments were changed more frequently than the former in an ensuing Monte Carlo energy minimization. The resulting structure was compact and folded with reported resemblences to the native structure. Methodology and results of this part show that techniques for one method are not independent set that cannot be used for others.

C. *Ab Initio* 3D Structure Prediction

Knowledge-based methods are successful; but not all sequences have a match in the database. Fold recognition methods are useful, but only if the fold is one among those that have already been characterized. Whereas a successful *ab initio* method is extremely valuable because it essentially absolves any need for references and is a breakthrough for protein folding. The approach used technically is as always done: Conformations are generated in such a way that they sample the conformational space, and a scoring function is set up so that it is able to match the native structure to the global minimum. These two are often aimed to be made interdependent so that the scoring function can bias the conformation search to take place closer to the global minimum. The sampling of any particular region on the conformational space is supposed to act as a feedback to the scoring function. Nevertheless, there is no reliable technique that directs the search neatly towards the native fold as more and more conformations are generated. In fact, the scoring function is often the one to blame as excellent models have been shown in CASP 5 (Jones, et al., 2003) to be ranked below other conformations. This means that an understanding of the interactions responsible for the stability and uniqueness of the native conformation is insufficient, essentially arriving at the protein folding problem in chapter 1.5.

Molecular Dynamics methods are often used to provide detailed conformational searches and energy assessments. Proteins are far from static (chapter 1.2) and are also cooperative meaning the entire tertiary structure is thought to form as one unit (chapter 1.5). MDS runs of proteins shed light on the interatomic forces that maintain secondary, supersecondary and tertiary structures as protein "evolve" over time (*ref.* chapter 1.3). Inferences on protein folding are often obtained with simulations involving just the C_{α} atoms (or any other subset of all atoms in the protein, called minimalist models) and this method is used for *ab initio* predictions too. A hierarchical (*meaning step-wise by rank*) strategy is often used (Pillardy, et al., 2001) and methods start with the sequence, form secondary structures first (prediction in 1D), followed by determining long-range contacts (prediction in 2D), and finally arriving at the tertiary structure (prediction in 3D). All other atoms are added to the final model to obtain the entire protein as described below in chapter 1.4.5 completing the protein. Monte Carlo methods describe an ensemble of conformations that, via Boltzmann distribution, relates to the population of folded, unfolded and native conformations. To come close to the real picture within a cell, of course, needs more study–some proteins need to associate into multimers to attain the biological conformation (Skolnick, et al. 1999) whereas others need chaperones to aid in folding (*ref.* the following chapter on protein folding). Several methods perform *ab initio* predictions and the CASP competitions have reported considerable rise in the number of these methods and their success rate since CASP 1. For some examples, *ref.* methods in literature (Moult, et al. 1986), (Bruccoleri, et al. 1987), etc. A more recent and "true" *ab initio* method is outlined below:

ASTRO-FOLD

Original authors: J. L. Klepeis and C. A. Floudas; Department of Chemical Engg., Princeton University, Princeton, New Jersey (USA) (Klepeis, et al. 2003).

Principle:

Stage 1: Local contacts are first modeled that will invariably result in the formation of helices in several segments of the target sequence.

Stage 2: Hydrophobic interaction modeling that would result in the evolution of β-strands that can be linked into β-sheets following the "maximal hydrophobic contact" optimization principle.

Stage 3: Further constrains are added on the system and loops are modeled.

Stage 4: Tertiary structure prediction involves the optimizations of several parameters such as the distribution of dihedral angles in the Ramachandran plot, etc.

D. Methods that use a Combination of the above Strategies for Prediction in 3D

There are several *ab initio* methods that borrow techniques from the methods of other classes, and this is because *ab initio* prediction is difficult. One of the major reasons for methods to *ref.* to information stored in the PDB is the acceleration of experimental advancements and the resultant "giant leap" in the number of solved protein targets owing to the protein structure initiative.

FRAGFOLD (Jones, 2001)

This has basically been classified as an *ab initio* approach: a method that uses information from just the sequence to predict protein structures. However, it is, as mentioned under "Prediction in 3D" introduction above, many of these methods also take the help of databases. A direct comparison of sequence of the target with sequences (in homology modeling) or structures (in fold recognition) of a database is probably not the source of decision making in *ab initio* methods. Thus, although "comparative modeling", "fold recognition" and "*ab initio*" are the 3 methods to predict structure, *FRAGFOLD is one of numerous examples that show the blurring of distinction between these approaches*. This is the reason FRAGFOLD is presented under this chapter.

Here, an outline of this method is provided to show how other strategies are interwoven. It first evaluates secondary structure formation tendencies and from that, obtains supersecondary structures. The model tertiary structure is then obtained from the overlapping description generated when all supersecondary structures have been described in the protein. It uses a simulated annealing approach to join the fragments. (Earlier version of) This method has been involved in predicting structures in CASPs. There are other methods that use fragment assembly: ROSETTA by David Baker and coworkers (Simons, et al. 1997) and Christian Sander and coworkers (Rost, et al. 1997).

Method:
   i. A multiple sequence alignment procedure obtains several homologues and aligns them with the target sequence. Supersecondary structures are preselected from the database of proteins such that they match literature descriptions and include α-hairpins, α-corners, β-hairpins, β-corners, βαβ unit and "split" βαβ units (for details *ref.* chapter 1.2 protein structures).
   ii. Then the aligned sequence as well as the target are all threaded into preselected supersecondary structures. The threading results are compared with an independent secondary structure prediction method PSIPRED (Jones, 1999) and the threading that contradicts structure prediction is discarded.

iii. From the above, a specific conformation is thus ascribed to every residue occupying a certain position in each of the supersecondary structures obtained. The generation of random conformations for the blind sequence during the conformation search process is done using these stored fragments for each residue.

iv. Every conformation of target sequence that results (using the above fragments for all involved residues) is checked for optimal arrangement of atoms. For this, the database is studied for atomic arrangements and interactions to set up a list of "optimal distances" and once this is accomplished, databases are not referred to further. These optimal distances are compiled for each pair of residues including their backbone N, Cα and C atoms as well as C$_\beta$ atoms and the generated conformation of the target is checked with respect to these values.

v. Those conformations that do not have steric violations as per the list of atomic arrangements are selected to function as the starting suggestions for conformational search. Then the various potentials present in the force field expression are optimized by their weights and the conformations generated from each run are ranked by the force field.

vi. The force field contains potentials for solvation, steric, short-range and long-range interactions, hydrogen-bonding and chain compaction. A later version removed the additional compaction potential, originally added to emphasize that only those conformations that lead to globular tertiary structure need to be searched. Therefore in the later version, the compaction was considered an implicit solvent effect.

CODA (Deane, et al.) combines FREAD (knowledge-based) and PETRA (*ab initio*).

E. Receptor Mapping (a drug design based approach to prediction)

Introduction: As mentioned earlier, the 3D structure of proteins that act as receptors for most of today's therapeutically used drugs remains unknown. Receptor mapping uses the chemical information from the various ligands (natural or drug) that bind to these receptors to build a model of the pharmacophore (the arrangement of groups of atoms on a ligand that is found to interact with a receptor; for details *ref.* chapter 2.3.2.B). This would help us determine the residues and their spatial orientation close to the binding pocket. This approach helps to refine loops and the position of secondary structures around the binding pocket.

Prerequisite information: Theoretically, an astronomical number of conformations are possible for a molecule, especially if it is as large as a drug molecule. The degree of freedom (i.e. the number of accessible conformations) is often limited by its neighbors–solvent molecules in solution, neighboring molecules of the same compound in a crystal, or the hundreds of surrounding soluble and insoluble components within a cell. But only a very small group (or ensemble) out of all of these possible conformations, interact with the receptor to elicit drug action–this ensemble is termed the biological conformation. In order to obtain the correct pharmacophoric pattern, the bioactive conformation must be studied. This is not possible without knowing the structure of the protein molecules (and to remind the reader that it is the current problem at hand-to determine this structure) and also not possible directly by experiments. The closest

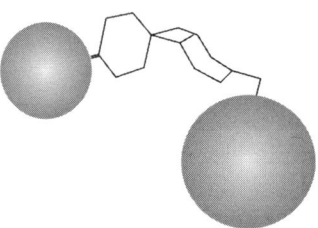

Some groups pose strong steric hindrance and can accommodate only very specific types and arrangements of proteins side chains around them.

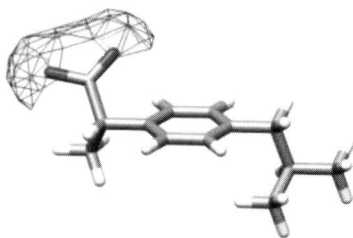

Some moieties exert strong electrostatic influence and need to be complemented by residue side chains with contrasting properties.

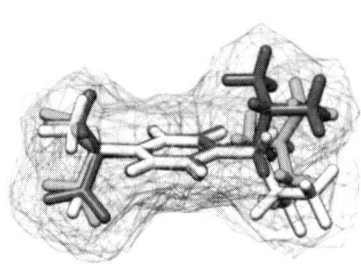

When 'circumscribing' the protein, a certain degree of flexibility must be allowed for the ligand to orient and flip around at the binding site.

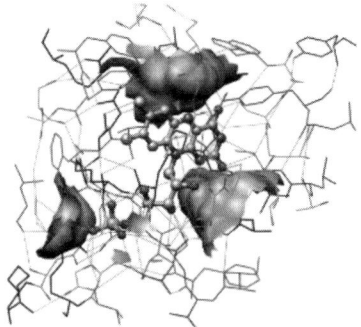

The protein (receptor) is constructed around the ligand. The predicted structure of the protein in this area can be refined.

Fig. 1.42: Schematic representation of the role of receptor mapping in structure prediction; known ligands can be used to refine the structure of a protein of unknown structure (for color version *see* Plate 1)

approach, experimentally, is to induce changes in the ligand and study its effect on receptor binding–provided the results are not complicated by pharmacokinetic effects and the biosignaling network. But, steric and electronic features of the bioactive conformation of drug molecules are needed. It is not possible to determine this bioactive conformation either from the ligand bound crystal structure of the protein, or from solution studies; reliable computational tools remain the sole option to obtain this conformation.

The following can be considered as prerequisites for mapping the binding pocket of a receptor whose sequence is known: *A class of drug candidates known to interact with the concerned receptor (ref. chapter 2.4.1 QSAR and 2.4.2 3D-QSAR) that:*

• Have distinct pharmacological pathway.
• Have a large variety of chemical structures.
• Act via the same mechanism.
• Bind to the same site.

- Have varying pharmacological potency ranging from 1 to 1000 on the relative scale.
- Have one rigid or at least semi rigid congener that can be used as a template to determine the pharmacophore (without this, the determination of the pharmacophore would require extensive statistical effort).
- Have *known* structure activity relationship.

This set is known as training set and usually contains 15 or more structures if one wants to obtain a good map of the receptor.

Steps: The following steps are performed to obtain the receptor map:

Conformational analysis to obtain the pharmacophore:
- All molecules in the training set are "searched" for all possible conformations that they can exist in.
- The search is performed by rotating about all single rotatable bonds in steps of a specific are the angle (say, 20°).
- The various conformations are checked for chemical relevance (i.e. van der Waals steric violation) and only sensible conformations are retained.
- For large molecules, a molecular dynamics simulation such as simulated annealing is undertaken to generate a set of well sampled conformations.
- The collection of conformation are analyzed and similar ones are discarded.
- From the structure activity relationship, the probable pharmacophore is marked (*ref.* chapter 2.3.2 B and chapter 2.4 for description and methodology).
- The structures are aligned by their pharmacophore and superimposed. The superposition might be manual, automatic, supplemented by energy minimization procedures, etc.

Calculating Molecular Electrostatic Potentials (MEPs)
- This is performed because drug-receptor interaction has both steric as well as electrostatic components.
- MEPs are calculated for those conformations that are found to have the correct pharmacophore arrangement from the above step.
- There are several ways to determine charge based on either topological analysis or quantum chemical analysis. These methods are detailed in Box 29 of chapter 3.2.3.A.
- Calculated charge densities are verified with experimental values such as dipole moments as reference, applicable for not-too-flexible molecules only.

Establishing Molecular Interaction Fields
In addition to the steric and electrostatic factors accounted for so far, the following properties are estimated:
- Hydrophobic areas, regions of charge transfer, H-bonding interactions, other polar interactions.

The general procedure to establish molecular interaction fields is as follows:
- Setting up a three-dimensional grid covering some region of space around the ligands
- Calculating potentials felt by a probe atom placed at the grid points from all atoms around it that it can come in contact with

- A specific probe atom is used to determine each of the above forces and appropriate formulae are used to calculate potential felt by the probe. For example, an aromatic CH probe estimates the strength of hydrophobic interactions.
- The presence of an interaction is determined within calculated limits. For example, the CH probe looks for an energy estimate of -1.5 kcal/mol as the strength of hydrophobic interactions
- Apart from accounting for a variety of interactions, similarities of ligands of different structure (that cannot be superimposed atom to atom in order to obtain a common pharmacophore) can be ascertained.

Deriving receptor maps

- Obtaining a common "field" or "contour" by comparing all pharmacophoric conformations and all probes for a certain drug family
- The (interaction) field is translated to a model of the receptor with appropriate amino acids (from the protein sequence) placed in order to fit the chemical properties demanded by the pharmacophore and probe
- The probe also helps to place the amino acids selected in their appropriate 3D positions
- The resulting model is sometimes called a pseudo receptor, as it is mainly incomplete (only the binding pocket is constructed to some extent)
- These separate pieces of information is then brought to order using sequence alignment, homology search, and structural information about the protein and the model is refined.

Validation: One of the most advantageous situations is when extensive experimental study has been done. As a selected number of rigid structures among all experimentally studied drug candidates are used for setting up the hypothetical receptor, its validity can be tested on the other drug candidates. If the theoretical model is able to calculate or atleast relatively rank the binding affinities of the various candidates correctly, then the 3D structure of the binding pocket has effectively been captured.

1.4.4 LOOP MODELING

As mentioned so far, the core-structures and the secondary-structures are known to be most conserved among proteins that resemble each other structurally despite being distantly related by sequence identity. Therefore, loops, especially the ones on the surface, are particularly difficult to model owing to their flexibility. However, these regions can never be ignored as they are by-far the most important segments involved in ligand **interaction** [ATP (Saraste, et al. 1990), NAD(P) (Wierenga, et al. 1986), calcium binding sites (Kawasaki, et al. 1995)] and **recognition** [antibody complement determining regions (Kim, et al. 1999), DNA binding (Tainer, et al. 1995)]. The characteristics of loops and their relevance to structure have been amply elaborated under chapter 1.2 and it was mentioned how function is characterized by structural differences of loop regions on the protein surface. It is evident that further application of built proteins to explore drug binding and pharmacological pathways is dependent upon the accuracy of loop modeling (Fernandez-Fuentes, et al. 2006).

A. *Ab Initio* Loop Modeling

This method involves connecting secondary structures by loops modeled using first principles that utilizing information on surrounding secondary structures and the core built so far. The sequence of the loop region is subjected to a conformational search. This is guided by a scoring function that calculates conformational energy. Some methods use Molecular Dynamics Simulations in addition (Fiser, et al. 2000) whereas others use a force-field to guide conformation analysis (Xiang, et al. 2002) The scoring function ranks loops prioritizing them primarily by energy, and in some methods, combined with additional parameters [such as in reference (Xiang, et al. 2002)] wherein r.m.s (root mean square) deviation of the first and last residue from the flanking residues of secondary structures is derived. It is a practice to break up a loop into fragments based on the frequency of their occurrence in the dataset and collect a set of "template" structures. These templates can be used to build loops (Offmann, et al. 2007). Already existing force fields are also employed to perform the ranking (*ref.* scoring functions discussed in part III chapter 3.2.3.B). The approaches used in these methods again deal with energy minimizations, conformational searches, efficiency of sampling the global minimum, correspondence of the global minimum to the native conformation, the use of force fields, etc that are common in protein folding investigations. Consequently, with sufficient conformational sampling, it has been shown that a loop structure close to the native state structure can be obtained.

B. Knowledge-based Loop Modeling

Knowledge-based methods are also known as database search or fragment search approaches. They collect and store all kinds of information about the surroundings of a loop of a particular conformation in proteins. As with any knowledge based approach, it is believed that the popularity of a certain structure is because it is optimal for the given surroundings. Databases aim to find out the presence of correlation between the stored environment and loop conformation. As the search for basis structures has already lead to using up homologous proteins from the database, the process of loop fragment searching strictly goes by the environmental information such as the flanking secondary structures, the amino acid sequence, the solvent exposure, the physicochemical properties of the residue side chains, etc. The conformation of the loop has been demonstrated to be strongly influenced by that of the residues that need to be connected by the loop. This is understandable, as the reverse–that loops are strongly influenced by the conformation of flanking secondary structures–has been discussed under chapter 1.2 on protein structure.

Example: SEARCH SPACE database

This method is presented here as an example to show how "knowledge" is accumulated, organized, retrieved and applied.

Authors: Narcis Fernandez-Fuentes, Baldomero Oliva*, András Fiser; Albert Einstein College of Medicine, New York, US; *Universitat Pompeu Fabra, Barcelona, Spain. (Fernandez-Fuentes, et al., 2006)

Purpose: Authors opine that the major limiting factor in *ab-initio* approaches, apart from the problem of sampling the global minimum and setting up a scoring function, is setting up an energy function that ranks the native conformation as the "best" among a generated set. Therefore, a knowledge based approach is used.

Method summary: All possible loop conformations in between α-helices and β-strands (these secondary structures are as defined by DSSP) in all protein structures are collected in the Search Space database. Out of these, loops that are incomplete (don't have backbone or C_β atoms) or that have high crystallographic B-factors (this indicates that the segment is flexible, and as discussed earlier, is calculated as an average for loop residues) are eliminated. With a search method that ranks appropriate loop candidates based on several parameters (length of the loop, the type of secondary structures that span the query loop) and by the geometry of the stem using various descriptions (distance between the anchor points, the hoist angle, packing angle and meridian angle). The best loops are prioritized. These loops are then transplanted into the protein and are eliminated if they produce high rms deviation at the stems, steric clashes for distance smaller than the 70% of the sum of the respective van der Waals radii (Tsai, et al. 1999), etc. The loops thus selected are then ranked by a tailor-made scoring function that compiles suitability by calculating the combined effect of sequence score, conformational similarity, main-chain dihedral angle propensities score, etc. in the form of Z-scores. Through these Z-scores, authors keep track of the performance of this knowledge-based method.

Database organization: The Search Space database is organized into 3 levels, narrowing down progressively from the type of the flanking secondary structures (helices, beta strands), through loop length (1, 2, 3 residues, ...) as determined by DSSP assignment, to the geometric criteria (described above). For proteins that do not have well characterized secondary structures, the parameters used are the distances between the end points that need to be connected, and van der Waal's radii.

C. Combination of Both

The disadvantage of *ab initio* methods is in the large number of conformations that need to be generated as an effort to sample the native state. If a database search can provide starting "suggestion" conformations so that search for the native structure does not require generation of astronomical number of random structures, there will be considerably less floundering around the confomational space. The method will also not be "messy" as sometimes happens with knowledge-based modeling wherein segments cut-and-paste from proteins that differ in domains, experimental method used to analyze it in the cell, resolution and refinement at which it has been deposited in the PDB, organism species from which isolated, etc. need to be extensively refined in the end. Loop regions selected from the database are inserted and re-optimized in the model protein. For examples *ref.* (Martin, et al. 1989). CODA (above) has also been used for loop modeling, so have Hidden Markov Models (Fernandez-Fuentes, et al. 2005). For the latter, the ArchDB database (Espadaler, et al. 2004) was used as the source of fragments.

1.4.5 COMPLETING THE PROTEIN

By now, readers must be quite familiar with the size of proteins which is why they are simplified to a set of pseudo-atoms. Structure is compared and assessed by these few points along the protein chain. Whatever the advantages of such representations, a collection of these points does not become the protein itself–after all, the simplification is only theoretical–and all the atoms must be completely arranged to call the biomolecule "a protein". A number of works aim to restore the full coordinates of proteins with the availability of part of this information. The need to "add" side chains to the backbone, or to add other backbone atoms first and then to add side chains, is encountered in several situations such as X-ray crystallographic or NMR determination of protein structure (as mentioned at the very beginning, in chapter 1.1), or here, in structure prediction.

It is well known that other than a cis-trans isomerization, there is not much else for the peptide linkage to do in order to generate diversity in atomic arrangement. Side chain conformations tend to exist in a limited number of rotamers which are dependent on the local environmental features like secondary structure, solvent accessibility and hydrogen bonding [(Tuffery, et al. 1997), (Schrauber, et al. 1993)]. Another method (Liwo, et al., 1993) completes the backbone atoms with the availability of $C\alpha$ atoms by arranging all N, H, C and O to produce the largest hydrogen bonded network (by matching peptide-group dipoles).

The addition of side chains can be done in several ways. One such method called MaxSprout (Holm, et al. 1991) involves the scanning of a database of protein structures for segments that satisfy the available backbone geometry information (for completing the backbone with the availability of just the C_{α} atom positions) and fitting the respective atoms. For arranging side chains, a "*side-chain rotamer library*" is referred from which chosen side chains fitted to the backbone using a simulated annealing procedure. In another method, (Bower, et al. 1997) that locates, from a rotamer library, a small number of appropriate conformations for the side chains, that can be further narrowed down by investigating steric hindrances after placing one conformer of each residue in the segment to be completed. Predictive accuracy was shown not to be limited to native backbone conformations but even to structures that can be theoretically generated. Although it has been reported that rotamers included in libraries give rise to fundamental Van der Waals clashes (Lovell, et al. 2000) structure refining to remove such clashes has shown to result in less errors (Bower, et al. 1997). Yet another method uses potentials of mean force to align peptide groups around the C_{α} atoms (Payne, 1993). At any rate, loop closure and side chain addition are major problems [(Tosatto, et al. 2002), (Xiang, et al. 2002)].

1.4.6 ASSESSMENT OF MODEL QUALITY

As mentioned earlier in different scenarios, the selection of and ranking of generated conformations such that the native structure is assigned the "best" model is the current challenge in structure prediction methods. Specialized programs are available for this purpose and, since CAFASP 4, are called "Model Quality Assessment Programs" if they are able to assess quality of a structure (and give a score) without the need for comparison with other conformations.

Quality assessment can be done in several ways. Some methods simply use a force-field potential to calculate energy of conformations to rank them from best to worst [(Sippl, et al. 2008), (Lazaridis, et al. 2000)]. Others check whether the distribution of φ-ψ values in the protein follows an "acceptable" pattern as found in high-resolution X-ray structures in the database (Laskowski, et al. 1996), (Hooft, et al. 1996) and these methods are used to correct errors in modeled proteins. Yet others cluster conformations and pull out the most appropriate model from the clusters. Or obtain consensus of several programs that check quality in various ways (Wallner, et al., 2003). MODCHECK (Pettitt, et al. 2005) and ProQ (Wallner, et al. 2003) are "true" MQAP methods (McGuffin, 2007). Despite all this, it is a widely accepted statement that there is no program that can select the best model in its resemblance to the native structure in a clear and unambiguous way [(Fischer, 2006), (McGuffin, 2007)].

1.4.7 DOMAIN BOUNDARY PREDICTION

Domain boundary prediction is an important step in both experimental and computational protein structure characterization. A domain is an independently folding unit and has been associated with the functionality of the protein. The determination of whether there is more than one domain, and for multidomain structures, prediction of the domain boundaries (given that a domain can be made up of one continuous segment of the polypeptide chain or several parts of the chain folding in and out) is principal–both in terms of applicability as well as the difficulty of the problem. For methods that predict all the possible secondary structures (composite structure prediction methods) successfully, their relative arrangements need to be correct to obtain the right fold and then the right domain boundaries. This can be imagined as resulting from two approaches that lead to the complete picture: the correct prediction of loops and the correct prediction of long-range contacts. These are two interdependent approaches separated for easy understanding and lead to one and the same result. If loops are accurately modeled independent of other parts, then automatically, the relative arrangements of secondary structures will fall correctly in place. The vice versa approach is when the relative arrangements of secondary structures are arrived at and then the interconnecting loops are brought to the optimum conformation. Tertiary structure prediction methods often work both ways. Sequence insertions also may occur at the domain boundaries making modeling more difficult than it already is because the template built by homology modeling and fold recognition may lose relevance. Two domain boundary prediction methods developed by the same group (Kim, et al. 2005) are outlined below wherein Ginzu is knowledge based and RosettaDOM is *ab initio*.

A. Knowledge based

Ginzu is a homologous sequence alignment based method that detects domains and computes their boundaries. It includes 2 protocols–a "template-based" and a "*de novo*" and is a part of the Robetta automated structure prediction server. It works in stages, stage 1 involving generation of sequence alignments by obtaining a consensus of several programs BLAST, PSI-BLAST, FFAS03 and 3D-Jury. From the matches obtained, Ginzu takes analysis to stage 2, wherein using Hidden Markov model based pattern recognition procedures, the PFAM database (Bateman, et al. 2002), containing information on the various protein sequences and their familial relations, is scrutinized. This stage results in suggestions for domain boundaries. Segments of the blind sequence that do not find counterparts in stage 1 or that are not assigned to domains in stage 2 are tentatively treated as linkers of domains. If these segments are 50 residues or longer, then in stage 3, they are BLASTed against the NCBI (http://blast.ncbi.nlm.nih.gov/Blast.cgi) non-redundant database of sequences for a final round of domain assignments (this is done by a program called "msa2domains" signifying that multiple sequence alignments–MSA–are converted to domain assignment information). Stage 4 involves deciding on "cut preferences"–deciding where to place the boundaries for domains–which involves combined analysis using several independent methods such as loop prediction by PSIPRED (Jones, 1999), assessment of distances, the ends of cluster obtained in stage 3, inclusion of a domain definitions (Taylor, 1999) as mentioned above, under chapter 1.2, etc complemented by *de novo* domain prediction by Ginzu from the clusters after MSA against PFAM database. Thus domains are suggested and refined iteratively (*meaning, in several successive steps*) obtaining a consensus assignment (the template-based part) and comparing it with self-generated domain delineation (the *de novo* part).

B. Ab Initio

Rosetta-DOM is an *ab initio* method and uses the query sequence only to predict domains and boundaries. Some 400 3D structure predictions are made and from these, the 200 most meaningful structures are selected. The domain among these 200 structures is defined (Taylor, 1999). A consensus boundary is obtained by looking for the most frequently occurring patterns and weighting these assignments. Additional parameters such as length of residues in domains are used to "smooth and polish" the predictions. Authors report the predictions to be "quite good" for a *de novo* prediction method. Ginzu's prediction is used when sequence alignments are possible and RosettaDOM in cases of low sequence similarity detection by Ginzu (*stage 1*: using BLAST, PSI-BLAST, FFAS03).

1.4.8 PROTEOMICS ROADMAP TO MEDICINAL CHEMISTRY–3

The student need not have any hesitation on whether familiarizing with the principles of protein structure prediction would benefit them as a medicinal chemist.

- In 1986, a comprehensive review reported less than 500 protein targets as being available for the the drugs of that time (Swindells, et al. 2002). There are 1,894 pharmaceutically relevant targets (listed in the Therapeutic Target Database at http://bidd.nus.edu.sg/group/cjttd/TTD_HOME.asp) as of March 2010. Out of this list, only a small subset of proteins has their structures determined experimentally.

- Making the model more reliable implies that the predicted model can be used in high throughput screening of combinatorial virtual libraries of drug candidates (*ref.* chapter 2.3.2.A2 *virtual library* in part II).
- Contact prediction is valuable in refining the non-bonded interactions in the protein. The better the non-bonded long-distance interactions and contacts are predicted, the better is the overall accuracy of prediction of protein structure.
- Non-bonded interactions are important to obtain the right tertiary structure of the protein. Tertiary structure dictates quaternary assembly of the protein and its biological function. The changes induced in protein conformation/properties due to the environment are key to the design of new ligands.
- Principles or "rules" that are obtained from attempts to reconstruct the 3D structure of the protein just from amino acid sequence follows the biological formation and function of proteins. Artificial proteins can be made that catalyze specific reactions following the mechanism of action of enzymes.
- The availability of the structure of many more biological from predictions targets makes the screening for new lead compounds more thorough.
- Knowledge of the behavior of proteins gives us a chance to modify natural proteins such as those of bacteria, viruses, prions (infectious protein particles), misfolded proteins that lead to precipitation in alzheimers or systemic amyloids, etc.

Bibliography

Recommended references: Proteins: Structures and molecular properties (Creighton, 1993); *Bioinformatics (Baxevanis and Ouellette)* Chapter 8 (Ofran, et al., 2005), chapter 9 (Wishart, 2005), chapter 12 (Barton, 2005); *Introduction to Protein Structure* (Branden, et al., 1999)

Websites

- Critical Assessment of protein Fold Prediction (CASP) http://predictioncenter.org/
- EVA (real-time continuous evaluation of protein fold prediction methods) http://cubic.bioc.columbia.edu/eva/
- SWISS-MODEL repository (Kopp, et al., 2004): contains 300,000 automated 3D homology models for sequences from Swiss-Prot and TrEMBL databases at http://swissmodel.expasy.org/repository
- Therapeutic Targets Database from national University of Singapore, at http://bidd.nus.edu.sg/group/cjttd/TTD_HOME.asp

1.5 *The Protein Folding Problem*

Now what form, Proteus? And how do thee manage it?

"'If everybody minded their own business,' the Duchess said,
in a hoarse growl, 'the world would go around a great deal faster than it does.'"

In "Through the Looking Glass", by Lewis Carroll

ORIGIN

The work of Christian Anfinsen and coworkers, in 1957, showed that an isolated protein sequence could fold into its native (local as well as global tertiary) structure independent of biological machinery guided only by physicochemical factors [(Anfinsen, et al. 1961), (Anfinsen, 1973)].

> **Did You Know? 6**
> **Anfinsen's experiments**
>
> *Anfinsen and coworkers experimented with ribonuclease, a 124 amino acid long enzyme. Its role is to cleave improper and "waste" RNA molecules. The binding with the RNA molecule results in the formation of two disulfide linkages that stabilizes tertiary structure of the protein. Although this was not known when Anfinsen performed his historical experiment, what he observed was that ribonuclease, when placed in denaturing solution, lost its 3D structure and when under renaturing conditions, gained it back. Removal of 2 mercapto ethanol (used to break the disulfide bonds of his enzyme) in the continued presence of denaturant urea brought back 1% activity. For his research, Anfinsen received the Nobel Prize in Chemistry in 1972.*

Since then it is known that certain globular proteins denatured by heat, extreme pH or certain chemical agents will regain native structure and biological activity if returned to conditions in which their native conformations are stable (in other words, if renatured). The native conformational states of proteins may usually be unfolded reversibly by adding denaturants, increasing or decreasing the temperature, varying the pH, applying high pressure, or cleaving disulphide bonds. The structure of the DNA was determined by Rosalind Franklin using X-ray crystallography technique (in 1952, on which Watson and Crick modeled the DNA structure in 1953) to be a simple double helix throughout. But a protein (the sperm whale Myoglobin), as determined by Max Perutz and Kendrew (Kendrew, *et al.* 1958) using the same technique, was found to be much more complicated in structure. Such a complex shape self-folding without any external help is indeed remarkable. Anfinsen *et al.* also calculated that the 8 cystines of ribonuclease could form up to 4 disulfide bonds in 105 ways. However, they observed that this happened only on urea denaturation of ribonuclease. After renaturation or spontaneous folding, only the native disulfide bridge pattern prevailed.

REVERSIBILITY

Another point to note–folding was observed to be reversible. This means each time the native structure is disturbed through denaturation there is a sure way the protein will regain it—indicating the presence of a thermodynamic bias or slope towards the native structure in conformational space. The presence of this "slope" is interpreted as follows: the native state IS the lowest energy conformation of a protein wherein all atoms are arranged in the most advantageous way in terms of interactions and any other conformation is not as stable as the native one under biological conditions. Only if this is true, the protein will find the native structure in a cell as 'hands-free cycling' downhill. Also, it is clear that the native structure is at the global minimum–that is, there could be several other conformations at various energy minima (called local minima) but not as low in energy as the native structure (the global minimum) (*ref. section 2.3.2.F*). It would be appropriate to think of the first inference from *Anfinsen's dogma* at this point—that this global minimum is achieved *per se* by the amino acid sequence without external biological help (that too, when protein structure is not a simple repetitive double helix). Research in this field has fascinated generations of scientists from all fields and is fondly called "*the protein folding problem*". We believe that this introduction highlights the strong interconnectivity among the various schools of thought on proteins and their behavior. Typically, one starts to answer a particular question, in turn generating several others and in an attempt to answer all those, ends with the original question. There is nothing discouraging about this–because during the answering process, a lot of information is generated.

THE PROBLEM

"The protein folding problem" is considered as one of most important bottlenecks in molecular biology (*ref.* Did you know). This fundamental problem has come to be known as the **Levinthal's paradox**. Cyrus Levinthal, in 1968 stated that if folding was a random process and a protein sampling each possible conformation in the shortest possible time (10^{-13} seconds: the time required for a single molecular vibration) would take 10^{77} years to sample all possible confirmations. However, a protein folds within seconds.

Box 7: The Levinthal's Paradox

Quoting, (Levinthal, 1968): "On the one hand, the existence of renaturation suggests that the native state is thermodynamically the most stable state under `biological' conditions. On the other hand, a chain has zillions of possible conformations ($\sim 2^{100}$ for a 100-residue chain, since at least two conformations are possible for each residue). Thus, the chain needs at least $\sim 2^{100}$ ps, or $\sim 10^{10}$ years to sample them all and to find the most stable fold. Then, how can the chain find its most stable structure within a `biological' time (less than minutes)?"

WHAT ARE SCIENTISTS LOOKING FOR?

As under section 1.4 on protein structure prediction, the overall problem was divided into two parts, one–of predicting the final structure, and the other–of folding, which is deriving the thermodynamic preference. The folding problem can be further analyzed thus: What is the physicochemical reason for the folded state to be most stable? Why is it that a sequence chooses the same native state each time? Given that unfolded state is more or less random, but still manages to 'wander on time into the folding pathway', what is the kinetics of this 'conformational rearrangement reaction'? Is there a rate limiting step, a transition structure, an intermediate like other chemical reactions and how do all these look? Do all, proteins independent of their class and topology, follow the same pathway? To sum it all up, *what is the mechanism of protein folding?* Most of the theories and observations obtained in attempts to predict structure (secondary and higher) from sequence form the foundation of understanding and modeling the physical and chemical interactions involved in protein folding. Once the covalently bonded sequence is available, all the different shapes and geometries taken up by the macromolecule are simply conformations–single bonds of the backbone and side chains rotated by varying degrees (except disulphide linkages, of course, which are covalent in nature).

APPROACHES

Predicting structure is based on either statistical or physical approaches. However these are not totally independent approaches. A protein is a huge molecule and its native structure is not just one single conformation as rigid as the hard plastic ball-and-stick models that we make from a model kit. There is always an ensemble of equivalent conformational states populating the unfolded, partly folded and native states.

Table 1.9: Approaches to obtain structure from sequence

Statistical approaches	Physical methods
• Knowledge-based: studies databases of existing structures	Derives rules to calculate the energy of a protein fold in various conformations
• Searches for rules based on the preferences of certain residues to form certain secondary structures	The energetically most favorable among all possible conformations can then be identified

IN THE CELL

The 3D scaffold of proteins, in addition to being formed by the folding process, must also be kept in position. The cell must therefore provide for not only the synthesis and fomation of protein structure, but also for the protein to maintain itself amidst the hustle-bustle of the cellular environment. An inquisitive student now thinks: Is the native fold uniformly stable (throughout the macromolecule) or are there parts of the protein such as the ligand binding site that are more stable than the rest? Is the answer the same for all the variety of folds in nature that we encountered among receptors, hormones, enzymes, etc. in chapter 1.2? Do receptors and enzymes differ in any way on this point? The Levinthal's paradox shows how protein folding is not random process and is driven by physical and chemical phenomena. Therefore, spontaneous (re)folding must follow a pathway; folding is not random since most proteins fold in 10^{-1}–10^3 seconds (Creamer, et al. 1994). So what drives folding? There are several theories, universally founded on the fact that the fully folded state is only about 20 kcal/mol more stable than other conformations (*ref.* Fig. 1.30A in section 1.2.1.E and its corresponding text). The chance for a protein to reach its folded state does not appear in front of it like a race track where it can fold in one straight sprint heading right for the fully folded conformer (for a more scientific and detailed view of this discussion *ref.* (Dill, et al. 2008) and its references).

HOW STRONG IS A PROTEIN'S FOLD?

From the results of the *Paracelsus challenge* (*ref.* section 1.4) and experimental data (distributed all through this section) it is clear that every amino acid along the entire sequence of a protein need not be conserved to generate the same fold. Substitutions spread out over the entire protein was found not to change rate of folding significantly for the same native structure (Dill, et al. 2008). Mutations in the form of deletions, insertions and substitutions that might change as much as 70% of residues most of the time (and as much as 90% in some cases) still do not affect the final fold of the protein. This suggests the presence of key residues in determining the native fold (maintaining 3D structure of the protein) and function (residues on the surface that interact with ligands) that are conserved (Scheerlinck, et al. 1992). It is a well known fact that folding occurs co-translationally in the cell – meaning a protein folds as it is being synthesized (i.e. even before its synthesis is complete). Two events followed:

1. Before Anfinsen's experiment, folding was thought to be induced by the ribosome
2. From the above, a theory followed that folding proceeds from the N- to the C- terminus.
3. Experiments performed later showed how folding was not necessarily directional
4. It was also demonstrated that the termini of a protein were not important to drive the folding process

Theories are constantly being updated to keep in par with experimental and theoretical results.

"I used to believe in forever . . . but forever was too good to be true."

Winnie the Pooh in "Winnie the Pooh", by A.A.Milne

THE POTENTIAL ENERGY DIAGRAM FOR PROTEIN'S CONFORMATIONS

Notwithstanding these observations, the fact that protein folding does not follow a *pathway* but more a *surface* is well known–a simple reason is that there are an astronomical number of unfolded conformations. With so many different "reactant" structures, it is not possible for all of them to follow the exact same pathway from start to finish. Secondly, protein folding is a process that represents massive arrangement and rearrangement within one configuration, rather than one reactant structure becoming a product structure.

The formation of certain contacts within the huge macromolecule becomes favorable for the overall folding process and this greatly reduces entropy as folding proceeds to completion. However, it is also clear from the above studies and more discussions to follow, that somewhere along the folding path, these various starting points begin to converge and hence exhibit common behavior (in terms of kinetics, thermodynamics, transition state characteristics, Intermediates, etc).

All the worlds a cell... and the proteins in it, the actors and actresses!

Despite the extensive research and modeling of the protein folding process and enormous amount of information from both the experimental and theoretical fields that have led to the derivation of several useful theories, protein folding remains an enigma. One of the fundamental reasons this knot exists and cannot be resolved is the complexity of biological systems. Even if a detailed mechanistic description of the folding process is established, it can be evaluated only in the "gas-phase" or probably in a bed of water molecules. Simulating protein folding by imposing on it the interactions and environment of a cell remains a fantasy; there is no current technique that can handle the thermodynamics and entropy of the protein's "home". For instance, biological selection of sequences and the way this modulates kinetics and thermodynamics is very complex. As rightly pointed out (Onuchic, et al. 1997), "organisms exist at different temperatures (the pig around 300K and the methanococcus at 350 K) and this leads to a big difference", even in simple systems such as a cluster of water molecules.

The protein folding surface (the conformational space of a protein—the free energy landscape discussed later in this section) is not always the same. Some proteins are fast folders and have just one minimum–the global minimum–and it is a "dream come true" for protein folders when such a surface is encountered.

Did You Know? 7

The quest for fast folders among biological proteins is a hugely debated topic and has elicited a flurry of research activities-both experimental and theoretical, as reviewed (Dill, et al. 2008).

In light of the shape of potential energy surface:

Box 8: On protein surfaces

"(If the surface had just one minimum)...Then protein folding would be a very enjoyable process indeed. The native fold would be easy defined by rolling down the energy surface until we hit the ground. Such a function has a built in global minimum...

At the other extreme there is the nightmare of a function shaped like an egg box with an enormous number of local minima, all of roughly the same depth as the global minimum. Imagine stumbling around blindly on such a rough surface, with no idea where to go. One might even stand on the global minimum without recognizing it, continuing an aimless search..." (Dill, et al. 2008)

Literature records that the protein's conformational space (containing all the number of conformations accessible to a polypeptide chain) is also limited by "the purpose" for which the protein exists; the less-than-infinite number of conformations searched by a chain before it folds (the folding pathway) is "inherited" by evolution (*ref.* Scheme 1.13: convergence and divergence in protein evolution in section 1.2.1 and Scheme 1.25 in section 1.5.9 on nature's selection of sequences). In other words, proteins have their own conformational spaces which they 'inherit' from the DNA in the form of its amino acid sequence! One does begin to wonder that probably, the existence of such complicated energy functions (the energy function is the mathematical expression of the free energy surface shape) among some proteins serves some so far unknown purposes which can be better exploited for drug design.

1.5.1 STRUCTURAL RELEVANCE TO FOLDING

Some general points in the relation between structure, sequence and function from these various sections of part I so far are presented here (note how some examples in nature lead to the derivation of contradictory statements)

Table 1.10: Some structure-sequence lessons from nature

Observations	Inferences
There are 515,203 known sequences (http:www.expasy.ch/sprot/) as of March, 2010 There are 1393 known folds in the PDB as of 2010 by SCOP (Murzin, et al., 1995) classification	Multiple sequences can form the same 3D
Proteins with non-homologous sequence usually have different native state structures Sequences that differ by ~ 50 % or so (Discussion 1.8: The Paracelsus Challenge) have completely different secondary structure compositions	Similar sequences have similar structure; different sequences lead to different structures (the question "how different?" remains)
The same proteins occurring in different species that have the same native structure and perform the same function can have low sequence similarities. For example, adenylate kinase in pig and in bacteria are only 20% similar	Different sequences can also lead to similar 3D structures
Residues with non polar side-chains towards the interior and hydrophilic sidechains at the surface are often conserved within the same homologous superfamily (Perutz, et al., 1965)	One must look for patterns in amino acids that possess similar properties, than look for patterns of distribution of a particular residue itself
"Certainly no protein is known to adopt alternative fully folded conformations. A protein invariably has the same three dimensional conformation, differing only in surface side-chains and loops, when crystallized in different ways and into different crystal lattices" (Creighton, 1990)	There is one and only one fully folded native state for a sequence of amino acids in biological conditions

The theory that can satisfy all of the above observations: There are some important residues (referred to as *key residues*) that are responsible for a protein to assume a certain structure. Disturbing these will change the native fold; conserving these will conserve the native fold. It is not sequence similarity as an overall percentage, that one must look at.

As discussed under protein dynamics, the atoms in a protein are under constant motion and interaction. It is this that gets the protein to fold in the first place. Some basic points related to this motion are in Table 1.11.

Table 1.11: Some structure-sequence lessons from computations	
Observations	*Inferences*
A folded protein is not a rigid structure like a piece of furniture that has been assembled and nailed together. It is flexible to some extent. "Even in the interior of proteins, most tyrosine and phenylalanine side-chain aromatic rings are flipping by 180° on the millisecond time-scale" (Boyer, et al., 2008)	There is always a collection or "ensemble" of conformations (*ref.* Discussion 1.7) located around the equilibrium.
The flexibility of a folded protein is not as great as that of the unfolded one	The unfolded state ensemble is much larger than the folded state ensemble
Some loops have no energetically favored conformation	The degree of flexibility influences folding and unfolding mechanism
Folding–unfolding activity is known to be greatest at the surface	Solvent interaction, enzyme activity, interaction with other proteins, etc. are causes for such activity
The overall 3D structure–at the teritiary level is known not to deviate too much from that determined by X-ray crystallography or by NMR methods (Phillips, et al. 1995)	
There are difficulties in delineating domain boundaries (chapter 1.2 on protein structure and chapter 1.4 on structure prediction	Domains are known to move and breathe (chapter 1.3 on dynamics)
The third type of protein motion in Table 1.8 under chapter 1.3 involves massive movements of about 10 residues or more at a time, over relatively long distances	This is defined as "flexibility"

1.5.2 BASIC TERMINOLOGY

> *I have seen a cat without a grin...but a grin without a cat!*
> *It's the most curious thing I ever saw in all my life!"*
> *Alice, in Lewis Carroll's Alice's Adventures in Wonderland.*

Complicated phenomena that are not based on (or cannot be explained using) the simpler and more fundamental ones that we learn in school and college are a good example of superstition, those that we really need to be cautious about. Definitions of some fundamental terms are refreshed in this section; readers are requested to *ref.* standard textbooks (Creighton, 1990), (Leach, 1997), etc. for details.

a. *Native state:* The preferred folded conformation of a protein in a certain condition; the native state of a protein in gas phase, in solvent, in biological environment, etc. are similar but not necessarily identical. One always refers to a group or an ensemble of conformations even in each environment.

b. *Transition state:* The structure occurring at the highest free energy point along the pathway; saddle point (*ref.* 2.3.2.F on *reactions*); the TS generally cannot be isolated because it is very transient (very unstable) owing to its very high energy content

c. *Intermediate:* A structure occurring at an energy minimum of higher energy (yes, it is still a minimum on the PE curve) than reactant or products and lying in the path connecting the two species; it can be isolated experimentally depending on conditions

d. *Heat capacity:* The changes in the protein that take place at constant pressure; the measure indicates how sensitive or rigid a protein's native fold is in terms of energy. Heat capacity has several definitions and usages (Prabhu, et al. 2005).

1.5.3 STAGES IN FOLDING

This section outlines some stages in protein folding and also explains some evolution and background behind these conclusions that correspond to the observations. These observations are obtained generally from experiments; more recently, with the advent of strong simulation techniques, theoretical investigations also give considerable insights to mechanisms (compare Figs 1.43 and 1.44).

A. The 'Ideal' Unfolded State

A "completely unfolded" protein is ideally one in which every residue is free to assume any conformation independent of other residues [of course, (1) without violating basic interaction rules such as van der Waals steric repulsion, and (2) without breaking covalent bonding]. This state is termed a "random coil" and is easy to imagine the sense in which this descriptor was used for loops that were difficult to classify (under section 1.1, secondary structures). The ensemble that is taken up by the protein complying to the above conditions have comparable free energies as there is no structure that is particularly favored (*ref.* Fig. 1.43). A bias is generated only when stable, advantageous interactions are encountered and this does not happen in the random coil state.

B. The Unfolded State with a Bias

Proteins denatured by some chemical agents are known to have TRULY random coiled structures. However, for other denaturants such as extremes of pH or temperature (in

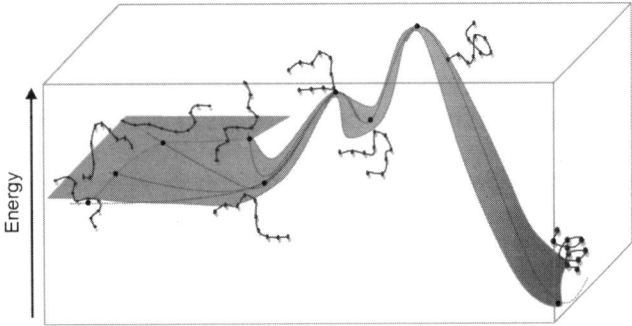

Fig. 1.43: The potential energy diagram of a protein in not a 2D curve

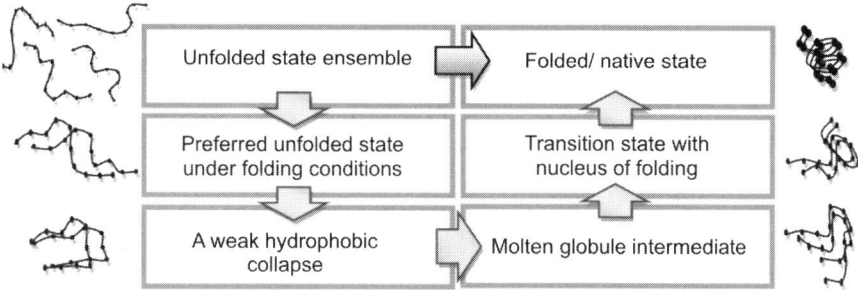

Fig. 1.44: Stages of folding: a hypothetical schematic overview

the absence of chemical denaturants), there appears to be BIAS in the randomness (there is not a TRUE randomness in structure). A protein is made up of residues of different properties whereas the medium surrounding the protein is uniform in its chemical properties (whether pH, polarity, temperature, or any other). In these conditions protein residues do not behave in the same way–some residues repel water and this repulsion *is not cancelled* by the solvation of certain others; repulsion in that residue still prevails and that residue will not be exposed to a hydrophilic environment. Similarly, solvation of the other residue also prevails and it will prefer to remain on the surface. The partitioning becomes unavoidable even if denaturing conditions are strong and there will be less disorder or randomness than in the *ideal* unfolded state. We saw that there is no structural bias in the ideal unfolded state → this is maximum possible disorder and can be achieved only in absence of solvent, i.e. gas phase. At any rate, the unfolded state (whether ideal or real) is capable of accessing a large number of conformations–at any instant of time an experimental solution of unfolded protein would not contain two molecules in identical conformation.

Box 9: The excluded volume effect

The ideal unfolded state itself is not totally random:

1. Its residues are covalently linked reducing their degree of freedom unless very high energy is pumped into the molecule.
2. One atom in a protein cannot enter the van der Waals radius of another.
3. Possibility of steric repulsion excludes several conformations from this ensemble of structures (this repulsion operates between immediate neighbors in the sequence as well as residues far apart in the primary structure that can come in close proximity in 3D space due to folding).

The three of the above reasons lead to the excluded volume effect – not all conformations are possible for a protein. So even theoretically, the number of conformations that a random coil can assume is not infinite.

C. The Molten Globule

The term "molten globule" is often used to describe the structure that is formed somewhere midway during the reversible transition between the folded and unfolded states of a protein. It is sometimes considered to be the transition state and sometimes regarded as being an intermediate (Onuchic, et al. 1997), (Abkevich, et al. 1994). This state can be compared and contrasted with the unfolded and the native states in the following ways:

- Unlike most other conformations, a folding protein spends relatively more time in the molten globule form owing to its relatively greater stability.
- The stability is much less than the native state but greater than other transient conformations.
- In shape, it is approximately globular. A long rope wound into a ball indicates compaction – the tighter the ball, the more it resembles a sphere. The molten globule is roughly spherical and reflects the much greater compaction achieved compared to the unfolded state.
- By volume, it is larger than the native state.
- Its energy content (enthalpy) is closer to the energy of the unfolded ensemble than to the energy of the native state.
- However, its secondary structure composition and some of its long range contacts resembles that of the native state.
- A cross section of the molten globule will not show clear distinction into a hydrophobic core and hydrophilic exterior (i.e. the protein's environment is not asymmetric). Almost all atoms in the molten globule are found to interact with the solvent.
- The molten globule rapidly transforms into the fully *unfolded* state and back without cooperativity (*ref.* section 1.5.4.B), but interconversion with the fully *folded* state is slow and co-operative (section 1.5.4.B).

> *"'I don't see much sense in that,' said Rabbit. 'No,' said Pooh humbly, 'there isn't.*
> *But there was going to be when I began it. It's just that something happened to it along the way.'"*
> *By Winnie the Pooh in "Winnie the Pooh", by Milne*

D. The Intermediate

The homogeneous molten globule is not found to be the most favored conformation in some proteins. It has been observed (Efimov, 1993) that in some proteins, the asymmetric structure with a small hydrophobic core, is preferred. Some authors therefore use the term 'compact intermediate' to denote these structures (Fink, 1995) and consider them to be the *preferred subset of unfolded protein structures* when placed under conditions that favor folding (conditions in which proteins are placed could favor folding, unfolding or equilibrium. Biological conditions of pH and temperature are found to strongly favor folding). As mentioned above (under 'molten globule'), partially-folded "passing-through" conformations are energetically unstable under all conditions relative to either the unfolded or native states. The folding intermediates of homologous (same-family) proteins have similar structures and yet can differ in other properties such as relative stability. For examples, hen egg-white lysozyme and α-lactalbumin are homologues. The intermediate state of the former is known to be stable under a variety of conditions, but the conditions that stabilize the intermediate of the latter are selective. Surprisingly, both proteins were found to adopt similar intermediates during the folding process (Radford, et al. 1995).

Did You Know? 8
Experimentally Observing an Intermediate

To experimentally observe an intermediate, it either has to be stable enough to live for a time comparable with the time of its formation (thus, it must be more stable than the unfolded state and precede the rate-limiting folding step), or it has to be quenched and trapped. The trapping is usually done either using the quench-flow hydrogen-exchange pulse labeling (with a subsequent nuclear magnetic resonance (NMR) investigation of the trapped product), or using the disulfide bond formation...........(Galzitskaya, et al. 2001)

Discussion 1.12: Other stages identified in folding

Using proteins that have sizes that are "average" for a protein folding study (100 – 200 residues), it has been demonstrated that stages additional to those above can be observed:

- The unfolded state forms, in a "burst" phase that takes a few milliseconds, a 'pre-molten' globule. This structure is attributed to have a partial formation of the secondary structures and a partial reduction of volume such as the several helix-coil transitions described in earlier sections [*see* (Eaton, et al. 2000) *for review*]. However, it has been clarified (Gutin, et al. 1995) that its formation is not a must (i.e. this is not an "obligatory prerequisite") along the folding pathway.
- A few more milliseconds resulted in the molten globule–another intermediate.
- From here on, detailed atomic interactions and local rearrangements start to occur and sometimes, proteins diverge into groups–slow folders and fast folders–based on the cis-trans isomer distribution, resulting adjustment of chain packing, non-native disulfide bridge formation, etc. (Eaton, et al. 2000) as detailed at various points throughout this section. Thus even though the next stage is the fully folded one, it can form anytime between a fraction of a second to hours.

It must be understood that the theories that support and contradict each other above proposing and characterizing various stages of folding with different names and attributes only try to segment the Levinthal's paradox into a series of "sub-problems" but do not explain how major conformational searches are cut-down and the protein quickly finds its native state at each of the various stages above. Other theories such as that by *Shakhnovich et al* (Abkevich, et al. 1994) have been postulated for this purpose, to the effect that the protein chain forms certain crucial contacts that are advantageous in terms of energy as well as entropy, and this is how enormous conformational search is avoided. This is described under the heading "theories that support models". These specific contacts could thus appear at any stage (collectively forming a 'nucleus' as described later) and this subset of contacts (not a "stage" during folding) is obligatorily to folding. It is suggested to appear midway during the rate limiting step of folding (signifying the TS) independent of the term various groups call it with (molten globule, etc.). The nucleus of folding (readers are reminded of previous section wherein the ASTROFOLD method (Klepeis, et al. 2003) used 5-residue segments to observe a 3-residue nucleus if the segment was made to form a helix) leads subsequently to the native fold in one step, wherein other contacts may or may not surround it and are found to occur with low probability.

1.5.4 FOLDING MECHANISMS

The term "folding mechanism" suggests a proposition which expects to explains, essentially, how a protein solves the Levinthal's paradox. It is *MORE THAN* the generalizations that suggest there are numerous unfolded states and how they narrow down to a few canonical folded conformations, or those that postulate that *probably* a certain experimental result corresponds to a structure that *might* resemble a certain intermediate *although* such a parallel was not found experimentally. Several key issues have been identified in delineating mechanism of folding. Fundamentally, one can never "see" the folding of protein molecules. In the quest to "pin Proteus down", one can only try to reconstruct the major events that occur during folding. The following example explains the situation, taken from a famous paper of folding (Onuchic, et al. 1997):

An α-helix is known to form within microseconds in any peptide of protein even if the folded state does not contain helices. Helices are also known to disappear as fast as they form. The question therefore arises as to the stage in which the helix becomes stabilized during the folding pathway. This neatly delivers to yet a relevant and related question–given that even in a folded state there is a continuum of conformations and their respective energies, how stable is a stable helix? Or another question that could arise is whether the formation of a helix is a prerequisite for folding even if the native state has no helices. It is known that the stability of the intermediate relative to the stability of the folded state influences the folding mechanism. But given the rapid equilibrium in solution, there is no way of delineating a clear mechanism. These are the usual limitations that theories encounter in any field of research and therefore, often, more than one theory is applied in computational models to handle the different levels of description.

Under this heading, three terms are explained: "energetics of folding" (only an outline: because the free energy funnel and the kinetics of folding are discussed in much greater detail under the respective headings), "Co-operativity of folding" that is essentially *THE* promising solution to the Levinthal paradox and "The folding transition state" that defines folding barrier and how its structure is inferred.

A. Energetics of Folding: Overview

A folded protein in a test tube has been denatured. After removal of the denaturing agent, "refolding" conditions are established. In this situation, once equilibrium is established,

i. Single-domain proteins follow two state kinetics–they exist in either the native or the unfolded states, and the intermediate is found among the unfolded.

ii. Multi-domain proteins usually unfold step-wise. Although domains are defined as independently folding/unfolding units within the polypeptide chain of a protein, there may be varying degrees of interactions between them

iii. Multisubunit proteins usually dissociate into submits first followed by the unfolding of the respective subunits. Simultaneous dissociation and unfolding may occur if the entire domain faces the surface of the quaternary structure rather than other subunits.

"It's so much more friendly with two."
Piglet in "Pooh's Little Instruction Book", by Milne

For single domain proteins, the equilibrium constant K_{eq} is given by:

$$K_{eq} = [N]/[U]$$
$$\Delta G^0_N = G^0_N - G^0_U = RT \ln K_{eq}$$

The ΔG^0_N above indicates the net stability of the folded state in this transition between the folded and unfolded states. Even under optimal conditions, the folded state is found to be marginally more stable that the unfolded by just 5 to 10 kcal/mol in terms of ΔG^0_N (gets a negative value). The K_{eq} value lies between 10^4 and 10^7. That is, for every unfolded conformation, there are 10^4–10^7 molecules in native state, and if one assumes a rate constant for folding of $1s^{-1}$ (spontaneous inter-conversions occur every second) then for all the protein to unfold, it would take 10^4 to 10^7 seconds (i.e. half-time $t_{1/2}$ of 2 hours to 80 days). Thus although most folded proteins must be spontaneously unfolding completely under all conditions, this spontaneous unfolding will normally be only transient, because the protein will promptly refold.

B. Cooperativity of Folding

As early as 1959, the helix formation of poly-α-amino acids was characterized to be a co-operative process with the Zimm-Bragg parameters σ (Zimm, et al. 1959) that referred to the *co-operativity factor* for the initiation of helix formation and *s*, the *equilibrium constant* indicating conversion of coil $\rightarrow$ helix transition (Chou, et al. 1974). The following discussion is all about cooperative folding.

Description: Once unfolding of a domain is initiated, it proceeds to completion. This statement is a simple rewording of the statement under *energetics of folding* above, that protein folding is a two-state process (populated states are either the folded or the unfolded). This implies that if unfolding is initiated in a native domain without any stops or stage, in one steady step, it ends up in the unfolded state ensemble (or the compact intermediate, which belongs to the unfolded state). At a molecular level, unfolding involves the breaking of a few essential interactions of the folded state, resulting in the "unzipping" of all interactions followed by the macro molecule falling apart. The vice versa happens during folding (these few crucial interactions comprise the nucleus, described later) and this is called "co-operativity". Breaking one or more of the interactions destabilizes the others increasing the free energy content of the once folded protein–with the folded protein already some-way along the upward journey of the roller-coaster pathway towards the transition state.

Identification: In a plot of the reaction coordinate versus population of folded proteins, a sigmoidal curve results as in Fig. 1.45A over a very short region of conformational changes, proteins suddenly fold, though this is not a *necessary* condition. It actually represents a large equilibrium constant for folding in the absence of denaturant such that the proportion of unfolded molecules is negligible initially [Sippl].

The Chevron plot [not discussed here; *ref.* (Creighton, 1990)] is a better indicator of co-operative behavior.

Box 10: Co-operativity—experimentally

Co-operativity of folding transitions is experimentally inferred if:
- Intermediate conformations are not substantially populated (independent of the principle used).
- The fully folded state should be distinct and unique in terms of stability when compared with any other conformation accessible to the polypeptide; proteins are known to fold completely into only one native state.
- The unfolding transition is abrupt. For example, in a pH titration of a protein, the acid induced unfolding occurs abruptly over a smaller pH range. Multiple ionizable groups within the protein interior, especially histidine residues (which are aromatic and hence in the hydrophobic core), can ionize only after the protein unfolds and ionize in concert.

The co-operativity factor, denoted in this text as "k_{co-op}" [based on the definition by (Höltje, et al. 2008)] needs introduction in this text. In Fig. 1.45B, let k_{5-10} be the equilibrium constant of formation of H-bond between residue number 5 and 10, and k_{6-9}, that for the H-bond between residues 6 and 9 and these two, the only interactions present in the folded state of the 12 residue peptide. *Entropic co-operativity exists* between them if the formation of one brings the interacting atoms of the other into geometric proximity, *giving extra help to the bond formation process.*

The cooperativity index between the two interactions is defined such that if $k_{co-op} > 1$, cooperativity exists (called **entropic co-operativity**), if it equals 1, the interactions are independent and $k_{co-op} < 1$ indicates that one interaction discourages the other (known as **anti co-operativity**). Entropic cooperativity is further presented in Discussion 1.13. Entropic co-operativity ($k_{co-op} > 1$) contributes to the "free energy of stabilization" of the folded state [equations not presented, *ref.* (Höltje, et al. 2008), (Creighton, 1990)].

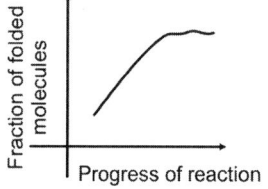

Steady change in conformation leading to a steady increase in fraction of folded molecules with all conformations being in equilibrium

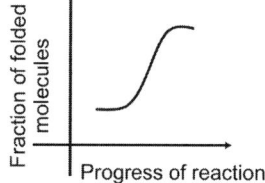

Sudden change in conformation in an all-or-none fashion leads to a sigmoidal increase in fraction of folded molecules indicating cooperativity

Fig. 1.45A: Sigmoidal curve for co-operative folding

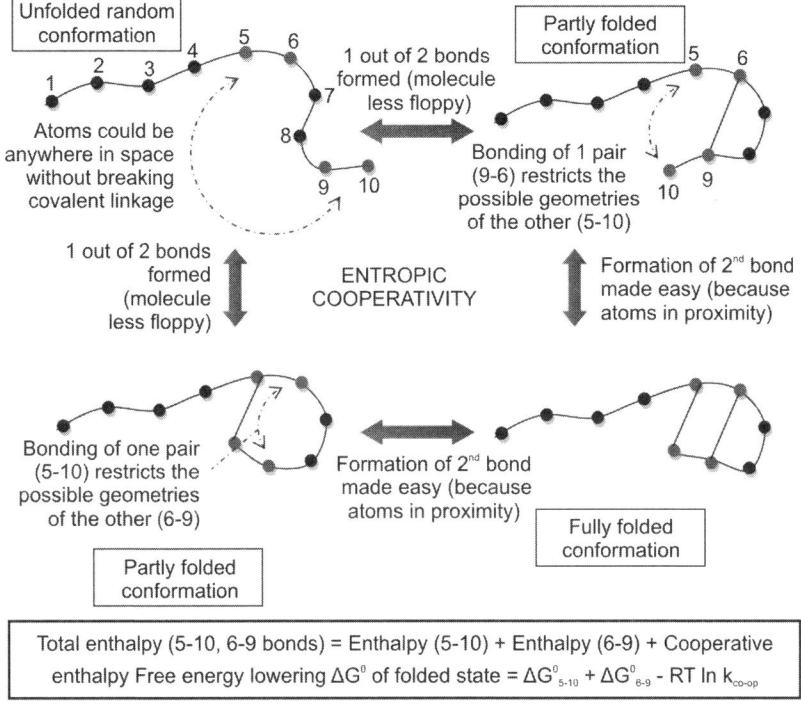

Fig. 1.45B: Entropic co-operativity in a 10-residue peptide

Did You Know? 9
Snapshots of the Experiments behind some Theories

Source of this theory—the experiments, how they are done, and their pros and cons:

- *This explanation of the cooperativity is based on experiments that either measures the stabilities of the disulphide bonds during folding or the contributions of individual interactions to stability using site-directed mutagenesis.*
- *In the latter method:*
  - a. *One residue that characterizes the folded state (generally apart in the sequence, but comes together after folding) is removed or changed. The measurement of the change in stability after removal of this interacting group is determined.*
  - b. *Site-directed mutagenesis is, however, complicated by the possibility of the mutant fold to assume a different native conformation, follow a different folding pathway, behave differently when unfolded, etc. that might result in a product that does not compare with the original situation of trying to compare the bark of dogs and cats—cats simply don't bark!*
  - c. *Removing a residue or a side chain (by substituting the residue) by mutagenesis will not create a void in the native-state—the protein conformation will shift a bit to make itself 'at home'.*
- *Using disulphide bond formation between cysteines as a marker is a relatively straightforward unique because the degree of bond formation can be controlled by varying the ratio of thiol (RSH) and disulphide (RSSR) reagents in the solution.*

Reasons for the Existence of Co-operativity

We know that the partly folded states are not favored during the folding transition owing to:

i. The presence of unfavorable contacts and interactions, or

ii. Uncompensated disruption of favorable ones, resulting in conformational strain.

Either of these is absent in folded/unfolded structure driving folding/unfolding to occur in one cooperative step. It must be noted that although strain results in cooperative folding, it does not influence the net stability of the folded state as the latter term is compared only to unfolded state and not to strained conformations. In other words, whatever be the height of the barrier, the difference between the folded and unfolded state (thermodynamic drive) gives the overall stability of the folded state. The following are other aspects that justify the existence of co-operativity among receptors:

i. The effect on entropy of more than one interaction within a single conformation are supra-additive–i.e. their combined effect is much greater than the addition of the effects of each interaction as an individual. This is called *entropic co-operativity* in the folded state.

ii. A protein's architecture and the sequence that goes with it is naturally selected and designed such that interactions become cooperative when folding. Thus whatever be the secondary structural composition, topology, class, evolutionary location of the protein, its folding is always cooperative (Freire, et al. 2004)

iii. Each interaction in the final folded conformation becomes more stable than when the same interaction occurs transiently in, say, the compact intermediate (remember, this belongs to the unfolded protein). With the presence of sufficient number of co-operative interactions, the free energy of the folded state will become lower than that of the unfolded protein-even if

   a. Each interaction is weak, by itself, and if

   b. The entropy of the final form is low (due to its highly ordered structure).

   The fully folded state is then stable, and the folding transition is co-operative.

iv. *Entropic co-operativity is minimal on the surface*: The contributions of individual interactions to cooperativity of the folded state vary–it has been accepted that there is no 'standard' value for the net stability within folded proteins of a particular interaction. The closest one can get to judging contributions of interactions is that the most rigid parts of the protein interior contribute the maximum to stabilization of the folded state (Sippl, et al. 1994). To be able to accurately state the contribution of various interactions, one must generate a large number of conformations of the protein and calculate their free energies.

Discussion 1.13: Entropic co-operativity

It is conceivable that the occurrence of an interaction between two atoms in a totally unfolded protein is dependent on the distance and approach of these two atoms. Consider the formation of hydrogen bonding between the backbone amine hydrogen of residues 5 and 6 with the backbone carbonyl oxygen atoms of residues 10 and 9 respectively. The approach of the bonding atoms of 5 and 10 is made much easier if a H-bond is first formed between 6 and 9 and vice versa owing to one H-bond bringing the other's atoms in geometric proximity. The favor in conformation is makes matters much simpler than adding the formation of 5–10 bond and 6–9 bond independent of each other (supra-additive effect).

The k_{co-op} value applies to both the involved interactions stated in the text under "identification" referring to Fig. 1.45B independent of the order of occurrence-the magnitude of the effect of interaction H-bond$_{5-10}$ on H-bond$_{6-9}$ is the same as that of H-bond$_{6-9}$ on H-bond$_{5-10}$. Co-operativity between any numbers of interactions can be treated in a cumulative manner. Different pairs of interactions might get a different k_{co-op} value. In the above example, if there exists a 3rd interaction between residues 7 and 8 (H-bond$_{7-8}$), although the k_{co-op} for the influence of H-bond$_{7-8}$ on H-bond$_{6-9}$ formation and vice versa would be the same, but this k_{co-op} value could be different form that between H-bond$_{6-9}$ and H-bond$_{5-10}$.

The co-op factors for each successive interaction are implicit in the final equilibrium constant determined between the unfolded and the fully folded state (with the latter having all the native interactions in place). If one thinks a little further, the main point behind this simplification is that the degree of freedom is greatly cut down for one H-bond (or ionic interaction or hydrophobic attraction or Van der Waals' interactions) with the formation of the other. This neatly delivers us to the doorsteps of the Levinthal's paradox–cooperative folding is one way in which random conformational search is avoided. Stretching this thought a little farther, the following generalization is obtained: that only those interactions that favor and result from cooperativity can be found in abundance within an unfolded sequence under folding conditions.

Simulation Model based on Co-operativity

CORE (COmplementary REgion) (Freire, et al. 2004) is a mathematical model and computer simulation that handles protein folding by energetically accounting for cooperativity. It is based on the theory that there exists a partly folded state that is higher in energy (and consequently less stable) than the folded and unfolded states. This is because of the destabilizing energetics resulting from the solvent exposure of unfolded regions and those folded regions of the partly folded state called "complementary surfaces". In addition to lowering the stability of the partly folded state (making it less likely to exist) the strain brought about by the solvent interaction is also attributed to increase cooperative folding behavior. Authors claim that the method could analyze the following:

1. The conditions in which partly folded states would accumulate,
2. The two-state kinetic behavior of the system, and
3. The role of solvent in folding and stabilizing the final fold.

C. The Transition State for Folding

The Transition State (TS) in protein folding is the cat-on-the-wall that lies await at the top of the reaction pathway between the unfolded and folded states, and comes rapidly tumbling downhill along the free energy curve to complete the transition (whether towards the folding or the unfolding process depends on the folding or unfolding favored conditions). It has the highest free energy and its structure is said to be distorted from the native structure in most aspects, and partly resembling the latter in some, compared to the native state. It is attributed to contain those essential contacts needed for folding, termed "nucleus" (described in detail later). The higher its free energy, the slower the reaction proceeds and is midway along the rate-limiting step. Much like the "Cheshire cat" in *Alice's Adventures in Wonderland*, it is this transient structure that shows the way for the reaction to proceed; it is hypothetical, as it can neither be isolated nor characterized directly.

Transition states can be characterized only by measuring the effect of certain changes on the rates of unfolding and refolding; the changes can be brought about either in the protein or in its surroundings. The following is a partial list of the properties of the TS:

- Under the same conditions, the same TS should be encountered in both the forward as well as reverse reactions.
- The TS continues to react to temperature in the same way as the folded state, measured in terms of heat capacity. The heat capacity of the TS also differs from that of the unfolded state and is closer to the folded state.
- If the TS has this same asymmetry (hydropholic-hydrophilic difference) in structure and comparable level of compaction as the folded state.
- Important long-range tertiary contacts of the folded state are present in the TS.
- From ligand-based studies, the binding pocket of the TS is established as being different from the folded state.
- The TS does not contain the native's co-operative folding property and packing.
- The lack of compaction of the TS to the level observed in the native state has also been deduced; the TS occupies greater volume relative to both unfolded and folded states.

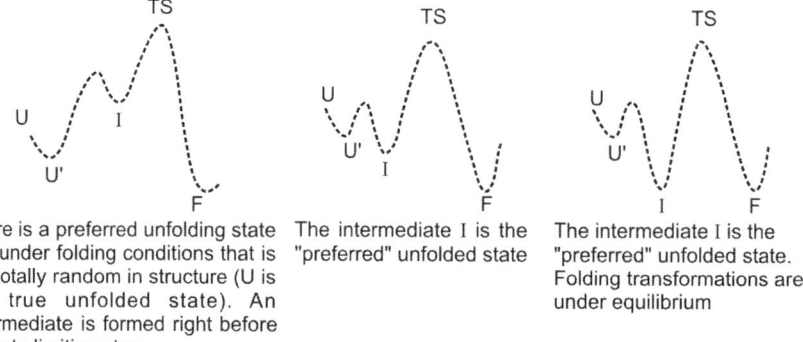

There is a preferred unfolding state (U') under folding conditions that is not totally random in structure (U is the true unfolded state). An intermediate is formed right before the rate limiting step

The intermediate I is the "preferred" unfolded state

The intermediate I is the "preferred" unfolded state. Folding transformations are under equilibrium

Fig. 1.46: A 2D potential energy curve indicating unfolded (U), intermediate (I), transition (TS), folded (F) states

- The heat capacity of the TS is not identical to the folded state because the core of the latter is much more densely packed than the former. A small change in this core region in the folded state makes the protein energetically susceptible to weakening of hydrophobic interactions and the core falls apart. The TS is less cooperative and hence does not have as high heat capacity as the folded.
- Major changes in conformation occur in the unfolded state before it starts to fold via the formation of the intermediate. However, there is no 'preparation' for the unfolding event.
- The free energy barrier to unfolding is also the high barrier overall for refolding indicating that this is the rate limiting step. It can be easily visualized that this is a result of co-operativity in the fully folded state.

D. Cis-Trans Isomerization

The rigid planarity of the peptide bond (see section 1.1 on protein structure) makes it susceptible to cis-trans isomerization. It is well known that:
1. The trans form is free of steric hindrance.
2. The *cis* form is hindered: model this using plastic ball and stick models and find out the atoms that clash: (*answer*-C_α atoms and side-chains of neighboring residues)
3. The trans form is energetically favored by about 10^3-fold (Brannigan, et al. 2002) over the *cis* form.
4. However, the cis form is not disfavored if the following residue happens to be a Proline (*model this on a computer–why?*)
5. When preceded by a proline, both geometric isomers end up having comparable free energies (the trans is favored only 4-fold).

Cis peptide bonds have been reported to frequent reverse turns on the surface of the protein (Creighton, 1990). It has been observed that in some cases, the molecules are essentially all cis or all trans in the folded form, whereas in other cases, both forms have been simultaneously observed in the folded state (Sippl, et al. 1994). The fully folded state is known to have a preference; the native states of some proteins prefer all cis, some, all trans, and some, a mixture, depending on which isomers increase stability. Thus, the effect of conformational stability on isomer choice indicates that isomer choice also has the same effect on stability of a certain conformation.

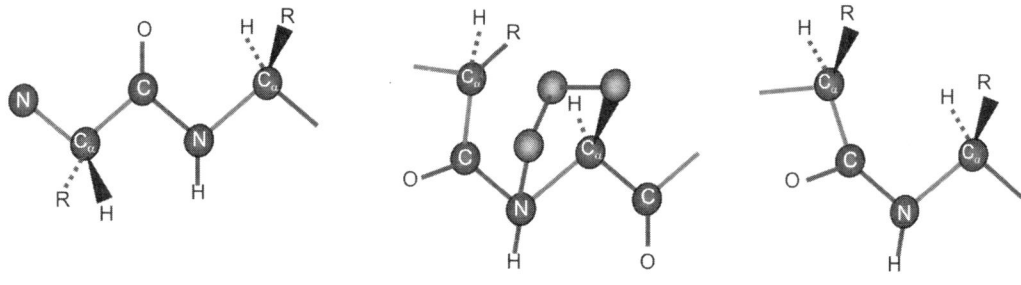

Trans peptide bond   Cis peptide occurring before a proline   Cis peptide bond

Scheme 1.19: Cis peptide bond, trans peptide bond and cis-bond before a proline residue

The cis-trans isomerization of Proline's peptide bond takes about 1 second and in the unfolded state (remember, this is a 'random coil'; the conformation of one residue is independent of the rest) there is no 'favor' or 'disfavor'. Consequently, some residues would flip to the cis form even if the native state requires all-trans conformations. This flip might not have any consequence on the unfolded state, however, under folding conditions, it becomes necessary that these residues flip back to the trans configuration (also remember: these are not conformations). Those conformations in which this flip has not taken place in the unfolded state fold without any delay contrary to those that have to flip back. Thus unfolded molecules can be segregate based on their folding times into "fast folders" (the U_f fraction) and "slow folders" (the U_s fraction)–the only difference between them lies in the need for isomerization (and not in the folding mechanism, pathway or TS). By probabilty, the larger number of Proline residues in the protein, the larger number of slow folders, and this has been identified experimentally (Creighton, 1990). However, this situation is not ideally linear. It has also been observed that some proteins can fold into a native-like conformation with one or more incorrect isomers. These proteins might have to partly or fully unfold to fold back to the correct native conformation.

Box 11: Role of Proline in Structure and Energy

Site-directed mutagenesis can be used again to pin-point the role of proline: Substitution of the proline residue by any other was found to abolish segregation into slow and fast folders, but the folded state was destabilized (cis configuration is favored only if the following residue is a proline. It appears as if prolines are inserted into proteins to introduce a "self-regulatory" mechanism that controls rate of folding of the protein from the inside.

1.5.5 ASSISTED FOLDING—CHAPERONES

We know that the protein is synthesized on the ribosomal RNA. There are theories that a protein starts to fold inside the ribosome even before synthesis is complete (co-translationally) and that the ribosome senses it (and decides where to shuttle proteins). Ribosome can manufacture proteins at the rate of 1–10 amino acids every second. But ribosomal participation is not a requirement as proteins fold and unfold all the time even in vitro. Thus folding is not dependent on the presence of a 'biological' environment. Thus, mutations induced in the genome can lead to a search for the *fittest* protein and, independent of this, each protein can come to an understanding with its environment through physical and chemical interactions. Our understanding is that proteins are capable of folding and unfolding themselves, as evident from computations (*in silico*) and experiments (*in vitro*) in which an individual protein is denatured. However, the mechanism of folding is influenced by some aspects of the environment and so is the structure of the native fold. At its "home" in the cell, the situation is a lot more complicated than in a test tube as one would have to think about the influence of the following, for a start:

- The primary solvent (water in the cytoplasm or lipids of the plasma membrane),
- The presence and simultaneous folding/unfolding of other macromolecules called *crowding* (Ellis, 2001), as the ribosomes do not synthesize just one protein at a time (intracellular macromolecular concentration may sometimes exceed 100 μM)

- Dissolved solutes and their concentration,
- Temperature (although this is maintained fairly constant in the warm-blooded homeotherms, one has to account for different conditions in other organisms such as bacteria, amphibians, etc.),
- pH and the protein's isoelectric behavior, and
- The assistance received by folding proteins from chaperones.

Although it does not require an intense training to serve dishes, it does take considerable amount of practice and guidance to skillfully move around and serve food and drinks in, say, a crowded disco–*especially without disturbing the dynamic customers, or bumping into other servers!* Similarly, globular proteins are capable of ending up comfortably in their respective native states, unassisted; chaperone assisted folding often becomes necessary in such crowded and hectic intracellular environment. Every functional (i.e. properly folded) protein is invaluable and every misfolded protein is disasterous. Cells cannot afford to have misfolding and this is not just because of wastage of resources. Proteins that do not fold correctly are known to aggregate. It is in order to prevent the risk of precipitation of these insoluble amorphous aggregates that chaperones are needed to protect a folding protein from steric/electrostatic disturbance of neighboring macromolecules. Folding proteins sometimes need protection even from exposure to heat or other changes in the cellular environment. As chaperones aid them in this way, they are also known as *heat shock proteins*. These assist in folding and maintenance of the folded conformation. There are various classes of chaperones and they usually act in succession:

1. The HSP70s, so called because they have a molecular weight of 70 kilodaltons, are the most important class of chaperones. They bind to the developing protein chain and protect those parts of the nascent protein that are particularly sensitive to premature reaction with the environment and therefore to malformation.

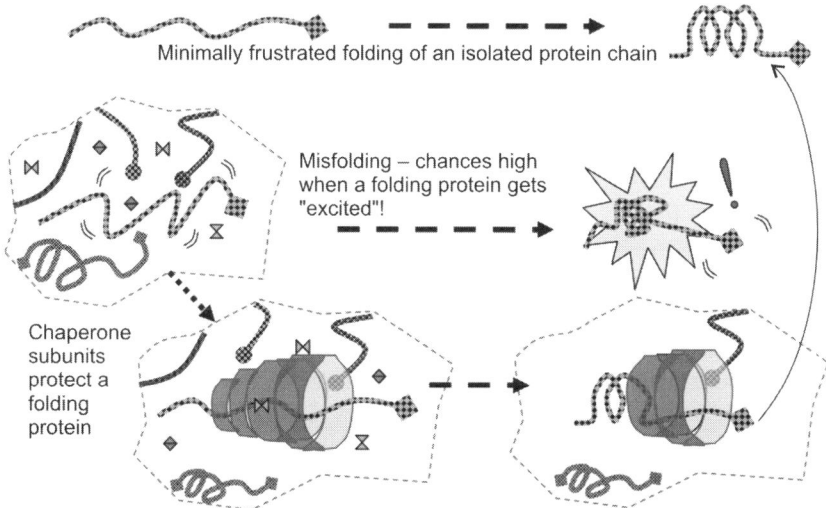

Scheme 1.20: The work of chaperones: Diagrammatic representation

2. These then dissociate from the protein and the protein chain is now ready to fold
3. The HSP70s molecules is now taken over by a chaperonin, a molecule shaped like a double ring, which fits round the protein chain like a cylinder so that the protein can fold undisturbed inside
4. The protein leaves the chaperonin only when it has achieved its folded state

For some proteins, chaperone assistance is a must. In these cases, chaperones either isolate them when folding or help to unfold kinetically trapped misfolds of the proteins giving them another chance to refold properly.

Did You Know? 10

The cylindrical folding cage of a chaperonin is known to open approximately every 10 seconds

1.5.6 PROTEIN FOLDING THEORIES THAT SUPPORT MODELS

"Did you ever stop to think, and forget to start again?"

Winnie the Pooh in "Winnie the Pooh", by Milne

In this section, several theories of protein folding that directly postulate how proteins fold, as well as those that explain related ideas and postulates have been presented. Protein folding models (described in the next section, 1.5.7) use one or more of these principles to investigate the energetics of folding via computer simulation.

1.5.6.1 Background

i. Most protein folding simulations operate with the approximation that 3D structure of proteins is determined by only its sequence and maybe water molecules in its environment, i.e. without the obligatory role of external factors. It is easy to understand that this is a major simplification for some proteins that require help from chaperones

ii. The Levinthal's paradox implies that all conformations of the polypeptide chain, except those that lead to the native state, are equally probable. Therefore in a protein conformational search, those interactions that lead to the native state's conformation should have greater influence on stability than others.

iii. (Harrison, et al. 1985) There is not just one path from the unfolded to the native state. Even if a protein needs to fold in a short time, it can take any of several similar paths. One therefore looks at an *ensemble* of conformations that following distinct yet similar pathways.

Folding scenarios: The conditions in which folding/unfolding parameters are derived can be divided into three categories:

• *Biological or folding conditions*: Investigation of kinetics that most interest us are under conditions that are as close to the native (biological) environment of the protein as possible (25–37°C, neutral pH, absence of denaturant). Behavior under these conditions are either observed in experiments, incorporated in experiments or inferred via extrapolation [*ref.* (Creighton, 1990), (Sippl, et al. 1994)]. These conditions do not just function to simulate home–they also strongly favor folding resulting in the native state being much more stable than the unfolded state. Folding intermediates are also known to be more stable than the unfolded state and thus accumulation of these intermediates become possible. The all-or-none or 'two-state transition' occurs (*ref.* 1.5.7)

- *Thermodynamic equilibrium*: Under these conditions, the stabilities of the folded and unfolded states are comparable. But even here, protein folding takes place (Kuwajima, et al. 1978), (Segawa, et al. 1984).
- *Equilibrium unfolding:* A gradual change is induced in the environment from those that favor folding to those that favor unfolding (using guanidinium hydrochloride or urea). In *equilibrium folding,* conditions are varied from strongly unfolding to folding favorable ones. Experimentally, the fractions of folded and unfolded molecules are measured.

1.5.6.2 Supporting Theories

Several tenets have been identified in literature by which proteins fold, some of which are discussed here:

A. *If Folding Starts with Random Structures, How Random is Folding?*

The possible conformations for a random coiled protein are very large in number. Each of the 1015 or so protein molecules in an 8 M urea- or high temperature-denatured protein solution that is contained in a test tube is probably in a different conformation at any instant of time. However, all of their energies are close to each other (independent of the method of denaturation), and all these distinct conformations become "thermodynamically indistinguishable" (Creighton, 1990). This is why we can place all of them in a single ensemble of the unfolded state. The folding that starts with each member of this ensemble will initiate in different ways, depending on the contacts that are immediately made possible by each conformation. At some point(s) along the process, these different structures converge and ultimately lead to the native structure. this convergence does not occur by a random conformational search, as per the Levinthal's paradox (Box 7).

Many small proteins are known to fold rapidly (Jackson, 1998), without any significant accumulation of folding intermediates under a wide range of conditions, including those that favor thermodynamic equilibrium as well as biological conditions that favor folding. As mentioned earlier, this is called two–state kinetics and is similar to the ***thermodynamic "all or none" transition*** in kinetics. This model of protein folding was first proposed very early on (Anson, 1945), but is believed to hold only for small, single structural domains of proteins; larger domains and multi-domain proteins often exhibit intermediate states. Studies on folding and unfolding clearly show that properties of the native state are restored or destroyed co-operatively. However, for some proteins, this mechanism was observed under both the above conditions (the reversible thermodynamic transition between the native and the denatured states as well as for the folding-favoring biological conditions) whereas for others, it was observed only under reversible (or equilibrium) conditions. The thermodynamic indistinguishability, therefore, might apply universally to all proteins–but under equilibrium conditions rather than biological conditions.

B. *The Hydrophobic Collapse Theory*

A key idea persisted in the 1980s that the primary sequence gave rise to secondary structures, which then formed the tertiary structure. However, towards the end of that period, the "folding code" (Dill, et al. 2008) was recognized to be distributed both locally in continuous stretches of the sequence and nonlocally all through. *A protein's secondary structure is as much a consequence of the tertiary structure as a cause of it* (Dill, et al. 2008). How this is made possible? Owing to the presence of hydrophobic amino acids.

The hydrophobic collapse (Fig. 1.47) refers to the spontaneous aggregation of hydrophobic side chains of amino acids in a protein in an attempt to get buried into its interior, when the entire protein is placed in an aqueous environment. It is brought about by the simultaneous pushing out of water molecules and the aggregation of hydrophobic moieties. Decrease in entropy of the folded protein (because it is getting organized into secondary and tertiary structure) is generally a major barrier to folding. But if we consider the folding to take place in the presence of water, the situation turns around. However, pushing out water molecules itself requires energy. The increase in entropy of the surrounding water molecules, after they have been pushed out, not only provides some compensation to the above factor, it also can compensate the energy required to displace water from the protein. Eventually entropy becomes the driving force for folding *ref.* Scheme 3.2 in part III.

Within the protein, aggregation of hydrophobic moieties lowers the energy of the protein (and also initiates the co-operative folding process). The release of energy is in turn used to displace water molecules and form secondary structures.

C. *The Significance of Partly-folded States*

As discussed under section 1.5.4A 'energetics', a protein folds and unfolds constantly in the cellular environment. We know so far that protein function–whether ligand

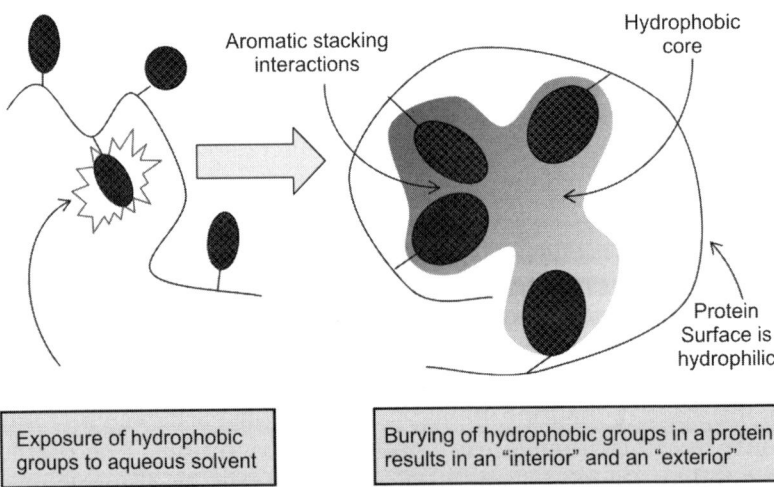

Fig. 1.47: A line drawing showing hydrophobic side chain interactions leading to collapse of a protein

binding, transport, interaction with other proteins, or any other depends on its existence as an intact and fully folded native structure. We also know that if a protein refuses to fold, or if it misfolds, it means trouble to the cell. However, it was discovered that *partly folded states have physiological significance* in some cases. This 'unfolding' that is being referred to here is not the transient conformations that protein passes through when it has equilibrated with biological conditions or the *breathing* of a protein (*ref.* chapter 1.3 dynamics). This partly folded state is a destination for the protein and plays some biological function:

- Pre-folded ribonuclease A, with four disulphide bonds intact and at least one incorrect cis-trans peptide bond isomer, is protected from cleavage by pepsin near its C-terminus exposing another region to cleavage by trypsin (Creighton, 1990)

- One of the cleaved fragments of dihydrofolate reductase inhibits the protein's refolding (Hall, et al. 1989) by interaction with the pre-folded protein

- We know that a protein can no longer perform its function once it has been unfolded (denatured).

However, there are **intrinsically unstructured proteins**, which are 'unfolded' in their native state, but still functionally active.

D. *Secondary Structure Formation*

The study of secondary structure formation under the purview of folding in larger proteins or of its formation in a peptide has always been considered when theories of folding are proposed. For instance, as early as in the 1950s, studies on the helix-coil transitions resulted in classical theories (Bryngelson, et al. 1989) that proposed that secondary structure formation can play an important role even before the protein molecule collapses. The theory was based on research on the conformations of peptide fragments (Becktel, et al. 1987) and showed that *EITHER*, Peptides have a weak tendency to form their respectively folded structure as in the protein, autonomously, *OR*, They form helices—even when their structure in the folded protein does not contain helices.

The idea behind a protein forming secondary structures at the start of folding is that these help to reduce entropy of the chain. By bringing together sequentially amino acid residues located close to each other along the primary structure, the chain is able to cut down entropy (i.e. the number of possible conformations) by reducing the floppiness of the chain. In other words, with such partial ordering, a large number of conformations of the chain that might not lead to any form of interaction between the different residues of the protein can be totally cut down. When the total number times residues come in contact with each other is increased, consequently, the probability of formation of the "correct" or native contacts is increased (because total number of possible conformations is reduced by secondary structure formation). This considerably reduces the configurational entropy of the chain (the entropy associated with the various conformations that a certain configuration can take up) even before hydrophobic collapse and co-operative effects come in place. This again serves as a solution to the Levinthal's paradox.

Box 12: Secondary structures in folding

One important discovery materialized out of further investigations of the formation of secondary structures in protein folding–the molten globule state of many proteins were found to contains considerable amounts of local α-helices, even when the final protein did not contain any (Hamada, et al. 1996). This showed that secondary structures are crucial, but not indispensible. Their main purpose is to stabilize the structure after water molecules are driven out (as mentioned earlier, decrease in entropy while folding is not favorable, but is compensated by increasing entropy of water molecules by removing the solvation sphere around the protein chain) by introducing H-bonds within the molecule.

E. *Folding in Large Proteins*

As mentioned, small proteins with single domains undergo only two-state kinetics – that is, they predominantly exist in either fully folded or unfolded states. For larger proteins, three steps can be observed and it is in this case that a clear intermediate or a molten globule can be ascribed. The former would generally contain the secondary structures of the folded protein whereas the latter would *ref.* to the state resulting from hydrophobic collapse. From here two paths are possible.

However, it is not clear whether these structures act as intermediates to the formation of the correct fully folded native state or they indicate misfolded structures in local minima that need to be overcome (Scheme 1.21) in order for the sequence to reach the native state.

F. *Glass Transition Temperature*

An outline of what happens at this temperature is presented here to familiarize readers with this concept. It demonstrates the effect of temperature on the protein molecule. On steadily lowering the temperature of a protein's surrounding, there is a sudden change in the dynamics of the protein at approximately 200 K. This has been experimentally demonstrated using several techniques such as X-ray Crystallography, Neutron Scattering, Mössbauer Scattering (*ref.* (Vitkup, et al. 2000) that contains a succinct summary). Dynamic breathing and random motions in a protein are suddenly

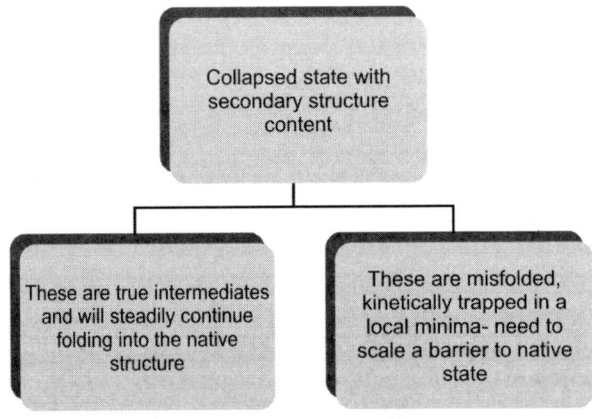

Scheme 1.21: Two possibilities from the collapsed state

frozen and only harmonic vibrations exist. The protein looses all functionality. In this state the anharmonic and long-range correlated motions that hold together protein tertiary structure in all its detail, are quenched. This is called the glassy state. This behavior observed in proteins is generally ascribed to certain liquids cooled to a specific low temperature at which they form glass. In proteins, in addition to intrinsic behavior of the polypeptide chain, solvent is known to play a very important role in bringing about glass transition. Change in temperature affects solvent mobility before it affects the mobility of the protein's atoms (the use of other specific solvents than water shifts the 'T_G behavior' to ~ 80 K). Theory goes that slowing down of solvent motion (called *caging*) restricts the flexibility of the protein chain and traps it from taking up other conformations. Numerous MDS studies have been performed to reproduce this behavior. At temperatures below T_G, few kinetic structures become accessible to the protein, one of them being the native state.

G. *Foldons*

When some large proteins are allowed to fold, they first form some smaller scattered units that are partly folded. These groups of secondary structures continue to exist in the native state. These are called *foldons*. These are formed because one part of the polypeptide chain requires crossing only a low energy barrier to lead to its folding. Thus, the protein handles its "time-bound folding problem" by breaking it up to smaller kinetically accessible parts. Some special architectures of proteins (nuclei) encourage this type of folding. Foldons have been observed experimentally as well as in computational simulations [(Abkevich, et al. 1994), (Panchenko, et al. 1996), (Radford, et al. 1995), (Maity, et al. 2005), etc.].

Did You Know? 11
Protein Foldons and the DNA

The foldons discovered in proteins by researchers were found to be comparable in size (though not an identical match) to the exons of the gene sequences for the corresponding proteins. Authors claim that this may be a reason why genes have pieces.

H. *Nucleation of Folding*

The Transition State–which is the highest free energy point along the folding and unfolding pathway–has been discussed to resemble the folded state in many respects. The TS has also been described to be located at the free energy *saddle point* (*ref.* section 2.3.2, Fig. 2.23). During folding, a multitude of folding-unfolding pathways originate from the unfolded-state ensemble and end in the native state by passing through the same TS. The TS is also considered to be the crux of whole process as it contains the essential contacts that lead to the folded state called "the folding nucleus". The following is an overview about the nucleus–how it is determined and how inferences about it determine theories and models–that is expected to occur midway between the folded and unfolded states. The study of concept of 'nucleus' can also be applied to the transition from the unfolded state to the native state via the molten globule.

The nucleus and the rate of folding: If one reflects sufficiently on this point, the question most likely to arise is, "if TS is so transient that one cannot observe it experimentally and if the intermediate is also relatively unstable that it does not accumulate, what is it that one can 'see' in an experiment?" The best one can do is, by the influence of site–directed mutagenesis on folding rates, zero-in on those residues indispensible for folding (of course, ensuring that the mutation has not affected the mechanism or the folded state). If the mutation induced shift in folding rate k_f = mutation induced shift in K, given:

$$\text{Equilibrium constant (K)} = \text{rate of folding } (k_f)/\text{rate of unfolding } (k_u),$$

then folding is the only process affected after mutation – this implies that the TS contains native contacts. Whatever be the change in K, if k_f remained unaffected after mutation, then the nucleus did not contain the native structure. The proposed 'nucleation' gives us another key to solve the Levinthal's paradox and to estimate the characteristic protein folding rates.

The nucleus-where is it? Several arguments have been proposed that the TS of a protein resembles its folded state (*ref.* "the transition state" under theories above) and the areas that resemble are collectively called the nucleus of folding. Efforts to characterize this nucleus have resulted in several approaches that mainly rest on this universal question. If the nucleus is very small including a bunch of specific and localized interactions or contacts, it can be captured only if we follow the evolution (folding / unfolding) of those few contacts over time (in other words, following the "reaction coordinate" as under section 2.3.2.F in part II). If a global and generalized reaction coordinate is used, a kinetic analysis would totally miss this nucleus, but such a coordinate would capture those nuclei that are large and spread out, "with structural inhomogeneities being a significant but secondary perturbation" (Creighton, 1990) [*ref.* Box 28 in section 3.1.3.B on the word 'perturbation'].

The nucleus– size and composition:
So, what is the size of the nucleus?
1. …quite large, comparable in size to the whole protein…. (Bryngelson & Wolynes).
2. …depends on the shape of the protein; the nucleus would be about one third the size of a single domain protein…. (Galzitskaya, et al. 2001).
3. (In lattice simulations)… is very small, perhaps containing only three or four key residues… (Abkevich, et al. 1994).
4. (Experimentally in chymotrypsin inhibitor CI2)… different residues participate to varying extents… (Fersht, 1995).
Research continues…

The Nucleus–Composition

How "specific" is its composition? The specificity of the nucleus is a descriptor of the difference in the types of interactions that contribute to it. For example, if it is made up of only hydrophobic interactions, it is highly specific and the energy of the various interactions is uniform. The main "aim" of the TS is to reduce entropy of the chain by forming contacts during folding. Hypothetically, if the nucleus is just made of

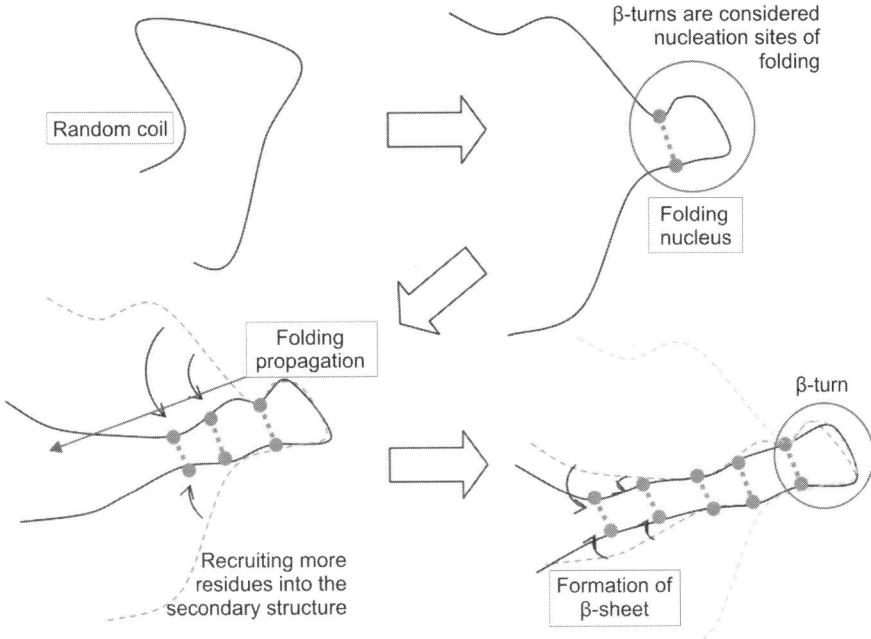

Fig. 1.48: Presence of a 'nucleus' during folding

hydrophobic contacts but still encompasses, say, more than one third of the protein, we have struck a gold mine! Thus when heterogeneity is small (when the contact energies are homogeneous), the extent of delocalization is a significant point.

Discussion 1.14: Experimental parameters

The ratio 'φ' (Onuchic, et al., 1996): An estimate of whether residues that interact in native state also interact in the TS. Sometimes φ values are used to estimate the participation of residues to the nucleus. It is assumed that the mutations do not alter the nucleus, the structure of the folded state or the unfolded state ensemble. To estimate φ, all the rates k have to be measured at (or extrapolated to) the same conditions, the `biological' conditions of zero denaturant concentration.

$$\varphi = \Delta \ln k_f / \Delta \ln K,$$

where k_f and K are as defined earlier. The Δ represents the difference between the corresponding values in the wild type (unmutated) (and mutation-induced protein.

If, after the mutation of a certain residue which comes in close contact with certain others in the 3D structure, φ = 1, then the shift in ln K_f equals the shift in ln K (that is, both are changed to the same extent,). When folding is affected, that means the concerned residue in the TS has already established native contacts.

• If φ = 0, there is no change in folding rate. This indicates an "unfolded" TS with respect to the mutated residue.

- If $\varphi \sim 0.5$, one of the following situations are attributed:
  a. Either the residue is at the surface of the nucleus (at the boundary between folded nucleus and unfolded regions)
  b. Or, the mutated residue belongs to a different nucleus in the TS (inside one of the alternative nuclei), indicating 2 folding pathways.
- If $\varphi < 0$, there is simultaneous decrease in folding and unfolding rates, and
- If $\varphi > 1$, there is simultaneous increase in folding and decrease in unfolding rates in opposite directions. For both the latter cases, there is possibility that the folding nucleus is not native-like. In the last case, one could imagine that the native state has a lower energy after mutation increasing unfolding barrier. These situations are rare and indicate changes elsewhere in the mechanism.

The ratio 'β' (Galzitskaya, et al. 2001): An estimate of the location of the TS as being closer to or farther from the native state. Experiments are conducted to determine unfolding (usually, but also folding) in various concentrations of denaturants. As mentioned, denaturants are known to act on the solvent-exposed residues and these residues are hydrophilic because the denaturants are dissolved in aqueous media. If δC represents change in denaturant concentration, (Matouscheck, et al. 1995)

$$\beta_T = (\delta \ln k_f / \delta C)/(\delta \ln K / \delta C).$$

- When β_T is close to 1, the TS solvent-accessible surface area is close to that of the native protein;
- When β_T is close to 0, the TS is rather unfolded.

Observed values of $\beta_T \sim 0.6$–0.8 for small proteins (average φ value ~ 0.3–0.4). The difference between the average φ and β_T values indicates that the TS has a comparable shape and degree of compaction, but not the exact same contacts, as the native state.

The nuclei of familial proteins: Proteins' 3D structures are known to be better conserved than their sequences. The nuclei of such spatially conserved proteins have been shown to be similar. But a contradiction has also been documented. Even a drastic change such as a circular permutation that results in a different topology has been demonstrated to sometimes contain very similar TS structures. The role of convergence and divergence of proteins (*ref.* Scheme 1.13 under section 1.2.1) in this respect is unclear.

The folded and unfolded phases: The nucleation idea helps to estimate the folding rates and the influence of changes in the protein as well as in the environment. One focuses on the events that occur mid-way between folded and unfolded states when folding and unfolding processes are at equilibrium (*ref.* section 1.5.6.1 on folding scenarios). When equilibrium is reached, we know that the rate of forward reaction (folding) and rate of reverse reaction (unfolding) are equal. The nucleus is thus identified with the TS located at the height of the energy barrier.

Discussion 1.15: Prediction of (unfolding time based on nucleation

i. The TS is modeled as a transient semi-unfolded (or semi-folded) state of a protein molecule (Galzitskaya, et al. 2001), such that the folded and unfolded phases exist within the same molecule.

ii. It is proposed that one part of the nucleus resembles the fully folded state and is called the 'folded phase', whereas the other part that is unfolded, containing loops that extend from the folded phase in various directions (called 'unfolded phase'). The folded and unfolded phases are thus parts of the same TS conformation.

iii. It is thus proposed that a greater "surface tension" exists at the unfolded phase surface; the folded phase has assumed a globular shape and therefore minimized its exposed surface area.

iv. The free energy barrier is said to be the barrier that the unfolded phase has to overcome to 'get into' the folded phase. In other words, the barrier of nucleation lies in the expansion of the boundaries of the folded phase throughout the nucleus in this transient semi-unfolded (or semi-folded) state.

v. It has been worked out and discussed that the size of the boundary is $\sim N^{2/3}$ for a chain N-residues long. Depending on the topology, the unfolded region may or may not contain random closed loops. The greater the occurrence of such closed loops, the larger the barrier to "convert" it all into the meaningful secondary structure of the fully folded state during folding. Their entropy thus adds to the existing surface energy of the boundary.

vi. The free energy of the boundary is a function of the size of the protein and has been estimated to be between $1.5N^{2/3}k_BT$ (when the unfolded region surrounding the boundary is covered by "random" loops) and $0.5N^{2/3}k_BT$ (when the boundary is free of such loops).

vii. Typically, the time taken by one residue to undergo rearrangement is approximately 1 nanosecond. Therefore one can estimate the time taken to overcome the free energy barrier be $\sim\exp(1.5N^{2/3})$ ns in the first of the above two cases, and only $\sim\exp(0.5N^{2/3})$ ns in the second case above.

viii. The above estimate has been verified to hold true to be the observed time for folding in proteins. Observed folding-unfolding time in mid-transition (at the point of equilibrium between the native and unfolded states) fits the theoretically predicted region. The quantity $\ln(\tau)$ lies in between $\ln(\tau) + 0.5N^{2/3}$ and $\ln(\tau) + 1.5N^{2/3}$ where τ refers to folding time. (Finkelstein, et al. 1997).

The τ for α-helix elongation by one residue is $\sim$ 10 ns as mentioned under the section on the structure of helix.

I. *Denaturation*

A number of experiments are carried out under various conditions as mentioned earlier that study kinetics and thermodynamics in systems that involve the addition of denaturants. How exactly do these denaturants bring about unfolding and how does the protein respond to such a change of conditions? Denaturation at various levels of proteins structure:

i. When protein subunits associate, they form quaternary structure. Denaturation at this level involves dissociation of these subunits followed by domain unfolding or, simultaneous unfolding and falling apart of the quaternary aggregate (if the domains are arranged such that they are solvent exposed and their unfolding is not hindered by other subunits/domains).

ii. Domains have always been described as independently folding 3D parts of a protein. At the tertiary level, they unfurl independently (at a very coarse level of understanding) disrupting covalent long-range interactions–the disulfide bridges–first. Next, long range interactions that keep the 3D structure together are disturbed, such as attraction between charged atoms of the side chain, any organized solvation sphere, dipole and induced dipole interactions, etc.

iii. As the secondary structure of the protein denatures, it approaches the unfolded state. Any regularity in structure or organization into shapes by coordinating with neighboring residues is abolished resulting in a random coil.

iv. Changes to the primary structure, of course, involve changes to the configuration rather than the changes in conformation dealt with here.

Chemical denaturation theories: So far, experimental results of folding and unfolding studies have been listed out and mentioned as those that formed the primary source of our current understanding of protein folding. Several theories of folding, unfolding and interaction have been postulated based on observations of these macromolecules in various conditions that favor folding, unfolding, and most importantly, equilibrium. These conditions have been brought about by various denaturants, especially chemicals (as these can be fine-tuned and reversed easily). The action of denaturants thus needs to be explained clearly. Some of the "chemical denaturation theories" are listed below.

Background: The experimental distribution of protein molecules between the folded and the unfolded states is given by the Boltzmann distribution that equates energy of the states with the probability of finding molecules in the respective states. Given the two-state kinetics that exists, the total molecules in the solution can be found in the folded and unfolded states with probabilities determined by the Boltzmann partition function. This has been described in detail under the mean field theory for fold recognition and folding (section 1.4). With increase in denaturant concentration, it is well known that unfolded protein fraction increases linearly (Fig. 1.45A). Why How? *Ref.* Discussion 1.16 [based on (Schellman, 1994), (Pace, 1975), (Schellman)].

Discussion 1.16: Chemical protein-denaturation theories

Denaturant binding model: Schellman

- The denaturant acts like a ligand and binds to specific sites on the protein
- (Much like how a curled up dog stretches out as you stroke it), with increasing denaturant concentration, more of these sites become available for binding: the site is not singular and localized

- The binding sites are not cooperative in their behaviour
- Protein unfolding is encouraged in the partly unfolded protein

Solvent exchange model: Schellman

- The denaturant interacts with the protein surface in non-specific way
- As concentration of denaturant increases, it might displace the protein surface-bound water molecules
- The water molecules are found at specific regions on the surface; therefore interaction converts from being non-specific to specific

Linear energy model (LEM): Pace

- The accessible surface area (ASA) of the unfolded molecule is greater by δASA than that of the folded one; the number of denaturant-exposed interaction sites is also greater
- With the addition of more denaturant, this difference (the δASA as well as the number of exposed interactions sites) increases
- One can obtain the change in stabilization free energy with increase in denaturant concentration.

1.5.7 THE INTERACTIONS THAT STABILIZE FOLDING

The sequence: With the advent of a plethora of theories on structure prediction (especially fold recognition) and protein folding, the ultimate test would be to synthesize new sequences to see if they fold and function in the way they have been designed to (mentioned also under section 1.5.12 on applications). From these ventures, it became clear that out of the astronomical number of combinations of sequences theoretically possible using 20 amino acids, natural proteins are a tiny subset that are meant to be only marginally more stable (5–10 kcal/mol) when fully folded, given that synthetic proteins can be designed to be much more stable, $\Delta G_N^0 = -22.5$ kcal/mol (–94 kJ/mol) [even as early as 1988 (Regan, et al. 1988)]. This is the first point to be remembered when studying the interactions that take part in the folding mechanism. The marginal stability is intended because proteins must constantly react to surroundings–metabolic and environmental–with conformational changes.

The side chains: Authors wish to make the readers familiar with yet another protein folding jargon–what's called *"the protein folding code"* (mentioned once in the previous section). This is the unwritten code of conduct among proteins that all scientists together wish to write–what makes proteins be the way they are. It refers to all the questions on protein folding, such as "how does the protein solve the Levinthal's paradox? What drives folding? Why does one sequence fold one way different from another?" addressed so far and so far and so forth, in a combined manner. The last question is important and yet, a very simple statement will suffice as an explanation–the difference between proteins lies in their side chains and not their backbones! But of course, this is not just one question, and all of us become 6 year olds asking a whole bunch of whys and hows... According to professor Ken Dill from the department of Pharmaceutical Chemistry of university of California at San Francisco, a renown researcher on protein folding, (Dill, et al., 2008) the protein's "folding code" is yet to be solved.

Water: The enthalpy (ΔH) and entropy (ΔS) parameters during folding and unfolding are temperature-dependent. This is because the folded state has very low heat capacity compared to the unfolded and a small change in temperature produces a much greater structural change in the folded than in the unfolded state ensemble. As discussed in chapter 1.3 and in part III, chapter 3.1, water molecules play an important role both by helping scale the entropic barrier to folding as well as by stabilizing folded conformations. Theory goes that the unfolded state owes its higher heat capacity to the temperature-dependent arrangement of water molecules around hydrophobic side chains which become solvent exposed in the unfolded state; they would naturally prefer to remain buried as in the folded state.

Hydrophobic interactions: (continued from the previous section 1.5.6) This is the main driving force and contributor to folding and the stability of the folded state is also due to the densely packed hydrophobic core. The theory was first propounded by Kauzmann (Kauzmann, 1959). Although most research groups agree that this is the principal driving force, how it is initiated in the random unfolded conformation is a point of considerable debate.

Box 13: Having side chains that fear water, submerged in water, serves a purpose

There is considerable evidence that hydrophobic interactions must play a major role in protein folding.

- The existence of hydrophobic cores indicates the necessity of non-polar amino acids to be driven away from water.
- Model compound studies show 1–2 kcal/mol (Wolfenden, 2007) for transferring a hydrophobic group from water into oily medium. This value is additive over several amino acids.
- Proteins are readily denatured in nonpolar solvents.
- Sequences that are jumbled but containing amino acids in the correct hydrophobic and polar patterning fold to their expected native state (Hecht, et al., 2004), even when no effort is taken to ensure packing, charge distribution, or hydrogen bonding…. (Dill, et al. 2008)

Hydrogen-bonding interactions: It is well known from the protein structure analysis section that backbone–backbone hydrogen bonds are important to maintain the structure (secondary as well as tertiary) of a folded protein. Several structure analysis methods are also based on this criteria (*ref.* section 1.2). H-bonds contribute about 1–2 kcal/mol (Fersht, et al. 1985), (Brannigan, et al. 2002) to overall stability, but only towards the end of folding.

Electrostatic interactions: These are felt over long ranges especially between protein and ligand (vide part III). When an independent protein is allowed to fold, residues with charged side groups are mostly located at the surface interacting with the aqueous environment. Although in some specific topologies like the Leucine Zipper (described under chapter 1.2) there are one or two crucial electrostatic interactions that define interaction and function, in general, the fold of a protein is not found to be greatly stabilized by electrostatics. The native state structure is not greatly influenced by pH (as long as it is close to biological or neutral range) or charge mutations (Shang, et al. 2007).

van der Waals interactions: This interaction is a result of several simultaneous forces. The hydrophobic interactions collapse the protein and this is followed by a Levinthal paradox–obedient conformational search resulting in other interactions that further drag the protein down the potential energy surface towards the native state structure. The globular shape assumed by a long linear chain is basically all about how to pack and van der Waals interactions–and both attractive and repulsive interactions are important (Brannigan, et al. 2002). Side chains are found conveniently staggered (as happens in *n*-butane conformations) in secondary structures; favored chain compaction take the baton from the hydrophobic collapsing force to run the next lap of the protein folding race. Helices and β-sheets are all-time-favorite ways for proteins to pack residues into secondary structures. Protein folding models later in this section postulate how local and global structures synchronize when folding.

Contribution of other interactions: The sum of the energetic contribution of all hydrophobic interactions does not reach the already meager 5–10 kcal/mol stability of the folded protein. Therefore the contributions of other intermolecular forces (Dill, et al. 2008) become significant. These lower the enthalpy of folding to make it more negative than that achieved from a simple aggregation of hydrophobic side groups. Traditionally, it was thought that these other interaction types contribute little, if not nothing, to the stability of the folded protein because they can be formed in the unfolded state with water molecules as well. More recently, however, this error that water can take up the role of other parts of the protein chain was pointed out (Creighton, 1990).

• Entropic co-operativity lowers free energy of each interaction more than the interaction with solvent

• Entropy of water is increased when protein folds.

• The transient interaction of water with protein is replaced by a stable interaction in the folded protein resulting in more negative enthalpy of the latter interactions.

• Close packed structure that remains so (water molecules are always diffusing and so do not close pack as a folded polypeptide chain does) has gained the favor of extensive van der Waals interactions also contributing to lower enthalpies.

It is important to know that these interactions in the folded state can also be found in the unfolded state although with lesser interaction enthalpies. The hydrophobic interactions are the most powerful for folding because it's the one thing that is absent in the unfolded state.

Effect of temperature: As mentioned earlier, the heat capacity of the unfolded state is much lower than that of the folded. At the transition state, the heat capacity approaches, but is not equal to that of the native. Heat capacity is temperature dependent, and so is the stability of the protein's folded state.

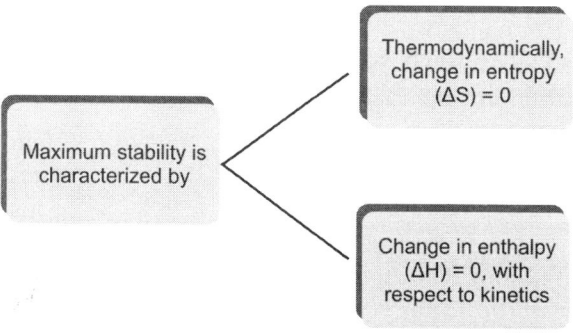

Scheme 1.22: Characterizing 'stability' of a protein

Maximum stability is characterized by

Thermodynamically, change in entropy (ΔS) = 0

Change in enthalpy (ΔH) = 0, with respect to kinetics

This stability (Scheme 1.22) decreases at temperatures both higher and lower to the optimal. There are specific differences between 'cold' and 'hot' unfolding that we wish to omit from this discussion. For detailed experiments characterizing the thermodynamics of folding, *ref.* (Privalov, 1989).

1.5.8 MODELS

Alice, in Lewis Carroll's 1865 novel Alice's Adventures in Wonderland, says:
"Would you tell me, please, which way I ought to go from here?"
"That depends a good deal on where you want to get to," said the Cat.
"I don't much care where —" said Alice.
"Then it doesn't matter which way you go," said the Cat.
"– so long as I get somewhere," Alice added as an explanation.
"Oh, you're sure to do that," said the Cat, "if you only walk long enough."

This discussion indeed amuses us at this point; modeling protein folding from first principles is not very different - however, with sufficiently long study, one hopes to eventually get to the global minimum...

In the same lines as the above quote, the aim of protein folding simulations is not to sample every possible conformation that a protein can take – in this case, one would ideally get to the native structure if one works on the problem "long enough". It is known that an all-atom Molecular Dynamics Simulation of folding performed for just 50 milliseconds of folding time would take 30,000 years using the most advanced computing resources!

1.5.8.1 Outline of Several Models

Under this heading, some well-known models that help readers to understand various approximations that operate in computational protein folding is presented. These models assume fast folding–i.e. the absence of intrinsically slow cis-trans isomerizations.

Template model: For about 100 years (till the 1940's), it was thought that proteins were made from a 'cast' or 'template'. This model became more sophisticated, with suggestions that the cast, or external driving force, came from the ribosome or other "foldases" (*ref.* section 1.5.12)

The jig-saw puzzle model – (Harrison, et al. 1985). Just as the conformation of each unfolded protein molecule is slightly different, the mechanism with which it folds is also slightly different. These different pathways are:

1. Unique in terms of rates,
2. Converge at the fully-folded conformation only, and
3. Are essentially irreversible.

The framework model – (Ptitsyn, 1973). Linus Pauling suggested that proteins would fold by forming local structures, steadily building towards greater complexity. In lectures delivered in 1951, published, (Linderstrøm-Lang, 1952) pathways for folding followed the hierarchical organization of protein structure.

The diffusion-collision model (also, hierarchical diffusion collision model) – [(Karplus, et al. 1994), (Myers, et al. 2001)]. Protein substructures (secondary or higher) form simultaneously and diffuse along the protein chain. As their conformations spread along the chain recruiting more residues (diffuse), their boundaries converge (collide) and form higher order structural arrangements. Eventually, the tertiary structure is in place. Some proteins, such as helical bundles, have been shown to follow a hierarchical diffusion-collision model. These elements then diffuse until they collide, whereupon they coalesce to form the tertiary structure (Dill, et al. 2008).

Hierarchic condensation model – (Krishna, et al. 2006). According to this theory, secondary structure formation can occur almost spontaneously by local conformational searches. Further assembly of the secondary structures results in tertiary structure formation. Other smaller units, such as the foldons, have been suggested (Abkevich, et al. 1994) as promoting access to the native state. Other works suggest "topomers" – unfolded states that are topology-wise canonical to the native (*ref.* section 1.5.12). Protein folding routes are not linear, but have a tree structure because of the hierarchy– at each node, several structures converge when assembled into more global structures (Abkevich, et al. 1994).

Nucleation model (Abkevich, et al. 1994) and its extensions (Nucleation-condensation model (Bychkova, et al. 1993), nucleation, rapid-growth model (Wetlaufer, 1973), nucleation-collision model–other ref.: (Fersht, 1995). These suggest the formation of specific contacts in the unfolded protein is crucial and is the 'nucleus' of the entire protein folding affair. More contacts are built from this and the chain rapidly takes up secondary structure formation along both directions similar to the fall of "stacked dominoes". The secondary structures grow bigger and form a diffuse Transition State Ensemble (TSE). These nucleate 3D packing and the formation of tertiary structure. As mentioned earlier, the size of the nucleus has been extensively debated. Specific β-turns and N-termini of helices have been indicated as sources of structure propagation. As the nucleation even is very local, the conformation of the unfolded state can be random. This model has received support from experiments conducted on small proteins (Fersht, 1995). The formation of a molten globule is the rate limiting step. Molten globule $\rightarrow$ folded state transition is rapid and irreversible under strongly folding conditions.

Network model, mass action model–This model was suggested based on kinetic equilibria observed experimentally. The huge number of possible unfolded conformations is in rapid equilibrium with each other and with a lesser number of partly folded structures (collectively called as, say, intermediate 1 as in Fig. 1.49). These are not stable and in turn equilibrate with each other as well as with others that

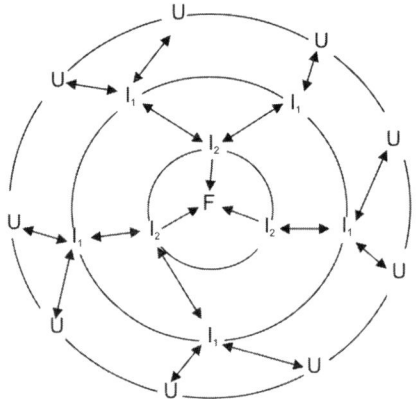

Fig. 1.49: Equilibration in network model

are closer to the fully folded state (in terms of shape collectively called as, say, intermediate 2). The final step that results in the fully folded native structure is rate limiting and this is where, independent of starting conformation of the unfolded state, all molecules of the protein share the common folding pathway.

Hydrophobic collapse model–(Robson, et al. 1971) Based on Kauzmann's description of the role of hydrophobic interactions this model was proposed and demonstrated on α-lactalbumin. Hydrophobic interactions and protein collapse leads to the formation of a condensed structure by a highly cooperative mechanism. This justified the lack of stable intermediates. An MDS investigation by Kollman and coworkers (Duan, et al. 1998) showed that a "molten globule" formed in about 200 nanoseconds. This structure then took 200–800 nsec of "quiet time" to settle. The fully-folded state was reached in 10–100 microseconds. The molten globule of this model is an intermediate; it was found to be very different from the unfolded state and closer (but not identical) to the folded structure in terms compaction and secondary structure composition.

Box 14: Summary of framework vs hydrophobic collapse model

- Hierarchical (local conformation → secondary structure long range interactions → domains → chain) vs
- Spontaneous (hydrophobic collapse → molten globule with high secondary structure content → continues folding)

The Dill model–This is often described as the "new approach" to protein folding that treats folding by the details in the shape of the free energy surface (invariably a funnel). Accordingly, there exist some pathways that the protein naturally folds by (that are kinetically favored by conditions of folding), and along these pathways, the protein may encounter intermediates. The intermediates have their barriers to formation. The high energy TS that these intermediates have to form make the walls of the funnel "rugged". The different molecules of the unfolded state ensemble take different paths that lead to canonical conformations. Thus, some randomness exists. The Dill model is therefore a hybrid of the stochastic (or the thermodynamic) approach and the predetermined (or the kinetic) approach.

The master equation model–Various stages of folding result in several states of molecules that can connect with others in parallel as well as in series simultaneously (*ref.* Scheme 1.23).

That is, a basic master equation can be defined, such as U → S1 → S2 → S3 → F wherein U (the unfolded state) results in F (the folded state) via 3 other conformational states S1 – S3. Here, U can form S1 even via alternative routes, and accordingly, U → A → S1 → S2 → S3 → F becomes another equation whereby A is an alternative state

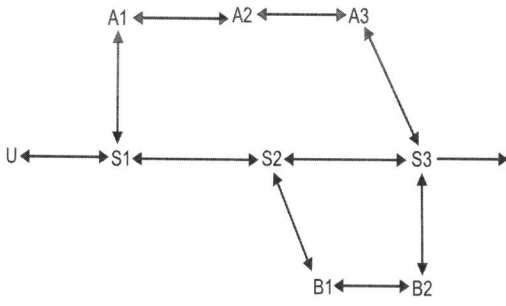

Scheme 1.23: Master equation model

that U can occupy that would eventually channel into the folding pathway. The model matches the experimental fraction of proteins that occupy various states. The TS occurs at approximately the middle of this equation. As expected, it is occupied by a very small fraction of molecules. *Note:* The structure of molecules in each state cannot be characterized as in the final folded state. Example: Folding in T4 lysozyme is sequential whereas that in cytochrome C is parallel (Dill, et al. 2008).

"...Why, you might just as well say that 'I see what I eat' is the same thing as 'I eat what I see'..." The Mad Hatter, at the tea party

in Lewis Carroll's Alice's Adventures in Wonderland

1.5.8.2 Simulation Strategy–Divide and Conquer

Many of the above models show how smaller units form first and assemble to larger ones. In a protein folding simulation wherein computationally a structure is folded, one or more of the models above are used (the use of one theory does not eliminate the use of others–protein can take any path to reach the folded form). Once the fundamental strategy is defined, the rules of the theory are worked into the force field and a simulation would help us visualize the conformational rearrange-ment that develops over time. Based on the interactions that result in favorable energies Scheme 1.24 is presented.

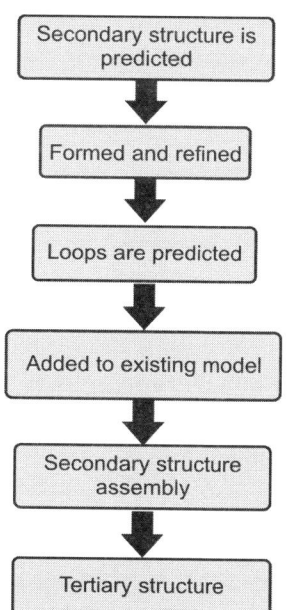

This is the "hierarchical" approach and is strongly supported by experimental literature (Rose, 1979), (Crippen, 1978). This approach will result in the generation of several conformations, many of which may occur in various local minima and the fully assembled model can be considered to be somewhere in the vicinity of the global minimum. One such protein folding algorithm has been set up by Dill and coworkers (Ozkan, et al. 2007) called the Zipping and Assembly Model/Mechanism (the ZAM). It is noteworthy that the models listed above are those created to fit experimental results. The ZAM is a simulation model–it includes force fields and is a computational recipe to calculate the conformation-energy relationship and the folding of a protein.

Scheme 1.24: Hierarchical approach in folding simulations

Discussion 1.17: Zipping and assembly mechanism

Authors: Ozkan SB, Wu GHA, Chodera JD, Dill KA; University of California at San Francisco (Ozkan, et al. 2007)

Introduction: To keep up with all the evidence that points to folding being hierarchical, the divide-and-conquer strategy is used to obtain the solution to placing the native structure at the global minimum. Smaller locally optimized decisions are made about specific secondary structures such as helical turns, β-turns, or small loops. The condition is that these structures must be formed within picoseconds to nanoseconds of the initiation of folding. The simultaneous search progreses throughout the polypeptide chain and structures that are found at within the mentioned time frame are termed "metastable" because they cannot exist independently. They are simply used for the next level of conformational search that involves their "growth". Stretching this further to span the next timescale, stable structures result and are closer to the native structure.

Principle: This method uses the all-atom AMBER96 force field and implicit solvent modeling which were found to be sufficient to guide the folding of a sequence. Usually 8-residue long segments are searched and compared by including neighboring residues or by combining with neighboring segments' conformations. The selected metastable conformations are "grown" in parallel and strong interactions are "locked" in place. This approach totally avoids extensive conformational searches and follows the "funnel" approach–a large number of possible conformations gradually and naturally end up converging on a few, with the formation of higher structural levels. This scenario also solves the Levinthal's paradox. Among the routes starting from the unfolded to folded states, some require extensive conformational search because each fragment cuts down entropy only to a very small extent. But authors report that the dominant folding routes explored by ZAM only involve very little conformational searching.

Summary: Small fragments search their respective local conformations faster than large fragments. Thus, search speed is governed by the calculated loop sizes [details on effective contact order omitted; *ref.* publications] that the chain must search at any step. The method has been used to identify routes to the native state from unfolded states by using all-atom force fields. It was found that fragments that did not resemble their respective native structures during early timescales of the simulation became "corrected" as the tertiary structure of the protein evolved.

1.5.9 ENERGY LANDSCAPING

The conformational space of the protein (i.e. the space containing all the conformations that a protein can take up) as it folds is often arranged by the respective energies of each conformation resulting in the protein's energy landscape. It is treated as a combination of the internal energy and the solvation free energy of a given protein as a function of the microscopic (atomic) degrees of freedom. This surface is funnel-shaped and hence the term "free energy funnel". This does not mean all proteins under the sun have the exact same surface–there are several types of (shapes of) funnels–it qualitatively implies that there are many high energy states (the ensemble of conformations is huge at high energy), but as temperature (and energy content of the molecule) reduces, and as greater order is created within the protein, the number of possible conformations is reduced (ultimately leading to the tiny ensemble representing the native state), giving the funnel-like appearance. Thus at high temperature, the protein is mostly able to access all including the high energy states and hence exists in the unfolded state (at the mouth of the funnel). There is always a balance between entropy, that opposes folding, and the tendency to obey the laws of thermodynamics and occupy the lowest energy conformation (Dill, 1990).

Progressive loss in entropy in Fig. 1.50, the distance between the horizontal lines represents diversity of conformations at each stage of folding. Compare: The four wide-spread red lines of the unfolded state ensemble and the variations in their corresponding conformations U^1–U^4 (difference in peptide structure as a whole)

- The two preferred unfolded state local minima conformations in violet U'^1 and U'^2
- The two grey lines representing structures belonging to the transitions state of the intermediate (structures labeled $I'^{1,2}$) (nucleus of folding is formed and remains undisturbed; changes in other parts)
- Even closer in line spacing and structural similarity, the two maroon lines marking the members of the transition state ensemble (labeled $TS^{1,2}$) (flexibility in the unfolded phase and rigidity in the folded phase of the TS)
- The closest and relatively most stable (least entropy in) the folded state of the native state ensemble (only breathing motions)

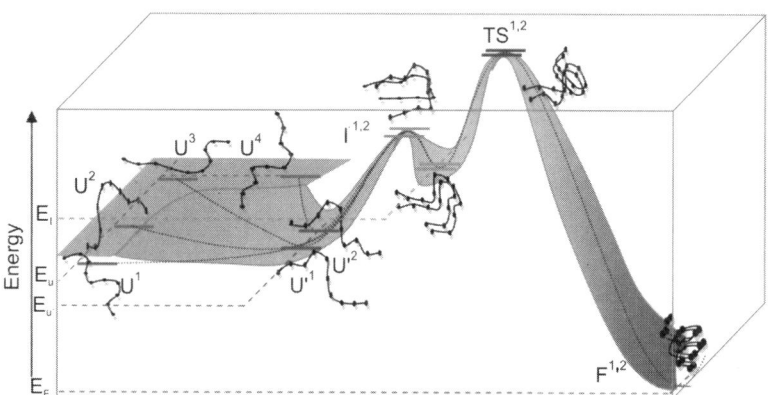

Fig. 1.50: The potential energy surface indicating the variations in conformations at selected points along the surface. Unfolded conformers (U^1–U^4) of approximately degenerate energy Eu form locally favored structures (U'^1, U'^2) of slightly lower energy ($E_{u'}$) at the start of folding. These latter conformations pass through a transition state (I'^1 or I'^2) and become stable intermediates of folding ($I^{1,2}$ of energy E_I). Next, the rate limiting transition to final folded conformer ($F^{1,2}$) of low energy (E_F) occurs by passing through the TS of folding ($TS^{1,2}$). At each stage from left to right, the variety of molecules (the diversity of the members of each ensemble) reduces, the unfolded molecule being most flexible and the folded, being most rigid, indicated by the spacing between horizontal lines that represent each conformer (for color *version see* Plate 1)

Thus there is no single folding "pathway" but a network of pathways that together form the "funnel". Proteins can reach the native conformation through any of these routes. The choice of the folding routes is dictated by the conditions of the system, which has been demonstrated experimentally by changing the denaturant (Sridevi, et al. 2004). As mentioned earlier (*ref*. Discussion 1.11 statistical mechanics description of the knowledge-based mean field approach-under 'fold recognition' section 1.4.3.B), to accurately characterize the shape of the energy surface, one would have to have numbers, for instance, on the fraction of molecules occupying a certain state at a certain level of energy versus other states at other energy levels–and this is termed the "*density of states*" and the all important "*partition function*" of statistical mechanics (as in the above section). To computationally calculate the entire surface of the whole protein in all its glorious diversity of atoms falls either just short of impossible (for reasons mentioned earlier) or just short of the scope of this primer [such as that accomplished by replica exchange methods (Sugita, et al. 1999)]. One popular shape attributed to proteins is the "rugged funnel". In this section, the theories on the basis of which this shape was derived and the implications of this shape in setting up computational simulations of protein folding are discussed.

Did You Know? 13

Sir Alan Fersht of Cambridge University used the following analogy to illustrate this model: if you blindfold a golfer and let him hit the ball in any direction he likes, the probability that he will hole the ball is almost infinitesimal. The same is true of a protein finding the right form by chance. However, if all parts of the golf course slope toward the hole, which is at the lowest point in the area, even a blindfolded golfer has a good chance of finding the hole…

A. The (Rugged) Funnel Landscape

The theoretical understanding of protein folding is based on the idea of the "energy landscape" and the description of its features (Bryngelson, et al. 1989). It is based on the principle of "minimal frustration" which means that there is only one solution when a sequence wants to fold–the native state–and this rests at the global energy minimum where it experiences least conformational strain. Discussion 1.18 delivers a condensed summary of the folding features following paths of the free energy funnel.

Discussion 1.18: The landscape of the free energy funnel of a protein

  i. Free energy landscape is a funnel because large numbers of degenerate conformations of the unfolded ensemble fold into one tiny ensemble of structures representing the folded state
  ii. The free energy surface is constructed from the internal energy of the protein (i.e. the energy calculated using molecular mechanics in vacuum as explained in section 2.2) adding perturbations (or corrections: *ref*. Box 28) due to solvent (van Gunsteren, et al. 1982).

iii. If only native contacts (contacts that will be present in the native structure of the protein) were formed, the funnel would be smooth. But, the walls of the funnel are rugged because atomic vibrations and other dynamic motions of the protein atoms form non-native contacts. Non-native contacts increase strain, make the molecule unstable and increase energy creating a barrier in the wall of the funnel. These contacts then decompose to result in native contacts and energy is lower than what the protein contained initially. This lowering in energy brings the system closer to the global minimum. The protein has to escape these kinetic traps (Cecconi, et al. 2005) during its descent to the bottom. These are termed as "hills" and "valleys".

iv. The protein folds down the funnel with a huge loss of entropy because the numbers of accessible conformations are drastically cut down owing to increase in protein structure organization.

v. The loss of entropy and lowering of energy is also brought about by lowering of temperature. At the glass transition temperature, the protein goes through an "irreversible transition" into a molten structure from which only those conformations lying close to the global minimum become accessible. In case a non-native structure results, partial unfolding and then correct refolding would become necessary on the part of the protein. This is not impossible: remember small change in energy very easily unfolds a folded protein owing to its high heat capacity.

vi. The free energy surface of folding is a funnel because the formation of native contacts is biased strongly against other interactions. This is due to entropic co-operativity. This induces the overall slope towards the native state.

vii. Some proteins fold slowly. This is because their surface contains regions that are flat – called "plateaus". As plateaus have no bias towards any conformation (they are flat), the protein has to cross the plateau by a random conformational search. Plateaus form an entropic barrier and not a kinetic one (Dill, et al. 1997).

viii. Although it appears as if the steep rugged walls of the funnel confuse the protein, this is actually not the case. Consider a totally smooth and flat surface with just one dip right at the centre corresponding to the native state. The protein encountering that dip will be totally at random and sometimes it might go round and round the flat surface without any guidance. To summarize, folding will be unpredictable. Funnels, and especially steep ones, guide proteins to their folded state.

ix. The physiologically active state is not just one lowest energy conformation but actually a whole "tribe of states" that can differ to varying levels- just by the rotamer (which is a very slight difference) or by the topology itself.

x. The factors affecting the protein as it folds are called order parameters and are as follows:
a. Solvent interaction with side chains
b. Fraction of native contacts formed

c. Resemblance of structure with the native conformation in terms of:
   i. Backbone dihedral angles
   ii. Secondary structure content (can be obtained from experiments)
   iii. Degree of collapse (excluded volume effect aims at lowering chain entropy)
   iv. Local conformation within secondary structures (such as kinks, caps, distortions, etc. For example, the defects in a helical structure is considered to result from the competition between compaction due to hydrophobic collapse and h-bonding due to desolvation).

Successful computational folding of a receptor requires clear definition of these parameters. *Other references:* (Clementi, et al. 2000), (Leopold, et al. 1992), (Onuchic, et al. 1997).

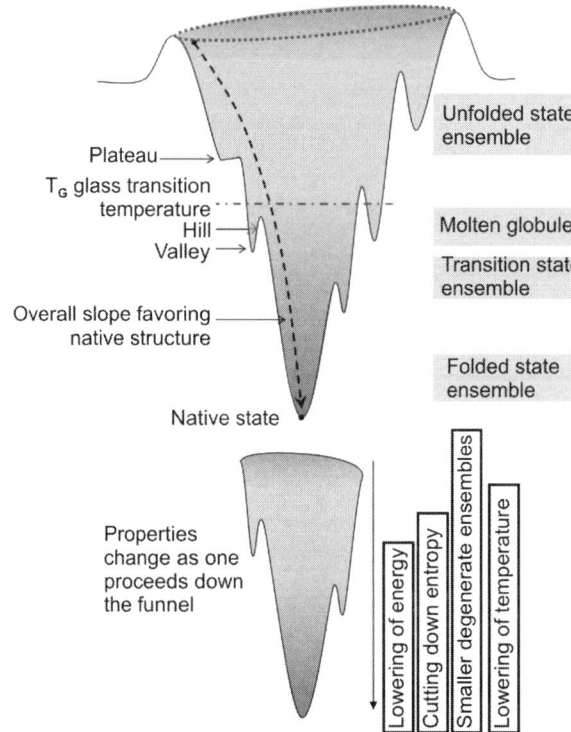

Fig. 1.51: Cross section of a rugged funnel indicating some of its properties

B. Types of Funnels

Although the rugged funnel was presented above in great detail, this is not the universal shape of the folding landscape. In the absence of isomerizations, the shape of the funnel depends on the native fold topology rather than the amino acid sequence (Hockenmaier, et al. 2006). Thus, homologous proteins share common folding features such as time, intermediates, TS, and pathway (funnel shape). The shape of the funnel connects the extent of conformational search (and hence time taken to fold) to the tertiary structure (which is in turn determined by the sequence). Free energy funnels of natural proteins come in the following shapes (Fig. 1.52):

i. *The simple funnel shaped like an inverted bell:* This is the funnel of fast folders. The unfolded conformation starts somewhere up the funnel and in one neat downhill path, ends up in the native structure. There is just one minimum–and of course, this is the global minimum. A few proteins are known to fold extremely fast– in microseconds or in just 100s of nanoseconds (Kubelka, et al. 2006). This observation lead to the construction of such a free energy funnel with the idea that there is probably no free energy barrier to the folding of these proteins [called downhill folding; *ref.* (Dill, et al. 2008)].

ii. *Funnels containing moats that act as kinetic traps (such as the rugged funnel):* Such funnels can be stratified, and each stratum characterized depending on order parameters.

iii. *Golf course funnel:* This is a billiards table or a carrom board with one pocket in the centre. The surface is essentially flat and ups-and-downs in energy are only random fluctuations about a mean. This flat "funnel" indicates a random conformational search made by the protein until it comes very close to the pocket. This folding is very slow in which one pathway is equally probable as the other.

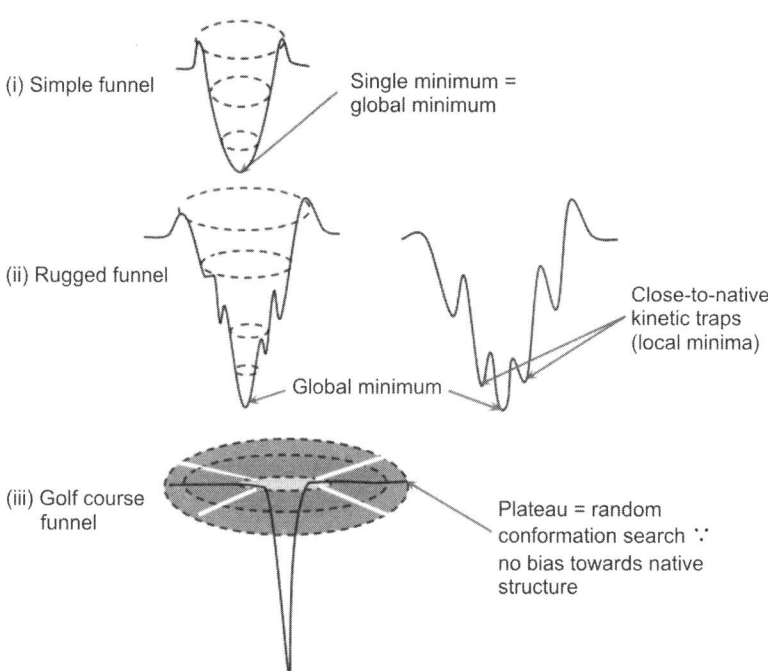

Fig. 1.52: A simple funnel, a rugged funnel and a golf-course

Discussion 1.19: Nature's choice of sequences for proteins

Sequences made of just 2 letters, but of fixed composition, were generated in several possible combinations and allowed to fold in a computer simulation (*ref.* section 2.1 on how this is done). It was observed that that arrangement of sequence that could result in the lowest energy global minimum was the fastest folder (Onuchic, et al. 1995). Further, at a temperature higher than the glass temperature, 50% of the sequences were already folded. The same kind of analysis on a polymer constructed of 3 letter codes (including one more type of monomer than the two used above) showed that well designed sequences did not lead to lowering of the global minimum, but, on the contrary, to the raising of the other states. This latter effect also leads to the increased stability of the folded conformer over others. If this is the case just for 2 or 3 types of monomers, it is not hard to imagine that extremely stable protein structure are possible with amino acids but have been purposely avoided in nature. Why?

There are thousands of amino acids in nature of which only 20 α-amino acids are used by the genome to make proteins. Now, if the 20 amino acids were to form 100-residue proteins, theoretically, 20^{100} proteins are possible. Proteins found in nature are hardly that diverse and therefore form a tiny subset of the universe (Scheme 1.25). The reason attributed to this natural selection is that sequence must be "foldable" under biological conditions (*thermodynamic foldability*) and in a timeframe that is of use to cells (*kinetic foldability*). Statistical mechanical treatment of sequence selection and combinatorial synthesis efforts to make foldable proteins (Schmid, et al. 1986) have brought out that "foldable" sequences must be stable at a higher temperature than the glass transition and the "other" random sequences need not follow this rule. Scheme 1.25 shows that the kinetically foldable molecules is a small group within the thermodynamically foldable one, depending on temperature. At higher temperatures, the preference of the native state decreases as other states become accessible, and so the protein remains denatured. For large multidomain proteins, the distinction between the two sets of sequences is not clear (Brannigan, et al. 2002). Biological proteins also need to be able to fold and unfold at the slightest stimulus from the environment (the folded state is only 5–10 kcal/mol more stable than others). Other references: (Creighton, 1990), (Clementi, et al. 2000)

1.5.10 SIMULATION MODELS

Computationally, structure, energy and recently, even rates (Gromiha, 2005) of folding can be calculated starting from the amino acid sequence. The computational models can be validated by calculating parameters that can be determined experimentally such as the φ-value discussed in previous sections by predicting a particular TS structure (White, et al. 2005). The reaction path parameters can also be assumed and parameters of the path calculated using these models. The parameters–the reaction path coordinate–can be assumed, such as fraction native conformation, fraction native contacts, radius of gyration, surface tension of unfolded regions, etc. (White, et al.

2005) (some of these were mentioned in MDS simulation in chapter 1.3). Similarly, the fact that structure is more conserved than sequence is theoretically re-produced when folding simulation of different sequences give the same 3D structure even amidst several approximations (Dokholyan, et al. 2002). As mentioned, the folded state is only ~10 kcal/mol more stable than the unfolded whereas the structures have total energies of the order of 10 million kcal/mol) (Fig. 1.30A).

The need for a great deal of accuracy is evident simultaneously increasing the computational cost. Scheme 1.26 shows a partial list of methods in protein folding.

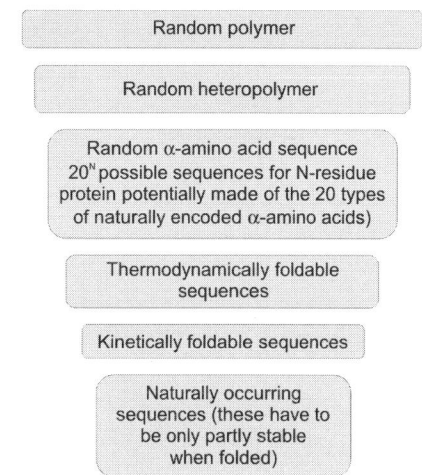

Scheme 1.25: A protein folder's view of the selection of 20 amino acids to recruit into proteins by the genome (at biological temperature *see* Discussion 1.19)

Atomistic Models

In these methods, the force field acts on all the atoms in a protein. One might wonder why other simplifications even exist; all atom simulations act on the complete protein and this is the method that will give the most accurate simulation of protein folding. The main drawback in such a simulation is that, as mentioned earlier in Scheme, a folding run that lasts for as short a period as 50 microseconds will take more than 30,000 years! Proteins are complex organic macromolecules and highly dynamic too. Protein folding simulations cannot ignore the role of water both as a solvent, to drive hydrophobic collapse and as a ligand to interact with specific sites on protein surface. So, millions of water molecules would be needed to fill up the box in which folding is simulated. All this makes simulations computationally demanding. Therefore simplifications are sought. However, an all atom simulation of folding for 10 microseconds has been accomplished (Freddolino, et al. 2008).

Minimalist Models

A few atoms representing all amino acids in the protein (maybe C_α, C_β, calculated pseudo-atom such as centre of mass of a residue, or just a series of linked beads ascribed with a certain property [(Buck, et al.), (Kolinski, 2004), (Sun, 1993), (Sippl, 1995)]. But these "representatives" of proteins can be subjected to detailed calculations because they are very simplified systems. In related papers one can observe detailed theories of physics such as mean field polymer and lattice treatments, spinglass theories, exact enumerations, etc. (Dill, 1999) The polymer in a minimalist model is not a protein, in the sense that anything less than the all-atom structure is not a protein. The behavior

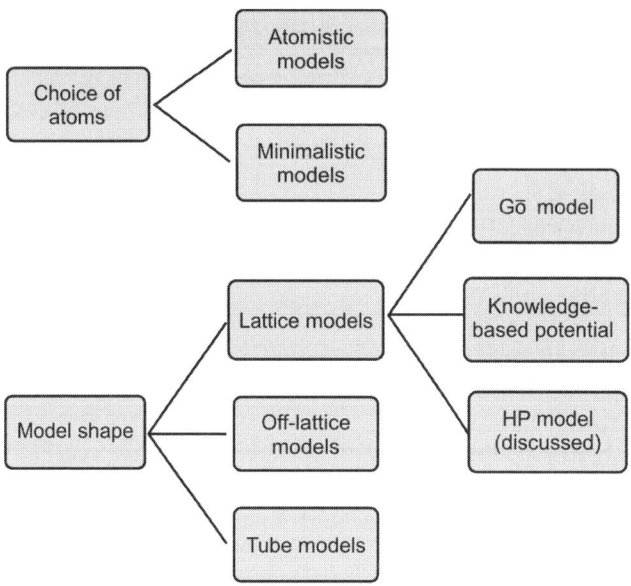

Scheme 1.26: Some protein folding simulation methods

of a chain of 100 beads must be "converted" to apply to a polypeptide chain of 100 residues. The latter's conformations must then be related to the location on the free energy funnel.

Lattice Models

These have been extensively developed and so far, as mentioned in the respective places, several important verifications and theories have been derived from such simplified simulations. A few classic examples are mentioned in Scheme 1.26. The HP model is briefly outlined in Discussion 1.20.

Discussion 1.20: The lattice (HP) model

The lattice models mentioned in the scheme above are the $G\bar{o}$, the knowledge-based and the HP models.

$G\bar{o}$ *models*–These simple lattice models scored the formation of native contacts with the aim of guiding folding towards obtaining maximum scores–ultimately resulting in the native state. This was one of the first computational folding models used on regular basis to investigate structure and folding developed in 1978 ($G\bar{o}$, et al. 1978) and used extensively since then (Hockenmaier, et al. 2006).

Miyazawa-Jernigan knowledge based potentials–(Miyazawa, et al. 1996) extracted information about the tendency of contact of the 20 residues with each other from the PDB setting up a 20 × 20 matrix of potentials. This *"knowledge-based"* contact potential was applied to guide the folding of proteins.

HP model–Lattice models as simple as containing just 2 types of "residues", namely the hydrophobic (H) and polar (P) (and hence called HP models, described further below), have given great insight into folding dynamics; developed by Dill and coworkers (Dill, 1985).

The HP Model

Original authors: KF Lau and KA Dill (University of California at San Francisco, US). (Lau, et al. 1989)

Method summary: This is one of the most simplified protein models, wherein the protein chain is made of just two types of monomers, namely, hydrophobic (H) and polar (P). The game of folding is played on a 2D square lattice where, without breaking the linkage that represents primary structure, a short protein chain is placed on the lattice. The "beads" (representing amino acids) are placed at the intersection of the grids in a random conformation, the only condition being that every bead in the protein occupies a position in the lattice. Only one bead can occupy each intersection point, both at the beginning of the folding simulation when placed in a random conformation and during the simulation when the chain is shuffled about the lattice to occupy various arrangements. Such a placement of beads such that only one bead occupies one lattice intersection at any instant of time, given that the primary linkage of the protein is not broken, is called *self-avoiding walk*. Self-avoiding walk has physical meaning–it is equivalent to the atoms of the natural protein not encroaching within each other's van der Waals radius. Each distinct "walk" represents a unique protein conformation. The lattice arrangement therefore takes care of the "conformation generation" part of determining the global minimum. The other part is to rank conformations based on energy determined by the contacts between monomers that are not adjacent in the primary sequence. As the occupation of the lattice by beads is varied, H-H contacts (contact between two non-adjacent hydrophobic residues occurring in adjacent lattice sites) are highly favorable; the

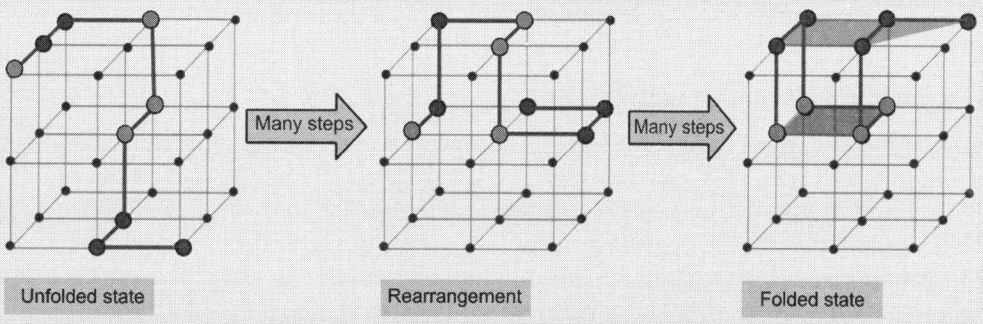

Unfolded state   Rearrangement   Folded state

Scheme: Folding on a cubic grid-a HP lattice folding simulation. Light grey spheres are "hydrophilic" and the other, "hydropholic". The most advantageous arrangement is achieved on the extreme right with "like" spheres found close together in space

scoring function marks every H-H contact energy score as "1". There can be HP sequence arrangements wherein, with such a simple energy scoring method, more than one lowest energy conformation can be obtained. Only those sequences of Hs and Ps that have one lowest energy conformation corresponding to the natural behavior of proteins to have only one native state are chosen for simulation. Authors report 24,900 unique-folding HP sequences for a chain of 20 beads (called a 20-mer) with each 20-mer capable of taking up 41,889,578 viable conformations on the 2D lattice.

This very simple model and its several variations such as the use of 3D cubes instead of 2D lattices are indeed very simple and yet give tremendous insight into the folding process.

1.5.11 KINETICS

"Either the well was very deep, or she fell very slowly, for she had plenty of time as she went down to look about her and to wonder what was going to happen next."

From Alice's adventures in Wonderland by Lewis Carroll.

In Fig. 1.53, the folding paths followed by 3 conformations of a protein are mapped.

Conformation 1: The pathway (yellow) encounters a small hill but succeeds in avoiding the peak of "mountain 1". Instead, it finds a valley formed by the mountains 1 and 2 that has relatively lower barrier height. Crossing 2 barriers (the "hill" and "mountain 1"), especially the second rate limiting one, makes protein molecules taking this route "slow folders".

Conformation 2: The pathway (blue) succeeds in avoiding any initial "hill"; it begins to climb "mountain 2" but then ends up circumventing the mountain. It meanders around to join pathway 1 at the valley. This is also a slow folder even if it encounters only one barrier.

Conformation 3: This molecule follows a pathway (black) of a typical fast folder with very little barriers—it is a straight run for the folded conformation.

A. Kinetics of Protein Folding

Folding is more rapid than a random conformational search, but a protein chain taking seconds to fold scan still search anywhere from 10^8 to 10^{13} conformations (Creighton, 1990). Experimentally, one can characterize the slowest step (the rate limiting step), the intermediates that accumulate at the rate limiting step, their TS, and perhaps the conformations and energetics of the most stable structures along the entire folding pathway. Summarizing facts obtained so far regarding the rate of folding,

i. Fast folders have more local contacts such as helices whereas slow folders have more tertiary organization such as into β-sheets….(*ref.* section 1.2)

ii. Rate depends more on the topology of the folded state (α-helix content, etc.) rather than the sequence

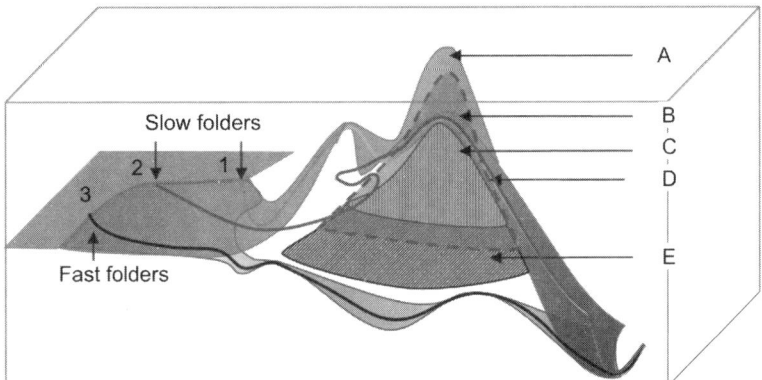

(A) "First Mountain", (B) Valley, (C) Cross section: Steep rise to a 2nd mountain,
(D) (red) Outline of 2nd mountain, (E) Base area of 2nd mountain

Fig. 1.53: The rate of folding depends on the path taken by the protein to reach the native state–a comparison among conformations 1–3 (for color version *see* Plate 2)

iii. There are programs that identify all direct folding routes from the unfolded state to the global minimum (Hockenmaier, et al. 2006)

iv. As mentioned earlier, methods have been developed that can predict the rate of folding of a given sequence based on several parameters such as the two written above.

B. Kinetics of Protein Unfolding

Unfolding is almost universally unfolding preceding it.

Creighton, 1990

Observations on the influence of various factors on the kinetics of protein folding are summarized in this section. Readers are referred to Discussion 1.21: *Understanding Kinetics* for a general overview. Unfolding is a cooperative process wherein the start of unfolding leads only to its completion in one smooth phase. This is a uniform behavior of all folded molecules-they all exhibit the same probability to unfold, the same rate constant of unfolding and a single rate limiting step, independent of the details of the experiment. This unanimity is probably because all folded molecules belong to a tight ensemble.

C. Kinetics of Protein Refolding

Contrary to protein unfolding which starts with molecules of similar conformation, refolding of proteins is not a uniform phenomenon. As mentioned earlier, molecules of the same protein might have different rates of refolding depending on the cis-trans isomerization of the peptide bonds preceding prolines (*ref.* above) that might have occurred in the unfolded state. Refolding can be summarized thus:

- The pre-folded state, which is the "most preferred unfolded state under refolding conditions", is not a random coil, as described above under *the intermediate*.
- The TS and the resemblance of its properties to the folded state.

- The ensemble of structures in the folded conformation, representing its conformational entropy (flexibility).

These inferences often underlie the setting up of protein folding models such as the network model that suggest rapid equilibrium among unfolded conformations making them as homogeneous in structure as the folded state. The rapid equilibration is possible only because the pre-folded state is not a random coil. The ensemble of pre-folded state conformation is much larger than the folded state ensemble, but is a smaller and better characterized subset of the random coil ensemble. Dynamic equilibrium between these conformations allows the unfolded state conformations to channel into the same folding pathway during refolding. Rate of refolding increases with increase in temperature, but only up to a certain limit. High temperatures, in accordance to the Boltzmann distribution, do not bias the folded state as other states become easily accessible to the folding molecule. In addition, this disturbance of folding is also known to be brought about by the difference in heat capacities of the folded and unfolded state.

Discussion 1.21: Understanding kinetics

Discussion contributed by Janarthanan Krishnamoorthy

Kinetics, like thermodynamics, is an important branch of sciences, which explains physical processes that evolve with time. For example, chemical reactions, growth of organisms, motion of an object, distribution of drug in body, etc. are all kinetic processes, and can be approached quantitatively using differential equations. If an object moves from one point to another, the velocity at each point it passes through need not be the same. The velocity measured at each point is called 'instantaneous velocity', in contrast to average velocity which considers only the magnitude of distance travelled (Dx) and the time taken (Dt) for it. 'Average velocity' (Dx/Dt) can be considered to represent 'instantaneous velocity' (dx/dt) if the time interval becomes infinitesimally small. In chemical reactions, mostly we are interested in predicting the nature of mechanism and rate of product formation. A systematic approach to unravel it would be:

- Proposing a mechanism
- Framing the required differential equations
- Solving the differential equations with or without steady state assumption
- Determining the kinetic parameters by model fitting.

Proposing a Mechanism

The mechanism gives the details of how product molecules are generated from reactants. Reactions may be reversible or irreversible, single or multiple step-based, linear or cyclic.

At the outset, we can only presume a mechanism; hence such proposals ought to be as realistic as possible to explain the physical system in hand. Simpler mechanisms are always preferred to complex mechanisms for a given system.

$$A \xrightarrow{k_{+1}} B$$

$$A \underset{k_{-1}}{\overset{k_{+1}}{\rightleftharpoons}} B$$

$$A \underset{k_{-1}}{\overset{k_{+1}}{\rightleftharpoons}} B \underset{k_{-2}}{\overset{k_{+2}}{\rightleftharpoons}} C$$

(A) Single step, irreversible and reversible reactions. (B) Two step equilibrium with an intermediate reactant (C) Four step cyclic equilibrium reaction

Framing the Differential Equations

Differential equations can be framed for the rate of every species involved in the mechanism. For a simple irreversible mechanism, the rate of change of A and B can be written as follows:

$$\frac{dA}{dt} = -1 \times k_{+1} \times (A)$$

$$\frac{dB}{dt} = +1 \times k_{+1} \times (A)$$

Here we see three components in the first equation, -1, k_{+1}, (A), all of which are multiplied together. To arrive at it, we start with the Le-Chaterlier principle, which states that the rate of forward reaction is proportional to concentration of (A); in other words, if (A) is higher, the forward reaction dominates compared to reverse reaction in the equilibrium $\frac{dA}{dt} \propto (A)$. Now we introduce a proportionality constant k_{+1} for equating the equation $\frac{dA}{dt} = k_{+1} \times (A)$. Finally, considering that the forward reaction is going to decrease the concentration of (A), we multiply a prefactor -1 to the RHS which becomes, $\frac{dA}{dt} = -1 \times k_{+1} \times (A)$. To clarify this further, we will consider the mechanism $(A \leftrightarrow B)$, here 'A' is associated with two reactions $A \rightarrow B$ (forward) and $A \leftarrow B$ (reverse), both of which affect the concentration of 'A', therefore the rate of change of 'A' is written as,

$$\frac{dA}{dt} = \underbrace{[-1 \times k_{+1} \times (A)}_{1} + \underbrace{(+1 \times k_{-1} \times (B)]}_{2}$$

The first part of RHS is the same as explained above, but the second part says that the reaction B–>A is going to increase the concentration of 'A', so a prefactor of $+1$ is multiplied to the corresponding rate constant k_{-1} and the corresponding reactant 'B'. Similar expressions can be written for more complicated species like (C) in two step linear equilibrium mechanism.

$$\frac{dC}{dt} = \underbrace{[+1 \times k_{+3} \times (B)]}_{1} + \underbrace{[-1 \times k_{-3} \times (C)]}_{2} + \underbrace{[+1 \times k_{+4} \times (D)]}_{3} + \underbrace{[-1 \times k_{-4} \times (C)]}_{4}$$

If there are more than one reactants then the reactants are multiplied together, as shown in the following model:

$$A + nB \underset{k_{-1}}{\overset{k_{+1}}{\rightleftharpoons}} C$$

The differential equations for (A) and (B) are:

$$\frac{dC}{dt} = \underbrace{[+1 \times k_{+1} \times (A) \times (B) \times (B) \times \ldots n\ times]}_{1} + \underbrace{[-1 \times k_{-1} \times (C)]}_{2}$$

Rewritten as:

$$\frac{dC}{dt} = \underbrace{[+1 \times k_{+1} \times (A) \times (B)^n]}_{1} + \underbrace{[-1 \times k_{-1} \times (C)]}_{2}$$

Solving the Differential Equations with or without Steady State Assumption

If there are 'n' species present in a mechanism, we need at least 'n' coupled differential equations to solve them. On solving these equations, we get an expression for each species in terms of time 't' as the only independent variable. Steady-state assumption simplifies the solving of differential equations, by reducing it to simple algebraic equations.

Solving under Steady-state Assumption

Steady-state assumption for a particular species means that its concentration does not vary with respect to time. The differential equation then can be equated to zero. The validity of such an assumption depends on the state of the system. For example, when a system is in equilibrium, the reactants, intermediates and the products are said to be in steady state. We will consider the mechanism (A↔B↔C), as an example to derive the appropriate expressions.

$$\frac{dA}{dt} = A' = -k_{+1}(A) + k_{-1}(B)$$

$$\frac{dB}{dt} = B' = +k_{+1}(A) - k_{-1}(B) - k_{+2}(B) + k_{-2}(C)$$

$$\frac{dC}{dt} = C' = +k_{+2}(B) - k_{-2}(C)$$

in matrix form the above equations can be written as

$$\begin{bmatrix} -k_{+1} & +k_{-1} & 0 \\ +k_{+1} & -(k_{-1} + k_{+2}) & k_{-2} \\ 0 & +k_{+2} & -k_{-2} \end{bmatrix} \begin{bmatrix} A \\ B \\ C \end{bmatrix} = \begin{bmatrix} A' \\ B' \\ C' \end{bmatrix}$$

Since we are assuming equilibrium $A' = B' = C' = 0$, then we have

$$\begin{bmatrix} -k_{+1} & +k_{-1} & 0 \\ +k_{+1} & -(k_{-1}+k_{+2}) & k_{-2} \\ 0 & +k_{+2} & -k_{-2} \end{bmatrix} \begin{bmatrix} A \\ B \\ C \end{bmatrix} = \begin{bmatrix} 0 \\ 0 \\ 0 \end{bmatrix}$$

Expressing all the species in terms of any one of the species (in our case 'A'), using expressions for A' and B' we have:

$$B = \frac{k_{+1}}{k_{-1}}(A)$$

$$C = \frac{k_{+2}}{k_{-2}}(B)$$

Substituting expression of 'B' into 'C' we get,

$$C = \frac{k_{+2}}{k_{-2}} \cdot \frac{k_{+1}}{k_{-1}}(A)$$

And finally using the fact (principle of conservation of mass) that the total amount of reactant is:

$$A_T = A + B + C$$

$$\therefore A_T = A + \frac{k_{+1}}{k_{-1}}(A) + \frac{k_{+2}}{k_{-2}} \cdot \frac{k_{+1}}{k_{-1}}.(A)$$

In the LHS taking out 'A' as common and rearranging, we have

$$A = \frac{A_T}{1 + K_1 + K_2 K_1} \text{ where } K_1 = \frac{k_{+1}}{k_{-1}} \text{ and } K_2 = \frac{k_{+2}}{k_{-2}}$$

Similarly, substituting the value of A in the expressions of B and C, we get:

$$B = \frac{K_1 A_T}{1 + K_1 + K_2 K_1}$$

$$C = \frac{K_1 K_2 A_T}{1 + K_1 + K_2 K_1}$$

The results shows that concentration of A, B, C will not vary with respect to time as there is no time variable 't' in the final expressions. Solving the same set of differential equations under partial steady state, (i.e. condition with only certain species concentration does not vary with time), is actually a subset of solving the same under non-steady state condition.

Solving under Non Steady-state Condition

Before we solve the previous case under non steady-state condition, we need to get familiar with two fundamental mathematical techniques.
1. Solving linear differential equation by variable separable method
2. Diagonalisation of a matrix.

Variable Separable Method

Consider the mechanism of (A→B), where the differential form of A is given as $\frac{dA}{dt} = -k_{+1}(A)$. This equation has only two variables (A and t) though the mechanism has three variable A, B, t. Such equations can be easily solved by separating one to the RHS and the other to the LHS thus, $\frac{dA}{A} = -k_{+1}dt$. Taking integration on both sides, we get:

$$\int \frac{dA}{A} = \int -k_{+1}\, dt$$

$$\ln (A) = -k_{+1}\, t + \text{constant}$$

we can determine the value of constant using boundary condition that sets $A = A_0$ at time $t = 0$

Using the above expression the profile of 'A' can be obtained by plugging different values of 't' and setting the constants k_{+1} and A_0 at arbitrary values. This method will not be applicable if the given differential equation has more than two variables and are combined linearly (added or subtracted). In such cases, we will adopt the following general methodology, which uses diagonalization of matrices.

$$\ln (A_0) = -k_{+1} \times 0 + \text{constant}$$

$$\therefore \text{constant} = \ln (A_0)$$

$$A = A_0\, e^{-k_{+1}t}$$

Diagonalization of Matrix

Given a square matrix as shown below, it is possible to represent it as a product of three matrices with middle matrix being diagonalized. Diagonolization is a process by which all the elements of a matrix except the right diagonal becomes zero. The elements of the diagonal matrix are called the eigenvalues and the matrix multiplied to the left of the diagonal matrix is called the eigenvector matrix. The matrix at the right of diagonal matrix is the inverse of the eigenvector matrix.

$$\begin{bmatrix} a1 & b1 & c1 \\ a2 & b2 & c2 \\ a3 & b3 & c3 \end{bmatrix} = \begin{bmatrix} A1 & B1 & C1 \\ A2 & B2 & C2 \\ A3 & B3 & C3 \end{bmatrix} \begin{bmatrix} \lambda_1 & 0 & 0 \\ 0 & \lambda_2 & 0 \\ 0 & 0 & \lambda_3 \end{bmatrix} \begin{bmatrix} A1 & B1 & C1 \\ A2 & B2 & C2 \\ A3 & B3 & C3 \end{bmatrix}^{-1}$$

The above matrices can be compactly written for better representation as

$$(a) = (U)(\lambda)(U)^{-1}.$$

Solutions for Coupled Differential Equations

Rewriting the coupled differential equations of previous mechanism (A ↔ B ↔ C), in a compact matrix notation (as mentioned above), (M') = (C)(M); where M', C, M are matrices of previously mentioned matrix expressions, but written from right to left. This form resembles the linear differential equation form encountered in '*Variable separable* section above. In fact the same integral approach can be adopted here and the solution for such matrix forms can be given as, $M = e^{[C]t} M_0$; where M, M_0 and C represents matrices. Please take note that the order of multiplication matters in matrix form, but not when terms are scalar in nature. The only difficulty in evaluating the above expression is the calculation of exponential of the matrix C though this can be expanded by Taylor series and evaluated up to second or third order. The better way is to diagonalize the matrix C and to proceed as follows,

$$(C) = (U) (\lambda) (U)^{-1}$$

$$e^{(C)t} = (U)e^{(\lambda)t} (U)^{-1} \text{ (Obtained using standard formula)}$$

$$\therefore (M) = (I)e^{\lambda t} (U)^{-1} (M_0)$$

Representing the elements of each matrix explicitly we have,

$$
\begin{bmatrix} A \\ B \\ C \end{bmatrix} = \begin{bmatrix} A1'A1e^{\lambda_1 t} + A2'B1e^{\lambda_2 t} + A3'C1e^{\lambda_3 t} & B1'A1e^{\lambda_1 t} + B2'B1e^{\lambda_2 t} + B3'C1e^{\lambda_3 t} \\ & C1'A1e^{\lambda_1 t} + C2'B1e^{\lambda_2 t} + C3'C1e^{\lambda_3 t} \\ A1'A2e^{\lambda_1 t} + A2'B2e^{\lambda_2 t} + A3'C2e^{\lambda_3 t} & B1'A2e^{\lambda_1 t} + B2'B2e^{\lambda_2 t} + B3'C2e^{\lambda_3 t} \\ & C1'A2e^{\lambda_1 t} + C2'B2e^{\lambda_2 t} + C3'C2e^{\lambda_3 t} \\ A1'A3e^{\lambda_1 t} + A2'B3e^{\lambda_2 t} + A3'C3e^{\lambda_3 t} & B1'A3e^{\lambda_1 t} + B2'B3e^{\lambda_2 t} + B3'C3e^{\lambda_3 t} \\ & C1'A3e^{\lambda_1 t} + C2'B3e^{\lambda_2 t} + C3'C3e^{\lambda_3 t} \end{bmatrix} \begin{bmatrix} A_0 \\ B_0 \\ C_0 \end{bmatrix}
$$

$$
\begin{bmatrix} A \\ B \\ C \end{bmatrix} = \begin{bmatrix} A_0[A1'A1e^{\lambda_1 t} + A2'B1e^{\lambda_2 t} + A3'C1e^{\lambda_3 t}] + B_0[B1'A1e^{\lambda_1 t} + B2'B1e^{\lambda_2 t} + B3'C1e^{\lambda_3 t}] \\ + C_0[C1'A1e^{\lambda_1 t} + C2'B1e^{\lambda_2 t} + C3'C1e^{\lambda_3 t}] \\ A_0[A1'A2e^{\lambda_1 t} + A2'B2e^{\lambda_2 t} + A3'C2e^{\lambda_3 t}] + B_0[B1'A2e^{\lambda_1 t} + B2'B2e^{\lambda_2 t} + B3'C2e^{\lambda_3 t}] \\ + C_0[C1'A2e^{\lambda_1 t} + C2'B2e^{\lambda_2 t} + C3'C2e^{\lambda_3 t}] \\ A_0[A1'A3e^{\lambda_1 t} + A2'B3e^{\lambda_2 t} + A3'C3e^{\lambda_3 t}] + B_0[B1'A3e^{\lambda_1 t} + B2'B3e^{\lambda_2 t} + B3'C3e^{\lambda_3 t}] \\ + C_0[C1'A3e^{\lambda_1 t} + C2'B3e^{\lambda_2 t} + C3'C3e^{\lambda_3 t}] \end{bmatrix}
$$

From the above equation we have obtained explicit expression relating A, B, C with the only variable time 't', and the rest constants like A1, A2, A3, B1,... which in turn are made up of different combinations of rate constants like k_{+1}, k_{-1}, k_{+2}, k_{-2}, etc.

Application in Enzyme Kinetics

In many of the enzyme kinetic problem, the main objective would be to elucidate the mechanism of interaction. Indirectly from the initial velocity or rate of product formation, it is possible to unravel the mechanism quite easily. We make use of previously explained methodology, to derive the classical Michaelis-Menten model for the following mechanism, $E + S \xrightarrow[k_{-1}]{k_{+1}} ES \xrightarrow[E]{k_{+2}} +P$. In the presence of inhibitors, similar such mechanisms can be proposed according to the nature of interaction. For example, the mechanisms for competitive, non-competitive, un-competitive inhibition with reversible binding are given as follows:

$$E + S \underset{k_{-1}}{\overset{k_{+1}}{\rightleftharpoons}} (ES) \overset{k_{+2}}{\underset{E}{\longrightarrow}} + P \quad \text{Competitive model}$$

$$E + I \underset{k_{-1}}{\overset{k_{+1}}{\rightleftharpoons}} (EI)$$

Non-competitive model (inhibitor binds to E even in presence of S)

$$E + S \underset{k_{-1}}{\overset{k_{+1}}{\rightleftharpoons}} (ES) \overset{k_{+2}}{\underset{E}{\longrightarrow}} + P$$

$$E + S + I \underset{k_{-1}}{\overset{k_{+1}}{\rightleftharpoons}} (ESI)$$

Un-competitive model (inhibitor binds to ES complex directly) tp E even in presence of S

$$E + S \underset{k_{+1}}{\overset{k_{-1}}{\rightleftharpoons}} (ES) \rightarrow E + P$$

$$k_{-2} \updownarrow + (I) k_{+2}$$

$$(ESI)$$

While considering irreversible mechanisms, only the forward reaction are devised omitting the reverse reactions.

Michaelis-Mentin Kinetic Model

The differential equations for the enzymatic reaction without any inhibitor is framed as follows:

$$\frac{dE}{dt} = -k_{+1}(E)(S) + k_{-1}(ES)$$

$$\frac{d(ES)}{dt} = +k_{+1}(E)(S) - k_{-1}(ES) - k_2(ES)$$

$$\frac{dP}{dt} = +k_2(ES)$$

We are interested in dP/dt, which is the rate of product formation (v). From the third equation, if we know the concentration of (ES), we can calculate 'v' easily. But it is very difficult to find (ES) as it is transient and difficult to measure experimentally. The other way around would be to express (ES) in terms of either (S) or (P) (concentrations). For example, when starch is hydrolyzed by amylase, iodimetry titrations can be carried to quantify the remaining starch substrate at different time intervals, or the hydrolyzed product, glucose can be quantified by colorimetric methods. To express (ES) in terms of (S), we will make use of a valid assumption that the concentration of [ES] does not vary with respect to time. So, we can write the second equation as:

$$\frac{d(ES)}{dt} = +k_{+1}(E)(S) - k_{-1}(ES) - k_2(ES) = 0 \qquad (E) = \frac{(k_{+1} + k_2)(ES)}{k_{+1}(S)}$$

(on rearranging). Now we know that (E), the free enzyme concentration is also difficult to measure, so we use the principle of conservation of mass to express (ES) in terms of (E_T) (Total enzyme is the sum of free and bound enzyme concentration),

$$(E_T) = (E) + (ES)$$

$$= \frac{(k_{+1} + k_2)(ES)}{k_{+1}(S)} + (ES)$$

$$= (ES)\left[\frac{(k_{+1} + k_2)}{k_{+1}(S)} + 1\right]$$

$$\therefore (ES) = \frac{E_T}{1 + \dfrac{k_{-1} + k_2}{k_{+1}(S)}}$$

Substituting [ES] into expression for 'v', we have

$$v = k_2 \frac{E_T}{1 + \dfrac{k_{-1} + k_2}{k_{+1}(S)}}$$

In the ratio $(k_{-1} + k_2)/k_{+1}$ in the denomenator is actually the sum of the rate constants of two reactions that dissociates [ES] back either to the substrate or to the product.

$$E + S \xleftarrow{k_{-1}} ES \xrightarrow{k_2} E + P$$

Whereas k_{+1} is the rate constant that brings about association of (ES): $E + S \xrightarrow{k_{+1}} (ES)$

Thus the above fraction is the ratio of sum of dissociation rate constants to the association rate constant. In general this is termed as k_D, the 'dissociation constant'.

$$v = k_2 \frac{E_T}{1 + \dfrac{k_D}{(S)}} = k_2 \frac{E_T(S)}{(S) + k_D}$$

The term $k_2(E_T)$ is similar to $v = k_2(ES)$, except for the difference that (E_T), is in the place of bound enzyme (ES). Which means 'v' is proportional to bound enzyme and if all the enzyme are present in bound form, then that is the maximum velocity that could be reached for the given (E_T).

$$v' = k_2 \, (ES)$$

in $(E_T) = (E) + (ES)$, if $(E) = 0$, (i.e. no free enzyme present), then $(E_T) = (ES)$ $= k_2 \, (E_T) = v_{max}$ substituting back into the expression for v

$$v = \frac{v_{max}\,(S)}{K_D + (S)}$$

1.5.12 PROTEOMICS ROADMAP TO MEDICINAL CHEMISTRY–4

A. Recent Endeavors

 i. A folding simulation of the villin headpiece (of 36-residues) in explicit solvent for ~1 μs was carried out by Kollman and coworkers. This supercomputer calculation resulted in a collapsed state that deviated from the experimental structure by ~4.5 Å (Duan, et al. 1998)

 ii. The villin headpiece was folded for 10 μs using an all-atom force field by Claus Schulten and coworkers (Freddolino, et al. 2008)

 iii. The folding@home project is an interesting method of carrying out all-atom simulation of villin on the screensavers of volunteer computers worldwide. It was developed by Pande and coworkers (Zagrovic, et al. 2002)

 iv. IBMs "blue gene" is a supercomputer built to study biomolecular behavior. The project is a collaboration among IBM, Thomas J. Watson Research Center, Lawrence Livermore National Laboratory, United States Department of Energy and the academia. The project was awarded the National Medal of Technology and Innovation by US President Barack Obama on September 18, 2009.

B. Pharmaceutical Applications

 i. Protein folding gives much greater insights to protein dynamic studies. Modeling induced-fit behavior of proteins enables us to predict drug affinity more accurately.

 ii. Detailed understanding of protein recognition and motion in the cellular medium helps us to simultaneously tackle a part of pharmacokinetics and drug delivery when studying pharmacodynamic behavior.

 iii. Being able to build protein behavior towards solvent, temperature, pH, denaturants, etc. from the behavior of its atoms completes a large portion of our understanding of biology. Further steps will lead us to prevention, correction and cure of a large number of diseases.

 iv. The above knowledge also helps us design new proteins for transport and delivery of drugs among other industrial applications in other fields.

 v. Artificial folding molecules are called *foldamers*. They are constructed by editing structures of known natural proteins or by creating new protein-like macro-molecules from non-biological monomers. The success of their design expands the creation of "new functional materials" with enormous applications as antimicrobials, (Hill, et al. 2001), (Hecht, et al. 2007), etc.

vi. Diseases of protein misfolding (also known as the most menacing diseases of our era) are the current focus of study that immensely benefit from the study protein folding; for an outline on the diseases and research, *ref.* Discussion 1.22.

Discussion 1.22: Diseases of protein misfolding

i. Fatal neurodegenerative diseases like Bovine Spongiform Encephalopathy (BSE) or the 'mad cow disease' and its human equivalent Creutzfeldt-Jakob disease (CJD) are caused by *prions*. Some related facts are:
   a. Prions are misfolded proteins that are triggered by a conformational change.
   b. The precise mechanism of the diseases is not known.
   c. The prions became an entirely new class of disease-causing agents.
   d. In general, nucleic acids were thought to be the specialists of genetic information and infection transfer. It was later discovered that nucleic acids such as the catalytic RNAs can catalyze reactions, a function till then attributed to proteins only. The possibility that prions, being proteins, carry genetic instructions (a role traditionally attributed to nucleic acids) completes the duality of functions to both classes of macromolecules.

ii. The family of amyloid diseases include:
   a. Alzheimer's disease results in loss of memory, thinking and language skills, and behavioral changes. The neurons become enveloped by a plaque of misfolded and precipitated β-amyloid protein. Drugs such as donepezil, galantamine, rivastigmine, tacrine, memantine, etc. have been investigated (Cummings, et al. 2002).
   b. Familial amyloid polyneuropathy is a condition (*amylum* means 'viscous') wherein the tetramer protein transthyretin misfolds. This gives rise to amyloid deposits that interfere with normal nerve and muscle function. These deposits are significantly reduced, and misfolding of the protein even prevented, if certain mutant monomers of the protein are incorporated into transthyretin. These findings suggest potential therapeutic strategies for amyloid and related misfolding disorders.

As in mad cow disease, a molecular understanding of the misfolding process may lead to treatments of the disorders.

Proteomics Research for Drug Design

Protein replacement therapy was historically the therapy for treating these conditions. Current treatment strategies are based on the use of ligands to stabilize the correct (native) state of the protein. These ligands are called *pharmacological chaperones*. These are specific to the misfolded disease-causing proteins designed based on available knowledge such as hydrophobic and polar patterning (Loo, et al. 2007). Analogues can be designed for a whole range of conditions based on these principles, such as cystic fibrosis, the amyloidoses, Parkinson's disease, Alzheimer's disease, metabolic disorders such as Gaucher disease, etc. (Ringe, et al. 2009), (Khanna, et al. 2010).

Part II
Drug Design and
Molecular Modeling

*If today's chemistry lets us turn things on or off by blocking or unblocking receptors
and enzymes, tomorrow's molecules will be able to balance complex metabolic
processes like growth and aging by fine tuning the regulation of genes and their
products.*

– Schlick, 2002

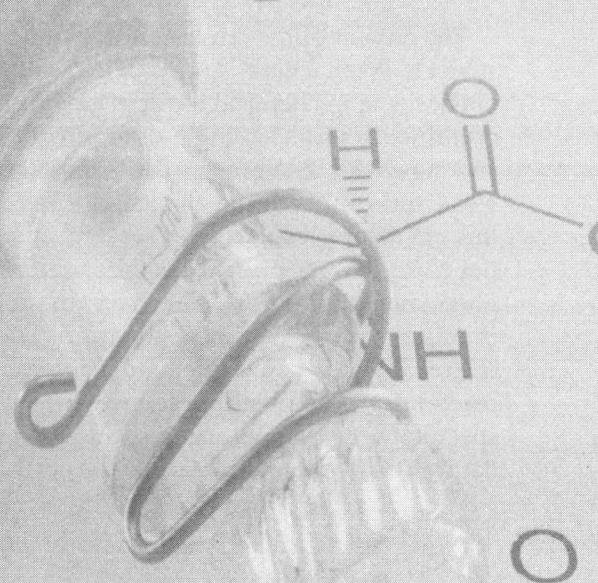

2.1 *Introduction*

This part deals with the study of some important principles of medicinal chemistry which form the foundation of drug designing. Strategies used to create or identify new chemical entities that promise to show pharmacodynamic properties have evolved over a long period of time and this evolution has been well documented in textbooks and other sources (Foye, et al. 2008). A repetition of this evolution is superfluous; however, this text intends to expose readers to a very recent technique–the use of computations.

Nature has evolved over billions of years. Over this time-frame it has built and perfected a "molecular language" by which organisms exist, survive, communicate, pass on traits to the next generation and evolve. The DNA, for example, is one long molecule that literally "speaks for" the identity and existence of species–it stores and expresses information ranging from the physical appearance, habits, and adaptations. We know that transcription and translation are the processes by which the information in the DNA and the RNA is used to synthesize the RNA and proteins respectively. The RNA, transcribed from the DNA, regulates DNA activity and also translates coding DNA regions into proteins. The transcription process (which is the conversion of DNA to RNA) and the translation process (which is the conversion of RNA into protein) in turn involve a host of other molecules. Though these are extremely complex processes, still they involve the elementary bond breakage–bond formation–weak interactions (such as hydrogen bonding, van der Waals repulsion, dipole effects, Coulomb charge interactions, etc.) that we have read about since high school. Thus, however, complex the biological process in question such as imagination and dreaming, fetal growth, the emotions, the senses of sight/smell, the movement of skeletal and smooth muscles, the recognition of those around us, etc. can be described as an organized interactions of elements (carbon, hydrogen, oxygen, etc.).

The advent of the study of biochemistry and molecular pharmacology as essential subjects in pharmacy and medicine reflect this trend of understanding biological phenomena in chemical terms. The infectivity of viruses is an example. A new strain of influenza virus having a different antigenicity requires a fresh search for vaccines and cure. The change in strain is initiated by mutations in the genetic material of the virus and results in the change of viral coat protein composition. The knowledge of this chemistry helps researchers look for the right vaccine (for prevention) or drug (for cure). In the same spirit of the above approach, which is to understand the biological phenomena in terms of chemistry, the cell can be considered as a pot with a soup of chemicals in it. One can easily appreciate the fact that in the presence of millions of chemically active molecules and macromolecules, all biochemical and pharmacological reactions proceed without interference. This is the language very special to biology–specificity of reaction and response. It is this "specificity in diversity" concept that nature has perfected ever since the earth was formed.

There are about 1.5 million species on earth (http://www.currentresults.com/). Each individual organism recognizes itself (the molecules of its own body) and what is foreign. Some life processes are universal–present in unicellular prokaryotes and complex multicellular organisms alike-such as respiration. In general, all components of the respiratory chain have equivalents in all organisms. Let us consider the cytochrome C respiratory protein; the results of the analysis of the cytochrome C proteins deposited in the protein data bank are presented in Scheme 2.1. In total 106 unique proteins were obtained from 56 different species. Although all these 106 proteins perform very similar functions in the 56 species, the proteins could be classified into roughly 24 types based on their structure. The differences are not uniform–they vary from very mild differences in minor segments of the proteins to very large differences in overall structure!

Such knowledge of similarities and differences in organismal chemistry forms the basis of action of antimicrobials, CNS drugs, anticancer drugs, etc. Most drugs directly or indirectly target proteins; the former ones bind to proteins reversibly or irreversibly to elicit action whereas the later group influence protein processes such as protein synthesis (transcription, translation) assembly expression levels, modifications (post translational) and degradation. Proteins are the "work horses of the cell"; a clear understanding of their physiochemical properties is an essential part of the drug design approach. Although there are billions of proteins in nature, their properties as macromolecules can be generalized under descriptive summary presented in part I. Accumulating data on proteins, natural substrates and invented drugs can form the basis of drug design provided an effective means of keeping track of all the information is available. We all know that computers are well suited to store, retrieve and analyze information from experimental and theoretical investigation. We can use computers to analyze an unknown situation and predict the outcome. Molecular modeling and

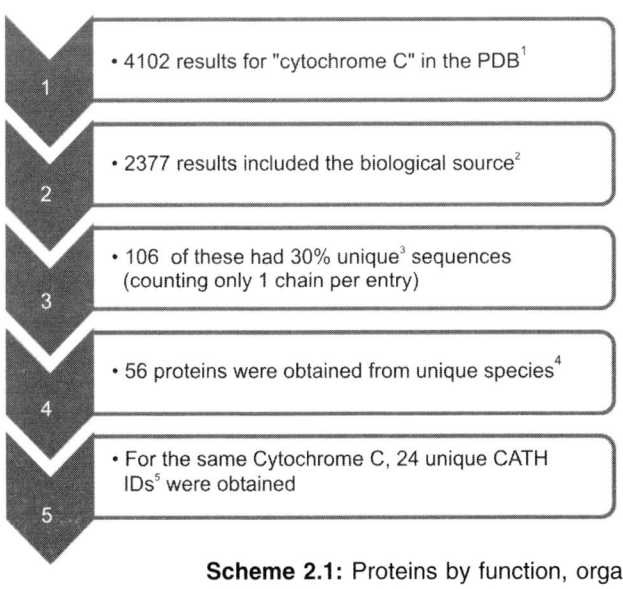

1. • 4102 results for "cytochrome C" in the PDB[1]

2. • 2377 results included the biological source[2]

3. • 106 of these had 30% unique[3] sequences (counting only 1 chain per entry)

4. • 56 proteins were obtained from unique species[4]

5. • For the same Cytochrome C, 24 unique CATH IDs[5] were obtained

[1]: the protein data bank; [2]: the species from which the molecule is isolated; [3]: *unique* after repeated entries of identical proteins were filtered; [4]: subspecies and varieties were not counted as different entires; [5]: CATH is a protein classification system and different CATH ID represents different structure

Scheme 2.1: Proteins by function, organism and structure

simulation software are used for such analyses. These further calculate chemical behavior as resulting from the physics of molecular interactions, i.e. the group of atoms of one molecule attracts or repels the group of atoms of another molecule. For the given pair of molecule placed at certain distance from each other, the sum of molecular interaction energies indicate whether the molecules favor each other or they repel. The software calculates these forces of interaction using mathematical relations built into it by those who programmed and developed it.

The advantage of using computers to handle any problem is well known, such as capacity to handle large amount of information, speed of processing, accuracy and the embraced application of procedures uniformly to all examples (one cannot expect the human mind to treat all cases alike). The drug design has stepped into a novel phase involving bioinformatics and computations which demands an understanding of the principles of medicinal chemistry in these terms, presented here.

2.1.1 Drug Design is a Truly Multidisciplinary Field

Natural products used for treatment have been extensively exploited as templates to obtain new drugs. Analyzing the steps to carry out the evaluation, isolation and characterization of the ingredient of natural source, chemists check whether the isolated compound is indeed the active ingredient, molecular- and cellular-biologists device specific tests that the compound has to pass in. The implementation of these tests is increasingly done on microorganisms (rather than on animals) and so step in genome experts and microbiologists. It is not sufficient to just know that a compound is active; today, establishing the (molecular) pharmacological pathway is essential, which brings in the valuable knowledge of a biochemist. Advances in the use of femtosecond laser spectroscopy, mass spectroscopy, chromatography and other analytical techniques are constantly used to improve the evaluation and study of reaction mechanisms and complexes. Promising drug candidates are then tested on animal models and then tested clinically: the work of pharmacologists. Formulation of the isolated chemical compound into a dosage form that can be administered to animals and humans involves pharmaceutics. Suggestions for promising drug candidates is generally obtained by analyzing natural sources such as plants, animals, minerals, sea life, etc. applying the expertise of plant and animal biologists and biotechnologists. So man mimics nature.

> *"To have computational chemists work in teams with medicinal chemists – that works best... there's this huge, huge demand (for persons with computational expertise)"*
>
> *(Lipinski, 2003)*

The most time-saving method is to obtain this knowledge from local inhabitants of regions all over the world. Natives who use local plants and plant parts over centuries know the exact remedy for many ailments. These remedies include knowledge of the part of the plant (flowers, leaves, stem, etc) or the method of preparation (infusions, brewing, etc). Most of this knowledge is folklore and must be recorded before it will fade. This discipline of collecting information from local inhabitants is referred to as *ethnopharmacology*, and is a mix of sociology, medicine, anthropology and botany. For example, *ref.* the history of aspirin is presented in "Did You Know" 14.

Did You Know? 14
About the development of aspirin

1. *Hippocrates (460–377 BC), the father of modern medicine, left behind written records of ache and fever healed by the powdered bark and leaves of the willow (Salix alba).*
2. *The therapy was in practice among several other local groups around the world such as the Native Americans, the Totenhoms of Germany, etc.*
3. *1828: 'Salicin' was first crudely isolated and named by Johann Buchner, Professor of Pharmacy at University of Munich.*
4. *1853: Charles Frederic Gerhardt tackled the acid's gastric irritation side effect by neutralizing it with acetyl chloride, forming acetylsalicylic acid*
5. *1899: Felix Hoffmann, a German chemist at the Bayer Corporation of Germany rediscovered Gerhardt's formula. The first non-steroidal anti inflammatory drug aspirin was patented on February 27, 1900.*

Carried out by optimal procedures and conditions, and predicting outcomes in order to take important decisions in and in-between every step listed above need computers. However, students in research should know how and what it means to apply computer software to calculate quantities in chemistry, biology, biochemistry, etc. without even so much as washing a beaker, and how this can cut costs, tremendously. It is important that the revolution that computational work has brought about in industrial research is felt and appreciated by education, research, and professional practice alike.

2.1.2 Some Terminology

> *'I quite agree with you,' said the Duchess; 'and the moral of that is*
> *—Be what you would seem to be—or if you'd like it put more simply—*
> *Never imagine yourself not to be otherwise than what it might appear to others*
> *that what you were or might have been was not otherwise*
> *than what you had been would have appeared to them to be otherwise.'*
> *'I think I should understand that better,' Alice said very politely,*
> *'if I had it written down: but I can't quite follow it as you say it.'*
> *'That's nothing to what I could say if I chose,' the Duchess replied, in a pleased tone.*
>
> *Alice's adventures in Wonderland, by Lewis Carroll*
> *Some definitions are definitely mindboggling!*

Disciplines

Structural biology	Obtaining a detailed structural resolution of macromolecules and relating structure to biological function
Computational biology	Computational enterprises to molecular biology problems
Genomics (comparative, structural, functional)	Search, comparison and characterization of the 3D structure and biological function of genes and gene products in various species

Proteomics	The study of protein structure and function
Pharmacogenomics	Ascertaining drug, dose and regimen based on the presence/absence/expression levels of specific gene markers measured by testing patients; using DNA chips
Allies of biomolecular sciences	Include biology, chemistry, physics, mathematics, statistics, and computer science
Computational chemistry	Solving problems in chemistry using computers
Bioinformatics and chemoinformatics	Umbrella terms used to indicate the above enterprises (Schlick, 2002)
Theoretical chemistry	Calculation of properties and parameters of molecules
Biochemical engineering	Integrates chemical engineering with biology and biochemistry–to participate in biological discovery or to create processes, devices, or therapies
Cheminformatics	Uses mathematics, mathematical statistics, decision-making theory, probability theory and computer techniques to solve various problems in chemistry; different from chemoinformatics (above)
Chemometrics	Data-mining correlations (between molecular structure and properties) using statistical techniques.

Techniques

Dereplication	To determine whether unknown substances cause the observed biological effect in a sample
High throughput screening	The automated testing of a large number of compounds for target protein–influencing activities (such as inhibition, activation, etc.) deploying specific assays
Simulation	The act of imitating the behavior of some situation or process by means of a computer program (it imitates the internal processes and not merely the results).

Terms

Algorithm	A sequence of steps involved in the method considered effective for solving a problem
Database/databank	An organized collection of data for storage and retrieval representing one or more multiple uses
Program	A sequence of instructions written in a language that the computer understands and executes
Software	Programs read and written by computers for digitally storing and processing data.

2.2 *Principles of Molecular Modeling*

"'I wonder if I've been changed in the night? Let me think: was I the same when I got up this morning?
I almost think I can remember feeling a little different. But if I'm not the same,
the next question is 'Who in the world am I?' Ah, that's the great puzzle!'"

From Alice's adventures in Wonderland, by Lewis Carroll

We cannot see the events taking place in the cell at the molecular level, even when we know which ligands are active in correcting which disease conditions and which biochemical step they influence. Experimental data give us information that is in pieces, and is scrambled. For example, in knock-out experiments genes corresponding to a certain protein (receptor, hormone, etc.) can be deleted from the genome. If the deletion does not affect a vital gene, then organism remains viable and can be safely bred. Such experiments can single out the receptor molecule responsible for drug action. Isolation, and crystallization of that receptor with the drug, can tell us where the ligand best interacts on the protein. But just because the protein crystallizes with the drug at a particular site, we do not know if this is the site that the same drug acts on when the receptor is in the cell. For example, one cannot expect the G-protein to crystallize in its bioactive form because the protein must arrange its transmembrane helices across a biological membrane. The X-ray analysis of a G-protein crystal is devoid of any lipoidal phase and will therefore not resemble the bioactive arrangement of the molecule.

Even for proteins that do not pose such problems explicitly, one cannot readily accept that the crystal structure is the bioactive structure. Alternatively, one can calculate the various forces acting between the drug and receptor and then verify this by structure-activity analysis. One can also use computers to construct the unknown receptor structure by using the scrambled experimental information. But the fundamental question is, "how do we tell a computer that knows only 0s and 1s, what a molecule is?" Thus was born molecular modeling.

On understanding these theories and implementing these techniques, if we are able to model a system that can give a wide variety of results very close to those obtained from experiments, we know that we are very close to understanding the molecule and its mechanism of action. The more varied situations it can correctly predict, the greater is the accuracy (recall the difference between accuracy and precision: accuracy is being able to give a result that is closer to reality/the correct value, whereas, precision is being able to exactly reproduce a result any number of times). For example, if computer software can accurately predict your name from your date of birth, and if it can do this for a large number of different people, then we know that our understanding of name-DOB relationship is very close to the truth.

For a more physical example, say, one wishes to study the time taken by an apple to fall to the ground from a tree. With sufficient study one lists out the variables needed for this prediction (i.e. is the height of the apple from the ground, etc.). Then when a computer program is ready to execute the relationship between variables and constants (the Newton's equation) one obtains the time of fall as a number from the calculation. This number can be verified by measuring time of fall directly. Now, if we wish to estimate the time of fall of a mango, we simply use the apple fall program because we know that the fall of a mango is comparable to that of an apple. What about the drop of a rubber ball under similar conditions? Although the 'time' output is comparable, one observes practically that a rubber ball rebounds to a certain height, where as this do not happen in the case of an apple or the mango. Can this difference be obtained from calculations such that, when necessary, variables concerning the material of the object are supplied (here, rubber), and the program can calculate the entire process of dropping and rebounding? Now, can this program be used to simulate the fall of the feather? One now observes that the feather takes much longer and a totally different path (i.e. not a straight line) to fall to the ground whereas the other three objects fall straight. Although the resistance due to air was ignored until this point, this feature is now included and the program can simulate more and more systems.

From this description, we realize that more we observe from nature the more information we can supply to the computer and more widely applicable and accurate the results will be. No system modeled in a computer can perfectly reflect biological action–computer simulations are, among several factors, mainly limited by:

- *Knowledge of the developer:* First, do WE know everything about biological action to be able to tell the computer to do as we say? (Computers do what we tell them to!)

- *Resources available to perform calculations:* What is the use if a supercomputer takes 10 years to complete a calculation?

For the first limitation, we must realize that a large number of experimentalists all over the world have generated enormous amounts of data- and simply analyzing this data for (e.g. cause-effect) correlations can give us a lot of insight into biological action-this is why we need bioinformatics (and several other fields mentioned under section 1.2). The second can be overcome by what are called "approximations" (heuristic and otherwise; see Did You Know? 15).

Did You Know? 15
Heuristic

An heuristic in the noun form is an intuitive or educated guess or a rule of thumb. An heuristic approximation is one that is arrived at to rapidly make a problem feasible. Archimides is said to have shouted "Heureka" when he discovered the principle of flotation in his bath. The word later became Eureka!

If any calculation is too heavy to perform within reasonable time frame, we substitute difficult parts of the calculation with simpler ones. These approximations are really useful when executed meaningfully—one can obtain reasonable results from a PC in a couple of minutes and continue with research. Three *axes* are often spoken of in molecular modeling and computational studies. The first axis is the size of the system (equivalent to the number of atoms), the second, the accuracy with which we wish to determine the result (this corresponds to the number of equations to be calculated) and the third, the time taken to study the event that is being modeled (Foye, et al. 2008). The third axis that refers to time signifies two aspects:

- If one wants accurate results for very large systems, one might have to even wait for a thousand years! Compromises in the expected accuracy (i.e. settling for less accuracy) are useful and often includes meaningful (heuristic) approximations. This aspect reduces the time taken to perform a calculation.
- Natural phenomena studied such as binding, folding, catalysis, etc. take place on a pico-, nano-, and micro-second time scales. However, for carrying out a high resolution calculation, a computer takes steps that are much shorter in time than one picosecond (further under chapter 1.3). Therefore the entire simulations must be extended to one million steps (1 picosecond × 1 million steps = 1 second) in order to match a natural occurring event. For this, the computer needs to allow the entire process to evolve and collect snapshots at regular intervals which result in millions or sometimes even billions of such molecular states. The sheer bulk of data generated by such studies prevents the modeling of milli-second time scale events even with current technology if one wants to model the system at high resolution (the solution to this problem has been explained elsewhere). *Ref.* Scheme 2.2 for details.

Molecular modeling applied to drug design demands the study of some of the fundamental and important approximations directly applied in procedures such as docking. These have immediate effect on the numbers that we believe are 'results' (remember computers cannot think for themselves!). More approximations are used as a part of advanced techniques that have specific applications in Computer Aided Drug Design and will be dealt with under those specific topics in this section. If we do not understand the underlying theory and blindly run programs and copy down numbers from the computer, just because they are available and because the tutorial says so, the situation is termed "garbage in, garbage out"; most of the numbers would make no sense! These are the mentioned in Table 2.1.

Biological action is elicited via molecules of all sizes. We know that molecules are made up of atoms. Each atom has a nucleus and some electrons. The most accurate picture of the molecule would therefore be obtained only if, in a computer, we can account for the energy and behavior of all electrons with respect to all nuclei. One glance at the pages that derive and explain the Schrödinger's wave

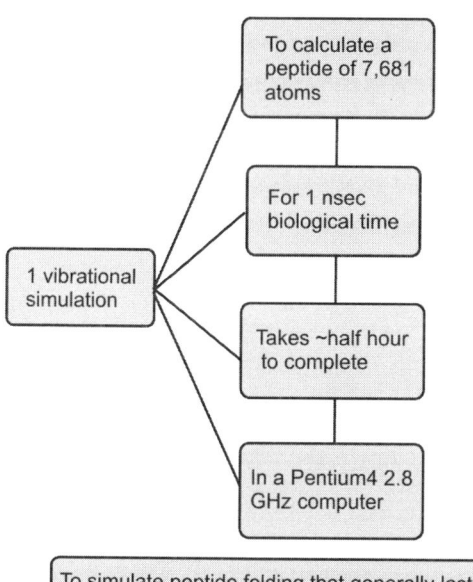

Scheme 2.2: Time taken for good computational investigations increases with the size of the molecule

Table 2.1: Various approximations used in drug design numbered as appearing in this section text

Approximation no.	Title	Remarks
1	Born-Oppenheimer approximation	Describe the ways in which a molecule is
2	Frontier orbital theorem	viewed as a collection of bonded atoms that
3	Molecular mechanics	was formed by reactions and is ready to react with other molecules. Therefore, they expand on the need and implementation of molecular modeling strategies
4	Static structure	Indicate approximations that compare and
5	Mimicry of natural behavior	contrast processes that are calculated in
6	Empirical average parameters	computations with those that occur in nature
7	Force fields running reactions	Explain how programs handle thermo-dynamic and other
8	Relative, not absolute	calculations and discuss whether these
9	Gas phase study	computational settings have a physical meaning

equation would tell us how complex it really is, not to mention that it can be solved only for the most simple of chemical systems (can you name some one-electron systems?). The equation also has the relativistic and the non-relativistic forms. The Heisenberg uncertainty is important to our understanding and it states that position and momentum of an electron cannot be accurately determined simultaneously (*ref.* Box 15).

Did You Know? 16
Calculation of Electronic Energy takes very Long

To calculate the electronic and nuclear energy of a "small molecule" such as pentane (n-alkane with 5 carbons), a Gaussian98 program would need about one minute's time. Performing this same calculation on an n-alkane with 20 carbons would need more than 15 minutes (how many electrons does the latter molecule have?). At this rate, one cannot even think of performing such a calculation on a "small protein" – a 100 residue protein has 200 carbons just in its backbone!

Box 15: Heisenberg uncertainty principle

The Heisenberg uncertainty principle can be written out in 2 ways:
$$DE \cdot Dt \geq h/4p \quad (OR) \quad Dx \cdot Dp \geq h/4p$$
Where h is the Planck's constant ($h/4p = 0.527 \times 10^{-34}$ Joule-second)

In words, the uncertainty in energy (DE) times the uncertainty in the time (Dt)–or alternatively, the uncertainty in the position (Dx) multiplied by the uncertainty in the momentum (Dp)–is greater or equal to a constant (h/4p). The significance is that irreducible uncertainties at the atomic level resulting from this principle are amplified exponentially when extended to the macroscopic level. However, this is only the case in those measurements for which the time interval is extremely short. For macroscopic quantities of 'everyday physics' measured at much larger time intervals (larger compared to the frequency of electrons), these effects usually do not contribute significantly (Barone, et al. 1993).

The implication of this principle is that electrons cannot be labeled. We cannot state that a particular electron "belonged originally to the p-orbital of oxygen" after bond formation between oxygen and, say, carbon. If the momentum (or the energy level it occupies) is known, the position of the electron becomes unknown.

2.2.1 THE BORN-OPPENHEIMER APPROXIMATION

This text is presented here in continuation with the Heisenberg Uncertainty Principle. It would be very convenient if energy of a molecule can be coupled in a simple way to the conformation or configuration of its atoms. And in order to perform something as this, we actually don't have to think twice. There is already a rule called the Born-Oppenheimer approximation that operates in molecular modeling. It states that nuclei will remain relatively fixed compared to the timescales of electronic vibrations. This implies that changes in nuclear positions will not significantly affect the behavior of electrons, as their negligible mass will allow them to instantly adjust to the change in position of molecules (think of a meeting addressed by an important person to a large number of volunteers: won't the volunteers be willing to get together at a new place if the leader wants to change the venue?). Thus electronic and nuclear energies are considered approximately independent and electronic energy can be described as a function of nuclear coordinates. This text does not intend to delve deeper into this point.

2.2.2 FRONTIER ORBITAL THEOREM

Instead of performing detailed calculations (mentioned in the above paragraphs) on *all* the electrons in a molecule, one can simply include the HOMO and LUMO of the concerned molecule if we are interested only in its reactivity. This is one of the important approximations that simplify the need for extensive and superfluous calculations. Although an atom can be completely described only by including all the electrons it contains, the reactivity is not greatly influenced by inner occupied orbitals. This is the Frontier Orbital Theorem. *Ref.* Discussion 2.1 below.

Discussion 2.1: The frontier orbitals

Background: The frontier orbitals are molecular orbitals (in contrast to atomic orbitals) and to understand their meaning, we need to brush up some fundamentals. Atoms form molecules, and molecules undergo chemical reactions (to form other molecules). The orbitals change accordingly:

Atoms   Possess atomic orbitals
Molecules   Posses molecular orbitals that are formed from atomic orbitals

An orbital is a one-electron solution to the Schrödinger equation. Atomic orbitals (AOs) combine to form molecular orbitals (MOs):

1. Such that the MOs are different from the AOs.
2. Such that there are as many MOs as there are AOs (i.e., one AO from one atom and one AO from the other atom are 2 AOs in total and give 2 MOs in total as in either figure below).

3. Such that there are bonding MOs (indicated as 'MO' in the figure below) which have lower energy than the lowest-energy-AO and anti-bonding MOs (indicated as MO* in the figure below) which have higher energy than the energy level of either AO.
4. Such that MO* is as high in energy as MO is low with respect to the AO energies.
5. By the Linear Combination of Atomic Orbitals (LCAO) approach, and
6. The two methods of calculating MOs are the valence bond approach and perturbation approach MOs.

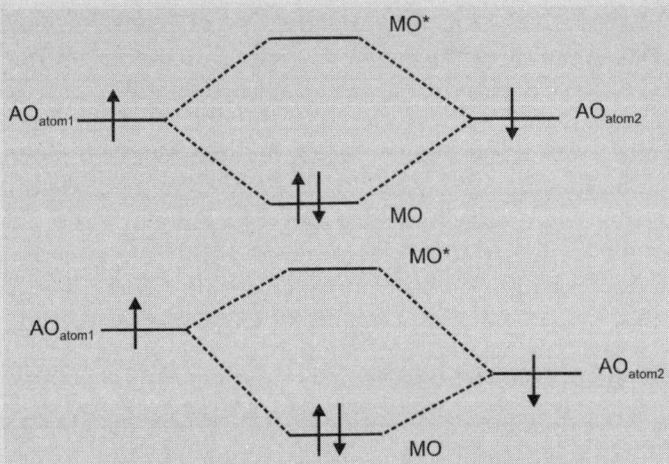

*MO diagrams for homonuclear and heteronuclear AOs combining to form respective MOs

7. Such that the electrons in the AOs fill the MOs following Hund's rule of maximum multiplicity, Pauli's exclusion principle and the Aufbau filling order (*ref.* standard textbooks in molecular modeling such as (Leach, 1997) for a summary these rules).
8. But, electrons are always indistinguishable–whether they belong to the AOs or to the MOs, they cannot be labeled (owing to Heisenberg's uncertainty).
9. And all the MOs formed need not be filled (i.e. in the ground state; several unoccupied orbitals in the ground state may become occupied when molecules are in their excited state).
10. And the highest MO that is filled is the Highest Occupied Molecular Orbital (HOMO) whether it is bonding MO or anti-bonding MO.
11. And the lowest MO that is empty (which is usually higher in energy than the HOMO) is the Lowest Unoccupied Molecular Orbital (LUMO)

Frontier orbital theory: The Highest Occupied Molecular Orbital (HOMO) and the Lowest Unoccupied Molecular Orbital (LUMO) are collectively called the Frontier Orbitals and considered to be the most important MOs participating in chemical reactions according to the Frontier Molecular Orbital (FMO) theory. The nature of the FMOs dictates reaction mechanisms. Molecules react to form products and a rearrangement takes place resulting in more stable MOs compared to reactant molecules.

In drug design: In a bimolecular reaction, each reactant (remember: each reactant is a molecule made up by the combination of atoms and has several MOs of its own) has a HOMO and a LUMO (so, there are 2 molecules, 2 HOMOs and 2 LUMOs); however, only the LUMO of one and the HOMO of the other determine reactivity. In other words, that HOMO (of reactant 1 or 2) and that LUMO (of the other reactant) that are closer in energy generally participate in the reaction. Reactivity between 2 molecules and the mechanism of reaction are often ascertained by just studying the shape (in terms of symmetry) and energy of the more appropriate pair of the 4 frontier orbitals. The statements are further clarified by considering ligand and protein as two reactants.

The study of the HOMO and LUMO of the ligand (substrate or drug) as carried out (Pang, et al. 2008), (Pichierri, 2002), (Mendieta-Wejebe, et al. 2008) gives us a deep understanding of the nature of the receptor and the way it complements the ligand. Going one step further, one can also understand the changes induced in the ligand and in the receptor in terms of electron density distribution, charge redistribution, etc. The study of these changes is important because a protein cannot be an enzyme of it simply complements properties of the ligand! (For greater clarity on this point, please *ref.* "applications" at the end of section 2.3.2F). It takes special

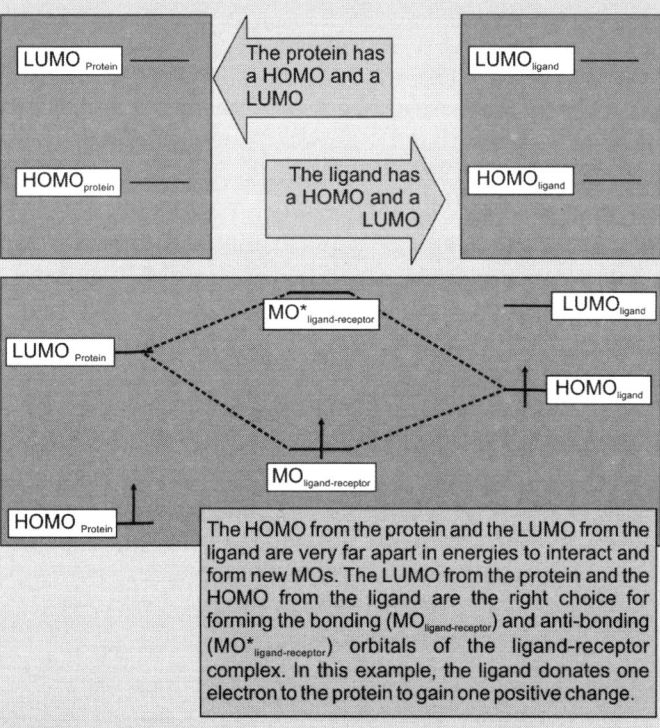

algorithms and software to calculate (Dixon, et al. 1997) and display (Stone, et al. 2009) the HOMO and LUMO for protein and ligand. Only three of several successful applications are mentioned above. The HOMO-LUMO of the receptor and ligand is shown in the molecular orbital energy diagram.

The protein CypA has a total of 4807 occupied molecular orbitals.
We considered the first 10 highest occupied molecular orbitals to be its HOMOs and
the first 10 lowest unoccupied molecular orbitals as its LUMOs
"From Two Rules on the Protein-Ligand Interaction" (Pang, et al. 2008?)

2.2.3 MOLECULAR MECHANICS

In order to model large systems, one needs drastic simplifications such as totally skipping the solution to the wave equation. What does this mean in physical sense? Let us think for a moment: (we do not have to look into thick old books for an answer, as think Box 2 shows).

Think Box 2

The name of the equation: Schrödinger wave equation
We also know: It is a Quantum Chemistry principle
That means: It should *ref.* to the wave nature of particles
What particles: It cannot be neutrons or protons—it has to be electrons because Q-chemistry is based on the Heisenberg Uncertainty principle (remember that this is what led to the idea of the "orbital" rather than circular "orbits").
Skipping any reference to the mentioned equation means we believe there are no electrons!

It is always useful to summarize the effects using equations. The potential energy in a molecule before *approximation 3* would be:

$$V_{tot} = V_{ee} + V_{ne} + V_{nn}$$

In words, the potential energy of a molecule is the sum of electron-electron (repulsive) energy V_{ee}, nuclear-nuclear (repulsive) energy V_{nn} and the electron-nuclear (attractive) energy V_{ne}. We know that what keeps atoms bonded is V_{ne} component (attractive). After *approximation 2*, as there are no electrons any longer, the equation would appear to be "$V_{tot} = V_{nn}$".

This does not make physical sense (Think Box 3): something is wrong! Removing the only attractive force, one has to artificially 'bring about bonding' in some other way, with some example from classical mechanics (we removed the quantum mechanics principle; classical or Newtonian mechanics refers to the physics of velocity, acceleration, etc., of 'everyday life' that was believed to be universally applicable before Einstein's $E = mc^2$ in 1905).

Think Box 3: Leaving out the electrons

"$V_{tot} = V_{nn}$". Does this make sense? That is, "the total energy of the molecule is simply the interacting energy of all its nuclei". The nature of internuclear interaction is repulsive. When there are electrons, the electron-nucleus attractive term in a molecule predominates. So attraction is greater than repulsion and the atoms stay bonded.

If there is only repulsion in a molecule, then there is no molecule–because in order to reduce repulsion, each nucleus would fly as far away from each other as possible!

Physically, how do two atoms of a molecule, held together in chemical bondage, act? They repel when compressed and attract when slightly pulled apart. They also vibrate maintaining an average distance between them, which is what we measure and call "bond length". The electronic (electron density based) explanation for this (and other) behavior of bonding atoms led to the derivation of wave/quantum mechanics. As we no longer want to deal with this, is there any system (from classical mechanics) that repels when pushed together, resists when pulled apart, and can be described by a simple equation? We need a simple system as our purpose is to reduce computational work when describing macromolecules like proteins. Surprisingly, yes and this is a spring! The potential energy term is $V = \frac{1}{2} kx^2$ – and this is the *third approximation* used by molecular mechanics. Comparing a chemical bond to "a spring" is not correct in many ways. Can you think why? Graphically, if a bond were a spring, its energy profile would take the shape of a parabola as in Fig. 2.1A, whereas in reality, the energy profile for a diatomic molecule resembles the one in Fig. 2.1B (for an interpretation of the shapes of the graphs, please *ref.* Discussion 2.2). This type of modeling aims to mimic the behavior of atoms with respect to each other without deriving these properties by applying quantum effects. This is the principal approach in molecular mechanics (For definitions and a scientific description of molecular mechanics, *ref.* (Leach, 1997)). Molecular mechanics is used in Computer Aided Drug Design to understand, visualize, estimate and predict interactions at the molecular level. With such an insight, one can design drugs that elicit specific response and have better control over the treatment of infections, diseases and disorders and make molecules do what we want. After the reign of the principle of "bacterial slavery" in the name of biotechnology in which we were able to trick the bacteria (by sneaking genes into their DNA!) to make them produce therapeutic products of our choice, we now aim to take over the unruly reaction pathways of human body responsible for disease.

After the application of the *third approximation*, namely, using molecular mechanics to estimate energy, the complete picture for drug design purposes is that of a huge mass of balls and springs (the protein) interacting with a tiny ligand to undergo change in conformation and structure, and induce similar changes in the ligand. Conformational change occurs at a much localized region in the protein-such as a few amino acids of the active site. Structural changes, in contrast, are more large scale (and affect helices, strands and turns that a protein is made of and even its overall shape). Structural changes include a large number of conformational changes distributed throughout the protein and these become responsible for the initiation of cell signaling and the cascade of events that can be found in standard biochemistry textbooks [recommended: Lehninger's (Nelson, et al. 2008)]. The central step is to determine if there is favorable interaction between ligand and receptor. *Ref.* Scheme 2.3 for an overview of the correlation between physics, biochemistry and computations, an understanding of which is needed for effective implementation of pharmacology.

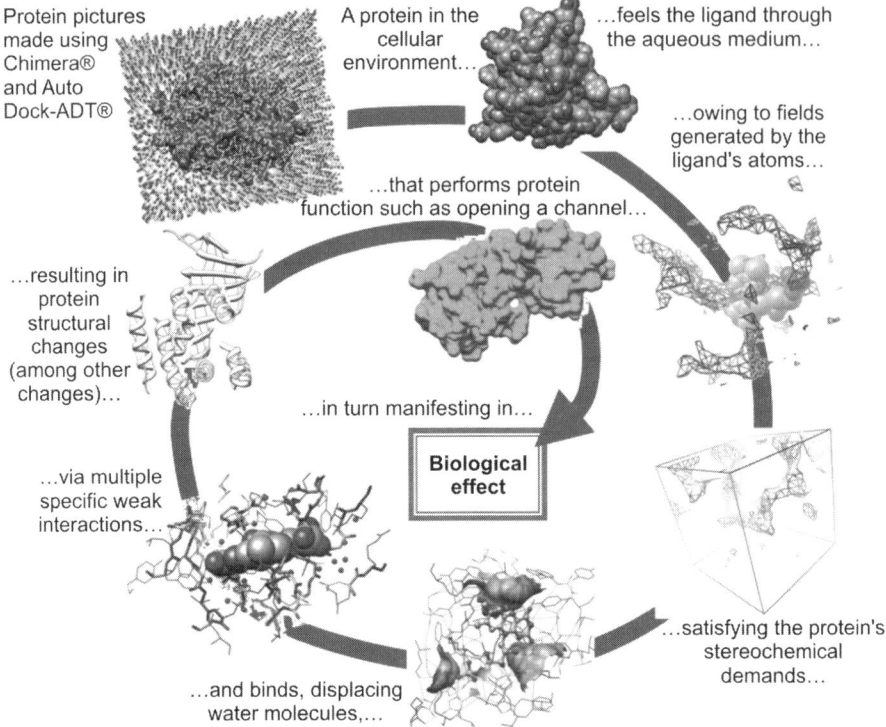

Protein pictures made using Chimera® and Auto Dock-ADT®

A protein in the cellular environment...

...feels the ligand through the aqueous medium...

...owing to fields generated by the ligand's atoms...

...that performs protein function such as opening a channel...

...resulting in protein structural changes (among other changes)...

...in turn manifesting in...

Biological effect

...via multiple specific weak interactions...

...and binds, displacing water molecules,...

...satisfying the protein's stereochemical demands...

Scheme 2.3: An overview of protein-ligand interaction (for color version *see* Plate 2)

Discussion 2.2: Discussion of Fig. 2.1

A mathematical expression is often used to describe natural phenomenon. By doing so, the validity and reproducibility of the observation can be verified. The vibration of atoms in a molecule and the corresponding changes in energy with the change in geometry is of paramount interest in designing drugs. Change in geometry implies changes in bond length, bond angle, dihedral angle, etc. These lengths and angles are collectively called 'parameters'. Considering the most simplified case, a homonuclear diatomic molecule can be used to study atomic motion (within the molecule). The arrangement of the atoms of a molecule that results in the lowest energy (*ref.* section 2.3.2.E for advanced details) is called the *equilibrium geometry* of the molecule (r_0). Any deformation from the equilibrium geometry increases potential energy content and drives the molecule towards equilibrium resulting in oscillation much like that of a pendulum. The deformation can be stretching resulting in increased r (indicated as r+ along the X-axis) or compression resulting in decreased r (indicated as r-along the X-axis). The parabola in Fig. 2.1A represents this situation and the vibration is said to be harmonic. Although such a description is simple and effectively describes vibration, the two atoms forming the molecule will never dissociate! Increases in r will only increase energy content of the molecule and intensify the drive towards equilibrium bond length but will never break the bond.

In order that the bond breaks beyond a certain degree of stretching (value of r), the energy profile of the diatomic molecule must resemble that shown in Fig. 2.1B. Deformations from equilibrium geometry (r_0) due to increase (r_+) in interatomic distance increases the energy content of the molecule, but only to a certain extent as in the former case. Excessive stretching of the bond (resulting in large interatomic distance r_{++}) results in bond breakage. In case of a homonuclear diatomic molecule (covalently linked by a single bond), both atoms dissociate with an electron each, and E tends to zero with increasing r (each atom feels the presence of the other lesser). At r = ∞ they do not feel each other and E = 0. Excessive compression increases potential energy to exceedingly large positive values.

In molecular modeling: When the distance between atoms is specified by the user, the above relation (in Fig. 45A for complex and B for simple molecule) can be used to calculate bonding and interaction. How does the user specify the distance? By providing:

In-silico constructed ligand	The bonding is only covalent and the molecule is small. Therefore, one can afford to handle it using the detailed equations in Fig. 2.1B
A protein file (a '.pdb' file) During the docking study of a ligand into a protein (receptor) active site.	These situations involve a protein that is huge in size (macromolecule) and has both covalent and non-bonded interactions

Equation represented by Fig. 2.1A and also Discussion 2.5 are used to describe covalent bonding (ball and spring, harmonic); various equations are used to estimate the weak interactions for the protein alone (structure) and the protein-ligand complex (docking).

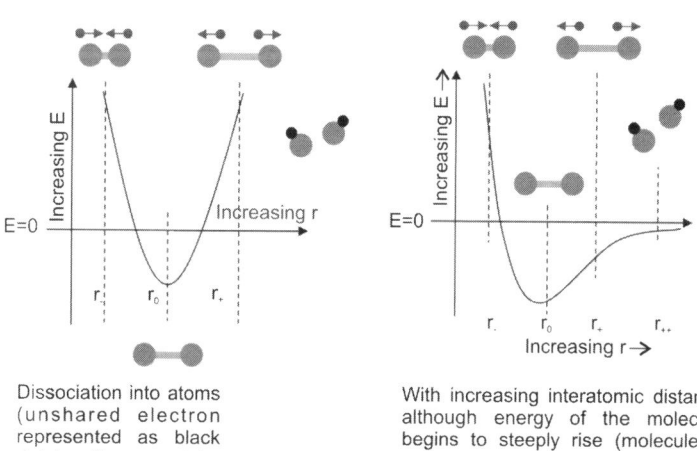

A

Dissociation into atoms (unshared electron represented as black dots) will never take place

B

With increasing interatomic distance although energy of the molecule begins to steeply rise (molecule is strained), at one point the 'bond' "breaks" (electrons are no longer shared)

Fig. 2.1: Describing the bond and its behavior

2.2.4 STATIC STRUCTURE

In drug design, one cannot be satisfied with finding out that a New Chemical Entity (NCE) works. For example, it is insufficient knowledge that the NCE elicits "an effect" on certain receptors which is most probably responsible for the synthesis or secretion or action of insulin or insulin-like-factors and therefore can be used for the treatment of diabetes. In a scenario where a lot of investment is at stake, such as at an R&D department of a pharmaceutical industry or in academic research, one would be ecstatic about any such NCE considering the manifold gains associated with patenting and marketing. But the work of theoretical chemists and biologists starts here, if they were not already involved in the discovery of the NCE. First, they enter the molecule into drug databases (several databases have been mentioned throughout this book) and upload the structure of the protein with or without the ligand for the future of bioinformatics. Next, investigation of how and why follow, the sole purpose of which is to use such success stories to predict other unidentified molecules based on properties and activities. Such 'knowledge-based' approach tremendously cuts down cost, time and uncertainty. In addition molecular modeling can enlighten the mechanism of action.

The basis of molecular modeling as described in the approximations 1–3 lies in converting inter-atom forces to the chemistry of molecules. To get to the biochemistry, one has to start incorporating theories of ligand-protein interactions. Two of the popular theories are the Lock-and-Key model and the induced-fit model [for definitions and comparison of the methods *ref.* Lehninger's (Nelson, et al., 2008), etc]. According to the former, the binding pocket of the receptor in terms of shape and property is likely to accept only certain ligands, whereas the latter, a more dynamic model, propounds that an appropriate ligand can induce some changes in the receptor active site in order to fit in. As always, the static model which is the simpler of the two is widely used for initial and simple investigations, bringing us straight to the fourth approximation (*ref.* part III on what the approximation means in virtual modeling) prevalent in drug design. The ligand-protein interaction is mainly due to:

- Steric approachability and steric fit to the active site

- Complementary properties that bring about a number of weak interactions (in part III on how weak interaction become so strong as to dictate binding affinity) hydrogen bonding, electrostatic interactions, charge transfer, hydrophobic interactions, aromatic-ring stacking interactions, induced effects such as attractive dipoles, etc.

2.2.5 MIMICRY OF NATURAL BEHAVIOR

We should not forget that when we state these interactions, we do not just mean they exist in nature (which is common knowledge) but we intend to make the models of molecules in the computer feel the influence of these interactions (at least they will pretend to hydrogen bond like actors on the silver-screen, which is sufficient for us). The catch lies in how to calculate strength of these interactions in the absence of electrons? The modeling needs to follow the condensation strategy:

Biology → described using chemistry → described in terms of physics → described in terms of mathematical equations,

And uses the approximations discussed in the preceding pages. The sum of these interactions is what determines the strength of 'best fit' between ligands and protein. Therefore, for each of the above interactions, equations and curves guide the computer to determine interaction energy at the specified geometry and structure. A collection of all the pros and cons of such a modeling is given in Discussion 2.4 and will be treated as the *fifth approximation* in this list. This forms the basis for converting geometry to interaction energy even in the absence of electrons. As mentioned earlier, the more one observes, the more details one can incorporate into the simulation and more reliable the results are.

Discussion 2.3: Understanding bonding

A bond between two atoms is generally represented by a line connecting the elemental symbols of the two atoms, whether amidst text or in a chemical structure of a molecule. In reality, what bonds the two atoms together? It is the properties and behavior of the subatomic particles. In a simplified situation, the distribution of electrons in an isolated atom is maximal around the nucleus and thins out with increasing distance as shown in diagram (i). In a chemical bond between two atoms, one might imagine a simple side-by-side overlap of two graphs of diagram (i) as shown in diagram (ii.a). This, however, only leads to repulsion between the two electron clouds. A more meaningful situation is portrayed in diagram (ii.b) indicating a maximum electron density in between the two bonding nuclei and this is the indication of bonding which is greater than the SUM OF the independent distributions around the two atoms. The electron cloud of atom 1 is attracted towards the nucleus of atom 2 and vise versa making all electrons indistinguishable after chemical bonding.

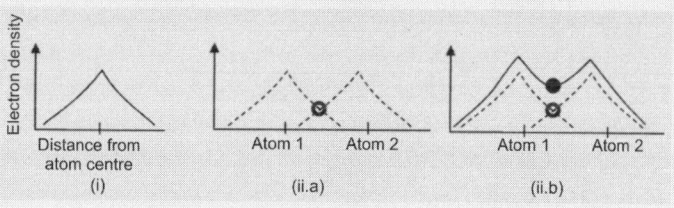

How mathematical expressions have been used successfully to model chemical behavior has been outlined in Discussion 2.4.

Discussion 2.4: From observations to simulation

This discussion stems from Fig. 2.1B. The single continuous curve can be expressed as in the figure below. At any distance r of the centre of atom 2 from that of atom 1 (the centre of atom 1 is fixed at r = 0), the energy of the diatomic molecule is the sum of the stabilizing attractive component (increasing E in the negative direction) and destabilizing repulsive component (increasing E in the positive direction). When the centre of atom 2 is brought closer to that of atom 1 from infinity the X-axis is read from right to left. Until a certain distance, the two atoms hardly feel each other and the net value of E remains 0.

Total energy goes from 0 to negative at approximately 2-times the Van der Waal's radius, when the London dispersion forces operate (attraction). This attraction predominates and intensifies with decreasing r. London forces are nothing but induced dipole–induced dipole attractions; i.e. the electron cloud of one atom 1 repels the electron cloud of atom 2 exposing atom 2's nucleus. The positively charged nucleus favors its exposure to the electron cloud of atom 1 for that instant. In the next instant, the electron cloud of atoms 2 comes back to its original position repelling that of atom 1, exposing atom 1's nucleus which is again favored (at the second instant of time). Such a synchronized exposure of nucleus of one atom to the electron cloud of the other is an interaction between two induced dipoles. This stabilizing attraction stops when the electron clouds of the two atoms come close enough to be unable to move away from each other. Overlap of 2 electron clouds results in exchange repulsion and a very steep rise in the repulsive component is evident. Equilibrium geometry (r_0; the distance of atom 2's centre from that of atom 1 corresponding to the lowest energy) is a balance between the two forces.

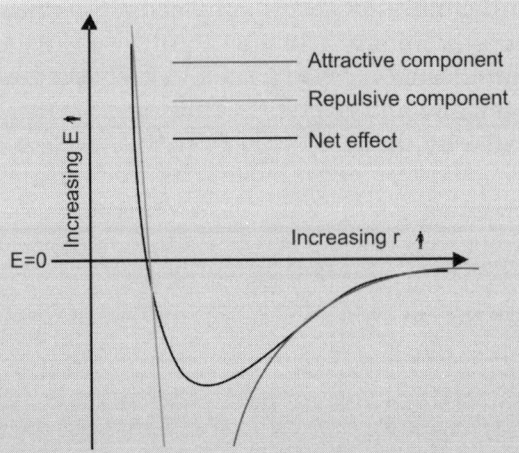

Adding up the attractive and repulsive component yields the total energy of the diatomic arrangement at any distance r. This curve is modeled by the *Lennard–Jones potential* in which the attraction is proportional to r^{-6} and the repulsion, to r^{-12} (A, C represent several terms put together):

$$V(r) = (A/r^{12}) - (C/r^6)$$

For this reason, the LJ potential is also called the 6–12 potential. The curve has been constructed using other potential equations as well. For example, the *Morse potential* is an exponential function (D_e is equilibrium energy; r_e is the equilibrium bond distance; r is current interatomic distance; A represents other terms):

$$V(r) = D_e [1 - e^{A(r-r_e)}]^2$$

And the *Buckingham potential* expression has an attractive component that resembles the LJ potential and a repulsive component that is exponential (A, B, C and D represent various terms in the fomula):

$$V(r) = (Ae^{-Br}/r^D) - (C/r^6)$$

Note that the above expression with V(r) on the LHS is in accordance with our earlier discussion–potential energy is calculated as a function of atomic coordinates (in other words, molecular geometry). A summary of several atomic interactions and its relation to the value of r is given (Cramer, 2005; Leach, 1997):

Charge-charge α $1/r$

Charge-dipole α $1/r^2$

Dipole-dipole α $1/r^3$

Charge-induced dipole α $1/r^4$

Dipole-induced dipole α $1/r^5$

Dispersion α $1/r^6$

van der Waals repulsion α $1/r^{12}$

Hydrogen bonding ~2.8 Å (generally)

Summary of protein-ligand interactions:

Mostly, the drug–receptor interaction takes place in aqueous medium (even if the receptors are anchored across lipid membranes). Accordingly, electrostatic interactions are felt initially and predominantly. The strength of the interaction is known to be influenced by the charges (q1 and q2) on the atoms, the distance of separation (r) and the dielectric constant of the medium (ε) generally written out as "E α q1.q2/ε.r" the following types are recognized:

1. Charge-charge (in the potential energy written above)
   a. Ionic (with integral charges)
   b. Polar (molecular charge is the sum of partial charges of atoms/groups)
2. Charge-dipole: E α $(z.\mu/\varepsilon.r^2)$ cos φ, wherein z = valence of the ion; μ = Dipole moment; φ = angle between dipole and the line joining the centre of the ion and the dipole
3. Dipole-dipole (whether attractive or repulsive depends on alignment of the dipoles and strength of interaction depends on the angle of orientation with respect to each other). E α $(A.\mu2.\mu1/\varepsilon.r^3)$ wherein A = 1 for parallel and 2 for head-to-tail dipole arrangement.

   The value of ε varies depending on the region in or around the protein where the interaction occurs. We know that 'ε' is ~ 80 in water (bulk), 1 in the gas-phase, is about 28 on the surface of proteins and ~3–5 in the interior. Instead of using a different value for each spot, ε is often expressed in terms of distance [*ref*. molecular modeling textbooks such as (Cramer, 2005; Leach, 1997; Rapaport, 2004) for details]. The potential energy relations show that the maximal range exists for charge-charge interactions and that the other two types operate at much closer ranges. Complex formation between drug and receptor leads to a favorable redistribution of charge in either molecule (depending on the polarizabilities). The redistribution of charge may lead to detectable conformational changes at times [oxidative decarboxylation of pyruvate to acetyl CoA by the pyruvate dehydrogenase complex in the citric acid cycle, or the pyruvate-thiamine pyrophosphate reaction catalyzed by pyruvate decarboxylase; *ref.* biochemistry textbooks such as Lehninger's (Nelson, et al. 2008) for the reactions].

4. *Charge transfer:*

   a. Some drug-receptor interactions also result in transfer of charge from one molecule to another. Charge transfer is generally not included in investigations, however some useful results have been obtained from those that were done on heavy metals (Sakharov, et al. 2009)

   b. The interaction involves transfer of electrons from molecular orbital of donor to the empty lower energy orbital of the acceptor

   c. These interactions have both distance as well as directional constraints.

Other types include:

5. Induced dipole (a charge or a dipole induces a temporary dipole in an uncharged molecule)

   a. Ion-induced dipole: $E \, \alpha \, (\alpha z^2)/(D^2 r^4)$

   b. Dipole-induced dipole: $E \, \alpha \, (A\alpha\mu^2)/(D^2 r^6)$
      Wherein α = polarizability, A = as before

   c. Induced dipole-induced dipole interactions are transient, fluctuating, and universal existing between non polar molecules as well.

6. These are London dispersion forces and become significant owing to the numbers in which these interactions exist though, individually, they are very weak.

   a. Potential energy $E \, \alpha \, (\alpha_1 \alpha_2 / r^6) \, (I_1 I_2 / I_1 + I_2)$ in which I1 and I2 are ionization potentials of interacting molecules or moieties.

   When atoms are brought into very close contact, their electron clouds overlap leading to strong repulsion

7. Exchange repulsion energy increases exponentially with decrease in distance
   Molecules and the complex formed between them can be described as a sum of several of the above interactions.

8. Equilibrium internuclear distances observed between bonded atoms is the sum of the van der Waal's radii of the 2 atoms.

   a. It result from balance between several of the above forces

   b. In bonding situations, these can be modeled by a single potential energy curve
      i. The Buckingham potential $E = (Ae^{-Br}/r^D) - (C/r^6)$
      ii. The Lennard-Jones potential $E = (A/r^{12}) - (C/r^6)$

   A very important weak interaction in biochemistry is hydrogen bonding.

9. Hydrogen bonds

   a. Are present in the protein (to maintain structure; *ref.* chapter 1.2) and formed between the protein and ligand (chapters 3.1, 3.2).

b. Can be calculated from dipole moments or partial charges (called coulombic H-bond determination) using the respective equations above, but introducing the directional constraints on the arrangement of atoms (*ref.* Fig. 2.7A and B in chapter 2.3.2.B1).

c. The presence of H-bonds can also be determined from distances and angles (called geometric H-bond determination) rather than from charges.

d. Need not be separately included in a description when van der Waals and electrostatic interactions are described well

e. Are many times formed between an acceptor and more than one donor group (called forked hydrogen bonds mentioned in section 1.2.1.D in the formation of β-bulges). Other references: (Kubinyi).

2.2.6 EMPIRICAL AVERAGE PARAMETER

Whatever be the height of knowledge one attains in pharmacy, chemistry, biology, etc. there are some fundamentals that one just cannot afford to forget. Among such details are one's name, address, the definition for atomic number, atomic mass, atomic radius, van der Waals radius, bond length, one's e-mail password (or where to look for it), etc. Thus we know that atomic radius is calculated for bonded atoms, the van der Waals radius, for non-bonded atoms, bond length is the distance between the centre of atoms chemically combined, and the values of the atomic and van der Waals radii depend on the way the atoms have chemically combined (whether covalent, ionic, etc.). When you think of all the bonds in a protein, it is useful to sit down and think of answers to the following questions:

• Is bond length the sum of the atomic radii of participating atoms (repeated from above)? *Ref.* Fig. 2.2. Except for inert gases, r in situation (i) is not practicable. Radius obtained from (ii) by halving internuclear distance of bonded atoms is atomic radius. Radius obtained in (iii) by halving internuclear distance of atoms that are in contact "through space" (called non-bonded atoms) is called van der Waals radius (by hard sphere definition; unfortunately, there are several definitions for van der Waals radii).

• Is the bond length between any two atoms a universal constant? In other words, is the inter-carbon bond length the same for C–C single, double and triple bond? The answer is "No".

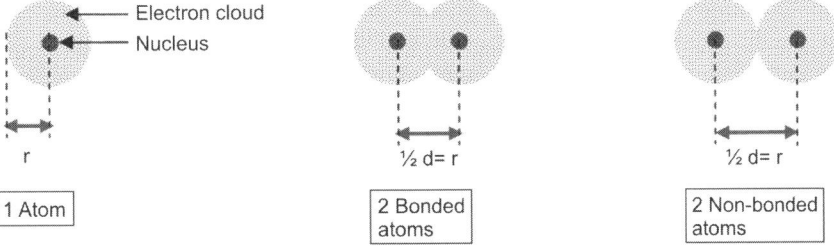

Fig. 2.2: Atomic and van der Waals radii

- How can you differentiate between a C–C, C = C, and C ≡ C situations of molecular mechanics when there are no electrons?

This is how…

In molecular mechanics, different electronic environments become springs of different lengths and tightness! From the first few chapters of your ominous "Textbook of Organic Chemistry", you would have learnt that the difference between the 3 situations of bonding lies (among other properties) in the bond strength and length. These two parameters (strength and length) are governed by the terms k and x respectively in our equation for potential energy, $V = \frac{1}{2} kx^2$ and this is the *sixth approximation. Ref.* discussion 2.5 (that is based on discussion 2.1) where it is discussed how changing terms k and x can model the energetic behavior of the 3 types of bonds. As mentioned under introduction of section 2.2, *approximations 4, 5 and 6* contrast natural and computational bonding-situations. For simplifying calculations, one simply uses information obtained by observing nature and measuring parameters such as bond strength and length to calculate the presence (or absence) of bonds after calculating energy content.

Discussion 2.5: Single, double and triple bonds

How can we differentiate between a single bond, a double-bond and a triple bond when there are no electrons? We saw how the dependence of energy on interatomic distance expressed mathematically (in Discussion 2.4) was used to calculate the energy content of the bonds in a molecule. Similarly, differences in the location of equilibrium bond length, the corresponding value of energy and the change in energy with varying bond lengths (slope of the 'walls' of the parabola) can be exploited to produce energy profiles having curves of different shapes. The following correspondences are evident:

The atom	Property of the "ball"
The bond	Property of the "spring"
The molecule	Sum of the potential energy calculated for properties of each pair of interacting atoms or bonds
Equilibrium bond length	The position of the lowest point in the parabola on the X-axis
Equilibrium bond energy	The position of the lowest point in the parabola on the Y-axis
Rigidity of the bond	The "tightness" of the spring represented by the steep/gentle slope of the walls of the parabola
Single bond	Long + loose spring of less negative energy
Double bond	Medium long + moderately tight spring of moderate energy
Triple bond	Short + tight spring of high energy content (more negative)

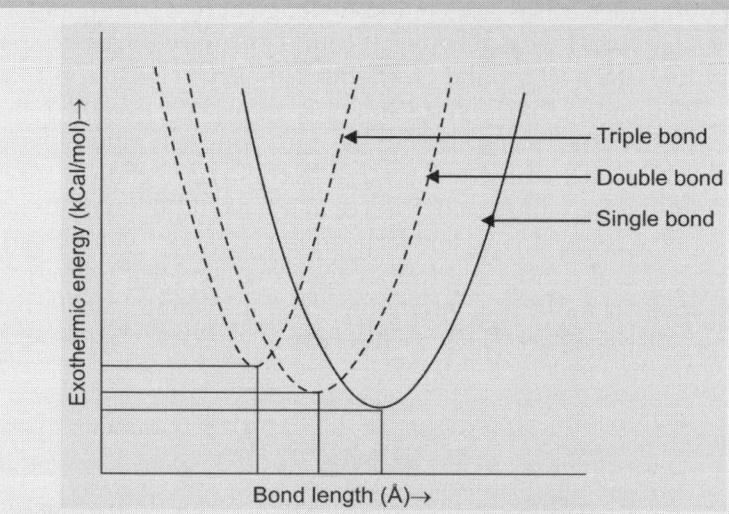

The mathematical expressions (and graph shapes) that best match the behavior of atoms bonded in the three situations are used. All three bonds are modeled as "springs". But there are different types of springs-loose, flexible, etc. A single bond is long and of lower energy than (not as negative in energy as) a double-bond (which is relatively more rigid) or a triple bond (more rigid than a double-bond). This difference is reflected in the mathematical expressions by changing the value of r0, the equilibrium bond length and k, the spring constant in the expression $V(r) = \frac{1}{2}k.(r - r_0)^2$. New values are substituted for k and r_0 in case of $N - C$, $N = C$ and $N \equiv C$. Similarly, for every unique atom-pair and bonding, appropriate curves are constructed with meaningful values for r_0 and k.

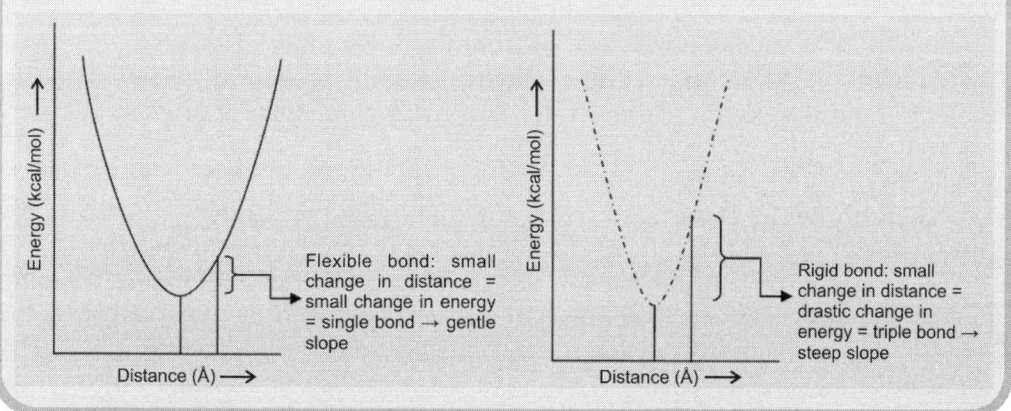

2.2.7 FORCE FIELDS RUNNING REACTIONS

So far, we have bits and pieces of our movie in place... we have found stage actors and their costumes (molecules as balls and springs), all the sentiments and scenes they have to act out (which arises from our knowledge of receptor-ligand interaction-the role of shape (steric) and weak (chemical) complementary forces, *ref.* part III) and some of the story line (the background biochemistry). What's next is to wrap it into a formula movie. The formula that governs how the atoms of a specified molecule are to behave towards each other incorporating the equations and values we have listed out so far results in what's called a *Force Field*. This is a technical aspect of this computational work-it is very important to have at least a rudimentary understanding of the operation, all the better if you can work out the equations yourself. This section attempts a superficial and conceptual (rather than mathematical) description of the *seventh approximation* in molecular modeling. The mathematical derivations are available in plenty of references [such as (Brooks, et al. 2009; Cramer, 2005; Leach, 1997)].

Did You Know? 17
Modern medicinal chemistry is not just about docking

The application of molecular modeling techniques to explain protein behavior is not a 'recent' trend. Example: research work at Agouron Institute, La Jolla, California in 1988. The binding of trimethoprim to E. coli dihydrofolate reductase was explained by

1. *Energy minimization, frequency calculations, protein conformational changes, entropy penalties to binding, docking*
2. *Using well characterized force fields that could handle all protein atoms (ref. chapter 1.5 for all-atom vs minimalist models)*
3. *Including explicit water molecules in the study and accounting for the importance of their presence........ (Dauber-Osguthorpe, et al. 1988)*

The current trend in Medicinal Chemistry is not to simply perform such calculations, but to streamline these and other techniques for routine use in new drug discovery.

The purpose of a force field is to prevent chemical blunders such as one atom penetrating the van der Waals radius of another resulting in some meaningless nuclear fusion (without the energy release as in a real hydrogen bomb, of course). The force field acts as the invisible shield of protection (like the ones that erupts in Japanese anime episodes) and can be understood to perform the following policeman duties:

- To keep atoms at chemically relevant distances (by slightly changing the arrangement provided by the user during docking or energy minimization)
- To make atoms exert meaningful forces on one another (involving charges, bonding, etc.), so that the forces can be numerically added up to give the potential energy of the system and manipulated according to further commands given by a human to the software.

A well constructed potential (is an expression where the potential energy has been added up well thoroughly) can identify most favored conformations. ***Note 1:*** Among all possible H-C-C-H dihedral angle arrangements in ethane, the staggered form will end up having the minimum (most negative) energy corresponding to the least conformational strain. For every degree of rotation of the dihedral angle, a certain potential energy value results as mentioned by the equation earlier and subsequently, ethane's potential energy diagram is a sinusoidal curve that one often sees in textbooks. If, for instance, a force field is constructed that does not contain the "dihedral angle potential" term, then all the above conformations of ethane would be calculated to have the same energy because the two conformations–staggered and eclipsed–do not differ by any other parameter. ***Note 2:*** Force fields calculate strain energy and not internal energy. *Ref.* under section 2.2.8.

Box 16: Summary of concept–energy and conformation

A list of equations are now available to judge the strength of interactions such as covalent bonding (single, double, triple), electrostatic attraction and repulsion, hydrogen-bonding, van der Waals repulsion, etc. A molecular modeling software now possesses the arrangement (geometry) and identity (C, O, N, H, S, etc) of every atom in the given molecule. The arrangement in terms of distance/angle/ dihedral angle is used to determine the strength of interaction from the curves.

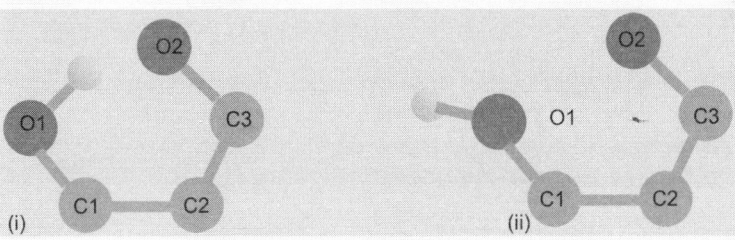

For example, Which of the following is the lowest energy conformation?

In case of conformation (i), the positioning of O1–H1–O2–C3 in terms of the H1–O2 distance and the O1–H1–O2 angle favors the formation of a hydrogen–bond. In case of conformation (ii), there is no interaction between its atom-pairs that additionally stabilize the conformation (i.e., in addition to covalent bonding). By how much energy (kcal/mol) is conformation (i) stabilized? According to H-bonding rules, if O1–H1–O2 is arranged in a straight line, the strength of the hydrogen bonding formation is maximum (~5 kcal/mol exothermic). H-bond strength decreases proportional to the alteration of this angle as [*ref.* section 1.2.2.1.F]:

180°–120°   Maximum strength (say, ~ –5 kcal/mol)
120°–100°   Moderate strength (say, ~ –2 kcal/mol)
100°–0°   Negligible bonding

For example, for an O1–H1–O2 angle of approximately 120° the strength of the H-bond is about –3 kcal/mol. In the specified example, only one H-bond is possible among the several non-bonded interactions. If the presence of more interactions is determined, their respective energies are added up. Favorable interactions make V_{total} more negative and unfavorable arrangements of atoms destabilize the potential energy resulting in less negative energies.

$$V_{total} = V_{stretching} + V_{bending} + V_{torsion} + V_{electrostatic} + V_{H\text{-}bondong} + \ldots$$

This expression converts geometric parameters into potential energy to estimate stability of molecular arrangements and is the Force Field. Detailed description and functions of force fields follow in the section 2.2.10.

Discussion 2.6: Specifying molecular geometry–the use of coordinates

Why do we need coordinates? To a reader freshly introduced to the use of computers in drug design, it is easy to wonder how software recognizes molecular geometry of ligand and protein to, as applied by the user. Using coordinates make changes, we can systematically specify the arrangement of various atoms in a molecule. Software will place specified atoms according to the instructions given in the coordinates and will generate molecules that can be viewed in 3D. Molecular coordinates are specified in two formats—internal and Cartesian.

Internal coordinates: In this format, every atom in the molecule is ordered with respect to a reference atom. The reference atom may be an atom physically present in the molecule or an imaginary "dummy" atom using which the atoms of a molecule can be ordered. For example,

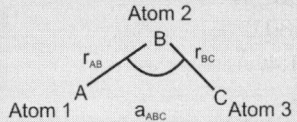

Internal coordinate format:
```
[line 1]  A
[line 2]  B A r_AB
[line 3]  C B r_BC A a_ABC
```

Example: H_2O
```
[line 1]  1 H
[line 2]  2 O 1 0.95
[line 3]  3 H 2 0.95 1 104.5
```

This is to be read as, linewise:
Line 1: place atom 1 which is 'H'
Line 2: place atom O. Connect it to H at a distance of 0.95Å from 'H' already placed as per line 1
Line 3: place atom H. Connect it to O maintaining a distance of 0.95Å from B at an angle = 104.5° from H.

If there was a fourth atom, the dihedral would be mentioned as follows:

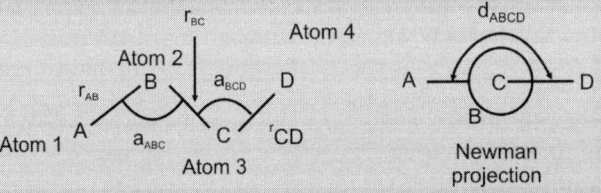

Internal coordinate format:
```
[line 1] A
[line 2] B A r_AB
[line 3] C B r_BC A a_ABC
[line 4] D C r_CD B a_BCD A d_ABCD
```

*Example: H_2O_2 *(trans**):*
```
[line 1] 1 H
[line 2] 2 O 1 0.95
[line 3] 3 O 2 1.47 1 94.8
[line 4] 4 H 3 0.95 2 94.8 1 180.0
```
Line 4: Place atom H (4th atom) at a distance 0.95Å from O (3rd), at an angle 94.8° from O (2nd) and dihedral 180.0° (trans form) from H (1st).

* The O–O bond length of 1.47Å and the H–O–O bond angle of 94.8° in H_2O_2 is taken from gas phase values

** The trans form of H_2O_2 is shown only as an example and does not suggest the true geometry

*** *Note:* When there is just one atom, its positioning doesn't matter. When there are 2, we need just one parameter–the distance. Three atoms lie in the same plane and 2 parameters–one angle and one distance–can characterize the position of all three. Finally, a fourth atom needs 3 parameters—in addition to mentioning a distance and an in-plane angle, the angle by which it deviates from the plane (the plane is already defined by the other 3 atoms) needs to be mentioned and this is the dihedral angle.

- Write out the internal coordinates for:
  1. Ethane,
  2. Ethylene,
  3. Acetylene.

Circular coordinates:
- *Euler angles* <pronounced "oiler">: Just as the Cartesian coordinates *ref.* to the X,Y,Z space, this type of circular coordinates *ref.* to the ρ, θ, φ space.
- *Global coordinates:* Special internal coordinates are available for describing the various conformations taken up by rings (e.g. conformations of 1, 3-dimethylcyclohexane). These are called circular coordinates such as the Cremer-Pople Global Coordinates.

Cartesian coordinates: The Cartesian coordinates system describes the position of atoms as discrete points in X, Y, Z–space. Therefore, the connectivity of atoms is not explicit. The fixed spatial coordinates have an external origin–i.e. the origin of the coordinates (0, 0, 0) can lie anywhere in, around or away from the molecule.

The ABC example written in Cartesian coordinates resembles:

```
A    10.5   10.5   10.5
B    11.5   11.5   10.5
C    11.8   10.0   10.5
```

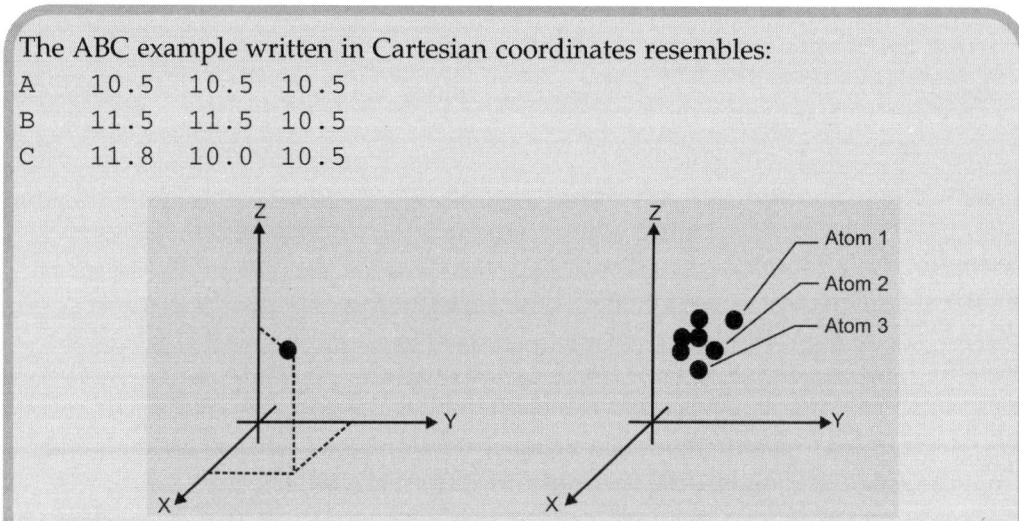

Both formats have their advantages and disadvantages (discuss this) (Hint: Writing internal coordinates for a peptide of 10 residues—this would contain about $10 \times 15 = 150$ atoms)!

2.2.8 RELATIVE, AND NOT ABSOLUTE

At this point, it is useful to summarize some of the concepts discussed so far. In general,

1. Experimentally, one can obtain the geometry of a molecule using X-ray crystallography, NMR technique, etc. This gives a suggestion for the relative positions of atoms in a molecule. The conformations in which the molecule appears is unique for that experiment and covers the few of all possible conformations (*ref.* part I).

2. The connectivity of atoms and the geometry of the molecule being available, a quantum mechanical calculation would yield some of the properties of the molecule including its orbitals, most preferred conformation, its vibrations along with frequencies and, most of all, its electron density map.

3. The electron density map mentioned in the above point is important as it shows why atoms that are bonded together stay together (Discussion 2.3). For simplicity we show this bonding using 'lines': H–O–H.

4. Quantum calculations give an accurate estimate of the internal energy of the molecule (the sum of rotational, vibrational and translational energy). This energy is the energy contained in the molecule owing to that particular connectivity and arrangement of atoms.

For macromolecules

1. What energy of a protein is relevant?
    a. A small protein contains 1000s of atoms and it is meaningless to calculate the electron density for all

b. A 100 residue protein can assume 3^{99} conformations. If the computer can sample one conformation in one second, it would take 3×10^{34} years to go through all of them

c. Why do we need the internal energy of the protein? From the drug design perspective, we only need to keep track of *changes* in energy and conformation before and after solvation, ligand binding, interaction with another protein, introducing metals and ions, introducing allosteric ligands, folding, etc.

2. For the above reasons, an absolute quantum description of a molecule is not necessary and electrons are not included any longer. However, energies still need to be estimated accurately. A much simpler way of calculating energy (changes) is

a. Setting up an average: 1000s of molecules in nature have been analyzed for their structure and geometry. Similar molecules are clustered together and an average is obtained in terms of geometric parameters such as bond length, bond angle, dihedral angle, charge, etc.

Did You Know? 18
Parameters and values

'Parameters' refer to quantities being measured such as bond length, bond angle, charge, etc. 'Values' are the numbers obtained after measuring. Example,

Parameter = bond length, Connecting atoms = CC, Molecule = ethane, and Value = 1.54 Å

Parameter = bond angle, Connecting atoms = HOH, Molecule = water, and Value = 104.5°

---

b. Comparing user-defined molecule with the average molecule in terms of their geometries

c. Identifying differences in parameters between the calculated average and the new user-defined molecules

d. Converting the difference in parameters into changes in energy

Consider the averages defined in (a) above - the 'average' is the set of molecules that define ideal binding conformation. This situation is stored by the software and is referred to by the force field. This is called the *basis set* (Note: the term "basis set" means something totally different when used in quantum chemical calculations). The use of a basis set is the *eighth approximation* simply because it applies averaged-out values for every bond in the molecule.

2.2.9 THE GAS PHASE STUDY

All the forces so far that have been acting on various atoms of the molecule have been from other atoms within the same molecule itself. One must realize that there has been no account of external forces. Can you name any external force that can act on molecules? Yes, the solvent. So, what is the physical state of the molecule that is being modeled so far? The absence of any "solvent effect" shows the absence of any solvent–meaning the energy of the molecule is being calculated in vacuum! If you think about it a little bit, one can also argue that the crystalline state of the molecule does not feel the influence of solvent. Indeed so, the interior of a crystal has been attributed to have a gas-phase like environment in this context. There are three states of matter-solid, liquid, and gas. In which state do you think the molecule is being modeled? The second point, therefore, is that there is no influence of other molecules of the same kind either. That means the molecule being modeled is not in the crystal (as this involves dense packing of like molecules) but in the gas-phase. Summarizing, the lowest energy conformation of a single molecule in the gas-phase is being modeled. How relevant can such a modeling be? Can it even be compared to the state of the molecule in a biological environment? We arrive directly to the *ninth approximation* that after modeling solvent effects and incorporating temperature corrections, the enthalpy or the entropy of the molecule (whether it be a protein or a ligand) is comparable to that in the biological environment. Please *ref.* part I and molecular modeling textbooks [such as (Leach, 1997)] for an outline on how the influence of solvent and temperature can be modeled, respectively.

Ironically, a *tenth approximation* would be that after nine such and several other approximations, it is believed that calculation of binding energies between ligand and protein gives an estimate of whether a lead/analogue can become a good drug candidate. For more details on the components of binding energy, *ref.* Part III section 3.1. It is for this purpose that the field of molecular modeling and Computer Aided Drug Design is still very young. When pharmaceutical companies invest anywhere from $2 to $5 billion for every drug's development and involve research that spans anywhere from 8 to 12 years, one can never be too cautious while investing in the development of a promising lead molecule or in cutting out analogues because they do not show a good profile. At any rate, modeling helps us in understanding molecular pharmacology, mechanism of drug action, protein-protein interaction, etc.

2.2.10 FORCE FIELDS AND CALCULATION OF POTENTIAL ENERGY

> *"Yes, we have to divide up our time like that, between our politics and*
> *our equations. But to me our equations are far more important,*
> *for politics are only a matter of present concern.*
> *A mathematical equation stands forever."*
>
> *Albert Einstein*

Backgroud

1. The atom is made up of electrons and nucleus. Adding these energies at a particular condition gives the energy possessed by the atom. Several atoms arrange themselves as molecules. We calculate internal energy, enthalpy and free energy for molecules and reactions between them. Whereas enthalpy and free energy are influenced by pressure, volume, entropy and other environmental factors, the internal energy is expressed as the sum of the electronic and nuclear energies of the constituent atoms in that particular arrangement found in the molecule. This internal energy is expressed as:

    Internal energy = rotational + vibrational + translational energy

    We also know that molecules possess kinetic and potential energies. How does this relate to the above? The kinetic energy arises from its translational and rotational motion. Increase in temperature increases molecular vibration, translation and rotation and therefore increases kinetic energy. Potential energy is due to bonding–the forces acting within the molecule among the atoms that compose it. It depends on the variety and arrangement of these atoms. Potential energy is dependent on the molecule's configuration and conformation (the bonding arises from the sharing of electrons). The Heisenberg uncertainty principle states that electrons are indistinguishable; the distinction between a molecule and others therefore lies in the nuclei and it is this nucleus that makes one atom different from another. We have arrived in a full circle back to where we started out for atoms: the sum of the electronic and nuclear energies gives the energy of the system.

2. Potential energy (PE) is very important to us because it is this that explains several relations between structure and function. When studying PE of molecules (the properties of molecules in relation to its structure) the atoms are often considered to be at rest. Therefore the Kinetic Energy (KE) component is zero. The total energy or, more importantly, the variations in the energy of the molecule is studied in terms of changes in PE.

3. There are three categories of methods by which potential energy of molecules can be calculated (the differences outlined in section 2.3.2.C)

   a. *Ab initio methods:* That dutifully calculate all the integrals involved when considering electronic behavior.

   b. *Semi empirical methods:* That substitute experimental data.

   c. *Molecular mechanics methods:* That use force fields, ignore electrons and calculate potential energy from Newtonian mechanics as discussed in this chapter.

The need for Force Fields and Outline of their Function

4. Molecular Mechanics (MM) oversimplifies chemical systems. Considering the atoms as "balls" and the bonds as "springs" makes all atoms and all bonds appear alike. Now, the identity of the various balls and springs need to be provided from an external source. For example, O, H, N, etc. are all "balls" and if the bond formed between any two of them is the same "spring" then one can never do chemistry. Even in plastic bench top models, atoms are provided in different sizes and colors so that they can be differentiated. There are provisions for the construction of single, double and other types of bonds. The number and arrangement of bonds is also varied for the varios spheres that represent atoms. Imagine a chemistry model kit in which all balls are uniform in size, black in color and with only one hole to attach the sticks and all bonds are single and white! In a MM software, the list of rules that differentiates atoms, the bonds formed between them, the connectivity of groups of atoms (configuration), the arrangement of connected atoms (conformation) and much more information is all stored in the force field. When atomic arrangements are subjected to the rules in force field, one is able to compare changes in energies resulting from structural or geometrical changes. The mentioned "rules" calculate the potential energy of the molecule; they are equations that convert interatomic distances and angles into energy.

5. MM knows no electrons (and no electrons means no bonding)–how can interatomic distances and angles be converted into energy? The equations calculate the influence of placing one atom next to another in terms of the preference of that atom in being next to the new one as observed in nature. In other words, the experimental and quantum mechanical information on the geometry–energy relationships of hundreds of molecules covering as many chemical classes as possible are collected. From this an "average molecule" is arrived at for each (meaningfully aggregated) class. This average molecule is stored as a reference; it need not exist in nature; it is only obtained by averaging the values (such as 1.545 Å, 1.543 Å, 1.546 Å) for every parameter (say, bond length between C–C atoms) in a chemical class of molecules (here, alkanes). A different parameter (tetrahedral angle of sp^3) will have a different average value (109.5°, etc.) in a different class of molecules (in this case, all molecules that have sp^3 carbons). This average is called the basis set.

6. Why all this information collecting, statistical averaging and classifying? Because a new molecule supplied by the user can simply be compared with the ideal value recommendations supplied by the basis set. If the value for a certain parameter is the same as in the basis set, the stored energy is used. For example, if the angle formed by two bonds of an sp^3 carbon in a user-supplied molecule (say indomethacine) is indeed 109.5°, then there is no dispute. However, if it has been erroneously inputed as 105° then there is increased STRAIN in the supplied indomethacine geometry. The strain arises from the 4.5° reduction in bond angle. The relationship between sp^3 carbon bond angle and strain energy is obtained from the study of molecules performed over all these years. For the sake of explanation in this text, imagine that 105° bond angle in an sp^3 carbon corresponds to 20 kcal/mol. This 20 kcal/mol is then added to indomethacine's potential energy by the force field. If there are any other parameters (such as other bond lengths, angles, dihedrals, charges, etc.) with deviations, all the resulting deviations are converted to strain energies with the help of equations stored in the force field and then added up. Thus, even in the absence of electrons, chemistry can be mimicked in the various balls and springs with the help of force fields. So far we have presented only an idea on what takes place in force fields. The next paragraphs will mention the parameters and their relationship with molecular geometry (the equations connecting strain/potential energy and parameters are already mentioned in Discussion 2.4).

Box 17: Force fields have several technical aspects

Each molecule possesses its own force field. This can be derived from spectroscopic studies of the molecules. In infrared spectroscopy, each pair of atoms vibrates with a certain frequency depending on the nature of the bonding and involved atoms. This is called natural vibration frequency. Any external force that causes disturbance in this vibration results in the atoms been shifted with respect to each other (stretched or compressed when considering bond length). However, this displacement is soon overcome resulting in the molecule always existing close to its equilibrium geometry. Because the comparison is only that of strain and not that of internal energy, the initial potential energy content of the molecule is set to zero. Molecules having similar geometries (such as "peptides" or "monosaccharides") are "disturbed" in similar ways and have force fields that resemble each other. This is why the force field can be 'averaged' over a class of molecules. Now it is evident as to why bonds are considered as springs. Actually, the force field is a matrix of force constants; in general there are ½ (3K-L)(3K-L-1) force constants which change for each molecule. Several approximations are used to calculate deviations from an averaged out force field. Technical discussions in this aspect are very interesting, but are beyond the scope of such an introductory text. For details, please *ref.* molecular modeling text books (Leach, 1997; Rapaport, 2004; Rappé, et al. 1997) or the literature of individual force fields such as CHARMM (Brooks, et al. 2009), etc.

Force Fields: Outline of Components

All the following potentials put together become a mathematical model that adds and subtracts energy depending on whether interactions are attractive or repulsive. It must be remembered that in a force-field, values are averaged over several molecules within a class and hence in all of the above cases, parts of equations may no longer be chemically relevant. For every term introduced, no effect must be counted twice.

*References for MM2/MM3: the home page at http://europa.chem.uga.edu/allinger/mm 2 mm3.html, (Allinger, 1977; Allinger, et al., 1989)

Note: MM = molecular mechanics, MM2/ MM3 = name of methods! These are different

The "molecular mechanics internal potential energy" of a molecule: The calculation of bond energies results in a set of ideal values that are stored by programs that calculate energy. These programs simply add up bond energies to obtain the heat of formation of the molecule and this heat of formation is considered the energy of the unstrained molecule. The potential energy calculated by some force field is added to the sum of all bond increments and the heat of formation (at 298 K) and this gives an impressive mimicry of natural effects. Nevertheless, the method is still straightforward and is clearly applicable only to molecules that combine atoms in a "straightforward way". When special electronic effects operate in a molecule (such as π conjugation) one cannot add in extra-stabilization. MM2 and MM3 force fields contain the delta increments for each bond and calculate heat of formations for molecules (although a narrow range: carbon, nitrogen, oxygen, hydrogen, halogen, sulfur, phosphorus) bonded in one of the following ways: sp^3–sp^3, sp^3–hydrogen, sp^2– sp^2, sp^2–hydrogen.

Simple structure parameters: Potentials are calculated between two, three and four atom arrangements such that one accounts for distance, angle, and dihedral, respectively. Geometries that did not resemble the average were considered to be strained or sterically hindered and the corresponding strain energy or steric energy were added. van der Waals interactions were incorporated together with stretching and bending deformations to obtain geometries with minimum steric energies. In this way, the force constants of bond stretching, angle bending, dihedral angles were included in the force constant matrix of the force field.

Coupling- interaction between structure parameters: The above terms such as bending, stretching, torsion, etc. are not independent of each other. For example, if the two hydrogen atoms in a water molecule are stretched with respect to the central oxygen, O-H bond lengths increases simultaneously, this allows a reduction in H-O-H angle as the like charges on the hydrogens would be farther apart and charge repulsion becomes smaller. Bond stretching is now coupled to angle bonding, modeling such connections between the various stand-alone terms in the expression for the potential a full molecule are done by individual expressions collectively called "cross term potentials". The above term is called the stretch-bend cross term potential. Six other potentials are, as incorporated in the MM4 force field, the angle bend-angle bend, type 1 torsion-bond stretch, type 2 bond stretch-bond stretch, torsion–angle bend, torsion-torsion, torsion-improper torsion, angle bend-torsion-angle bend, improper torsion-torsion-improper torsion cross term potential. Further interrelation between these were added in order to increase detail in a force fields description–these are called coupling terms that indicate non-bonded interactions. For example, *van der Waals* interaction includes dispersion and exchange repulsion or *electrostatic interactions or hydrogen bonding*.

Electrostatic interactions: In physical chemistry one would have come across the fact that charges and partial charges on atoms depend on the medium in which they are placed. Although charges can be separated well by water, chloroform or benzene do not possess this property to the same extent as water. The property being refered to is denoted by the dielectric constant of the medium. Vacuum has an arbitrary dielectric constant of 1 and all other media are expressed relative to this value. The dielectric constant ε also depends on the temperature. Electrostatic potential is calculated as a function of the partial charges q1 and q2 separated by distance ρ in space: $V_{el} = 332.06$ q1.q2/$(\varepsilon.\rho)$ expressed in kcal/mol.

van der Waals interactions: van der Waals interactions involved the inability of atoms to penetrate each other's radii. Several situations model this behavior in several ways as two atoms approach each other as mentioned in Discussion 2.4.

Electronic effects: One can go deeper and deeper; the addition of the following equation in the force fields describes electronic effects:

$$V_\phi = 1/2 \, [k_{tor1} \, (1 + \cos_\phi) + k_{tor2} \, (1 + \cos 2_\phi) + k_{tor3} \, (1 + \cos 3_\phi)]$$

because cos ϕ, cos 2ϕ, cos 3ϕ terms represent interaction between bond dipoles, hyperconjugation and anomeric interactions, and bond staggering respectively. *Dipole-dipole interactions:* Parallel dipole moments repel each other, perpendicular ones ignore each other and antiparallel ones attract each other. Jean's formula is used. *London dispersion forces and exchange repulsion interactions:* These occur at a slightly larger distance than the above forces and involve interactions of the electron cloud via induced dipoles. To induce a dipole in atom, in real world, the electron cloud should be loose enough to accommodate movement. Thus this depends on *polarizability* of the involved atoms or molecules and these values are incorporated. London dispersion forces are slightly attractive from a statistical point of view.

Caution 1: For reasons that are beyond the scope of this book, the individual parameters in the force field have no physical meaning as they become closely interdependent on other terms. In other words, isolating each contributing term in the force field equation and analysing the significance of the values obtained makes no sense. One cannot reason from a molecular mechanics calculation why molecular property has a particular value. A single parameter cannot be isolated from the force field and therefore cannot be transferred from one force field to another. Different force fields with different values for each parameter can lead to the same result once added.

Caution 2: It is easy to understand that the strain energies can only be compared for different conformations of the same molecule, but not for different molecules. In order to do the latter one would have to calculate the energy in total. For example, in MM2 and MM3, energy of the unstrained is calculated for each group of atoms and each bond resulting cumulatively in the heat of formation at 298 K. PE cannot be measured because any method that is used to measure it actually measures the total enthalpy that contains the total energy (KE+PE) of which PE is only a part.

Caution 3: It was mentioned that only conformations can be compared and that too only computationally in MM methods as force fields are used to perform calculations. Sometimes, with several in-depth substitutions (such as corrections for resonance energies in pi-conjugated systems) added to the expression for heat of formation at 298 K, the resulting energy will not simply be the strain energies that need to be compared between different conformations of the same molecule. In fact, they become comparable to the energies obtained from experiments and can also be used to compare different molecules, of course, as long as they belong to the same class as described by the force field.

Classification of Force Fields

1. *Class one:* force fields containing only length-angle-dihedral relations and simple terms. It is easy to calculate very large macromolecules using this field and is therefore used in specific cases
2. *Class two:* Contain explicit coupling terms in the force constant matrix. Small organic molecules can be handles very well as done by MM2 and MM3. Application: in calculating dissociation and enthalpies of reactions of type A + B → C (i.e., different configurations/classes of molecules).
3. *Class three:* Special chemical effects such as hyperconjugation, anomeric effect, etc. are included as done in MM4.
4. *Class four:* Improved electrostatic description covering also polarization of electric charge. These are also called polarized force fields.

Discussion 2.7: The TRIPOS force field

The TRIPOS force field function is the following expression:

$E = \Sigma E_{str} + \Sigma E_{bend} + \Sigma E_{oop} + \Sigma E_{tors} + \Sigma E_{vdw}$ (+ optional terms)

The optional terms = $\Sigma E_{ele} + \Sigma E_{dist\_c} + \Sigma E_{ang\_c} + \Sigma E_{tors\_c} + \Sigma E_{range\_c} + \Sigma E_{multi} + \Sigma E_{field\_fit}$

Each term is as follows:

1. E_{str} = energy of a bond stretched or compressed from its natural bond length. $E_{str} = \Sigma_{all\ bonds}\ 0.5 \times k_{b,i} \times (di - di^0)^2$. Here, d_i is the length of the *i*th bond (Å); d_i^0: the equilibrium length of the *i*th bond(Å); $k_{b,i}$: the bond stretching force constant (kCal/(mole.Å²)

Table 2.2: Examples of commonly used force fields

Name	Remarks
AMBER (Assisted Model Building with Energy Refinement)	A versatile force field often used in protein dynamics. It also has united atom and all-atom versions; developed by Kollman and coworkers (Cornell, et al., 1995).
CFF (Consistent Force Field) at http://struktur. kemi.dtu.dk/kjr/	To get geometries, conformations, vibrational spectra, strain energies of complexes and crystals with consistent accuracy, developed by Kjeld Rasmussen and coworkers (Jonsdottir, *et al.* 2000)
CHARMM's (Chemistry at HARvard Macromolecular Mechanics)	A versatile force field used for protein dynamics and to solve other thermodynamic problems. Also has all-atom and extended/united atom versions; by Karplus and coworkers (B. R. Brooks, et al. 1983)
Dreiding Force Field	A force field for 37 atom types (first four rows of the periodic table) (Mayo, et al., 1990)
ECEPP (Empirical Conformation Energy Program For Peptides)	For organic molecules and peptides; the united atom version is UNICEPP. Develop by Scharega and coworkers. (Arnautova, et al., 2006)
MM2, MM3 (MM4 also)	For organic and small molecules; one of the very early force fields developed by Allinger and coworkers (Allinger, 1977; Allinger, et al., 1989).
MMFF 94 (Merck Molecular Force Field)	Aims to calculate variety of parameters for a wide range of organic molecules including proteins; based on MM2 force field; ~ by Merck Research Laboratories (Halgren, 1996), http://server.ccl.net/cca/data/MMFF94
OPLS (Optimized Potentials for Liquid Simulation)	For MDS of liquids and solutions and includes TIP (Transferable Intermolecular Potentials) for liquid water (Jorgensen, et al., 1996).
Tripos force field	A versatile force field for protein and other organic molecules; incorporated in sybyl package (Clark, et al. 1989)
UFF (Universal force field)	Generate force field for 126 atom types of the entire periodic table (Rappé, et al. 1992)
Yeti force field	Modeling biomacromolecules, components of AMBER and CHARMM, better hydrogen bonding potential (Vedani, 1988)
Some other force fields	Empirical force field, UB-CFF (Urey-Bradley CFF), Quantum Mechanical Force Field (QMFF), etc.

2. E_{bend} = energy of bending bond angles from their natural values.

   $E_{bend} = \Sigma_{all\ angles}\ 0.5 \times k_{\theta,i} \times (\theta_i - \theta_i^0)^2$; where: θ_i = the angle between two adjacent bonds (degrees); θ_i^0 = the equilibrium value for the *i*th angle; $k_{\theta,i}$ = the angle bending force constant (kcal/(mole)(degrees)^2)

3. E_{oop} = Energy of bending planar atoms out-of-the plane.

   $E_{oop} = \Sigma_{all\ trigonal\ atoms}\ 0.5 \times k_{oop,i} \times d_i^2$; where: d_i = the distance between the center atom and the plane of its substituents (Å); $k_{oop,i}$ = the out of plane bending constant (kcal/(mole)(degrees)^2).

4. E_{tors} = torsional energy due to twisting about bonds.

$E_{tors} = \Sigma_{all\ torsions}\ 0.5 \times V_{\omega,i} \times [1 + S_i \times \cos(|n_i| \times \omega_i]$; where, $V_{\omega,i}$ = the torsional barrier (kcal/mole); S_i = +1 for staggered minimum energy and –1 for eclipsed minimum energy; $|n_i|$ = the periodicity; ω_i: the torsion angle.

5. E_{vdw} = energy due to van der Waals non-bonded interactions.

$E_{vdw} = \Sigma_{all\ non\text{-}bonded\ atom\ pairs}\ E_{ij} \times \{[1/a_{ij}^{12}] - [2/a_{ij}^{6}]\}$; where, E_{ij} = the van der Waals constant (kcal/mole) = $(Ei * Ej)^{0.5}$; $a_{ij} = r_{ij}/(R_i + R_i)$; r_{ij} = the distance between atoms i and j (Å); R_i = the van der Waals radius of the *i*th atom (Å). Note the 6–12 form of the equation resembling LJ potential as under Discussion 2.4.

Optional terms (mathematical expressions not given):

E_{ele} : Energy due to electrostatic interactions.

E_{dist_c} : Energy associated with distance constraints.

E_{ang_c} : Energy associated with angle constrains.

E_{tors_c} : Energy associated with torsion angle constraints.

E_{range_c} : Energy associated with range constraints.

E_{multi} : Energy associated with multifitting.

E_{field_fit} : Energy associated with fitting fields.

Box 18: CHARMM energy function

Not all potential energy functions contain all energy terms. The CHARMm energy function can be expressed by the equation:

$E = \Sigma E_{bond} + \Sigma E_{ang} + \Sigma E_{oop} + \Sigma E_{tors} + \Sigma E_{vdw} + \Sigma E_{ele} + \Sigma E_{cons} + \Sigma E_{user}$

1. Internal energy terms: Bond length (E_{bond}), Bond angle (E_{angle}), Torsion (dihedral) angle ($E_{torsion}$), Out-of-plane (improper) torsion (E_{oop})
2. Nonbonded (external) energy terms: Electrostatic potential (E_{elec}), van der Waals interactions (E_{vdW})
3. Extra energy terms: Constraint energy (E_{cons}), User-defined energy (E_{user})
4. Not included by default: hydrogen-bond expression.

2.3 Computer Aided Drug Design (CADD)

"Now, here, you see, it takes all the running you can do, to keep in the same place.
If you want to get somewhere else, you must run at least twice as fast as that!"
The Queen, in Alice's adventures in Wonderland by Lewis Carroll

Decades of simultaneous world-wide research coupled with miracles in technology and communications have tremendously advanced our understanding of biology. However, this advancement comes of some use to most people only when it improves the quality of living. It is important to realize the impact that such a molecular-level understanding of life can have on health and community. Even the current largely incomplete understanding has helped us prevent, cure or at least understand in detail the "curses" on mankind such as plague, malaria, leprosy, cholera, influenza, HIV, Alzheimers, etc. The discovery, development, and production of new drugs stand as a pinnacle among the applications of chemical sciences and still aims to contribute to those areas with unmet medical needs.

Whatever be the technique involved in drug design, however recent it may be, and however complicated, it is the establishment of the relationship between molecular structure and biological activity that has ever made the rational and purposeful steps towards drug design possible. A glance at the history of structure-activity relationship and the evolution of the modern day understanding of factors that govern pharmacokinetics and pharmacodynamics is essential. The review of history is divided into *selective examples from early times* and *generalized techniques of recent years*.

Selective Examples from Early Times

- *1869, Crum-Brown and Frazer:* Molecules with widely different pharmacological properties, when converted to quaternary ammonium compounds, behave as muscle relaxants: "muscle relaxant activity required the quaternary ammonium group"

- *The generalization was further developed:* Specific chemical groups, or nuclei, were responsible for specific biological effects: "one chemical gives one biological action"

- *Discovery of acetylcholine:* A natural neurotransmitter and activator of muscle contraction was a quaternary ammonium compound: Crum-Brown and Frazer's hypothesis was disproved as opposing effects of relaxation and contraction were caused by the same chemical group

- *The receptor:* Paul Ehrlich (Nobel Laureate, 1908, in Medicine), after observing staining in bacteria, proposed that chemical compounds act on other chemical compounds in the body having side chains with complimentary properties. The "other" compound in the body was called the *receptor*–and Ehrlich became the father of the *Receptor Hypothesis*

- *Selectivity:* Adrien Albert (from Australian National University) modified Ehrlich's postulates developing the idea of "selective toxicity"

- *Steric factor:* The same quaternary group eliciting opposing effects was explained by H.R.Ing: that both acetylcholine (natural neurotransmitter) and tubocurarine (the muscle relaxant in curare) acted on the same receptor, however, the former fitted better, activating the receptor whereas the latter, due to its improper fit owing to larger size, did not allow the acetylcholine to interact
- *Utilizing the steric factor:* It followed that chemical compounds that blocked the effect of neurotransmitters larger in size, but had the same chemical groups
- *Physicochemical property:* Sulfanilamide and PABA have different functional groups; however PABA was capable of reversing the antibacterial action of sulfanilamide. This was possible only if both compounds had the same steric and electronic properties despite the difference in functional groups (i.e., at physiological pH, the ionized forms of both compounds have a similar electronic configuration and the distance between the ionized acid and the weekly basic amine group is also very similar): Thus functional groups influence physicochemical properties and exert biological action.

Some Generalized Techniques of Recent Years

The rise and fall of High Throughput Screening (HTS) as a single major source of leads: HTS is a technique that suddenly launched to fame. The screening of a large number of molecules increased the probability of finding a valuable lead. It cannot be considered an 'intelligent' and highly target oriented technique; the analysis of a large number of samples (here, experimentally; one can also use virtual screening techniques, computationally) boosts the chance of identifying a drug if the experimental methods used to identify the compounds are effective.

Ultra High Throughput Screening followed: Whereas HTS was performed on ~20,000 compounds per week, uHTS typically involves >100,000 compounds per day, sometimes even with samples that contained mixture of compounds.

> *In total, we screen ~10^8 individual enzyme reactions in only 10 hours,*
> *using <150 μL of total reagent volume (by the "drop-based microfluidics" method)*
>
> *Agrestia, et al., 2010*

- Coupled with combinatorial synthesis, this became a boon for the pharmaceutical industries that were desperate in search of new leads. In the turn of the millennium, the technique was at its peak with companies relying for a promising hit solely on its outcomes
- It took several years of practice and follow-up to realize that the risk of failure was very high if one allowed this technique to monopolize lead discovery:
  - Mixture of compounds gave false results
  - Positives needed to be confirmed
  - Storing samples for confirmatory tests lead to disintegration
  - A large number of molecules caused false positive results because of non-specific binding
  - Several valuable leads might be lost because the screening tests were not tailored to recognize their presence.

- Ultimately, some works even suggested that HTS might slow down, rather than accelerate, the drug discovery process

Virtual screening: The availability of some information on large number of molecules as a result of the large-scale analysis by HTS encouraged bioinformatics and statistical approaches. Simultaneously, research in two directions progressed:

- Distinguishing drug from non-drug
- Predicting macroscopic effects from the molecular level

The general steps involved in this technique are outlined in section 2.3.2.A1.

Current strategies: The hurdles that need to be cleared in eliminating failures early and generating unique compounds with promising PK-PD (pharmacokinetics-pharmacodynamics) are too many to be cleared by single computer-aided drug design software. Currently, it is well recognized that success lies in adopting strategies that include a multipronged approach to the identification of leads. Careful integration of in vivo, in vitro and in-silico techniques such that the results obtained from one investigation acts as a feedback in carrying out others. The stress is therefore both on 'intelligent design' and speed.

Selected references: (Crum-Brown, et al. 1869), (Meyer, 1899), (Overton, 1901), (Albert, 1951), (Ing, et al. 1952) (Hammett, 1935), (Hammett, 1970), (Taft, 1952), (Hansch, et al. 1962), (Hansch, et al. 1964), (Armstrong, 1999), (Oprea, 2002), (Gribbon, et al. 2005), (Agrestia, et al. 2010)

2.3.1 THE BACKGROUND

The field of rational or systematic drug design (versus synthesis of compounds that mimic desired properties) was born from the work of Gertrude Elion and George Hitchings of Burroughs Wellcome. They won the Nobel Prize in Physiology or Medicine in the year 1988 for engineering drugs by modifying the deoxyribonucleotide bases. Since then, we have been successful in characterizing only a handful of natural products. Yet, as of today, this technique of modifying natural substrate structures to yield starting structures for the development of drugs has resulted in a quarter of the pharmaceuticals in the market. This technique involves molecular-level knowledge of the receptor-ligand partnership and has become heavily dependent on the use of *in silico* techniques. However, it is an undeniable fact that this interaction is far too complex to be predictable by a few scattered rules derived every now and then. In order to use *in silico* techniques constructively for drug discovery numerous aspects need to be systematically factored in, either as "error" or as another step to include in the protocol. *A few examples are:*

- Entropy and the dielectric constant are just two examples of subjects continuously debated among experts
- Beyond ligand-receptor interactions, there is the complexity of multiple binding modes, accessible conformational states for both ligand and receptor, affinity vs. selectivity, plasma protein binding, metabolic stability (site of reactivity and turnover), absorption, distribution and excretion, as well as *in vivo* vs. *in vitro* properties of model compounds

- Even if successful, such software could not provide generally applicable models due to the inability of statistically trained models to provide trustworthy forecasts for unknown (previously-not-seen-by-the-model) classes of compounds.

The sources of natural products were used as such in olden days without the isolation and identification of the active chemical entity, in the form of tinctures, pastes, galenicals, etc. But such traditional formulations face the following problems:

- Plants grown in different geographical regions contain different ratios of the active ingredients
- Not only seasonal variations, but also diurnal variations affect the presence and distribution of active ingredients
- Active compounds secreted by plants in one season will become unavailable in the other seasons
- An ever increasing demand among the growing population cannot be satisfied unless production is done at a commercial scale
- The control of the presence of unwanted extraneous matter is difficult unless the active ingredient is isolated in a chemically purified form. The standardization of herbal formulations is one of the biggest challenges in pharmacognosy
- Formulating chemical and biological tests to check the standard of these formulations is also difficult. Standardization of herbal formulation is a major challenge
- An administration of plant formulations without isolation of active ingredient does not help much in delineating the disease and the drug molecular pathway. For effective lead discovery and optimization, the influence of each chemical entity on receptors must be studied.
- So the active constituents are isolated and modified for minimal side affects and maximal therapeutic benefit.

A. Stages in Drug Design

In order to understand the stages of drug design, one must first recognize that there has been one major shift in the principles of medicinal chemistry amidst several minor ones.

"In a marriage of biotech and high tech, computers are beginning to transform the way drugs are developed, from the earliest stage of drug discovery to the late stage of testing the drugs in people"

Andrew Pollack, New York Times; 10 Nov 1998

Today, computational techniques form the core of (sub)structure–based drug design.

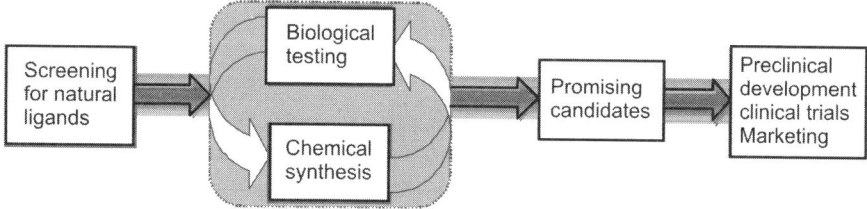

Fig. 2.3A: Traditional drug design cycle

The internet, the introduction of high-performance computing and the development of data management software have greatly facilitated the access to large amounts of data. Therefore there has been a major shift in drug designing and lead identification strategies to include computations in two major ways:

- For *data mining*–as done in bioinformatics–where the huge amount of data generated by various research groups are analyzed using chemometric methods for trends and correlations between various aspects in chemistry and biology
- For *design*–physical and statistical inferences are employed to perform simulations of existing systems (natural molecules, etc.) so as to be able to create new systems (new daughter molecules, etc.) with novel applications.

The newly emerged strategy in medicinal chemistry incorporates computations in every way as shown in Fig. 2.3B.

Structure based drug designing can be categorized into 4 distinct but not necessarily sequential stages:

Stage I: *Target-identification* involving experimental investigation of pharmacological pathways and informatics identification of suitable protein or nucleic acid targets

Stage II: *Target structure determination and optimization.*
      These two stages involving the identification of protein targets and characterization of their properties has been dealt with in Part I and therefore is only mentioned here for completion

Stage III: *Lead identification* that searches for new lead molecules that can be eventually developed into drugs

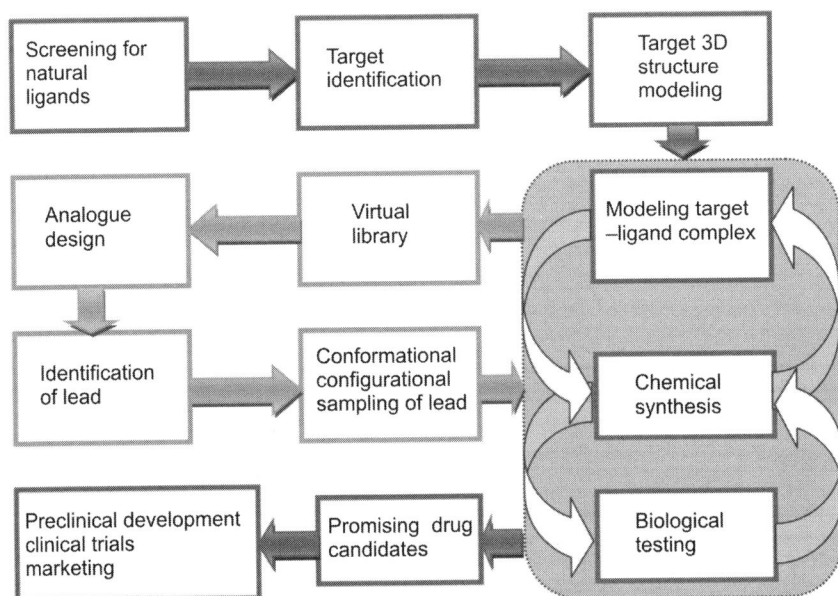

Fig. 2.3B: Structure-based drug design cycle

Stage IV: ***Lead optimization*** that searches for the balance between modifications to the structure of the lead and improvement in its drug-like properties

Successful identification of new lead molecules has been in the spotlight for further development for decades. From early days of the 1960s, with steady efforts, information accumulated giving way to knowledge-based generalizations. The leads selected using this strategy were popular in the late 1980s and were already close (in physical properties) to what was desired, especially for the drugs intended to be orally active. Advancements in high throughput screening, combinatorial chemistry, gene expression and analysis techniques contributed to this leap in theory. The desire for maximal extraction and testing of all the different molecules present in a sample of soil or plant extract increased giving rise to protocols such as those wherein drugs were dissolved in DMSO (dimethyl sulfoxide) for *in vitro* testing. Thus even very insoluble drugs could be tested. The experimental activities that take place during the various stages of drug design are listed in Table 2.3, for an idea. Discovery of a promising lead alone does not assure a good outcome.

Table 2.3: A partial list of experimental techniques used in drug design

Chemical	Biological	Drug design
HTS	Chemical library synthesis	Stage I
Enzyme-receptor assay	Synthetic chemistry	Stage II
Bioassay in cell lines	Series SAR	Stage III
In vivo animal models	Scale up synthesis	Stage IV

The identified lead has to be optimized for its action (agonist, antagonist, partial agonist, etc.) and side effects. The ***lead optimization*** step involves design of new possible candidates using the lead as template. It heavily involves study of the target structure, the role of the target in the natural cellular mechanism and its interactions with the natural substrates; the study of receptor-ligand complexes in terms of its nature, strength and reversibility; establishing trends in ligands that access the selected target (structure activity relationships) and the study of experimental results such as observed binding constants of available ligands with the identified target. Development of robust analogues is followed by *in vitro* study using cells and tissues, followed by study in animal models, preclinical lead development, clinical trials and monitoring the lead after introduction into the market as a drug.

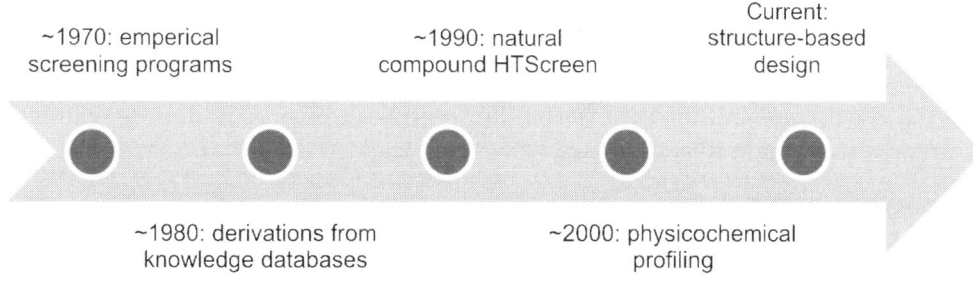

Scheme 2.4: A timeline showing the major techniques that identify and handle drug candidates

B. The Lead

Experimental as well as theoretical investigations contribute to lead discovery. This is followed by extensive development into candidates (analogues) that can exert various effects on an organism to varying degrees. Experimental methods are used to determine the agonist and antagonist activities of various ligands in specifically devised bacterial culture tests. Done on a large scale where 1000s of microtitre wells are cultured with treated bacteria everyday, this technique is a High Throughput Screen.

Lead discovery can be done in the following ways (Silverman, 2004), (Williams, et al. 2002):
* *Random search and screening*
  - By collecting materials from nature (such as plants) that have diverse chemistry, flora and fauna and isolating characteristic compounds (such as secondary metabolites) or generating compounds by combinatorial synthesis
  - The characteristic compounds are tested for various parameters such physicochemical properties (acid-base property, polarity, lipophilicity, etc.), structure, molecular weight, elemental composition, microbial response, resemblance to existing ligands/biomarkers, etc.
  - All molecules that are within specified limits are screened for activity in specific tests (microbial- or cellular-level/tissue-level/organism-level)
  - Sometimes a molecule may satisfy all the general requirements for a drug candidate and may lack result in specific tests. The search for the disease that can convert a promising molecule into a drug candidate (without a disease to cure, the molecule cannot be called a drug candidate) is sometimes called *irrational drug design*.
* *Non-random search and screening*
  - Compounds are collected/generated as above
  - screening for the presence of compounds that elicits strong response in an experimental test (such as an intense fluorescence spot that indicates the up-regulation of the expression of a certain protein owing to the presence of specific ligand)
  - This is actually a 'targeted random search and screening' because a specific number of tests are set up and the presence of a response indicates candidates for a certain disease condition.
* *Drug metabolism studies*
  - It is well known that several excellent pharmacodynamic drug candidates lose the limelight when their pharmacokinetic profile is analyzed
  - Study of metabolites and metabolic pathways can provide suggestions for converting them into prodrugs or for new leads.
* *Clinical observations resulting in "useful" side effects*
  - A poison is a drug in overdose. Side effects of certain known therapeutic agents can give way to novel uses for the same drug and also suggestions for leads that can be developed into more specific drug (example aspirin, sildenafil).

- *Rational lead discovery*
  - Step one: identifying cause for disease
  - Step two: identifying receptors that need to be titrated with agonist/antagonist
  - Step three: the natural substrate of receptor is the initial lead compound that nature has developed over 3 million years' time
  - Step four: analogue design.

> *"To invent, you need a good imagination and a pile of junk."*
> Thomas Edison

Inspiration for lead molecules is generally obtained from the natural substrate of the targeted receptor or from natural compounds. The following facts contribute to and result from the use of natural products in led discovery and optimization process:

- Unmet therapeutic needs drive new drug discovery
- The remarkable diversity of chemical structures in nature
- The variety of biological activities that lead to a range of naturally occurring secondary metabolites
- The utility of bioactive natural products as biochemical and molecular probes
- The development of novel and sensitive techniques to detect biologically active natural products
- Improved techniques to isolate, purify, and structurally characterize the active constituents of the above
- Advances in solving the demand for bulk supply of complex natural products
- The success of herbal remedies in the global marketplace.

So far it is clear that to explore the diverse chemical structures biosynthesized by various natural sources, one must venture into undisturbed abodes of nature such as forests, mountains and the depths of oceans. Steps necessary for development of lead from natural sources:

- Sourcing, sample acquisition, processing, and storage of specimens
- Evaluating biological activities of samples
- Identifying the biologically active natural product(s) in active samples
- Selecting an optimizing lead compounds for further development.

Design of complex drug molecules is only a first step; the molecules must be synthesizable and the synthesis must be feasible at large scale. Biomolecules are known for their selectivity and specificity. Reactions that can control the stereochemistry of products such as the Jacobsen and Sharpless epoxidations and the Evans aldol reaction are extremely useful in synthesizing just one stereoisomer when the molecules has as many as five chiral centers (National Research Council, USA: Committee on challenges, 2003). Revolution in synthetic organic chemistry during the 19th century enabled the production of a large variety of analogues of natural leads and also the active constituents of natural sources itself. Molecules that were hoped to be more efficacious agents could be tested, and became available in large-scale and all-through the year.

Requirements of a Lead

> *"Science is a wonderful thing if one does not have to earn one's living at it."*
>
> *Albert Einstein*

Qualities expected of molecules to make them prospective drug candidates are high biological activity, high specificity, minimal toxic effects, good bioavailability, high chemical stability, efficacy, meeting the ADME requirements (good pharmacokinetic profile), good solubility profile, cheap to synthesize, easy to analyze, manageable into a formulation, marketability (presence of a medical demand), novelty/patentability, pharmaceutical acceptance/patient compliance in consuming the formulated drug (regarding taste, odor), etc. Some of these expectations such as the solubility profile can be easily tested *in vitro* at very early stages of drug manufacture. However, detailed and expensive investigations are required to estimate parameters such as bioavailability. Establishing correlation between structure and biological activity/availability of a molecule is often done and termed *structure activity relationship*. The correlation is also investigated between physicochemical properties and bioavailability. Except for a limited number of drug classes, the specific physicochemical properties/structures that reflect *in vivo* behavior are not understood sufficiently to predict success and eliminate failures at an early stage of drug development. With the discovery of every new molecule, information is constantly added; bioinformatics techniques aim to make sense of the structure–physicochemical property–biological behavior so that failures can be weeded out prior to investment of extensive money, time and resources. One of the early attempts in drug discovery and design is the *Lipinski's rule of five*. It was derived by manually observing the features that were common among the successful molecules out of a high throughput screen in 1997 (*ref.* Discussion 2.8). Of course, as the quantity of data increases, this is no longer possible; current trends invoke the use of data fitting and pattern recognition by computers in the form of chemometrics and artificial neural networks, respectively (*ref.* chapter 2.4).

Discussion 2.8: Lipinksi's Rule of Five

Christopher. A. Lipinski became famous with his "Rule of Five" that was published in 1997 from the extensive study of a database of drugs in the Pfizer Global R&D facility in Connecticut, USA. His derivations were based on the observation that most medication drugs are relatively small and lipophilic molecules. His guidelines predict that poor absorption or permeation of an orally administered compound is more likely if it meets the following criteria:

- More than 5H-bond donors (sum of N–H and O–H groups)
- More than 10 H-bond acceptors (sum of N and O atoms)
- A molecular weight of more than 500 daltons,
- An octanol-water partition coefficient value (log P) greater than 5
  - As calculated by ClogP program (Leo, 1993)
  - Which translates to a Moriguchi log P value of greater than 4.58

– Reflects the fact that aqueous solubility is needed for dissolution in body fluids and lipophilicity, to permeate across biological membranes.

Some of the above points might not be applicable when other routes are used for administering the drug. Even via the oral route, there are exceptions, some of which are as mentioned:

- For CNS drugs, lower molecular weights and fewer hydrogen bond donors/acceptors are preferred than that stated in the standard rule
- Antibiotics and antifungals do not fit into this rule because they are not absorbed but are directly transported from the GI tract
- Natural products, especially plant products, are recognized as xenobiotics by the body and are therefore effluxed and excreted
- Cyclosporine, macrolides and yet other classes of drugs are orally well absorbed in spite of their high molecular weight.

To evaluate drug-likeness better, the rules have spawned many extensions, for example (Ghose, et al. 2006)

- Partition coefficient log P in –0.4 to +5.6 range
- Molar refractivity from 40 to 130
- Molecular weight from 160 to 480
- Number of atoms from 20 to 70.

"At Pfizer, we basically do not buy, and combinatorially do not synthesize, compounds that break 2 parameters in the Rule of Five... the most difficult parameter to control is lipophilicity"

Lipinski, 2003

C. What to expect from CADD

Some of the success stories of CADD that led to molecules that are of great importance are mentioned:

AIDS Therapy

Drugs that inhibit the two viral enzymes HIV protease (HIV: human immunodeficiency virus) and reverse transcriptase for treating Acquired Immune Deficiency Syndrome (AIDS). Design of such drugs was made possible by the availability of X-ray coordinates of the respective receptors.

A key enzyme in functioning machinery is identified. Here, the viral protease is responsible for the virus to mature, reproduce, and become infectious. Its inhibitors (indinavir, etc.) have a straightforward prospect in becoming a drug.

- Reverse Transcriptase (RT) inhibitors block the action of the RT enzyme required by the virus to make DNA from its RNA. Two types are:
  a. *Nucleoside analogues (AZT, etc.):* These resemble DNA nucleosides in overall structure. With sufficient study, an enzyme can be tricked. The RT enzyme incorporates the nucleoside analogues (which can never play the role of a real

nucleoside) into its DNA, jumbling the information content of the DNA being synthesized.

b. *Non-nucleoside RT inhibitors (nevirapine, etc.):* These are designed to be competitive inhibitors of the natural substrate in binding to the active site of RT enzyme.

A combination therapy is often followed as the virus is very likely to grow resistant of the drug due to mutations in the HIV enzymes. Combination therapy ensures that different stages of synthesis and assembly of the parts of a virus are affected.

Anticoagulants

The design of potent thrombin inhibitors in treating a variety of clotting-related diseases and conditions. This example shows 3 salient aspects of design:

* From the crystal structures of known thrombin inhibitors, Merck scientists built a variety of inhibitor analogues wherein a certain region of the known was made hydrophobic so as to bind stronger to the corresponding region of the enzyme. This is one of the typical protocols in CADD: changing structures to induce desired interaction between receptor and ligand.
* With further modeling, a smaller subset of these candidates showing advantageous pharmacokinetics is identified. In this case, some structures were compact: it is known that this helps oral absorption (Schlick, 2002).
* Theoretical design is a powerful tool in drug discovery process and helps to suggest drug analogues and synthesis methods to experimentalists. The most potent inhibitor from these modeling studies was tested experimentally and reported to demonstrated good efficacy in animals (Schlick, 2002).

Other examples of drugs that were developed with significant computational assistance include the antibacterial agent norfloxacin (Kyorin Pharmaceuticals), drugs for treating glaucoma (dorzolamide by Merck), Alzheimer's (donepezil from Eisai), and migraine (zolmitriatan by Wellcome and Zeneca)

Table 2.4: Online resources–database of drugs and related molecules	
Available Chemical Database (ACD)	http://www.mdl.com/products/knowledge/index.jsp (Drugs that satisfy Lipinski's RO5)
Comprehensive Medicinal Chemistry (CMC) database	http://www.mdl.com/products/knowledge/index.jsp {Based on (Hansch, et al. 1990)}
World Drug Index (WDI)	http://www.scientific.thomson.com/products/wdi/
MDL Drug Data Report (MDDR)	http://www.mdl.com/products/knowledge/drug-data_report/index.jsp
GPCR drug databases	http://www.jubilantbiosys.com/products.htm http://www.inpharmatica.co.uk/GPCR/Index.htm http://www.gvkbio.com/informatics/dbprod.htm http://www.aureus-pharma.com/Pages/Seminars/seminar_abstracts.php
Kinase targets	http://www.jubilantbiosys.com/products.htm http://www.gvkbio.com/informatics/dbprod.htm http://www.eidogen-sertanty.com/products.html

Toxicity and metabolism	http://www.mdl.com/products/pdfs/metab-tox_broc.pdf
	http://www.lhasalimited.org/index.php
Maximal Common Substructure (MCS)	http://www.simulationplus.com/classpharmer/classpharmer.html
	http://www.scitegic.com/products_services/pipeline_pilot.htm

Predix pharmaceuticals (Liszewski, 2006): Lead candidate for the treatment of anxiety and depression was discovered and optimized totally utilizing CADD techniques. They report that candidates reached clinical trials in less than 2 years since initiation of research, that <6 months was spent on lead optimization with a total of only 31 compounds synthesized! Strategy:

Modeling 3D structure of serotonin receptor → complexed receptor modeled with serotonin → active site identified → virtual screening → 78 virtual compounds → lead compound. Such a success is obtained only by the team effort of computational and medicinal chemists.

D. Requirements of the CADD Approach

- The need for coordinates of the protein being available or accessible by a computer is a prerequisite for any of the steps involved in CADD. Coordinates of proteins can be accessed from the protein data bank online at www. rcsb.org/pdb. The contents of this website have been presented in Discussion 1.4 in section 1.1.3 (part I) and a description of the PDB file has been summarized in Discussion 2.9 below.

- It is true that sometimes when coordinates of proteins are not readily available, one can model its structure using standard techniques such as homology modeling (*ref.* section 1.4.3A). This is a cumbersome process that needs time and dedicated work along with expertise.

- Protein coordinate files obtained from the protein data bank are called PDB files. The presence and role of water molecules at the binding site can be viewed. This reminds us that much of the binding energy involved in the protein- ligand interactions is initially spent in displacing these interacting water molecules.

- The ligand coordinates are also needed; some ligands being relatively small can be built using software; however, there is a limit in constructing small molecules on the computer, even if the built-in molecular fragments are available. For example, a steroidal structure will be difficult to build when only "atoms" are available to start with. However, most software has the built-in coordinates of the cyclopentano-perhydrophenanthrene ring to use as a framework or scaffold on which side chains can be added.

- If the next step that is going to follow will involve energy minimization, the exact conformation of the side chain atoms need not be modeled. But, if the specified structure of ligand is going to be used directly for, let's say, docking, then one has to take a lot of pains in specifying a conformation that is accurate to the distances, angles and dihedrals.

- Software packages are marketed with extensive default settings. It's relatively easy to perform a calculation using these settings that is sometimes incapable of providing a meaningful result.
- Little effort is also made in most packages to provide an analysis of error in estimating physicochemical properties and energies. Therefore, interpreting the results need experience and understanding of the principles on which the software is based.

Discussion 2.9: The PDB file format

An introduction to the PDB (protein data bank) at www.rcsb.org/pdb was given in Discussion 1.4. Every coordinate file deposited in the PDB is a Cartesian coordinate file that contains lots of details ordered in a particular format. Software that display and calculate structure are 'taught' to read this format; these look for data arranged in rows and columns (as in the exam marks of a class of students) that start with or contain specific key words. It is useful to know the PDB file format as this helps us to look up specific information about the protein, ligand or the experiment. It also helps us to modify the files to suite specific needs.

The format (compare with the example of 2CAB.pdb that follows)
Each file written in the PDB format contains (predominantly) a header, a coordinate block and the end lines. The header contains a lot of information such as

- The name of the protein, PDB ID code assigned to the protein, the biological source, mutations from wild-type if any, synthetic amino acids if any, post-translation modifications if observed and other non-standard amino acids,
- The authors who deposited the structure, the date it was deposited,
- The references to research for which the protein structure was obtained,
- Details of the experimental method used to analyze the molecule(s), the supporting computations that were employed to obtain coordinates and the procedure used to refine them,
- Number and details of the chains in the proteins, the amino acid sequence, secondary structure (helix, sheet and turn) elucidated after refinement of coordinates.

The coordinate block (also known as the 'Atom block' as every line starts with the word ATOM) contains the following data arranged into columns:

- The word 'ATOM', followed by the atom number (maximum of 6 digits allotted = 6 columns of numbers; highest number = 999,999), maximum of 2 characters for the atom ID and 2 characters to label alternative atom positions in case of uncertainty in experimental determination (= 4 columns), 3 letter residue representation (= 3 columns) , 1 character for chain ID, 4 characters allotted for residue number (a maximum of 9,999 residues can be labeled), followed by X, Y and Z coordinate values to a maximum of 99.999 preceded by a '–' sign if applicable and separated by an empty space (3 groups of 8 columns each), charge if applicable (= 5 columns including decimal), X-ray B-factors (=5 columns), PDB-ID, line number in the file (=5 columns).

- The ending of a chain is indicated by the 'TER' key word ; the ending of a model, by the ENDMODEL key word; a new model is indicated by the MODEL 1 heading above the corresponding atom block
- The protein atom coordinates are followed by the coordinates of heteroatoms – these include ligand, water, metal atoms, etc. that are in close contact with the protein
- CONECT information is mentioned for unusual bond length and is specified for the following molecules and purposes:
  - Intra-residue connectivity within non-standard heteroatom residues (excluding water)
  - Inter-residue connectivity of heteroatom groups to standard groups (including water) or to other heteroatom groups
  - Disulfide bridges specified in the SSBOND records have corresponding entries here.
- MASTER is a single line that summarizes the number of lines in the coordinate block for a specific record, such as helix, sheet, etc. (it serves for bookkeeping).
- The entire PDB file ends with the END key word

The above specific ordering of information, column-wise as well as row-wise, indicates how software searches for information from a PDB file. It was noted in Discussion 2.6 that connectivity of atoms is not evident from Cartesian coordinates. Yet, a protein's PDB file opened using molecular modeling software has its atoms displayed and connected. This is because the software has been programmed to recognize the presence of, say, N, CA and C in consecutive rows, to categorize them as the backbone atoms and connect these atoms. Similarly, CB, CG, CD, CE occurring in the 'atom type' column after the atom numbers all represent side chain carbons (C-beta, C-gamma, C-delta, C-epsilon). When we choose to undisplay the side chain atoms, these along with other atoms categorized as belonging to the side chain are hidden from view. Thus even if Cartesian coordinates consider atoms as points in space, depending on other information furnished in the file, the software is 'taught' to recognize identity (CA = carbon, O = oxygen, PRO = proline) and generate connectivity.

Contd...

Example: 2CAB.pdb

```
HEADER     HYDRO-LYASE                            05-OCT-83   2CAB      2CAB   3
COMPND     CARBONIC ANHYDRASE FORM B (CARBONATE DEHYDRATASE)          2CAB   4
COMPND   2 (E.C.4.2.1.1)                                             2CAB   5
SOURCE     HUMAN (HOMO $SAPIENS) ERYTHROCYTES                         2CAB   6
AUTHOR     K.K.KANNAN,M.RAMANADHAM,T.A.JONES                          2CAB   7
REVDAT   3   17-JUL-84 2CABB    1        REMARK                      2CABB  1
REVDAT   2   30-MAY-84 2CABA    3        REMARK FTNOTE ATOM          2CABA  1
REVDAT   1   02-FEB-84 2CAB     0                                    2CAB   8
SPRSDE       02-FEB-84 2CAB         1CAB                             2CAB   9
REMARK   1                                                           2CAB  10
```

```
REMARK   1 REFERENCE 1                                                  2CABB   2
REMARK   1  AUTH   K.K.KANNAN,M.RAMANADHAM,T.A.JONES                     2CABB   3
REMARK   1  TITL   STRUCTURE, REFINEMENT AND FUNCTION OF CARBONIC        2CABB   4
REMARK   1  TITL 2 ANHYDRASE ISOZYMES. REFINEMENT OF HUMAN CARBONIC      2CABB   5
REMARK   1  TITL 3 ANHYDRASE I                                          2CABB   6
REMARK   1  REF    ANN.N.Y.ACAD.SCI.          V. 429      49 1984        2CABB   7
REMARK   1  REFN   ASTM ANYAA9   US ISSN 0077-8923              332      2CABB   8
REMARK   1 REFERENCE 2                                                  2CABB   9
REMARK   1  AUTH   K.K.KANNAN                                            2CAB   12
REMARK   1  TITL   STRUCTURE AND FUNCTION OF CARBONIC ANHYDRASES         2CAB   13
REMARK   1  EDIT   R.SRINIVASAN                                         2CAB   14
REMARK   1  REF    BIOMOLECULAR STRUCTURE,       V.   1    165 1980      2CAB   15
REMARK   1  REF  2 CONFORMATION, FUNCTION AND                           2CAB   16
REMARK   1  REF  3 EVOLUTION                                            2CAB   17
REMARK   1  PUBL   PERGAMON PRESS, NEW YORK                             2CAB   18
REMARK   1  REFN             ISBN 0-08-023187-X               983        2CAB   19
REMARK   1 REFERENCE 3                                                  2CABB  10
REMARK   1  AUTH   K.K.KANNAN                                            2CAB   21
REMARK   1  TITL   CRYSTAL STRUCTURE OF CARBONIC ANHYDRASE               2CAB   22
REMARK   1  EDIT   C.BAUER,G.GROS,H.BARTELS                             2CAB   23
REMARK   1  REF    BIOPHYSICS AND PHYSIOLOGY OF        184 1980          2CAB   24
REMARK   1  REF  2 CARBON DIOXIDE                                       2CAB   25
REMARK   1  PUBL   SPRINGER VERLAG, BERLIN                              2CAB   26
REMARK   1  REFN             ISBN 3-540-09892-5               981        2CAB   27
REMARK   1 REFERENCE 4                                                  2CABB  11
REMARK   1  AUTH   K.K.KANNAN,M.RAMANADHAM                              2CAB   29
REMARK   1  TITL   STRUCTURE, REFINEMENT, AND FUNCTION OF HUMAN          2CAB   30
REMARK   1  TITL 2 CARBONIC ANHYDRASE-*B                                2CAB   31
REMARK   1  REF    INT.J.QUANTUM CHEM.QUANTUM   V.  20     199 1981      2CAB   32
REMARK   1  REF  2 CHEM.SYMP.                                           2CAB   33
REMARK   1  REFN   ASTM IJQSDI   US ISSN 0161-3642           936        2CAB   34
REMARK   1 REFERENCE 5                                                  2CABB  12
REMARK   1  AUTH   K.K.KANNAN,M.PETEF,K.FRIDBORG,H.CID-*DRESDNER,        2CAB   36
REMARK   1  AUTH 2 S.LOVGREN                                            2CAB   37
REMARK   1  TITL   STRUCTURE AND FUNCTION OF CARBONIC ANHYDRASES.        2CAB   38
REMARK   1  TITL 2 IMIDAZOLE BINDING TO HUMAN CARBONIC ANHYDRACE B AND   2CAB   39
REMARK   1  TITL 3 THE MECHANISM OF ACTION OF CARBONIC ANHYDRASES        2CAB   40
REMARK   1  REF    /FEBS$ LETT.               V.  73     115 1977        2CAB   41
REMARK   1  REFN   ASTM FEBLAL   NE ISSN 0014-5793          165         2CAB   42
REMARK   1 REFERENCE 6                                                  2CABB  13
REMARK   1  AUTH   K.K.KANNAN,B.NOTSTRAND,K.FRIDBORG,S.LOVGREN,          2CAB   44
REMARK   1  AUTH 2 A.OHLSSON,M.PETEF                                    2CAB   45
REMARK   1  TITL   CRYSTAL STRUCTURE OF HUMAN ERYTHROCYTE CARBONIC       2CAB   46
REMARK   1  TITL 2 ANHYDRASE B, THREE-DIMENSIONAL STRUCTURE AT A         2CAB   47
REMARK   1  TITL 3 NOMINAL 2.2 ANGSTROMS RESOLUTION                     2CAB   48
REMARK   1  REF    PROC.NAT.ACAD.SCI.USA        V.  72      51 1975      2CAB   49
REMARK   1  REFN   ASTM PNASA6   US ISSN 0027-8424           040        2CAB   50
REMARK   1 REFERENCE 7                                                  2CABB  14
REMARK   1  AUTH   B.NOTSTRAND,I.VAARA,K.K.KANNAN                        2CAB   52
REMARK   1  TITL   STRUCTURAL RELATIONSHIP OF HUMAN ERYTHROCYTE          2CAB   53
REMARK   1  TITL 2 CARBONIC ANHYDRASE ISOZYMES B AND C                   2CAB   54
REMARK   1  EDIT   C.L.MARKERT                                          2CAB   55
REMARK   1  REF    ISOZYMES-MOLECULAR STRUCTURE V.   1    575 1975       2CAB   56
REMARK   1  PUBL   ACADEMIC PRESS,NEW YORK                              2CAB   57
REMARK   1  REFN             ISBN 0-12-472701-8               979        2CAB   58
REMARK   2                                                             2CAB   59
REMARK   2 RESOLUTION. 2.0 ANGSTROMS.                                  2CAB   60
REMARK   3                                                             2CAB   61
```

```
REMARK   3 REFINEMENT. INITIAL REFINEMENT WAS DONE USING CORELS        2CAB   62
REMARK   3 (O. HERZBERG, J. L. SUSSMAN, J.APPL.CRYSTALLOGR., V. 16,     2CAB   63
REMARK   3 P. 144, 1983).  FURTHER REFINEMENT WAS PERFORMED USING THE   2CABB  15
REMARK   3 KONNERT-HENDRICKSON RESTRAINED LEAST-SQUARES PROGRAM.        2CAB   65
REMARK   3 DURING THE REFINEMENT PROCESS THE GEOMETRY WAS ADJUSTED      2CAB   66
REMARK   3 PERIODICALLY ON A VECTOR GENERAL DISPLAY.                    2CAB   67
REMARK   3 THE FINAL R-VALUE IS 0.193.                                 2CAB   68
REMARK   4                                                             2CAB   69
REMARK   4 COORDINATES FOR FOUR AMINO ACID RESIDUES AND THE ACETYL      2CAB   70
REMARK   4 GROUP OF THE AMINO TERMINUS ARE NOT PRESENT HERE.           2CAB   71
REMARK   5                                                             2CAB   72
REMARK   5 HELICES E1 AND E2 WERE ASSIGNED DEFAULT TYPE 1 (ALPHA).      2CAB   73
REMARK   6                                                             2CAB   74
REMARK   6 FURTHER REFINEMENT IS IN PROGRESS AND IT IS EXPECTED THAT    2CAB   75
REMARK   6 THESE COORDINATES WILL BE REPLACED WHEN THAT PROCESS IS      2CAB   76
REMARK   6 COMPLETED.                                                  2CAB   77
REMARK   7                                                             2CABA   2
REMARK   7 RESIDUE 74 IN THIS ENTRY IS IDENTIFIED AS GLN.  HOWEVER,     2CABA   3
REMARK   7 CHEMICAL SEQUENCE AND RECENT DIFFRACTION STUDIES ON AN       2CABA   4
REMARK   7 INHIBITOR COMPLEX INDICATE THAT IT SHOULD BE ASP.           2CABA   5
REMARK   8                                                             2CABA   6
REMARK   8 CORRECTION. ADD REMARK 7 AND FTNOTE 5.  ADD FTNOTE NUMBER    2CABA   7
REMARK   8 TO RESIDUE 74.  30-MAY-84.                                  2CABA   8
REMARK   9                                                             2CABB  16
REMARK   9 CORRECTION. INSERT NEW PUBLICATION AS REFERENCE 1 AND        2CABB  17
REMARK   9 RENUMBER THE OTHERS.  CORRECT TYPOGRAPHICAL ERROR IN         2CABB  18
REMARK   9 REMARK 3.  17-JUL-84.                                       2CABB  19
SEQRES   1   261 ACE ALA SER PRO ASP TRP GLY TYR ASP ASP LYS ASN GLY    2CAB   78
SEQRES   2   261 PRO GLU GLN TRP SER LYS LEU TYR PRO ILE ALA ASN GLY    2CAB   79
SEQRES   3   261 ASN ASN GLN SER PRO VAL ASP ILE LYS THR SER GLU THR    2CAB   80
SEQRES   4   261 LYS HIS ASP THR SER LEU LYS PRO ILE SER VAL SER TYR    2CAB   81
SEQRES   5   261 ASN PRO ALA THR ALA LYS GLU ILE ILE ASN VAL GLY HIS    2CAB   82
SEQRES   6   261 SER PHE HIS VAL ASN PHE GLU ASP ASN GLN ASP ARG SER    2CAB   83
SEQRES   7   261 VAL LEU LYS GLY GLY PRO PHE SER ASP SER TYR ARG LEU    2CAB   84
SEQRES   8   261 PHE GLN PHE HIS PHE HIS TRP GLY SER THR ASN GLU HIS    2CAB   85
SEQRES   9   261 GLY SER GLU HIS THR VAL ASP GLY VAL LYS TYR SER ALA    2CAB   86
SEQRES  10   261 GLU LEU HIS VAL ALA HIS TRP ASN SER ALA LYS TYR SER    2CAB   87
SEQRES  11   261 SER LEU ALA GLU ALA ALA SER LYS ALA ASP GLY LEU ALA    2CAB   88
SEQRES  12   261 VAL ILE GLY VAL LEU MET LYS VAL GLY GLU ALA ASN PRO    2CAB   89
SEQRES  13   261 LYS LEU GLN LYS VAL LEU ASP ALA LEU GLN ALA ILE LYS    2CAB   90
SEQRES  14   261 THR LYS GLY LYS ARG ALA PRO PHE THR ASN PHE ASP PRO    2CAB   91
SEQRES  15   261 SER THR LEU LEU PRO SER SER LEU ASP PHE TRP THR TYR    2CAB   92
SEQRES  16   261 PRO GLY SER LEU THR HIS PRO PRO LEU TYR GLU SER VAL    2CAB   93
SEQRES  17   261 THR TRP ILE ILE CYS LYS GLU SER ILE SER VAL SER SER    2CAB   94
SEQRES  18   261 GLU GLN LEU ALA GLN PHE ARG SER LEU LEU SER ASN VAL    2CAB   95
SEQRES  19   261 GLU GLY ASP ASN ALA VAL PRO MET GLN HIS ASN ASN ARG    2CAB   96
SEQRES  20   261 PRO THR GLN PRO LEU LYS GLY ARG THR VAL ARG ALA SER    2CAB   97
SEQRES  21   261 PHE                                                   2CAB   98
FTNOTE   1                                                             2CAB   99
FTNOTE   1 RESIDUES 30 AND 202 ARE CIS-PROLINES.                       2CAB  100
FTNOTE   2                                                             2CAB  101
FTNOTE   2 CYSTINE 212 IS MODIFIABLE BY MERCURIALS.                    2CAB  102
FTNOTE   3                                                             2CAB  103
FTNOTE   3 HISTIDINE RESIDUES 94, 96 AND 119 ARE ZINC LIGANDS.         2CAB  104
FTNOTE   4                                                             2CAB  105
FTNOTE   4 HISTIDINE RESIDUES 64, 67 AND 200 ARE IN THE ACTIVE SITE.   2CAB  106
FTNOTE   5                                                             2CABA   9
FTNOTE   5 SEE REMARK 7.                                               2CABA  10
```

```
HET     ZN      1       1       ZINC(II) CATALYTICALLY ACTIVE METAL ION   2CAB 107
FORMUL  2   ZN    ZN1 ++                                                  2CAB 108
HELIX   1   A TRP    16  TYR    20  1 CONTIGUOUS WITH HELIX B             2CAB 109
HELIX   2   B TYR    20  GLY    25  5 CONTIGUOUS WITH HELIX A             2CAB 110
HELIX   3   D SER   130  LYS   137  1 ALSO DESIGNATED AS 3/10 HELIX       2CAB 111
HELIX   4  E1 PRO   155  ASP   162  1 CONTIGUOUS WITH HELIX E2            2CAB 112
HELIX   5  E2 ASP   162  LYS   168  1 CONTIGUOUS WITH HELIX E1            2CAB 113
HELIX   6   F PRO   181  LEU   185  5                                     2CAB 114
HELIX   7   G SER   219  LEU   229  1                                     2CAB 115
SHEET   1 S10 LYS    39  ASP    41  0                                     2CAB 116
SHEET   2 S10 VAL   256  SER   259  1 N ASP    41  O ALA    258           2CAB 117
SHEET   3 S10 PHE   191  GLY   196 -1 N THR   193  O ARG    257           2CAB 118
SHEET   4 S10 SER   206  CYS   212 -1 N TRP   209  O TYR    194           2CAB 119
SHEET   5 S10 GLY   140  GLY   151 -1 N VAL   143  O THR    208           2CAB 120
SHEET   6 S10 ALA   116  ASN   124 -1 N VAL   120  O ILE    144           2CAB 121
SHEET   7 S10 SER    87  HIS    96 -1 N HIS    94  O HIS    119           2CAB 122
SHEET   8 S10 SER    65  GLU    71 -1 N HIS    67  O HIS     94           2CAB 123
SHEET   9 S10 THR    55  VAL    62 -1 N ILE    60  O HIS     67           2CAB 124
SHEET  10 S10 GLY   171  PHE   176 -1 N ALA   174  O ILE     59           2CAB 125
TURN    1  T1 ASP     8  ASN    11    REVERSE TURN                        2CAB 126
TURN    2  T2 PRO    13  TRP    16    TYPE I (3/10)                       2CAB 127
TURN    3 T2A LYS    34  THR    38    REVERSE, HELIX IN ISOZYME C         2CAB 128
TURN    4  T3 TYR    51  ALA    54    TYPE I (3/10)                       2CAB 129
TURN    5  T4 VAL    62  SER    65    REVERSE TURN                        2CAB 130
TURN    6  T5 GLY    81  PHE    84    TYPE I (3/10)                       2CAB 131
TURN    7  T6 VAL   109  VAL   112    TYPE II (3/10)                      2CAB 132
TURN    8  T7 ASN   124  TYR   128    TYPE I (3/10) RES 126 PRESENT       2CAB 133
TURN    9  T8 LYS   137  GLY   140    TYPE I (3/10)                       2CAB 134
TURN   10  T9 VAL   233  ASP   236    TYPE I (3/10)                       2CAB 135
TURN   11 T10 LEU   251  ARG   254    TYPE I (3/10)                       2CAB 136
CRYST1   81.500   73.600   37.100  90.00   90.00   90.00 P 21 21 21    4  2CAB 137
ORIGX1      1.000000 0.000000 0.000000        0.00000                     2CAB 138
ORIGX2      0.000000 1.000000 0.000000        0.00000                     2CAB 139
ORIGX3      0.000000 0.000000 1.000000        0.00000                     2CAB 140
SCALE1       .012270 0.000000 0.000000       -.02494                      2CAB 141
SCALE2      0.000000  .013590 0.000000       -.33832                      2CAB 142
SCALE3      0.000000 0.000000  .026950        .62129                      2CAB 143
ATOM     30  N   TRP     5      42.880  24.335 -26.897  1.00 26.34        2CAB 144
ATOM     31  CA  TRP     5      42.763  24.948 -25.567  1.00 21.17        2CAB 145
ATOM     32  C   TRP     5      43.736  24.127 -24.683  1.00 18.16        2CAB 146
ATOM     33  O   TRP     5      44.078  23.041 -25.124  1.00 18.08        2CAB 147
ATOM     34  CB  TRP     5      41.312  24.793 -25.118  1.00 19.57        2CAB 148
ATOM     35  CG  TRP     5      40.754  23.414 -25.020  1.00 17.77        2CAB 149
ATOM     36  CD1 TRP     5      40.067  22.688 -25.966  1.00 17.51        2CAB 150
ATOM     37  CD2 TRP     5      40.824  22.526 -23.877  1.00 16.84        2CAB 151
ATOM     38  NE1 TRP     5      39.710  21.460 -25.504  1.00 16.10        2CAB 152
ATOM     39  CE2 TRP     5      40.178  21.345 -24.201  1.00 16.43        2CAB 153
ATOM     40  CE3 TRP     5      41.422  22.651 -22.618  1.00 16.54        2CAB 154
ATOM     41  CZ2 TRP     5      40.084  20.255 -23.333  1.00 15.22        2CAB 155
ATOM     42  CZ3 TRP     5      41.324  21.599 -21.735  1.00 15.65        2CAB 156
ATOM     43  CH2 TRP     5      40.683  20.414 -22.087  1.00 15.70        2CAB 157
ATOM     44  N   GLY     6      44.078  24.638 -23.542  1.00 16.90        2CAB 158
ATOM     45  CA  GLY     6      44.982  23.892 -22.644  1.00 15.17        2CAB 159
ATOM     46  C   GLY     6      44.871  24.491 -21.247  1.00 16.22        2CAB 160
                              .  .  .
                              .  .  .
                              .  .  .
```

ATOM	2027	N	PHE	260	23.729	15.234	4.378	1.00	19.45	2CAB2141
ATOM	2028	CA	PHE	260	23.788	15.296	5.838	1.00	19.37	2CAB2142
ATOM	2029	C	PHE	260	23.805	16.688	6.432	1.00	19.61	2CAB2143
ATOM	2030	O	PHE	260	23.828	16.737	7.695	1.00	21.81	2CAB2144
ATOM	2031	CB	PHE	260	25.177	14.654	6.232	1.00	18.32	2CAB2145
ATOM	2032	CG	PHE	260	26.318	15.459	5.665	1.00	19.13	2CAB2146
ATOM	2033	CD1	PHE	260	26.645	15.322	4.303	1.00	18.99	2CAB2147
ATOM	2034	CD2	PHE	260	27.070	16.337	6.441	1.00	18.98	2CAB2148
ATOM	2035	CE1	PHE	260	27.705	16.029	3.744	1.00	20.00	2CAB2149
ATOM	2036	CE2	PHE	260	28.129	17.055	5.885	1.00	18.48	2CAB2150
ATOM	2037	CZ	PHE	260	28.464	16.905	4.529	1.00	17.85	2CAB2151
ATOM	2038	OXT	PHE	260	23.852	17.699	5.777	1.00	19.99	2CAB2152
TER	2039		PHE	260						2CAB2153
HETATM	2040	ZN	ZN	1	37.388	16.243	−14.458	1.00	8.37	2CAB2154
CONECT	753	751	752	2040						2CAB2155
CONECT	774	772	773	2040						2CAB2156
CONECT	950	949	952	2040						2CAB2157
CONECT	2040	753	774	950						2CAB2158
MASTER		86	10	1	7	10	11	0	6	2010	1	4	21	2CABB 20
END										2CAB2160

Contd...

Discussion 2.9: The PDB file format

Applying this Knowledge

We can edit the PDB file to our convenience; XYZ coordinates of specific parts of the file can be removed/retained as desired and such editing comes of use for the following manipulations:

• Remove water molecules
• Separate the ligand and protein (for docking studies)
• Cut out one segment of protein

For display purposes, the above segments can be hidden or undisplayed using the molecular modeling software itself. However, for energy minimization, addition of charge and other quantitative operations wherein all atoms in and around the molecule are included, it is useful to create separate PDB files of individual components appropriately labeled.

Other Formats

There are other file-formats such as the mol2, the Gaussian, the mmCIF, etc.

• The mol2 format is generally used for organic small molecules
• The XYZ format simply lists the element and the coordinates without connectivity or additional chemical information
• The mmCIF format is the input/output format for CHARMM energy calculations
• The Gaussian format is an internal coordinates format mainly used for small molecules

Some formats such as the FASTA and the BLAST list out only the protein sequence without any structural information. These files are used to store and search through large number of sequences for similarity matching.

2.3.2 THE TECHNIQUES

"I start where the last man left off."
Thomas Edison

Computational drug design strategies can aid researchers in accomplishing several steps along the drug design process thoroughly and in a cost-effective manner. Some examples of these steps are identifying targets, investigating binding sites in a protein, generating relevant molecules, evaluation of their drug-likeness, docking these candidates into target active site, ranking the docked conformations according to their binding affinities, elucidating binding mechanisms and finally, by using the inferences from several of these steps to optimize the leads and analogues for improved pharmacokinetics and pharmacodynamics.

As mentioned above, in-silico techniques have made the development of new drug candidates a faster and low cost process.

The economically-driven pressure to deliver the "first-in-class" drug on the market has forced the pharmaceutical industry to embark in a costly, yet untested, drug discovery paradigm: Hunting for the new gene, the new target, the new lead compound, the new drug candidate, finally hunting for the new drug.

Oprea, 2002

The use of complementary experimental and informatics techniques increases the chance of success in many stages of the discovery process. Traditional development process has resulted in high attrition rates with failures attributed to poor pharmacokinetics (40%), lack of efficacy (30%), animal toxicity (11%), adverse effects in humans (10%), etc. For the pharmaceutical industry, success is a trade-off between good science and good business. For example, extensive study of toxicity and pharmacokinetic performance in relation to molecular structure lowered the 40% failure (which was in 1993) to 11% by 2000. (Tsaioun, et al. 2009).

Discussion 2.10: Target Identification

Computers have become an indispensable tool in medicinal chemistry and have shifted the very course of drug discovery and design strategies. Drug design has become:

1. Rational,
2. Intelligent, and
3. Most importantly–target oriented, the word target used in two senses:
    i. Aimed to cut down failures in the early stage of research, and
    ii. Based on the structure and function of the exact target protein

The role of computers thus lies mainly in structure based design drug (*ref.* Fig. 2.3B and the 3D-structure of the target protein is vital for this purpose. Identification, sequencing, and structural elucidation of the biological target for a drug is one of the prerequisites of in-silico strategies in lead discovery and optimization. This is the first stage in rational structure-based drug design–and

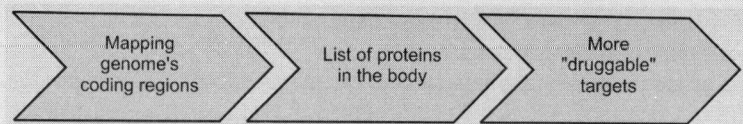

Fig.: Steps in target identification

that is why "target identification" is discussed under this chapter of part II of this book rather than presenting this view under part I on proteins. However, we wish to avoid plunging into the "techniques" used in this stage of drug designing beyond what is presented in part I of this book. Other parallel endeavors such as the human genome project greatly encouraged this because the mapping of the human genome was mainly performed on the genome's coding regions (*ref.* Discussion 1.2 under chapter 1.1). It is these coding regions that are transcribed into RNA and translated into proteins. Thus, if the nucleotide sequence of coding regions is known, one can guess the RNAs that will be transcribed from the gene of interest and eventually arrive at the list of possible sequences for proteins. Some of these proteins might be so-far-undiscovered hormones, receptors, enzymes, mediators, carriers, etc. that can act as "druggable" targets. The discovery of the protein's sequence can lead to prediction of its structure (vide chapters 1.3 and 1.4 under part I) which can be used for drug design. This is shown in figure above.

Thus, several categories of target can be identified:

1. Receptors – that are influenced by agonists and antagonists
2. Transporters – that can be blocked by uptake inhibitors
3. Ion channels – that can be blocked from operating

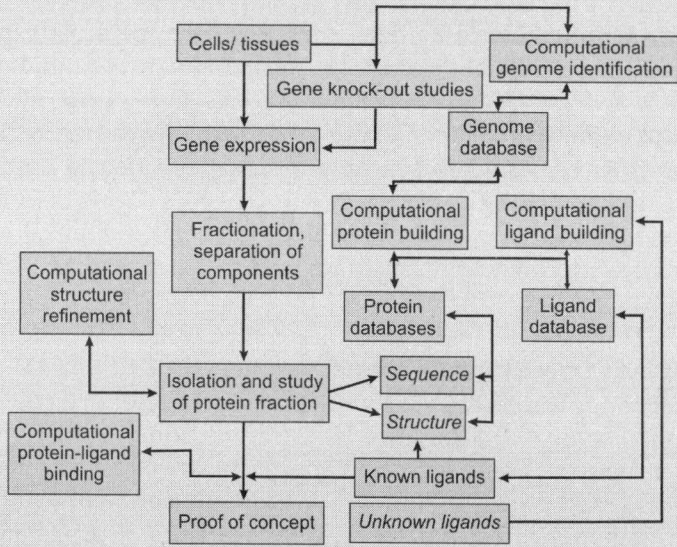

Scheme: Depicting the tangled web of experimental and computational shuttling of data

4. Enzymes – that can be inhibited

5. The DNA – that can be blocked or cleaved.

Thus, the gene also serves as a target; the identification of new genes can not only lead to a gene product (RNA or a protein) target, it itself, i.e. that particular segment of the DNA, can also serve as a macromolecular target. The physiological justification for the choice of a target macromolecule can take place before or after the target identification. In other words, the study of a specific biochemical step in a reaction cascade can lead to the isolation and identification of a target, or, the location of the target using genomics and proteomics can lead to the verification of the role of the target in the pharmacological pathway of the disease or disorder. Thus, for identifying proteins, as well as for following up on their structure and action, computations and experiments go hand in hand. This is depicted in the Scheme

A. Lead identification → Characterization → Generation

Lead identification refers to the recognition of the presence of a lead amidst several 'non-drug' molecules in a high throughput screen and this maybe done using theoretical or experimental methods. The members of a High Throughput Screening (HTS) library may have been obtained from samples of nature, from combinatorial synthesis, or a virtual construction. There is no systematic means to arrive at identifying a drug. Assays to test activity maybe set up to capture leads when screened experimentally for a particular disease or disorder. Whether *in vitro* or *in vivo*, these may leave out compounds that are active on other biological targets. Alternatively, screening assays maybe set up to obtain ligands that have good ADME properties (experimentally, called barrier assays; theoretically, called pharmacokinetic prediction). But the potency is not assured. Theoretical lead identification techniques are the fastest and least expensive way to narrow down the list of chemical molecules to meaningful drug candidates. One would need to completely understand and apply the characteristics of a drug, pharmacodynamic as well as pharmacokinetic, in relation to drug structure, and recognize how these differ from non-drugs. This is a topic of extensive research and debate been over decades; although the overall characteristics of a drug are increasingly being discovered, scientists do not have a well defined answer on how 'non-drugs' from a mixed database can be completely eliminated (techniques further discussed under section A1. Virtual Screening).

With the availability of the 'characteristics of a drug', a different approach would be to generate leads. However, this description is incomplete and theoretical lead discovery (as opposed to lead development) becomes rather difficult (QSAR and molecular modeling cannot be applied); newer techniques more suited for drug development have evolved. Computationally, building new leads can be done both by virtual screening (described under sub-topic Fragment-based approach) as well as using the target protein as a template (discussed under section A2. de Novo Design) eliminating the need for search through million-member databases. Characteristics of drugs are studied from drug databases and tested on databases of molecules used for HTS. The latter databases explore the conformational and chemical space of basic structures found in nature or those used for combinatorial synthesis. It is likely that among successfully identified leads (called 'hits') some are already drugs existing in the market! A bilateral exchange of information between the experimental and theoretical spheres of research is essential for successful drug design. Information already discovered over the years from experiments is used to correlate macroscopic effects with molecular structure. Computational insights on new molecules guide their synthesis, testing and formulation.

Discussion 2.11: Rational drug design

One of the approaches in rational drug design:

  i. The biochemical pathway and mechanism underlying a certain disease or disorder is known
 ii. The exact reaction cascades that need to be influenced to set-right the disease/ disorder and the molecules involved is known
    • Aim of the research is known
iii. Leads that can influence one or more of these reaction cascades is sought by generation of large number of molecules
    • Structural diversity hopes to capture all possible drugs with varying activity
    • Hopes to fulfill the aim of the research

Unmet medical demands drive the exhaustive sampling procedure. Testing the efficacies of various molecules will lead us to useful drugs.

Successive filtering of compounds based on several rules and properties can help to avoid in the product library:

• The presence of large numbers of halogens in the products
• The presence of highly flexible unsubstituted, unbranched alkyl chains
• The formation of compounds that exceed the maximum accepted number of rings, or ionisable groups
• False positive/negative such as molecules that would definitely bind to but also destroy proteins: Michael acceptors, ketones, aldehydes, and all manner of suicide inhibitors (Oprea, 2002).

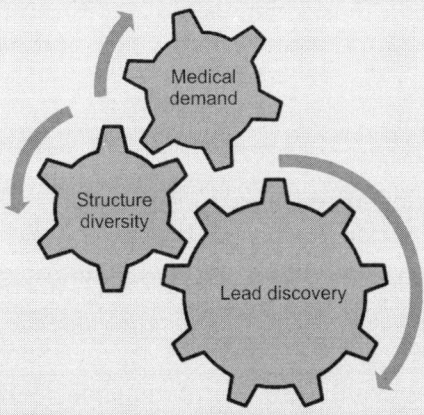

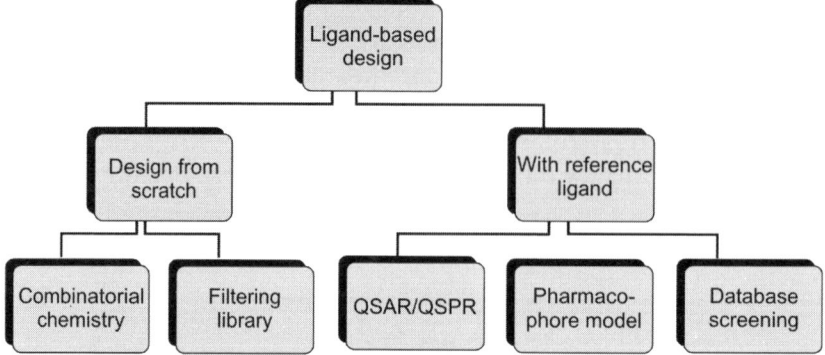

Scheme 2.5: Techniques used in ligand based design

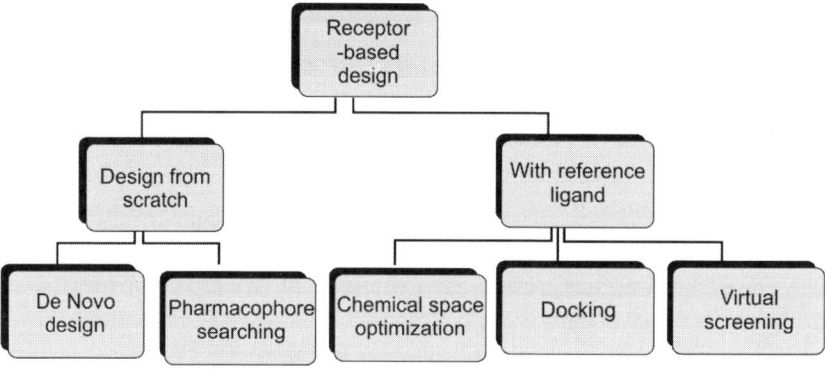

Scheme 2.6: Techniques in receptor based design

Virtual lead discovery includes various interrelated techniques:
- Ligand-based design–the design of new leads given the structure of successful ligands (such as the use of virtual screening techniques in section 2.3.2.A).
- Receptor-based design–the design of new leads given the structure of target protein, active site alone or as a whole such as de Novo drug design techniques in section 2.3.2.B.
- (Quantitative) Structure activity relationship and (Quantitative) structure property relationship discussed partly under section 2.3.2.B and partly under chapter 2.4 on chemometrics.

Information from experiments on series of related compounds are valuable:
- High throughput screening
- Property profiling–studying successful and unsuccessful candidates in the light of ADME, toxicity (combined into ADME-Tox or ADMET) and physicochemical characteristics
- Combinatorial chemistry, solid phase and parallel synthesis.

Several rules are applied for rapid property profiling to eliminate failures early such as
- Lipinski's rules (Discussion 2.8),
- *Veber rules:* Which states that the number of rotatable bonds (NROT) is an important parameter, a maximum of 10 or lower for oral bioavailability (Veber, et al., 2002),

- And other rules: Polar surface area correlates directly with the sum of H-bond donors and H-bond acceptors in a molecule (Oprea, 2002); passively absorbed molecules with a PSA of 110–140 $Å^2$ are thought to have moderate and <110 $Å^2$, low, oral bioavailabilities.

Whether research is carried out theoretically or experimentally, the lead identification stage of drug design is not as well defined as the stages that follow it because:

- Thousands of compounds need to be sampled (computation and experimental)
- Too much time and resources cannot be spent at such an early stage of drug design (computation and experimental)
- Sometimes samples are available only in μg quantities (experimental)
- There are chances of missing a good lead if the assays that test for it are not aptly designed (computation and experimental)
- Mixture of chemically diverse compounds need to be screened (computation and experimental).

Lead Characterization

"If you have the correct computational filters and good assays in place,
you can get the advantages of HTS while minimizing the downside of poor physicochemical properties"

Lipinski, 2003

GDB–13 is a database of 970 million chemical structures (at http://www.dcb-server.unibe.ch/groups/reymond/gdb/home.html) has been set up can be estimated using C, N, O, S, Cl, by applying simple chemical constraints (valency, chemical stability, synthetic feasibility, etc.) and limiting the atoms in a molecule to a maximum of 13 (Blum, et al. 2009). With robust characterization of drugs, one must be able to identify them from "other" molecules in even such a random database and even without any target structure. Such rules that aid in including pharmacokinetic predictions in the early stages of drug discovery helps caution drug developers on possible failures. One would agree that if this knowledge is available even before wet-lab synthesis, a lot of resources will be saved. This implies that prediction of pharmacokinetics must be done based only on the structure of molecules, as 3D structure would be the only information available at such an early stage of drug design. *In-silico* predictions of pharmacokinetics are done in two steps: *In-silico* prediction of property using structure, AND, correlating pharmacokinetics with property. One must calculate the confidence that can be placed on predictions by prior testing using known examples. Several characteristics of the lead need to be thoroughly investigated, some of which are briefly presented here. Success elevates the molecule to the next stage; failure gives way to optimization and more screening

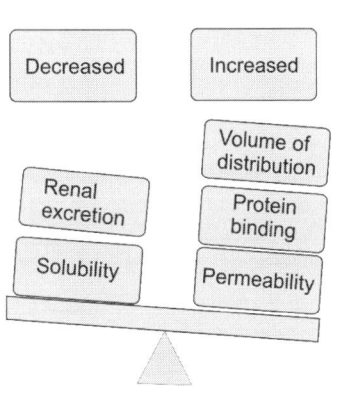

Fig. 2.4: Effects of increasing lipophilicity of a drug candidate

- Lipinksi's rule of 5, polar surface area, molecule flexibility, log D, pKa, solubility
- Information from combinatorial synthesis, cellular study and specific binding assays
- Pharmacokinetic barrier assays using membrane, pH, enzymes, etc.

Table 2.5: Estimation of *in vivo* drug performance when given orally	
Organ/ compartment encountered by the drug	*Tests (in vitro or in silico) performed to predict drug behavior*
Stomach, intestine	pH profile, stability in buffer, solubility, degradation by enzyme
Blood	Protein binding assays, stability in plasma
Intestine, liver, blood, kidney	Metabolism and resulting products
Distribution to site of action	Permeability across Blood Brain Barrier, log D, transporters, aqueous channels

Lipophilicity

Log D: Is used when partitioning across of ionized and unionized species is due to pH
Log P: Is used when all solute is neutral
Commonly used parameter is the octanol/water partition coefficient estimated at pH 7.4 ($logD_{74}$)

Software that predict the lipophilicity of compounds (i.e. log P and log D) are available and are considered to be reliable. *Ref.* list in Box 19.

Knowledge-based method: The computer is made to correlate the log P and the structure of a large number of known molecules. After this training, it is made to predict the log P of another set of molecules, also of known log P. If the prediction is satisfactory, (i.e. if predicted and known values are similar), the validation process is complete. This software can be used with confidence to predict log P values for unknown molecules of similar type.

The fragment-based approach: The contribution to log P of fragments of several thousand ligands (of known log P) is stored in a database. The log P of a new structure is predicted by diving the structure into meaningful fragments and summing the contributions of each fragment. Log D prediction is also done in similar manner.

Box 19: Some existing software that predict molecular properties
In an academic scenario, we are familiar with some of these software (in paranthesis): www. daylight.com (ClogP), www.schrodinger.com(QikPro), www.simulations-plus.com(ADMET Predictor), www.acdlabs.com (logP DB), www.accelrys.com (DSMedChem Explorer), www.cambridgesoft.com (ChemDraw), www.molinspiration.com (Molinspiration property calculator), www.logp.com/main.html (Interactive analysis LogP program *includes Lipinski numbers*)

The n-Octanol/Water is refered to as a standard system because of their
- Membrane analogous structure
- Hydrogen bond donor and acceptor property
- Practical insolubility in water

- Lack of desolvation on transfer into organic phase
- Very low vapor pressure
- Transparency in the UV region
- log P values available to fill a large database

Lipophilicity follows the famous additivity principle of π values (C. Hansch, 1964)
- $\pi_X = \log P_{R-X} - \log P_{R-H}$
- The lipophilicity parameter π is an additive, constitutive molecular parameter
- Violation to the additivity principle:
  - Intramolecular hydrogen bonds
  - Ortho effects (phenols)
  - Polysubstituted aromatic compounds
  - Conjugation (electron push-pull effect)
  - Heterocycles
  - Cyclophanes.

Depending on the dataset, technique, algorithm, etc. the software–predicted values is known to vary. As mentioned earlier, the properties of molecules in a drug database is easier to predict than in a screening database (from which leads have to be discovered) that contains a lot of non-drug-like molecules. There are practical limitations–a drug cannot be transported across the water-octanol interface (or across the cell membrane) faster than it diffuses to the interface. The relationship between log P and transport constant log k is non-linear, the rate of transport from one medium to the other limited by the rate of diffusion of the solute in question to the interface. This is applicable to both highly lipophilic as well as highly polar solutes. Other expressions that relate to lipophilicity are:
- In some models, Δ log P which is the difference between octanol-water and cyclohexane-water partitioning is used, for example, to correlate blood-brain barrier penetration of H_2-receptor antagonists with lipophilicity.
- Combinations of other properties also describe lipophilicity. For example, the sum of the van der Waal's volumes and the hydrogen bonding capability parameter describe lipophilicity and desolvation behavior.

pK_a

- pK_a indicates ionizability of molecules. When molecules consist of more than one ionizable side group, it can have different pK_a values at the various side groups. This results from the fact that the molecule can exist in various tautomeric forms as the pH changes
- Prediction of possible tautomers and the respective pK_a values of the relevant side groups can be performed by software
- Many of the software mentioned above under calculation of lipophilicity can also calculate pK_a
- Although such information is only partly useful for lead identification, details such as the pK_a of ionizable side groups is of great use during lead optimization, synthesis,

formulations and predicting biological activity (see Table 2.5 above for an example of oral drugs).

Solubility

- Varies with structure and physical conditions
- Low solubility limits absorption and causes low oral bioavailability
- Molecular properties for solubility and permeability are often opposed
- Good solubility is essential for Intra Venous formulations
- Solubility affects absorption only if <10 µg/ml
- Expressed as a function of pK_a and log P
  - Log P is used when molecules do not ionize, or do not ionize in the prevalent physiological pH.

Permeability

Types: Passive diffusion, endocytosis, active transport, paracellular permeation, efflux transport

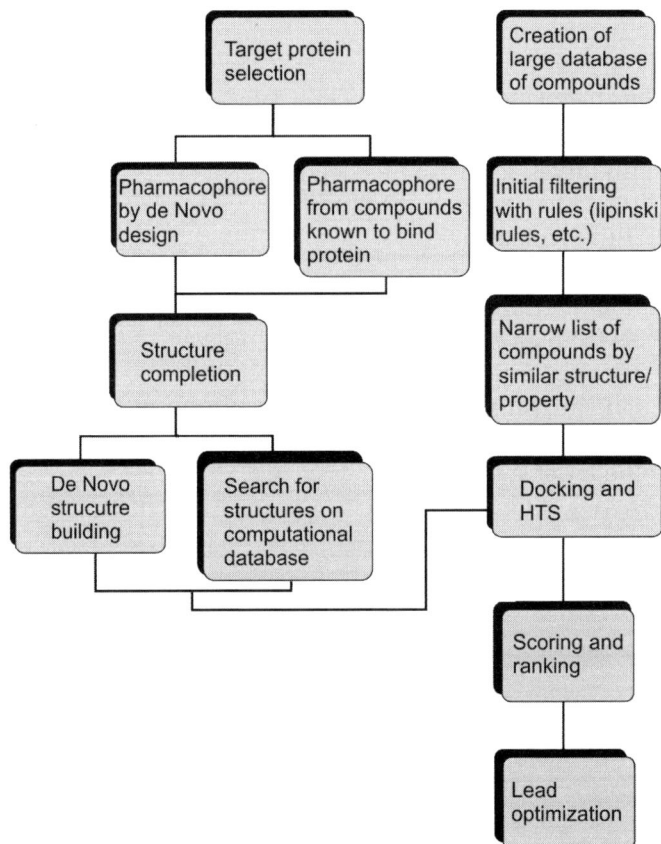

Scheme 2.7: Steps prior to lead optimization

- Prediction of intestinal absorption and permeability, oral bioavailability, Caco-2 permeability (Caco-2 is a standard cell line that behaves similar to human membranes), active transport, efflux by P-glycoprotein, crossing the blood brain barrier (BBB), plasma protein binding (PPD), metabolic stability, the Parallel Artificial Membrane Permeability Assay (PAMPA), interactions with cytochrome P450s and toxicity can be carried out computationally.
- It is evident that as one climbs higher in the levels of biological organization, the simultaneous interplay of numerous factors becomes complex. Permeability (the three types mentioned above) is a property investigated at the "tissue" or "organ" level whereas the investigation of lipophilicity, solubility, etc. was only at the molecular level.
- *In-silico* predictions are most reliable when similar molecules are present in the datasets used for training and for validation.
- Permeability predictions help in prioritizing specific structures from a list of analogues during the lead development phase. The better ranking molecules are investigated in depth, first.
- Software that calculate permeability can be found at www.simulations-plus.com (GastroPlus for the intestine and ADMET Predictor for the jejunum), www.chemsilico.com (CSHIA), www.schrodinger.com (Qikpro), etc.
  – Log P and polar surface area have been deduced as good descriptors.

Prediction of Pharmacokinetic and Toxicity (PKT) Behavior

Prediction of Absorption, distribution, metabolism and elimination (ADME) from the molecular structure gives scientists a head start in weeding out failures. Many drugs with excellent potency as well as ADME properties fail due to high toxicity. So the prediction of PKT (pharmacokinetic and toxicity, also known as ADMET and ADME-Tox) properties is an intense topic of research.

A thorough understanding of the structure–PKT relationship of molecules requires spanning all levels from atoms to organisms. This can be accomplished by a complete quantum mechanical (atomic level) calculation of an organism (and just think about this!) or, in a much simpler way, by establishing cause-and-effect correlations (using chemometric methods) at every stage of increasing complexity. The former method is only a joke and the latter method though approximate, is the only practical solution. However, the current state of research is not sufficiently advanced to predict PKT behavior even for developed leads. It cannot be used to resolve a database containing a mixture of drug and non-drug molecules.

The more one observes → the more information there is to input into a computer → the more reliable the results obtained.

Box 20: VOLSURF

VolSurf (Cruciani, et al. 2000)
This is a progam that predicts ADME properties based on pre-calculated models that cover:
- Drug solubility
- Caco-2 cell line absorption
- Blood-brain barrier permeation
- Distribution in the body.

It calculates 3D molecular fields and then converts them into simpler molecular descriptors such as:
- Size and shape (volume, surface area)
- Polarizability, polarity and hydrogen bonding
- Hydrophobicity
- Distribution of hydrophobic and hydrophilic patches on the whole molecule (Interaction Energy Moments, Amphiphilic Moments) of molecules.

Relevant information is accumulated from *in-vitro* studies (including studies using cell line), *in-vivo* experiments (animal models, etc.) and *in-silico* modeling (such as property prediction, docking, etc.). This information is collected from literature if available or by conducting simple, short and inexpensive experiments for this very purpose. Computational predictions involve molecular modeling (chapter 2.2) and chemometric (chapter 2.4) techniques. Some of the important aspects that can be used to differentiate the 'drug' and the 'non-drug' have been discussed above (such as lipophilicity, pK_a, etc.). How these properties influence bioavailability (which is a PK parameter) is also mentioned in Table 2.5. The ability to predict PKT of a molecule and the ability to distinguish the drug from the non-drug are major and interdependent topics of research. Extensive data collection and processing over the years (and still continuing) is stored in databases. Examples:
- CMC (Comprehensive Medicinal Chemistry)
- MDDR (MACCS-II Drug Data Report)
- WDI (World Drug Index).

Box 21: Software predicting PKT properties

Some software predict Pharmacokinetic - Toxicity properties such as CLOGP (www.daylight.com), Bioprint (www.cerep.fr), GastroPlus (www.simulations-plus.com), IDEA (lionbiosciences.com), TOPKAT (www.accelrys.com), etc.

A1 *Virtual Screening*

"The trick is to have quality in the original screening library."

Christopher A Lipinski (Lipinski, 2003), Pfizer Global R&D

On how to weed out failures early in drug design process

As mentioned earlier, computational selection and modeling of lead compounds can be considered a better starting point in the lead development process using rational drug design, compared to random and non-random high throughput screening techniques.

Virtual Libraries in Virtual Screening

Virtual screening techniques have been developed to predict ways in which libraries of compounds might interact with proteins and to prioritize the order in which they should be tested. These fall into two categories:
- Methods where a small molecule is docked into a specific site on a protein; and
- Those where compounds are selected on the basis of their similarity to the physical properties of a known ligand.

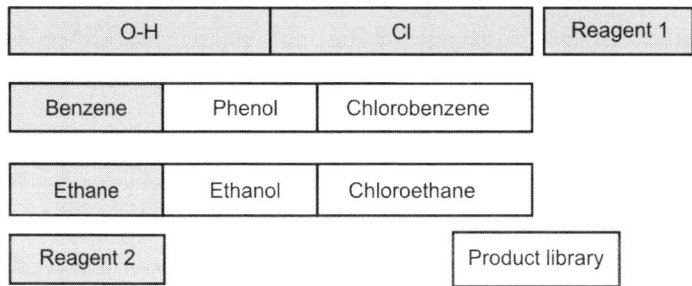

Fig. 2.5A: Simple combination of two classes of 'reagents' to generate a library

Literature suggests that these methods can give 10–100 fold improvements in finding initial hits over simple High Throughput Screening strategies (Alvarez, et al. 2005). Millions of compounds and hundreds of rules have evolved to predict drug activity over more than a century of research. The earliest of correlations showed that log P, molecular weight and number of hydrogen-bond forming groups influenced bioavailability of drugs (given orally). Lipinski's rule of 5 was coined later to estimate good oral bioavailability. It is used even today although several classes of drugs such as antibiotics and antifungals did not fit these rules (because these are transported and not absorbed into the body). The Rapid Elimination of Swill (REOS) approach was used to eliminate a large number of false positives by excluding molecules with the highly reactive side groups that bind non-specifically. Virtual libraries contain products obtained by combining classes of reagents. Each "reagent" contains several groups that combine to give the compounds stored in a library.

For example:

Generation of libraries involve 3 steps in general as shown in Scheme 2.8: Reagents containing reactive groups → products are generated (step is called enumeration) → 3 classes of reagents containing 100 groups in each will generate a 100 × 100 × 100 = 1,000,000 compound library.

A diagrammatic representation of how a combination of groups can produce varied products, some of which might violate the rule of 5 is shown in Fig. 2.5B. The violating

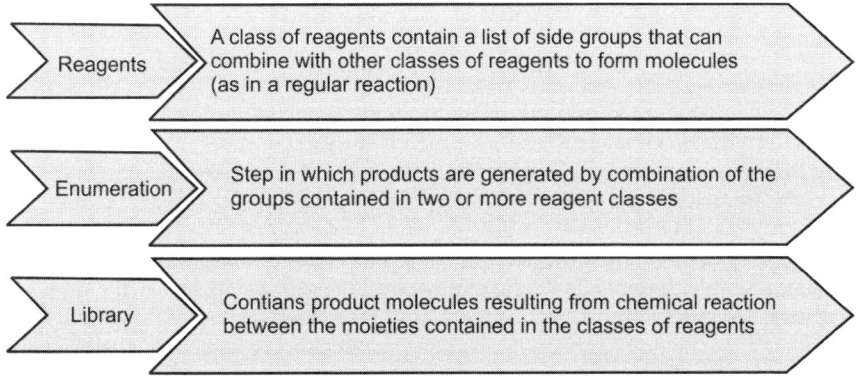

Scheme 2.8: Steps in generation of virtual library

	B1 1 O, 1 N-H,1 Cl, 1S + etc.	B2 1 O, 1 N-H,1 Cl + etc.	B3 1 O, 1 N-H, 1S + etc.	B4 3 Cl+ etc.
A1 1 Bz, 1 I				✦
A2 1 CPPP	✦	✦	✦	✦
A3 1 cHx, 2 I	✦	✦		✦
A4 4 N-H, 1 O-H	✦	✦	✦	

Fig. 2.5B: Restricting products that violate Lipinski's rule of five at the 'selection of reagents' stage. Products that are sure to violate the rule can be predicted (shown as clashes). {A1-A4 = members of reagent A, B1-B4 = members of reagent series B, O = oxygen (H-acceptor), S = sulphur (heavy atom), Cl = chlorine (heavy atom), I = iodine (heavy atom), N-H = amine (hydrogen donor), O-H = hydroxyl (hydrogen donor), Bz = benzene (aromatic, hydrophobic, bulky), CPPP = steroid ring (bulky), cHx = cyclohexane (bulky)}

compounds (indicated by 'clashes' in the table) can be predicted as being too hydrophobic, too heavy or with too many H-donors. One can program the generation of the library of products to avoid unproductive combinations. A much smaller and controllable database of products can be better used for *in-silico* screening.

Ligand-based virtual drug screening involves searching of structure and properties among thousands of ligands. The properties are those that characterize ligands, as mentioned under the introduction of this chapter. Search for structures in a database that match a given structure can be performed in 2D or in 3D. An example would be dextropropoxyphene vs. morphine wherein a two dimensional study of the former structure will not show even a trace of its resemblance to morphine; the resemblance become evident in a 3D structure [*ref.* Goodman-Gilman (Hardman, et al. 2001) or other standard text-books for structures].

Box 22: Note on log P

The properties predicting good oral permeability in the Lipinski's rule of 5 excepting *log P* can be calculated from the list of reagent groups itself, i.e. the total number of H-bond acceptors and donors, and the molecular weight. For example, the total number of H-bond acceptors of a product molecule in the library can be accounted for by simply adding the O and N atoms in each of these groups. If a member of reagent A has one N, that of reagent B has one N and one O, and that of reagent C has one N, the product will have four H-bond acceptors. Calculation of *log P*, however is not additive. It depends on the nature of all the groups present in the final molecule. In other words, the entire product molecule has to be formed in order to estimate *log P*. So, estimation of *log P* can be done only on the members of the library and cannot be predicted from the members of the various reagents.

One can use the above principle in reducing the size of the product library by filtering out groups sure to form products that will violate the rule of 5. It is easier to calculate and filter out 300 molecules (100 in each reagent set) than to look through 1,000,000 molecules formed in the library. Literature (Oprea, 2001) reports a way to circumvent the log P problem (*ref.* Box 22) and filter out groups based on hydrophobilcity calculations. So the products generated in the library will not have large molecular weights (Linusson, et al., 2000), (Weber, et al., 1995). The *parsimony principle* of lead choice states that the less the molecular complexity of the resulting lead molecule, the better it is for optimization. In the turn of the millennium, drug libraries screened to find good hits for a new target (protein) contained millions of molecules. But detailed analysis eventually revealed that *more* is not necessarily *better*. The need for intelligent data processing increased and studies directed towards the proper understanding of drug and non-drug was imminent. The results of such investigations lead to the identification of some structures that indicated false positives. Some examples are (McGovern, et al. 2002) (Roche, et al. 2002):

- *Privileged structures:* Some structures fit a lot of receptors. The leads developed from these structures might appear to be specific to one narrow class of proteins, but may elicit action on several other receptor types simply because it may be coupled strongly to the latter's effector pathways in other tissues. These structures are a definite target for success and a starting point for a series of manipulations to incorporate specificity and efficacy.

- *Drug-like molecules:* Based on some fundamental theoretical principals, some molecules may well satisfy the requirements of a drug. These molecules might even show some action in target assays during high throughput screening. However, they do not have committed molecular pharmacological pathway and will not elicit the desired action.

- *Promiscuous binders:* Just as there are orphan receptors (stray proteins that do not seem to have specific substrates) there are stray molecules that bind everywhere and to everything. These are nonspecific and could cause false positive results in HTS.

Discussion 2.12: Scenarios in high throughput screening

High Throughput Screening is a large scale experimental endeavor that aims to screen groups of compounds for specific activities. The results of the screen are based on a aseries of in vitro tests that are either performed on cell lines, in glassware, on microorganisms, etc. as demanded by the test and the activity being tested for. Literature (Oprea, 2002) recognizes 3 scenarios in virtual screening employed by companies:

HTS: Scenario–1:

1. 'Reagents' are combined to generate the library of complete, meaningful candidates (that are not random fragments of chemical structures and among which those that qualify will ultimately pass onto lead development stage)

2. Molecules in the library are screened by docking onto a target protein to investigate affinity and potency of the candidates

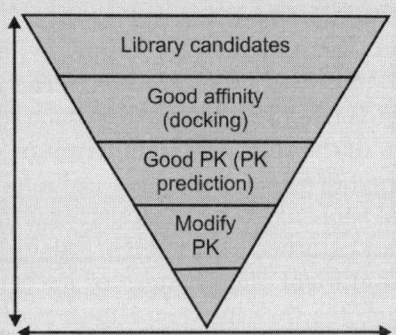

3. The docking will result in ranking of the molecules based on an in-built scoring system. Molecules with high calculated binding affinity with the receptor are ranked higher
4. The molecules that have 'satisfactory' affinity (as fixed by scientists working on the project) is followed by a pharmacokinetic filtering
5. As mentioned earlier, those molecules that satisfy both filters will be advanced to the optimization stage with preference to pharmacokinetic properties.

HTS: Scenario–2:
1. Reagents that will be used to set up the library are first screened to check if they will result in Lipinski's Rule of 5 compliant products (this is pharmacokinetic filtering)
2. Satisfactory reagents will be combined to generate a relatively small library. The members of the library are expected to have not-too-bad pharmacokinetic profile

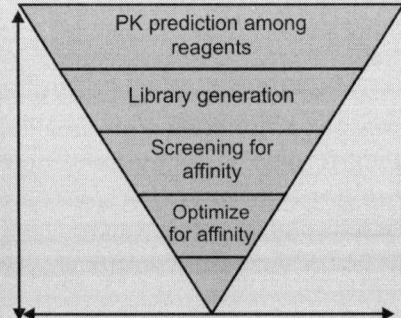

3. Candidate molecules from the library are docked and filtered further by affinity
4. Molecules that satisfy the needs of a lead will advance to the next stage and be optimized first for affinity.

HTS: Scenario–3:

1. At every stage, which includes enumeration and library screening, both affinity evaluation and PK predictions are carried out
2. When reagent selection prior to enumeration is included in the above, one gets a head start at zeroing in on the promising lead present in this set of molecules
3. This scenario may also incorporate other rules such as flexibility prior to enumeration
4. This is a fast and intelligent strategy to accelerate lead identification.

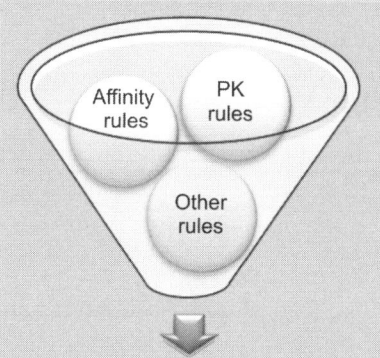

Failure to identify a lead in all of the 3 scenarios mentioned is followed by the generation of a new library by changing the reagents. Some problems that need to be addressed by any screening strategy are:

- Is docking (affinity evaluation) and PK evaluation sufficient?
- Are the cut-offs for binding energy values and PK values appropriate?
- Are any other aspects of drugs amenable to investigation at this pre-optimization stage?
- How large is "too large" for a library? (literature discusses that a simple increase in the number of molecules does not increase the chance of identifying a lead and that small libraries are more effective)
- Should affinity or PK receive the greater importance? (It is possible that increase in lipophilicity by cutting down hydrogen bonding may abolish some receptor specificity and vice versa.)

Fragment Screening

Fragment-based screening is the screening of a database of ligand fragments against a target protein, contrary to the HTS methods that dock completely formed molecules on proteins. The research paper that discusses this technique uses experimental (X-ray crystallographic) method to study the protein–fragment complex. In scenarios 1 and 2 above, affinity was evaluated only after the generation of the molecular library. In scenario 3, although affinity prediction may be performed prior to library generation, the affinity is not assessed by docking onto target protein as done by this method, but is only predicted by the presence of favorable groups.

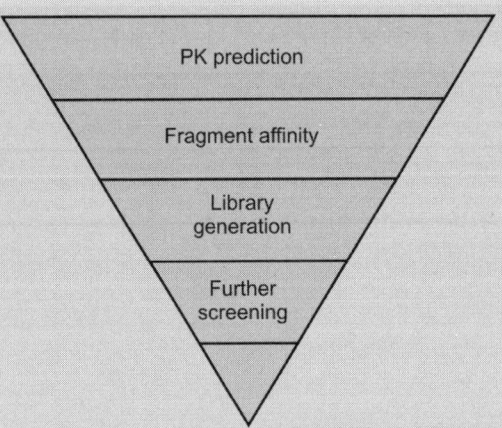

The basis for this approach is to avoid the use of fully formed molecules as the manipulation of large molecules in the binding pocket of proteins during docking is clumsy and time consuming for an initial (pre-optimization) investigation. Therefore, an initial "docking" is performed on fragments rather than on molecules. Only those fragments from the database of reagents that the target protein can accommodate are used for the generation of the virtual library. If the protein's active site can accommodate more than one fragment, these are placed at relevant distances and connected with appropriate bridging groups when the library is generated.

A "rule of 3" has been coined from the study of molecules that emerged successful in this experimental-cum-computational study to aid the generation of fragments for docking onto target proteins:

- Molecular weight is < 300
- Number of hydrogen bond donors is ≤ 3
- Number of hydrogen bond acceptors is ≤ 3
- ClogP is ≤ 3
- NROT (number of rotatable bonds) is ≤ 3
- PSA is ≤ 60

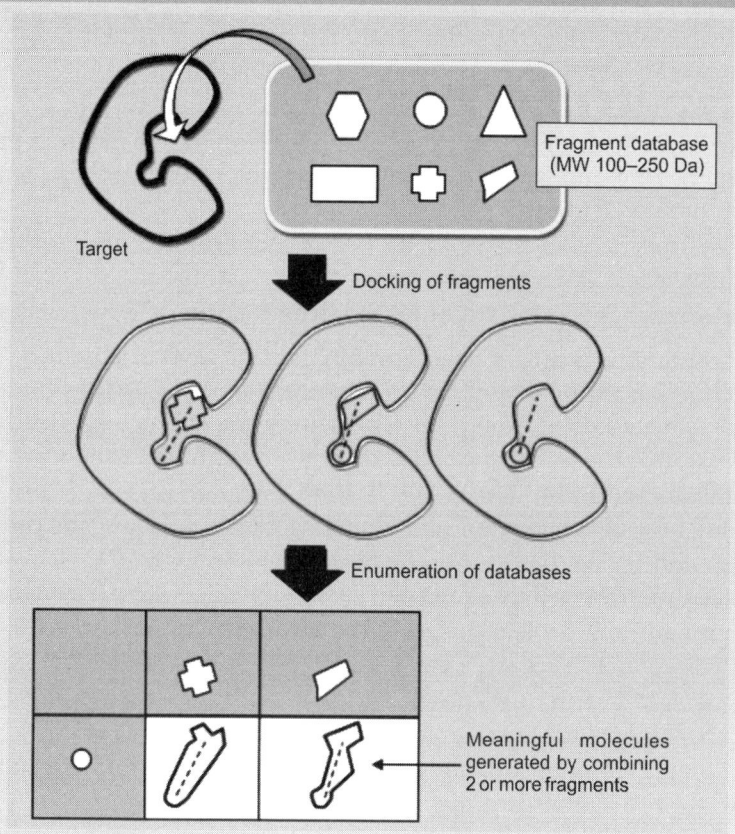

The efficiency of binding of fragments is assessed in terms of strength in relation to fragment size (equations not discussed here). The fact that the use of fragments for screening avoids the generation of a plethora of molecules that may be false positives is a point that is still debated.

> *"The rule of five was designed to assist decision-makers in drug discovery:*
> *"Out of these 2, or 5000 (virtual) hits, which ones should I study further?" and,*
> *based on the above, the answer is: "The ones that are Rule of 5-compliant" ..... (Oprea)"*

Other references: (Oprea, et al. 2001), (Harvel, et al. 2008), (Clark, 2002).

A2 *de Novo design*

Arriving at a lead molecule by generating and filtering databases, though is a non-random approach, depends to a large extent on chance. Even though rules based on the target structure or a successful ligand guide the construction and filtering process, these are mainly aimed at increasing the rate of success in a diverse database of molecules. In contrast, de Novo drug design is an approach in which the ligand is built from "first principles", i.e. only from steric fit and chemical complementarity with the protein. It is a standard procedure to base drug design research on existing information and explore new side chain modifications or discover new applications. But we can imagine that research is brought to quite another level when one discovers:

1. A whole new protein molecule that has never been targeted so far,
2. A whole new chemical entity that can be used as a lead (not to mention the enormous patentability of ring and side chain possibilities the configurational space that can accompany such a creation)
3. A whole new mechanism for prodrug being converted to drug, especially if the prodrug has better ADME than the drug
4. A whole new mechanism for targeting the drug to a specific site, say, a tumor, etc.

Given that situations 3 and 4 need combination of several advanced techniques, and that situation 2 is more an aim than a situation, let us consider situation 1, which essentially translates to drug design for a protein in the absence of a lead: what is the solution? This utilizes the technique called de Novo design. The following are involved protocols in this method (not necessarily in that order):

- To determine how much current knowledge is available about the protein:
- The location and tissue distribution (is the protein accessible?)
- The native orientation (are there hidden regions that cannot be accessed at all? For example, a membrane protein has only the intracellular and extracellular surfaces exposed)
- Is the crystal/NMR structure known and the coordinates available? (you need to start with coordinates for any computational work)
- If the coordinates are not available, at least, is the sequence known? (One can build coordinates from the sequence. *Ref.* section 1.4.3A)
- Is the function of the protein known even approximately? (either from experimental work or from the structure)
- The structure of a protein can be used to search for possible binding pockets in the form of cavities, clefts, channels, bays or concavities. Any of the above information comes in handy
- A study of the most likely binding pockets with respect to type and orientation of atoms will help to construct a pharmacophore
- A study of the shape of the pocket will give us an idea of the bulk and overall shape of the ligand that needs to be designed (which suggests the possible rings and chains that can be used).

Technically, a calculation of volume and charges on the protein will suggest the potential atoms and groups that can be used for lead design. If the aim of the design is simply getting a molecule to bind to the protein, one doesn't have to go into the details of the catalytic mechanism as one needs to do if the molecule is supposed to act as an inhibitor, activator, etc. of protein function. In either case, the target binding site can be attempted to be filled with appropriate atoms shifted around to match the potentials in a best way, sterically and with respect to the weak interactions. At the same time it should still be possible to synthesize a real molecule that contains these atoms in the required relative orientation. There are 2 strategies implemented (*see* Figs 2.6A and B).

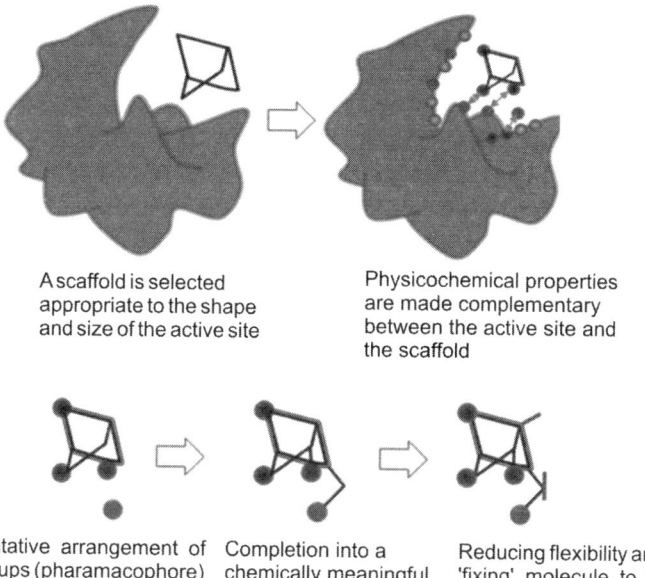

A scaffold is selected appropriate to the shape and size of the active site

Physicochemical properties are made complementary between the active site and the scaffold

Tentative arrangement of groups (pharamacophore) on a scaffold

Completion into a chemically meaningful structure

Reducing flexibility and 'fixing' molecule to its bioactive conformation

Fig. 2.6A: Inside-out strategy

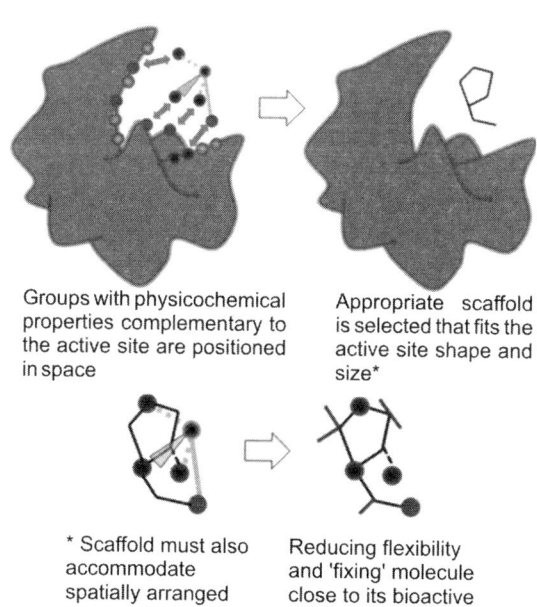

Groups with physicochemical properties complementary to the active site are positioned in space

Appropriate scaffold is selected that fits the active site shape and size*

* Scaffold must also accommodate spatially arranged groups

Reducing flexibility and 'fixing' molecule close to its bioactive conformation

Fig. 2.6B: Outside-in strategy

The Inside-out Strategy

- After mapping properties of the binding pocket and calculating its volume, the steric factor is dealt with first.
- A suitable scaffold is selected to fit the pocket shape and volume.
- The scaffold should also be able to reach the pocket easily if the pocket is located at the end of a channel shaped like a tunnel.
- The scaffold is placed at its best orientation in the binding pocket and side chains are added satisfying the steric fit and the complementary chemical properties (to ensure the presence of weak interactions)
- The strategy owes its name to the direction of adding atoms: from the scaffold to the pharmacophore.

The Outside-in Strategy

- After mapping properties of the binding pocket and calculating its volume, the weak-interactions factor is dealt with first.
- The atoms are positioned in the binding pocket at correct distances and angles from it counterparts on the pocket surface making the pharmacophore
- Suitable scaffolds are tested to best fit the pharmacophore arrangement
- The entire molecule should, of course, face no steric hindrance regarding its approach to and interacting with the active site
- In this strategy, atoms are added from the outside towards the scaffold.
- It is easy to imagine that with the outside-in strategy, the limiting factor may be in finding a suitable scaffold that doesn't disturb the pharmacophore arrangement and simultaneously fits the pocket. In either strategy, the scaffold has to complement the environment's properties also to some extent, as it is not totally shielded from the protein's influence. Other methods of construction are also recognized: such as incremental construction technique, etc.

If one now goes back to the 4 'situations' of novel research stated above at the very beginning of 2.3.2.A2, the de Novo drug design strategy is used when the protein discovered is new and untargeted. It can also be used to find out if any novel and totally different molecule can be a good drug candidate for acting on a particular receptor for which other leads are available and have been developed. De Novo design can also be used for the design of active prodrugs, evaluating its cleavage into the corresponding drug by investigating thermochemical parameters of the cleavage reaction. In the 4th situation, the prodrug is bound to a delivery moiety and administered to the body. The delivery moiety is designed to have high specificity and binding to a structure that is unique to the drug delivery site. The prodrug + delivery group binds to this structure via the latter, gets cleaved to the prodrug at the site to be administered, the prodrug binds to a second protein at the target site or closer to it and gets cleaved again, this time yielding the drug. This way, the targeted delivery of the drug molecule can be accomplished. The pharmacophore can also be used to map the receptor as described in section 1.4.3 E and this is the inverse of de Novo design.

Ongoing research includes:
- Streamlining the miscellaneous design and optimization strategies to obtain the best of them all
- To utilize the various strategies in a way as to save time and weed out failures early on
- To synchronize experimental and computational research
- To investigate (*in silico*) only those compounds that are synthesizable
- Intelligent design of reagents for libraries such that only meaningful "drug-like" compounds are created
- To increase the resolution between drug-like and "random" molecules.

Question Box

Can you give examples of drugs that have been designed de Novo? Can you give examples for drug research in "situation 4", stating the problems and limitations of such designing?

B. Lead Optimization

"Before beginning a Hunt—It is wise to ask someone
what you are looking for before you begin looking for it."
Winnie the Pooh in "Pooh's Little Instruction Book", by Milne.

Leads discovered using virtual screening and de novo design methodologies needs to be optimized to produce candidates with improved bioavailability and low toxicity. Pharmacokinetic property optimization is a rather complex undertaking that is likely to require changes in those molecular determinants that are responsible for binding affinity and specificity, e.g. hydrogen bonds (that are directional). It was recently argued that even hydrophobic interactions have some directionality. The following structure modification strategies (available in detail in reference books such as [(Kubinyi, 1995; Wolff, 1994): Burger's]:
- Conversion of ionizable groups to non-ionizable ones
- Increase in lipophilicity
- Isosteric and bioisosteric replacement of groups (see text below)
- Esterification of carboxylic acids
- Reduction of hydrogen bonding and polarity
- Introduce intramolecular hydrogen bonding
- Reduction of size
- Addition of non-polar side chains
- Formulation into a prodrug
- On the whole, modifications to structure must aim to influence hydrophobicity, molecular size, and hydrogen-bond capacity (Oprea, 2002).

Bioisosteres are functional groups that not only possess similarities in physicochemical properties, but also exhibit equivalent effects biologically. As molecular recognition is fundamentally the result of interaction between complementary electron density distributions, groups having similar size, volume and electron density are bioisosteres. These are specific to the biological system being discussed.

During the optimization process hydrogen bonds and side groups are added increasing molecular weight, log P, etc. This process when performed on a regular molecule will reduce drug-likeness. But, as it is performed on a simple lead molecule that is deficient in drug-like properties, optimization leads to an improvement of properties. The selection of an appropriate lead for optimization as discussed in the previous section is the most important step in the drug design process. Although it will go through modifications in the optimization stage, most parts of the lead (and its corresponding properties) will be conserved. Optimization step can be purely *in silico* or can include investigation of/results from *in vitro* and *in vivo* assays for receptor binding, inhibition, functional effects, kinetics, efficacy, potency, dose responses, duration of effect, etc.

Data is accumulated in steps by tenacious investigations. For example, it was established that for strong-binding ligands of up to 15 non-hydrogen atoms, the free energy of binding is approximately 1.5 kcal/mol for each non-hydrogen atom (Kuntz, et al. 1999).

"[If the lead selection is poor, in the optimization phase], would be like trying to go back and reconstruct the foundation after the house has already been built"

Lead optimization involves introducing changes to the lead molecule so that one can get a viable candidate to make into a drug. Chemical modification of a known ligand to derive a series of analogues from which SAR is derived represents the major means by which NCEs are developed in pharmaceutical research. Such known ligands are usually natural substrates such as a hormone, transmitter or secondary messenger for the target molecule. With the availability of a lead compound, a refinement of the lead structure generally involves one or more of the following steps:

- Identification of the pharmacophore
- Alteration of the length and arrangement of alkyl groups
- Modifying the functional group via isosterism and bioisosterism (classical and non classical).

Poor solubility and permeability is acceptable for compounds of high potency; however, when potency is low, good solubility and permeability becomes essential (Lipinski). A single intramolecualr hydrogen bond can increase permeability 10-fold (Lipinski, 2003). Such rules are best applied early in the drug design process. The addition or change of substituent and/or heterocycle during lead optimization is done following the indicator variables in a QSAR relation. For example, solubility, expressed as a function of log P and pKa, is reflected by the terms pKa, Hansch (π) constant, Hammett (σ) ionic substituent constants, molar volume and molar refractivity. Details rules are needed for sure success because sometimes compounds with poor properties might be the only starting point for optimization. General strategies are:

- Too many hydrogen bond donors on a drug $\rightarrow$ too little membrane permeation and low bioavailability

- Too few H-bond donors/ acceptors → binding is not specific
- Hydrophobic binding influences entropy of a reaction
- Entropy is governed by hydrophobicity, water release and conformational change
- Hydrophobic lead is not good because hydrophobic ligands react with a variety of proteins → low therapeutic efficacy and more side effects
- Flexibility of ligand is beneficial if the ligand is being designed to
  - Bind to more than 1 member in a class of proteins
  - Bind to proteins that mutate naturally such as the viral coat proteins
- Drug molecules can give the same affinity but can widely differ in the mechanism of binding
- Binding affinities of 1–10 µM range and potency improvement up to 10^5 times is required before considering drug candidates
- Balancing potency, selectivity, toxicity and bioavailability
- Data generated during secondary screening = (i) IC_{50} (ii) K_i information (iii) chemical structure
  - Helps in elucidation of bioavailability, structure modification suggestions and pharmacokinetics
  - However, no mechanism can be inferred
- Quantitative estimate of attractive forces such as H-bonding, van der Waals interactions and ionic bonds, hydrophobic interactions and stoichiometry are needed for accurate lead optimization

In the turn of the millennium, drug libraries (screened to find good hits for a new target protein) contained millions of compounds and this was also the number of compounds synthesized in a year in a company. The source of these drugs was HTS which is known to yield large molecules (that are also more lipophilic). Therefore, despite the large numbers, the success of a hit was rather low: around 1 per 100,000 compounds for enzymes (considered the easiest of targets). A shift in lead identification and development strategies was much needed and today, both phases include simultaneous investigation of PK and PD properties. Lead optimization is generally guided by Scheme 2.9.

Selective references: (Gribbon, et al. 2005; Di, et al. 2003; Marrone, et al. 1997).

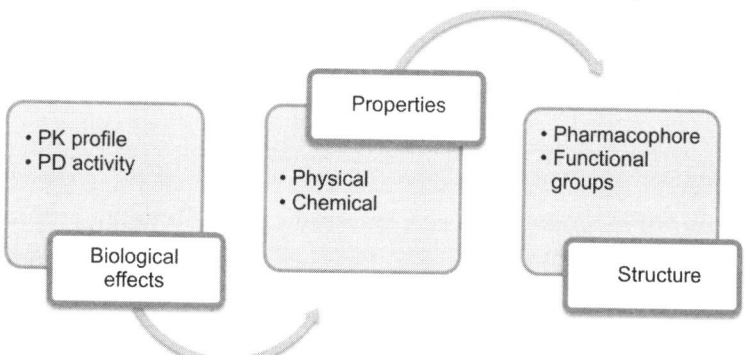

Scheme 2.9: Levels of complexity in a typical drug design scenario and the quantities involved under each

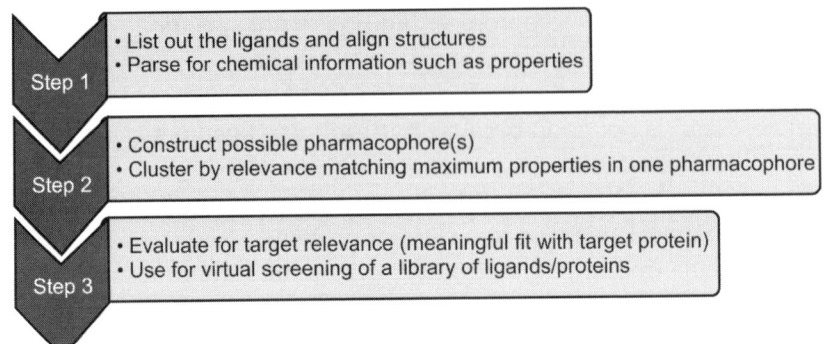

Scheme 2.10: Generation of pharmacophore models: The workflow

B1 *Identification of Pharmacophore*

The relevant groups in a molecule that interact with a receptor and are responsible for the activity are collectively called the *pharmacophore*. In other words, it is an ensemble of universal chemical features that characterize a specific mode of action of a ligand in the active site of the macromolecule in 3D space. Other atoms in the analogue are sometimes called *auxophore*. The framework or core "ring" of the analogue is often termed the *scaffold*. The pharmacophore is not a real molecule or chemical entity- it is just an arrangement of atoms at certain distances, angles, etc. such that chemically meaningful structures made by connecting them will react with the concerned receptor. It is primarily of pharmacodynamic relevance; it can also contribute to the improvement of pharmacokinetic properties of the drug. The constructed pharmacophores are valid for the existing molecules as well as for the unknown ones. They can be manipulated to yield candidates with selective affinity with the target. Pharmacophore generation is a simple method that can be used to screen large virtual libraries and are constructed in 3D. Some software (LigandScout) support multiple features per heavy atom to broaden the scope of a single model (enabling users to assign two hydrogen bond acceptors and one donor feature on the same atom). A popular book compares novel leads to a water-bed where adjusting the properties of one part can affect those of another.

The identification of the bioactive conformation is crucial. If the exact conformation is known (from an available ligand) rigid analogues can be designed. Otherwise, certain degree of conformational mobility is maintained in the analogue. Energetically favored conformations of a ligand taken up when crystallized with a protein (determined by X-ray crystallography) might not resemble the bioactive one as in the case of the protein as well. Small molecules in solution are flexible, and in a crystal, are rigid. When it comes to identifying biological conformations, experimental help is limited. A computational approach would sample all possible conformations that a ligand of study can take up and search through them for the presence of the pharmacophore.

List of interactions that are generally mapped on the pharmacophore is presented; these are known to have specific properties as in Table 2.6 such as distance constraints and directionality in space (Fig. 2.7B).

- Hydrogen bond donors and acceptors
- Positive and negative ionizable area
- Hydrophobic regions
- Aromatic ring
- Metal binding spots
- Excluded volume.

Table 2.6: The properties of specific drug-receptor interaction mechanisms

Interaction	Property
Hydrogen bond	Direction and distance constraints
Hydrophobic interactions	Distance constraints (and some direction)
Ionizable areas	Distance constraint
Active site excluded volume	Steric hindrance from protein atoms

The properties have to be modeled as such to obtain a good estimate of affinity

- Distance constraints represent the relation between two points, one located on the ligand side, one on the macromolecular side.
- Direction constraints represent the relation between two atom groups, one located on ligand side, one on macromolecular side. Groups form a rigid reference geometry, which acts as the basis for a directed vector.

Table 2.7: Partial list of distance ranges (Å) wherein some interactions are felt

Aromatic interaction with positive ionization	3.5–5.5 Å
Aromatic interaction with ring (parallel)	2.8–4.5 Å
Aromatic interaction with ring (orthogonal)	2.8–4.5 Å
H-Bond interaction	2.2–3.8 Å
Hydrophobic interaction	1.0–5.9 Å
Iron binding location	1.3–3.5 Å
Magnesium binding location	1.5–3.8 Å
Negative ionizable interaction	1.5–5.5 Å
Positive ionizable interaction with negative ionization	1.5–5.5 Å
Positive ionizable interaction with aromatic ring	1.0– Å
Zinc binding location	1.0–4.0 Å

Example: Hydrogen Bond Constraints

Hydrogen bonding is most likely only for certain arrangements of the donor atom, acceptor atom and hydrogen in the middle. For example, the default angle range for sp^2 hybridized heavy atoms is 50° cone angle in Fig. 2.7A.

Flexible H-bond interactions, as occurring at sp^3 hybridized heavy atoms, are represented by a *torus*. The default angle range for sp^3 hybridized heavy atoms is 34°. It has also been worked out that ~0.4 Å and ~20° suite most macromolecules (Mills, et al. 1996).

If we assume that the amide or the hydroxyl groups (H-donor) is present on the protein, then the truncated cone or the torus (respectively) would be a part of the pharmacophore. When the pharmacophore is built from the target protein, it is called

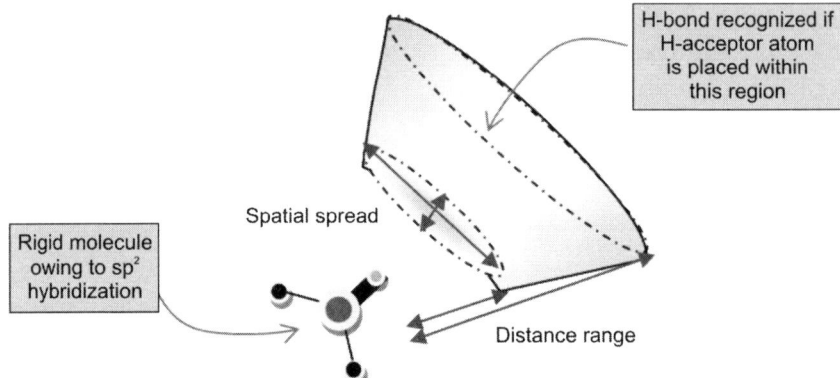

Fig. 2.7A: An sp² hybridized amide nitrogen has a truncated-cone shaped H-bond space

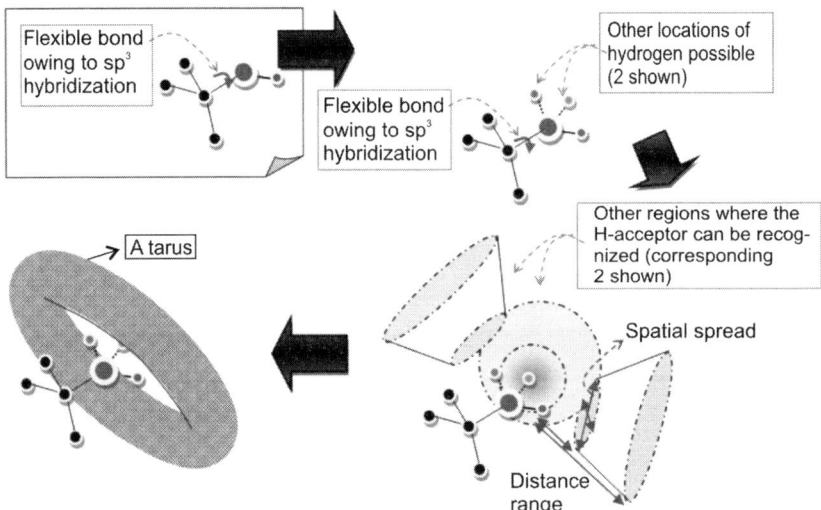

Fig. 2.7B: The derivation of how an sp³ hybridized–OH oxygen has a torus-shaped H-bond space

receptor-based pharmacophore modeling. If we assume that the H-donor is on a ligand that is known to bind to a certain protein (either because it is the protein's natural substrate or because it has been proven in past investigations to do so) then we expect the protein's H-acceptors to be in the H-bond space depicted above. The *ligand-based pharmacophore* built based on this known ligand will contain the H-bond space around it similar to that contained by the template ligand. In other words, H-donors (amide or hydroxyl) of the pharmacophore will lie close in space to the H-donors of the known ligand.

Alignment is a major technique used in pharmacophore modeling, whether it is performed on ligand molecules to generate a common pharmacophore, or using a built pharmacophore to identify matching ligands from a database. Standard alignment algorithm are used (alignment in general is outline as a part of homology modeling in section 1.4.3.A). The alignment can also be performed for *structure matching* (molecules' atoms are aligned and superimposed) or *feature matching* (in which properties such as hydrophobic spheres, etc. of various molecules are aligned and superimposed). *Pairwise* alignment is often done where one atom (feature) from the reference and another atom (feature) from the dataset are checked at a time for similarity. The reference is an already existing ligand or the pharmacophore; if neither exist, the reference is one of the molecules of the dataset, randomly selected. Pharmacophore represents the electron density distribution recognized by the receptor that results in conformational changes in the protein (where applicable) and secondary messengers. A range is always specified to determine whether the aligned atom/property overlap between the reference and the molecule in the dataset. This range is called *tolerance*.

Pharmacophore generation from a list of molecules is also similarly treated. If every atom or feature lies within the tolerance of all other counterpart atoms or features within the dataset, the average of atoms/features is taken and the pharmacophore is generated. Such a construction results in a *'shared feature pharmacophore'*. A more thorough investigation would search through several conformations of all molecules in a dataset. This implies that a conformational search is carried out on the molecules of the dataset, with the number of conformers obtained from each molecule depending on the number of rotatable bonds in the molecule. Although this is the best way to carry out a search for molecules compliant with the pharmacophore, it is time consuming and computationally exhaustive. New techniques constantly emerge [for example, (Yamaguchi, et al. 2005)] that tackle the problem using divide and conquer policy. A note on the ***binding site hypothesis***:

- This is the inverse of the pharmacophore hypothesis
- In this, the counterparts of the pharmacophore is mapped and similarity among ligands are tested by their fit with this counterpart
- This principle is not very appropriate for lead identification, optimization or screening because it includes greater uncertainty than the pharmacophore model (it models the counterpart of the pharmacophore which could accupy a region in space; the protein also has some flexibility in conformation)
- This principle is successfully used in 3D QSAR (*ref.* chapter 2.2.4). This hypothesis is mentioned with reference to distance and directional constraints of H-bonds in Figs 2.7A and B.

Discussion 2.13: "Pharmacophore model" for improved pharmacophore kinetics

(Penzotti, et al. 2002) A pharmacophore fitting a protein's active site is most comfortably associated with drug activity and pharmacodynamics. However, proteins also play a role in drug pharmacokinetics as the enzymes of the alimentary canal, as proteins of biotransformation, as efflux transporters, etc. and these proteins can be fitted with the pharmacophore as well. Determining the chemical substructures present in drugs that attract the attention of, say, P-glycoprotein (P-gp) efflux transporter will provide valuable information that can be used for lead optimization. P-gp is infamous for its power to recognize xenobiotics and effluxes drugs belonging to a wide variety of seemingly unrelated classes. It is overexpressed in cancer cells and has been targeted by multi-drug resistance reversal agents to aid cancer therapy [*ref.* standard textbooks such as Goodman-Gilman (Hardman, et al. 2001)]. The following structural similarities were identified: the presence of aromatic ring structures, amphiphilic nature, polarizability, etc. The role of H- bond acceptors has been very well documented; two patterns in H-acceptor arrangements have been identified (type I and type II). A QSAR model was also developed for P-gp subtrates (stouch, et al, 2001)

Results from the study:
- A large fraction of data generated could be resolved into substrate and non-substrate molecules
- The final informative ensemble selected to obtain best results contained 100 pharmacophores
- Features in the ensemble pharmacophore = h-bond acceptor, donor, and one or two hydrophobic groups

The model correctly classifies 50–60% of the P-gp substrates and greater than 80% of the non-substrates.

Methodology Overview

Features	• HBA/HBD, hydrophobes, -ve/+ve charges aromatic groups
Ph-phore	• Each ph-phore can combine of 2/3/4 features (2/3/4 point ph- phores)
Constraints	• Each ph-phore can contains max. 2 hydrophobic features
Conformers	• Max. 100 conformers generated/ stereoisomer drug in the dataset
Label	• Each ph-phore is labeled by 1 bit string called "molecular signature"
# Compds	• 144 structurally diverse compounds gave 3 million ph-phores
Ranking	• Based on ability to discriminate between substrates and non-substrates
The model	• Avg of several max. info content ph-phores gives the "ensemble model"

Terms: HBA/HBD: Hydrogen bond acceptor, Hydrogen bond donor; -ve/+ve: negative/positive; Ph-phore: pharmacophore; Max.: maximum; Info: information; Avg: average; #: number of

Box 23: About CATALYST, software for pharmacophores

Catalyst develops 3D pharmacophore models from a group of molecules that may have diverse structures and activities. The hypothesis includes features of the molecule that are likely to be important for binding to the receptor. These features (or molecular descriptors) include:

- Chemical function, location and orientation in 3D space, tolerance in location, weight (feature importance.

The feature importance is ascertained by the following interactions:

- H-bond acceptor and donor properties, hydrophobicity (due to aliphatic and aromatic groups), positive charge and ionizable areas, negative charge and ionizable areas, aromatic rings

HipHop is a module that:

- Identifies binding features for drug-receptor interactions, uses only active ligands, generates alignment of active leads, uses multiple conformers, can be further used for 3D-QSAR analysis

HipoGen is a module that:

- Performs activity-based pharmacophore modeling, uses both active and inactive ligands to set up hypothesis, used to "predict" or estimate activity of new ligands

B2 *Quantitative Structure Activity Relationship*

This section outlines the drug design application of quantitative structure activity relationship. The turn of the millennium witnessed the approval of about 40 new drugs annually, by the FDA (Gottlieb, et al. 1998), US being the largest consumer (~50%) of drugs prescribed in the world. These drugs target cancer, heart disease, AIDS, Alzheimer's, Parkinson's disease, migraine, arthritis, and many other disease conditions. This might be a small number compared to the ever existing need for advanced pharmaceutical agents and treatment regimens. However, the amount of experimental and theoretical information generated in the 8 to 15 years of research taken to arrive at these molecules is invaluable. For example, the SAR for a novel series of compounds can be derived by radioligand binding assays or functional assays involving biochemical responses or gene reporter systems experimentally. However, if a series does not exist for a new lead molecule, or if the disease condition is new, theoretical studies come in handy. The study of the properties of the molecule itself is as important as the study of its mechanism and effects. Knowledge of the molecule is mainly the understanding of its physicochemical properties which arise from the functional groups within it. Some of these properties are: acidity–basicity, water solubility, partition coefficient, crystal structure, stereochemistry.

An example would be structure activity relationship in steroids (*ref.* Goodman-Gilman for this, and more, examples). Analogues with bad PK fail at the very end of the drug design phase consuming extensive time and resources all through (Prentis, et al. 1988). Establishing an SAR and selecting only those analogues that fit into this series is a safer bet for investment. In a *series SAR* evaluation, a lot was invested early in the drug design stages but still the candidates failed PK and safety. A lot of time and resources were expended. So another addition to the investigation was the search for drug-likeness in the form of SPR (Structure-Property Relationship). Drug-like properties were those properties found commonly among the successful drugs in the analogue database. Solubility, permeability and stability *in vitro* reflected

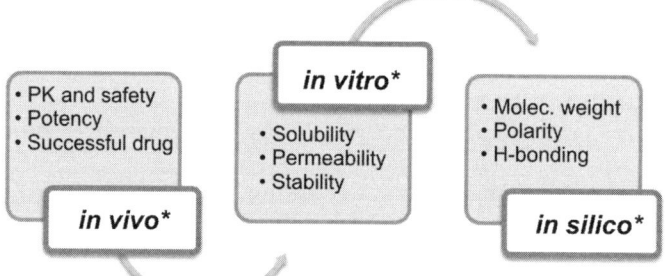

Scheme 2.11: The 3 avenues of investigation in drug design

pharmacokinetics and safety *in vivo* derived from molecular weight, polarity and hydrogen bonding *in silico*. Study at all these 3 levels is called *pharmaceutical profiling*. Compare with Scheme 2.9 under section 2.3.2 B *lead optimization*. This information supplements pharmacodynamic studies of mechanism of drug action.

How does one use SAR and SPR information?
• Prioritize compounds and select the best analogue(s) for the next stage
• Eliminate failures early in the development process (*fail fast, fail cheap*)
• Thoroughly investigate conformational space to get meaningful starting structures
• Predict *in vivo* behavior

These are statistical tools are used to calculate properties and activity. SPR is needed because low potency high bioavailablity is better than high potency PK failure. SPR modifies molecule size, H-bonding, polarity, ionizability, flexibility, etc. Modified structures might improve one property but retard another; it might also decrease activity.

Discussion 2.14: QSAR in daily terms

It is important to understand what is being done in Quantitative Structure Activity Relationship in order to appreciate its use and also to be conscious of its pitfalls. For this, as practiced frequently throughout this book, let us think about an everyday example. Let us temporarily ignore the "Structure" and the "Activity" in QSAR and simply think in terms of quantitative relationship; let the topic of the current discussion be "good impression". Our task is now to try to construct a formula for good impression.

What is the advantage of having a formula?
1. We have a ready-to-use expression and do not have to think from zero every time we wish to impress someone
2. We have a quantified relation between good impression and its components
3. We can understand what are the aspects involved in good impression
4. As we have quantified the relationship, we can also understand which aspects contribute more and which less.

Putting forth the question to a group of student, "what are the components of good impression?" we got the following answers:

Good impression = Appearance + mannerism + achievement + presentation + looks + talk + voice + dress + feel + politeness + punctuality + dominance + the number of cars in a particular parking lot per day taken for as many days as responses to the above question

This expression is not quantitative. In order to make it so, we need to do the following:

1. On the LHS, we need a numerical score for good impression
   - Say, a score from 1–10 which is taken in the rows of the dataset.
2. To ascertaining whether each term is related (either in a positive or in a negative way) to the LHS
   - This is done using Principal Component Analysis (*ref.* under chapter 2.4). The descriptors appear as columns in the dataset. From the above, we know that the number of cars in a particular parking lot is not related to the LHS, so we can remove it, though here, we keep it.
3. To optimization of what terms to keep in the RHS
   - We know that appearance = looks + talk + dress. Having all four terms in the expression overweights "appearance" by a factor of 2. This confuses the weights that will be assigned to other quantities and so we remove the repetition.
4. A dataset of various good impression scores collected with respect to the various terms (descriptors)
   - We need a good survey of how people rate the contribution of each term to good impression. The larger the size of the survey, the better we can assign weights to the terms.
5. To weight the various terms
   - Multiply each term with a constant to increase or decrease its contribution or 'importance'.
6. Optimizing the weights so as to reproduce the good impression score
   - Keep changing the constants on the RHS so that the trends in the data under each column reflect the scores at the start of each row.

So we arrive at:

Good impression $= k_1$ (appearance) $+ k_2$ (mannerism) $+ k_3$ (achievement) $+ k_4$ (presentation) $+ k_5$ (feel) $+ k_6$ (politeness) $+ k_7$ (punctuality) $+ k_8$ (dominance) $+ k_9$ (the number of cars per day in a particular parking lot for n days) $+ k_{10}$

The k_{10} is added so that the data can be made to fit easily to the LHS.

The dataset we collected looks thus:

Serial no.	Good impression score (1–10)	Descriptor 1 Appearance (/100)	Descriptor 2 Mannerism (/100)	Descriptor 3 Achievement (/100)	...	Descriptor m (/...)
1	10	99	99	45		
2	5	50	45	10		
3	1	1	0	10		
:	:	:				
n						

After solving for the QSAR equation, we arrive at the following results/inferences:

1. $k_1 = k_2 = 1$ meaning appearance and mannerism get equal and highest score from the above data (we can see this from some of the values shown in the table)

2. $k_3 = 0$ does not seem right because we know (and so do the people who voted in this survey) that achievement plays some role in impression created by the person. But we observe that achievement simply drops out because it is not consistant—why? Remember that the question "what are the components of good impression?" is a vague question. We did not specify whether the situation is a job interview or in impressing a girl/boy or any other. Therefore, people have assumed their own situations and the ratings did not correlate. The problem should be well defined in order to obtain the best answer.

3. $k_8 = -1$
   a. Negative weight means that people have weighted *dominance* as a trait that reduces good impression score
   b. The value (irrespective of the sign) is 1 signifying that dominance has as bad an effect on the score as appearance and mannerism have in improving the score

4. $k_9 = 0.9$
   a. We know that the cars in a parking lot on m successive days are not related in any way to good impression; however the result is a strong and positive correlation!
   b. We must understand that after all these are numbers—the trend in the data of this descriptor might have matched the trend in the scores column in this dataset; thus we must be able to interpret the result—we cannot blindly trust that there is relationship when any statistical analysis indicates so.

The readers are requested to correlate the above points with a QSAR study in medicinal chemistry.

C. Energy Minimization/Geometry Optimization

This section covers:

1. The principle	What is energy minimization?
2. The algorithms	How is it executed?
3. The types	Varying levels of accuracy
4. The structure-energy balance	Why do we need to perform minimization
5. Finding the global minimum	How to solve problems using minimization

6. The real-life parallel to the energy-minimized state

The pros and cons of minimization

7. Applications in research

Where to use minimization

C1 *The Principle*

Method overview: in general terms

The starting structure of the molecule is specified using either internal coordinates or Cartesian coordinates (*ref.* Discussion 1.6 under chapter 2.2). If specified in the latter format, a list of bond length, angles and other parameters including connectivity of atoms is extracted by the software whereas in the former format, these values can be directly obtained from the input file. In most software, the positions of only the heavy atoms are specified by the user. The software uses the atom identity and connectivity information from the input file to complete valencies of heavy atoms. This is done by adding hydrogens and electron lone pairs. Electron addition also needs to satisfy the total charge of the molecule as specified in the input file. The added atoms/groups/ electrons are placed around the heavy atom in accordance with the atom shape (tetrahedral, trigonal, linear, etc.). The geometry of the molecule at this starting stage is thus very crude. One can then perform a *single point calculation* (to calculate the energy of the current conformation). Further, one can also arrive at the (energetically) most stable conformation, and this procedure is called *energy minimization* or *geometry optimization* (discussed in this section). The procedure is called energy minimization, indicating that the search is for the lowest energy conformer, or geometry optimization, indicating that the search is for an optimum geometry of the molecule in which it is least strained. The terms used in force fields are recalled and summarized from chapter 2.2.4 in Scheme 2.12. The structure/conformation arrived at is called global minimum.

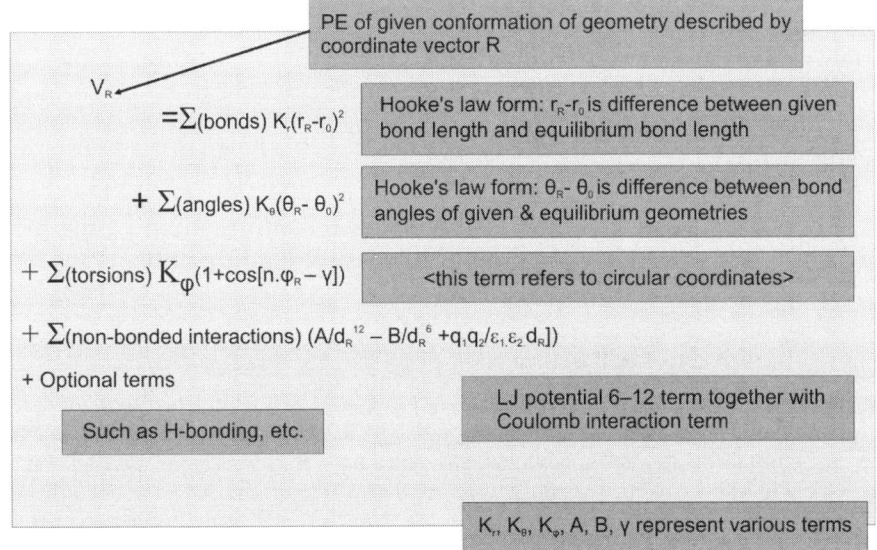

Scheme 2.12: Summarizing force fields terms

The most important aspect to remember is that potential energy V is a function of the geometry of the inputted molecule and is also written out as V(R) in many works. The literal form is $V_R - V_0$ showing that the potential energy calculated is the difference between that of the given structure and the equilibrium structure. But V_0 is set to 0 and V is simply $V_{(R)}$ or V_R is recognized as *strain energy* (recall the 'conformational energies' of various cyclohexane conformations in organic chemistry textbooks express only 'strain energies' and not absolute energies). The force field compares the inputted structure and the equilibrium values for parameters stored in its tables. Differences in values of various parameters are converted to strain energy (using equations as discussed under Discussion 2.4 in chapter 2.2) and added up. Geometry optimization aims to continuously change conformation and recalculate energy so that one can pick out the lowest energy conformation among all those analyzed. In other words, V_R is brought to a minimum for the given molecule.

Method overview: Other aspects

- How is it performed: How to pick the lowest energy conformation of (or How to energy minimize or how to optimize the geometry of), say, benzene? One can easily guess that this involves consecutive change of conformation and calculation of energy. In other words, it is a series of single point calculations performed after new conformations are generated by making slight changes in the atom positions. The first half of the problem (i.e. generation of new conformations) is discussed under "conformational search" under C2A. Several methods tackle both parts of the problem in the same algorithm–such methods are described in C2B. The entire process comes to an end when a conformer with reasonably low energy satisfying other conditions of the research is arrived at.

- The types: All molecules need to be energy minimized if constructed or edited in an empirical way; for example, a sulphate group is added to benzoic acid simply using the modeling software, or, one hydrogen atom is simply changed to fluorine, or an aspartate residue in a protein is mutated to glutamate. Depending on the size of the molecule and several other factors, energy minimization can be performed using very accurate theoretical calculations or using the 'ball-and-spring' molecular modeling methods. For details, *ref.* section C3.

- How do you know that the resulting conformer is indeed the lowest in energy? The word "lowest" indicates a comparison among all conformations of the molecule. Theoretically, one would have to sample all possible conformations. Why? *Ref.* Box 24:

Box 24: How does one know if one has the lowest energy?

Imagine that you are asked to pick out the lowest numbered ball from a box that contains balls with numbers painted on them. If you cannot see into the box and if you do not know what numbers are painted on the balls, when would you know that you have reached the lowest number? One will know this for sure only when all the balls from the box have been picked out. Even if one ball remains in the box, there is some chance that *that* ball will have the lowest number! Although this is the case for geometry optimization, it is not practical to sample *every* conformation of a molecule however small.

- This problem referred to in Box 24 is called finding the global minimum. The ways in which such an investigation would be useful is mentioned in subsection C4 and the techniques used for the purpose are discussed under subsection C5.

- It results that for a flexible molecule, one can never be sure that the expected geometry (the conformer expected to have lowest energy) and the optimized geometry (the conformer that actually results from a minimization) are the same as these are not unique isolated structures of a molecule that are just waiting to be discovered. These are just one of the many possible conformations that all together form a continuum. For example, the staggered form of ethane is just one of the infinite conformers possible. If the two hydrogen atoms that lie at $\varphi = 180°$ (anti) to each other in a Newman projection are considered, then hundreds of conformations are possible between $\varphi = 175°$ and $\varphi = 185°$ and the conformer with $\varphi = 180°$ just happens to be one of them. If the molecule is, say, dichloroethane instead of ethane, the staggered form with $\varphi = 180°$ would be more unique owing to a clear demarcation based on energy. Subsection C6 outlines similar insights that such calculations provide us with.

It is absolutely necessary for readers to understand the meaning of 'degrees of freedom' (*ref.* Discussion 2.15) and its implications on optimization.

Discussion 2.15: Degree of freedom of molecules

It would be useful to introduce the crucial concept of degrees of freedom of molecules in the following way:

There is nothing like the freedom of bachelor life, yet, people do get married! Whether they are happier married than when single is part II of the topic debated, and that depends on the constraints imposed on them after the wedding in comparison to what they experienced prior to it…

Bearing in mind that we talk chemistry, and not social behavior, the above statement can be further expanded. Atoms and molecules are free to move about (this is called translation) and roll-over (this is called rotation) in space–but not to an infinite extent. We are intuitively aware that free atoms have the greatest mobility in space, and atoms chemically combined into molecules are only ranked next. But what exactly is the difference? Physics tells us that the total degrees of freedom n of a molecule of N atoms is 3N. It can be split up as follows:

Freedom of Atoms

Consider an atom placed in X, Y, Z space.

1. It can move about freely along the 3 directions (X, Y and Z)
2. It makes no difference if it rotates along the X, the Y or the Z axis because it is spherical in shape
3. It cannot vibrate; the only possible vibration is expansion/contraction–the atom cannot alter its own atomic volume because its electrons and nucleus attract each other too strongly and have already reached an equilibrium

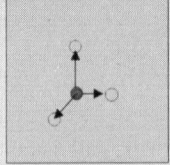
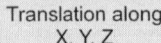
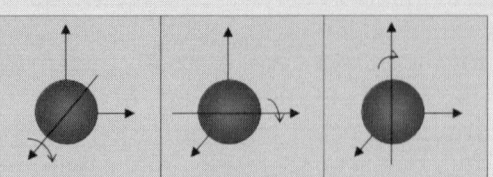
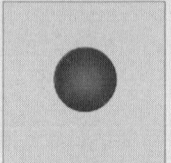

Translation along X, Y, Z	Rotation along X, Y, Z (corresponding axis depicted in foreground of each figure) – makes no difference!	It has no vibrations

(***in the figures in this discussion, filled circles represent original atom and empty circles represent a new position/orientation after rotation/vibration/translation as applicable)

Degrees of freedom of an atom = 3 translations + 0 rotations + 0 vibrations = 3

Total number of degrees of freedom $n = 3N = 3 \times 1 = 3$ (thus this has been verified)

The degrees of freedom that have been eliminated from the counting have low effect on total energy (with some exceptions such as at high temperature).

Degrees of Freedom of Diatomic Molecule

Instead of one atom, in the above situation, if there is a diatomic molecule, the following results:

1. It can move about freely along the 3 directions (X, Y, and Z) as one unit
2. Placing the molecule along the Y axis, it can rotate along the X and the Z axis; rotating along the axis of the bonding does not make any difference
3. It can vibrate along the Y axis (this is called stretching vibrations)

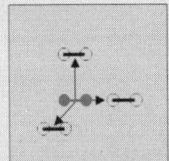
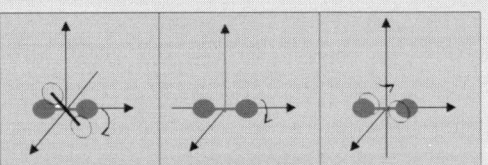
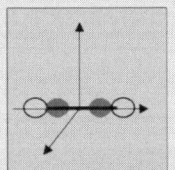

Translation along X, Y, Z	Rotation along X, Y, Z (axes depicted as above) – rotation along Y makes no difference!	Stretching vibrations along Y axis

Number of translational degrees of freedom = 3

Number of rotational degrees of freedom = 2

Total $n = 3N = 3 \times 2 = 6$

Therefore, number of vibrations = $6 - 3 + 2 = 1$ (which is bond stretching).

Degrees of Freedom of Triatomic Molecule

Let us first work out the number of translations, rotations and vibrations, and then visualize it:

Number of translational degrees of freedom = 3 (always, X, Y, Z)

Number of rotational degrees of freedom = 2 or 3 (if the 3 atoms were linear as in CO_2, there would be 2 rotational degrees of freedom for identical reasons as above; if the atoms are not linear as in H_2O, there would be unique rotation along Y axis as well)

Total $n = 3N = 3 \times 3 = 9$

Therefore, number of vibrations for linear triatomic molecule = $9 - 3 + 2 = 4$

And, number of vibrations for non-linear triatomic molecule = $9 - 3 + 3 = 3$

To avoid redundancy in explanations, let us consider only the non-linear triatomic molecule situation and put into words what was derived above:

1. It can move about freely along the 3 directions (X, Y and Z) as one unit
2. It can rotate along 3 axes
3. It can vibrate in 3 ways

Graphically this is represented as:

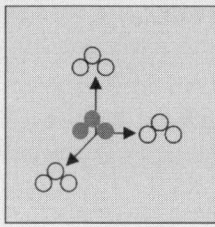 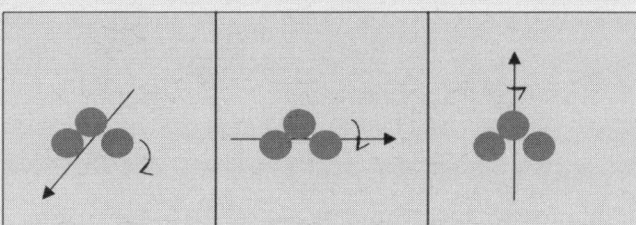

| Translation along X, Y, Z | Rotation along X, Y, Z (axes depicted as above) |

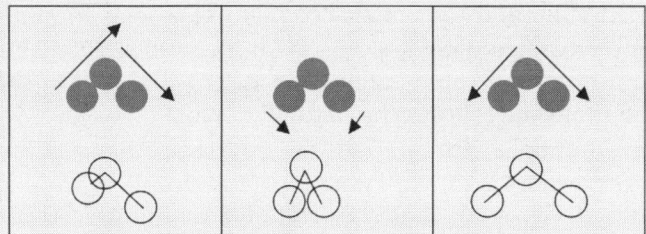

The 3 vibration modes for non-linear triatomic molecule

Degrees of freedom for a medicinal chemist:

1. The total n = not $3N$ but $3N–6$

Why should a medicinal chemist know about the degrees of freedom of a molecule? In mathematical terms, the degrees of freedom are the dimensions of a phase space. When only potential energy is considered in situations such as calculation of the progress of a reaction, calculation of enthalpies of bond formation and breaking, calculation of binding affinity, calculation of conformational strain, etc. one excludes rotational and translation motion. As supported in IR studies, bond formation and breaking primarily involves vibrations. Thus in this context the number of degrees of freedom is 3N–6 (or 3N – 5 for linear molecules) and not 3N as stated above.

2. The total n = dimensions of the PE surface

The potential energy surface of a non-linear molecule of N atoms has 3N–6 dimensions. Each dimension follows a certain degree of freedom of the molecule (each mode of vibration). The potential energy surface of H_2 has 3N–5 = 1 degree of freedom. Thus the PE surface of H_2 is only a 2D curve with inter-atomic distance being the only degree of freedom plotted (Vs energy which is the second dimension). For further details, *ref.* subsection 2.3.F analysis of reaction path.

Also, the calculation of the binding energy that is released when a ligand binds a protein also includes penalties for the reduction of the degrees of freedom of the ligand and of the protein after binding (*ref.* part III section 3.1.3, especially part A of the subsection).

3. Complexity of a problem increases with increase in *n*

The greater the number of atoms in the molecule, the greater the number of dimensions the potential energy function possesses and more investigations are needed along these various dimensions to arrive at the minimum energy structure. The human mind cannot perceive more than 3 dimensions in an image. A protein's PE surface has thousands of dimensions! As geometry optimization attempts to find all of the energetically preferred conformations of a molecule, there is a need for techniques to speed up the search process in this 1000-dimensional space (techniques such as those in Discussion 2.16 in this chapter).

Energy minimization proceeds in cartesian space–along the X, Y and Z coordinates. Each atom is shifted along the coordinates of this space so as to minimize the forces acting on it. So for a molecule with N atoms, each *i*th atom needs to be shuffled along X, Y and Z to minimize the forces acting on it. It follows that the optimization coordinates for the molecule follows the path N (x_i y_i z_i).

Energy minimization takes into account the degrees of freedom possessed by the molecules. From Discussion 2.15, we know that a molecule with N atoms has 3N–6 degrees of freedom. An N-atom molecule can also be minimized along its internal coordinates (rather than its Cartesian coordinates) by changing its dihedral angles (rather than its X–Y–Z coordinates).

*The X, Y, Z-coordinates of an atom *ref.* to the coordinates of the atom's centre

C2A *Conformational Search*

As discussed under C1. *Principle*, geometry optimization is the process of choosing the lowest energy conformer by performing several single point calculations on various structures taken from the conformational space of a molecule. This conformational searching is also a part of dynamics simulations discussed in chapter 1.3. There are two ways of sampling the conformational space. The methods used to generate these

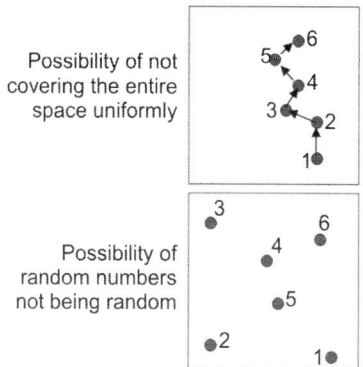

Possibility of not covering the entire space uniformly

Possibility of random numbers not being random

Any point in the conformational space (corresponding to a particular conformer of the molecule) can belong to the minimum

Fig. 2.8: Sampling of the conformational space using deterministic (top) and stochastic (bottom) methods. *See* Scheme 2.13

multiple starting geometries can be classified into deterministic and stochastic methods (Saunders, 1987); (Saunders, 1989); (Ferguson, et al. 1989); (Saunders, et al. 1990); (Lipton, et al. 1988).

Conformational search and step size: the Diatomic molecule—a model example
Optimization of the geometry of a diatomic is trivial. We know that a diatomic molecule has only 1 degree of freedom = the 'bond length'. For the current discussion, the potential energy function is modeled as a parabola (and not the more complex curve shapes of the morse potential, etc. as in Discussion 2.4). There is one lowest point and we wish to discover the geometry (here, bond length) pertaining to that point or at least a few points on either side of it as in Fig. 2.9A. A random structure starting anywhere else along this line can be "brought into" the trough, the area of interest, by generating several conformations with varying bond lengths, calculating the corresponding conformation (potential) energy using the expression $E = \frac{1}{2} kr^2$ (where r is bond length) and varying r. Thus, we map the downhill progress of the energy function until we have points on either side of the minimum. In this example, two bond lengths, one

Deterministic methods
- Systematic change in atom positions and exploration of conformational space
- Change in the atom positions in order to change conformations is brought about by varying the torsion angles of rotatable bonds systematically
- The new conformation is a variant of the orignal conformation

Stochastic methods
- Random conformations generated so that the entire conformation space is sampled
- Change in atom positions is induced by change in Cartesian coordinates or in torsion angles using random numbers
- New conformation is independent of the original one (there is no relation between any 2 conformations because random numbers decide the generated geometry)

Scheme 2.13: Conformational search methods

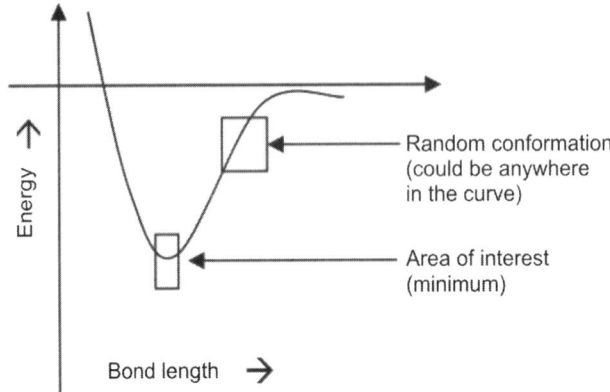

Fig. 2.9A: A conformation at a minimum is of chemical interest

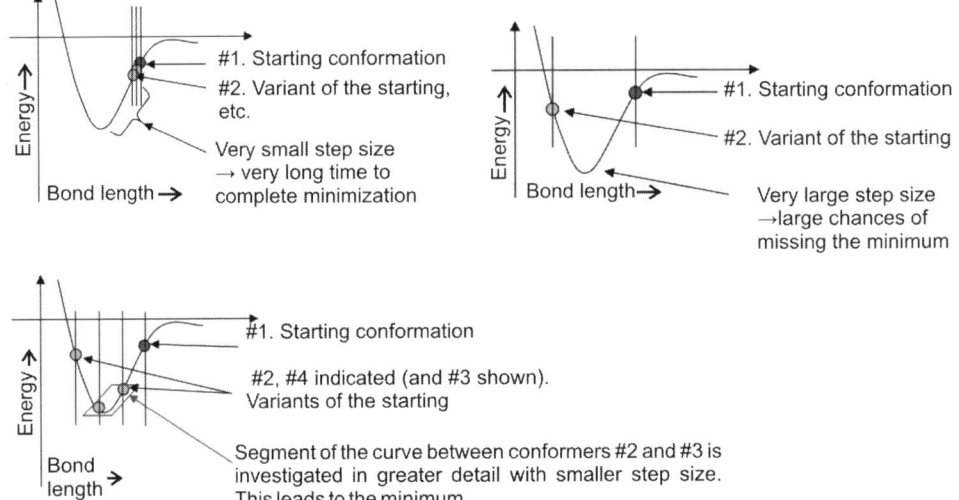

Fig. 2.9B: Small (top left), large (top right) and ideal (bottom) step size in generating conformations

much greater than the other, could correspond to similar energies (as shown in the Fig. 2.9B on the top right).

One thing which we cannot know is the "step size"–should the bond lengths be varied by 2 Å, 0.5 Å or 0.01 Å? Remember, we do not know how the curve (i.e. the function) will vary with respect to the changes made. We can only generate conformations and calculate energy. The technique in general is to start with step size that is not small or too large (Fig. 2.9B). In the former case, the calculation becomes too time consuming and in the latter case, one might miss the energy minimum. These are explained in the Fig. 2.9B. In the first case, the calculation would consume extensive time and resources for nothing and in the second case, the calculation would complete rapidly, less conformers would be generated (here, only 2) and one would assume that #2 is the energy minimum as #2 < #1 in energy!

The diatomic case is only a model case. With the points listed here in mind, a look at the strategies used in energy minimization in Discussion 2.16 will give us greater understanding.

C2B *The Algorithms*

> *"Begin at the beginning and go on till you come to the end: then stop."*
>
> *The King in "Through the Looking Glass", by Lewis Carroll*

Steps: Software that is performing a minimization task will change the conformation of the molecule by degrees to generate new meaningful structures. The energy of the newer conformation is calculated next. If the new energy is lower than that of the originally specified conformation, the induced change in geometry is retained. Otherwise a change is induced in a different way. In either case, fresh conformational change is introduced and the energy calculation repeated until a change in conformation does not produce any further lowering in energy.

Generating the conformations: There are several strategies used by software to couple inducing all possible yet chemically meaningful conformational changes with the tracking of the energy minimum (called conformational search) as outlined in Discussion 2.16.

How energy minimizing algorithms work: These detect the minimum closest to the starting structure, and cannot differentiate a local from a global minimum (*ref.* Discussion 2.16 for further clarification of this point and for the algorithms that are generally used). As mentioned earlier under principle, several conformers are generated and their energy calculated. This process is iterative until the potential energy is steadily "brought to a minimum" (figuratively speaking) as indicated by:

- The energy [given by E(R)] and structure (summed up by the vector R) remaining fairly constant from iteration to iteration.
- The first derivative matrix near zero [when a function–here, potential energy – displays a peak or a trough, the first derivative does not change much (~0)].

In order to ensure that the minimized structure is indeed located at a minimum, the second derivative matrix is calculated (this eliminates location of a maximum or a saddle point; *ref.* section 2.3.2.F reactions) and is further verified by the normal-mode vibrational *frequency calculations* (*ref.* section 2.3.2.E thermochemistry for frequency calculations and II.2.3.F reactions to understand what normal-mode analysis is and how this helps in identifying a minimum). Most molecular modeling software provide for the computation of vibrational spectra. This is summarized as a flowchart in Scheme 2.14.

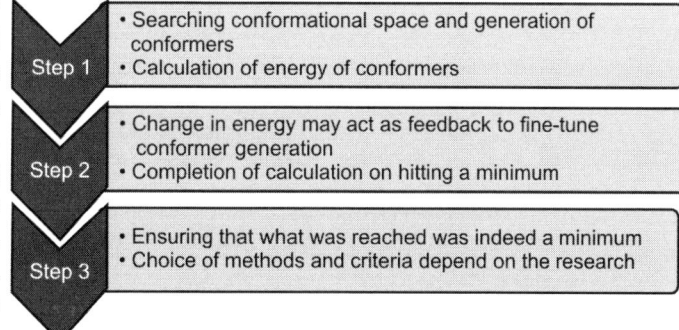

Scheme 2.14: Steps in geometry optimization process

Discussion 2.16: Algorithms for energy minimization

These can be classified as first derivative techniques (steepest descent method, conjugate-gradient method, etc.) and second derivative techniques (Newton-Raphson, etc.)

Steepest Descent Method

- In the potential energy profile of a molecule, chemically meaningful structures occur at the equilibrium geometry, i.e. the conformations, corresponding to the energy minimum. This means when starting with a random geometry and undertaking a systematic search to locate the equilibrium geometry, one is guided by the direction of change in energy as one always needs to search for a minimum
- The minimum is a point of maximum negative energy in the neighborhood of points along the line, i.e. a trough. It is characterized by the following features:
  - The rate of change of energy is 0 at the minimum;
  - And therefore, the first derivative with respect to potential is 0
- The steepest descent method calculates the first derivative of energy and looks for ~ 0 values.

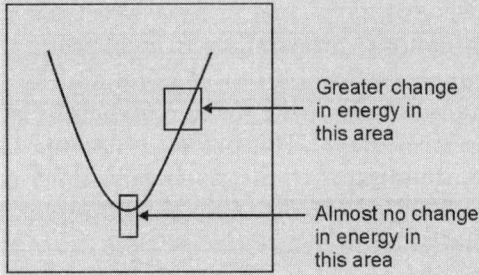

Fig.: The minimum has less change in a function than other areas

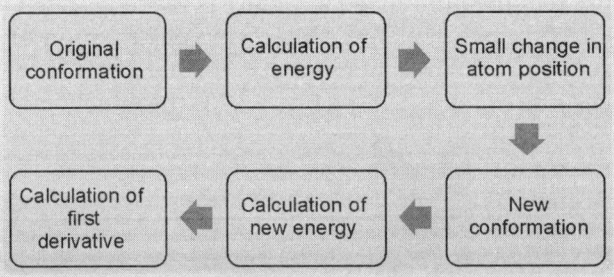

Scheme: Steepest descent energy minimization

- If the calculated first derivative is
  - ≠ 0, then the process of generating new conformations and calculation of first derivative will continue
  - ~ 0, and if the preset conditions for locating the minimum is fulfilled, the method stops.

This method is fast in going downhill but slows down close to the minima. Therefore it is used as an 'initial' search method to quickly arrive close to a minimum, and once there, is followed by other faster minimization methods.

Conjugate-gradient Method

- The method proceeds only in the direction of the minimum; any conformational change that is made in the molecule is made only in that direction

- For this, the method involves the accumulation of gradient data from the previous step. With each iteration, this accumulated data is used to guide the direction of progress.

- *Gradient optimization means:* Atoms are moved so as to reduce the net forces on them; the minimized structure has small forces on each atom.

- Conformational changes proceed steadily in the direction of the energy minimum. This is considered one of the best methods for large molecules; although memory requirements are greater, convergence of criteria (to indicate that the search is complete) occurs faster.

- The "path" taken to perform the minimization in the conformational space is not just a vector (as in the steepest descent method), but a combination of vectors called a *gradient*. The condition imposed on the path is that it must lead to a combination of vectors (gradient) having the least added up forces.

- The overall gradient (the "path" mentioned above) is obtained by adding up the contributions along X, Y and Z direction; the contribution along each of these 3 coordinates is called a *component*. Each cartesian component (whether along X, Y or Z) of the gradient of the molecule (with conformation vector R) is the first derivative of the potential energy E(R) with respect to that component (X, Y or Z). Gradient components along X, Y and Z combined give the overall gradient.

Newton-Raphson Method

- This is a second derivative method. It is very accurate but uses a lot of computational effort. It involves calculating the gradient as well as the curvature of the function and the root mean square gradients of the forces on the atoms (a force on the atom shifts the atom to a new position. New conformations are achieved in this way). The second derivative of the energy is calculated with respect to the coordinates of the atom, and this is known as the *Hessian*. It is this which guides optimization process.

- The first derivative of the potential energy function informs us of the rate of change of energy, but not of the direction in which the change proceeds. In other words, the first derivative is 0 both at a minimum and a maximum. However, the second derivative is positive when approaching a minimum and negative when approaching a maximum (*ref.* standard textbooks in calculus).

- The number of dimensions along which the first and second derivatives must be calculated increases when there are more atoms in the molecule. It is not suitable for large systems and maybe used when these have been pre-optimized using a more approximate method.

The *quasi-Newtonian methods* are used that approximate the matrix of derivatives taking several steps that are computationally less demanding. The *univariate search method* goes along one of the 2 axes only and is slow in searching for the minimum.

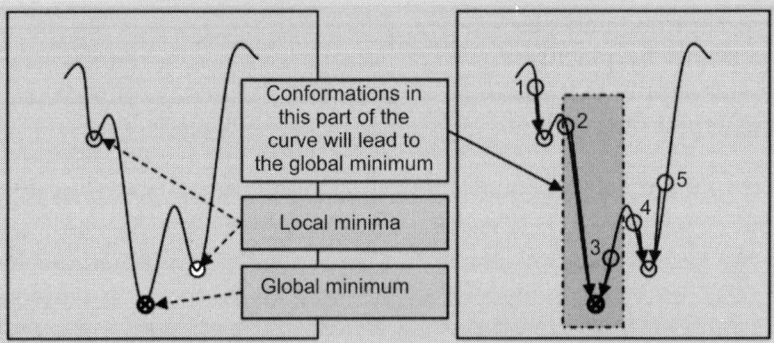

Fig.: The local minima and the global minimum

Consider the potential energy profile of a certain molecule–there are several local minima where the conformation of the molecule could have favorable interactions. However, this conformation is not the lowest energy conformation. The global minimum indicated (of which, generally, there can only be one) has the best arrangement of atoms in the molecule. Although a 'true' energy minimization procedure would imply that the global minimum of the compound is reached, the algorithms described in this discussion can only go DOWNHILL searching for the closest minimum. The empty circles labeled 1–5 indicate various starting geometries for the molecule. Note how the closest minimum is attained regardless of the direction (left-right) or the availability of greater minima (the methods are not even aware that there are other minima) as indicated by the arrows. This is because there is no way of going uphill in a systematic manner (i.e., no way to overcome an energy barrier or in other words, no way to systematically generate more strained conformations) so as to reach a maximum and then go downhill to the next minimum. Other techniques are used (*ref.* Simulated Annealing discussed next in section C2.c of this chapter) that can overcome energy barriers in order to sample the global minimum.

Note: The minimization can also be performed by optimizing the dihedral angle degrees of freedom, rather than the Cartesian coordinates.

C2C Non-derivative methods for Optimization— Genetic Algorithm and Simulated Annealing

Section contributed by Janarthanan Krishnamoorthy

In usual context 'optimization' refers to finding the solution for a function containing a set of parameters, by performing minimization of the difference between the ideal solution (calculated value) and the observed solution (experimental value). Many of the physical problems can be formulated in mathematical terms with unknown but determinable parameters. For example, if the growth of a plant with respect to its environment has to be studied, then we can list all the factors related to growth such as sunlight, water, minerals, air (oxygen and carbon dioxide) and systematically fix all factors except one and observe the growth pattern. As an example, we can start with seven plants by placing them in a well lit, spacious environment, but varying only the water supply that each plant receives. After 10 days of experimentation, we tabulate the height of the plant as a measure of its growth.

Table 2.8: The growth measured at the end of 10 days seen varying with quantity of water

Label	Water (mL/day)	Growth (cm)
1	0	0
2	3	10
3	5	12.5
4	10	15.38
5	15	16.67
6	30	18.18
7	70	19.18

We see that the quantitative relationship between growth and water is not linear but the curve reaches saturation by the 30th ml. The mathematical form for this non-linear curve can be obtained through detailed modeling; instead we can also write its equation from the shape of the curve, here we identify it to Michaelis-Menten model.

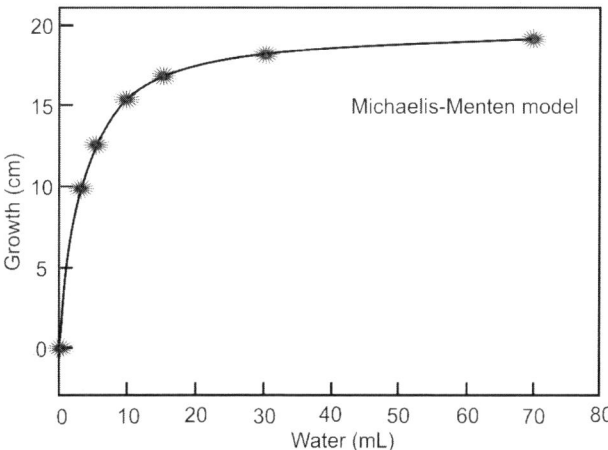

Fig. 2.10: The growth of plant fitted with Michaelis-Menten model using a and b as 20 and 3 respectively

$$\text{Growth} = \frac{a \times \text{water (ml)}}{b + \text{water (ml)}}$$

Equation: Michaelis-Menten model: Growth is the dependent variable and water is the independent variable, the parameters 'a' and 'b' are the constants.

As the variable 'growth' (y) is dependent on the variable 'quantity of water' (x), the former and the latter are called as dependent and independent variable respectively. The terms 'a' and 'b' in the above model are called as the constants or parameters. In fact, these constants represent a quantitative measure for the combination of other growth influencing factors i.e, sunlight, minerals, air. If we want to find the values for 'a' and 'b' from the given experimental data, we reformulate the problem as an optimization one and use 'Genetic algorithm' (GA) or 'Simulated annealing' (SA) to find the solution. Finding parameters is a simple case, much complex problems like finding the suitable growth condition for a bacterial fermentation culture to maximize yield involves optimization of multiple factors (carbon, nitrogen source, oxygen, temperature, pH etc.), and are routinely solved by optimization techniques. In the following discussions, we use the above example to understand the principles of GA and SA algorithms.

Genetic Algorithm (GA)

As the name suggests, the algorithm works analogously to how the microscopic organisms adapt/evolve with respect to its environment. If a colony of bacteria is grown in a small scale (50 mL) in the presence of Ampicillin, only few will develop the ability to degrade the antibiotic by synthesizing the enzyme 'Penicillinase'. This enzymatic resistance is attributed to its genotypic ability to mutate, cross over and reproduce successfully for several generations. The same principle is adopted in Genetic algorithm based simulations. For above case, we are interested in finding optimum values for 'a' and 'b' that represent the data better. So we define 'a' and 'b' as two genes and its combination/concatenation as 'chromosome' or potential solution to

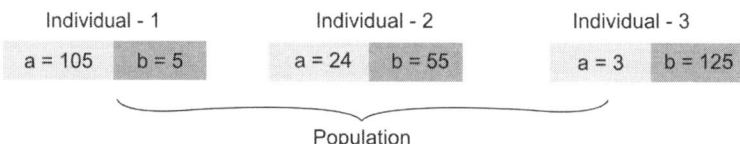

Scheme 2.15A: Three individuals with random values for 'a' and 'b'. Many such individuals constitute the population

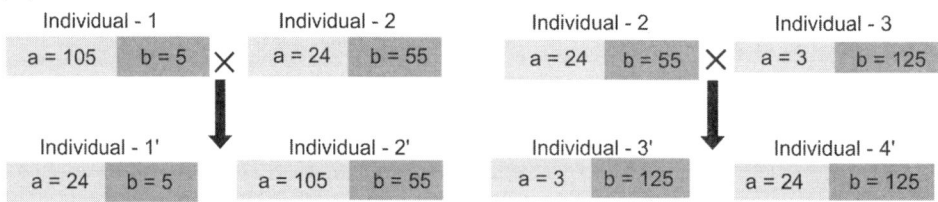

Scheme 2.15B: Individuals are crossed over among themselves, resulting in translocation of genes from one chromosome to another

Individual - 1"		Individual - 2"		Individual - 2"		Individual - 3"	
a = 23	b = 4.5	a = 115	b = 50	a = 1.2	b = 59	a = 21	b = 130

Scheme 2.15C: Mutation of gene values for the above crossed over individuals

the problem. At the outset, we generate a 'population' or pool (say 500) of such chromosomes with random values for 'a' and 'b'.

Subsequently, we allow crossing over of each chromosomes or individuals in the population by use of a random operator/function.

Following this, the existing gene values are mutated by another random operator/function.

A model function is used to evaluate the fitness of each chromosome i.e., how good this individual is in representing the correct solution. So we use Michaelis-Menten model, values of a, b for each individual and evaluate the 'y' value to tabulate the results below:

Table 2.9

x	$Y_{1"}$ a=23 b = 4.5	$Y_{2"}$ a = 115 b = 50	$Y_{3"}$ a = 1.2 b = 59	$Y_{4"}$ a = 21 b = 130	Y_{expt}
0	0.00	0.00	0.00	0.00	0.00
3	9.20	6.51	0.06	0.47	10.00
5	12.11	10.45	0.09	0.78	12.50
10	15.86	19.17	0.17	1.50	15.38
15	17.69	26.54	0.24	2.17	16.67
30	20.00	43.13	0.40	3.94	18.18
70	21.61	67.08	0.65	7.35	19.18

We see that individual '1' has 'Y(calc)' closer to 'Y(expt)' values. In the following step, we define 'objective function' as the sum of the square of difference between 'Y(calc)' and 'Y(expt)' for each 'x' value; this value is also called as 'chi square' or 'sum of squared residuals'. The lesser the value for objective function, the better that individual is; such individuals are allowed to proceed to the next generation. Based on the fitness value (i.e objective function value), each individual is allowed to reproduce. More offsprings are generated for the chromosome with better fitness value. The offsprings mentioned here are the chromosomes that are exact replica of the parent chromosomes.

$$\text{Objective function} = (1 - \frac{Y\text{calc}}{Y\text{expt}})^2$$

Equation: Objective function: The Y(calc) is calculated using Michaelis – Menten model; the Y(expt) is the observed experimental value.

This marks one generation; several such generations need to pass till a converged global minimum value is achieved for the objective function. The following table explains how the objective function and parameters converges with progression in optimization.

Simulated Annealing (SA)

SA is similar to GA, borrowing its principle from naturally occurring event called 'Annealing' seen in metallurgy. When the metals are heated to high temperature and cooled slowly, well ordered crystals without 'defect' would form, while rapid cooling, would result in defective and disordered amorphous form. This suggests, to achieve global minimum in the overall energy of a system, smaller continuous steps rather than large discrete steps are required for transitions. Similar approach is adapted in simulated annealing to achieve globally minimum solutions for a given problem. Most of the gradient based optimization techniques have a serious problem in common, that is, if the problem is not well designed and starting values for the arbitrary parameters far away from the actual solution, they are prone to get stuck with locally minimum solutions rather than reaching the globally minimum solutions.

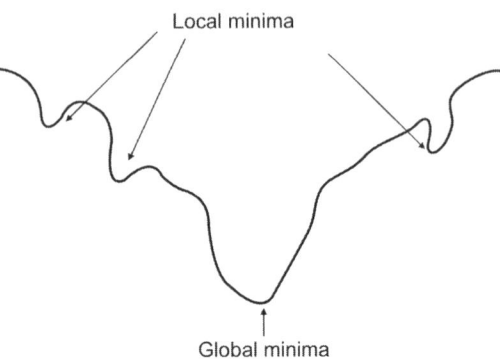

Fig. 2.11: A continuous function with many local minima and one global minimum

SA overcomes this problem, by using random operators, similar to the mutation and cross-over operators used in GA. These operators are temperature-dependent and enables the optimization to jump over the 'local minima' to reach the 'global minimum'.

Using the same example used for GA, we will see the working mechanism of SA. In SA, we consider a and b as entities which define the overall 'state' of the system. If a and b minimize the energy or the 'objective function' of the system, then it is bound to get to 'crystalline' state, else the undesired amorphous state with increased energy would result.

Table 2.10: The tabulated value corresponds to a single randomly picked individual among a population over different generations. As the number of generations increase, we see that the fitness value decreases and convergence to a global minimum value is achieved. The 'a' and 'b' value obtained in the last generation, compares well with the model fitted values 20, 3 obtained through another method (Levenberg-Marquadt algorithm).

Generation	a	b	Fitness value
1	347	145	30.2887
10	546	0	8486.9824
20	1	332	5.9590
100	75	10	16.7397
200	35	5.7	1.4660
450	19	2.98	0.0141
475	19.8	3.05	0.0012
500	19.9	3.01	0.0002

- The algorithm starts with an initial higher temperature (~3000K) for a randomly generated state. The random values of a and b define the state of the system at that temperature. The fitness or the objective function will be evaluated at this temperature for this state. Following this, a random operator will vary the values of both a and b to generate a new state; the degree of variation is again dependent on current temperature. The energy of this new state is evaluated, if its energy is lesser than the previous or 'old' state, the new state will be accepted. On the other hand, if the energy is higher, the new state may or may not be accepted based on the probability evaluated at this temperature.

$$\text{Pr obability} = e^{-\frac{(E_{i+1}-E_i)}{kT}}$$

Above Equation: Probability based on previous (*i*) and current (*i+1*) state at a given temperature. 'k' is the Boltzman constant.

- This unique feature in SA, where higher energy states are accepted under certain probability, allows the states to escape from getting trapped in local wells. The probability depends on the temperature of the state; at higher temperature, the higher energy states are accepted equally well as lower energy states, but as the temperature decreases, the acceptance probability of such states also decreases.

- On acceptance of new state, the algorithm proceeds with the subsequent lower temperature. The complete process starting from fitness evaluation, generation of new state, fitness evaluation is repeated again for this new temperature. After several iterations, when the temperature reaches user defined minimum, the algorithm terminates.

On the other hand, if the new state is rejected based on the calculated probability, then new randomization is performed at the same temperature, this step will go on for several times till a new state meeting the acceptance criteria is found.

The gradual decrease in temperature may be carried out in a (1) linear or (2) exponential manner. For both the schemes, user has to define the initial (T_{max}) and final temperature (T_{min}), along with the number of step ($Cycle_{max}$) required to make this transition.

$$T_{next} = T_{current}/\mu$$

Equation: The linear and the exponential scaling schemes for decreasing the temperature; here μ is a constant with value >1

$$T_{next} = T_{current} + \frac{\ln\left(\frac{T_{max}}{T_{min}}\right)}{e^{(cycles_{max}-cycle_{current})}}$$

References for Section 2.3.2.C2C

1. Genetic algorithm, http://www.iitk.ac.in/kangal/resources.shtml
2. Simulated annealing, http://www.gnu.org/software/gsl/manual/html_node/
3. Simulated annealing, http://www.gromacs.org/Documentation/
Materials and references: (Höltje, et al. 2008; Foye, et al. 2008; Leach, 1997)

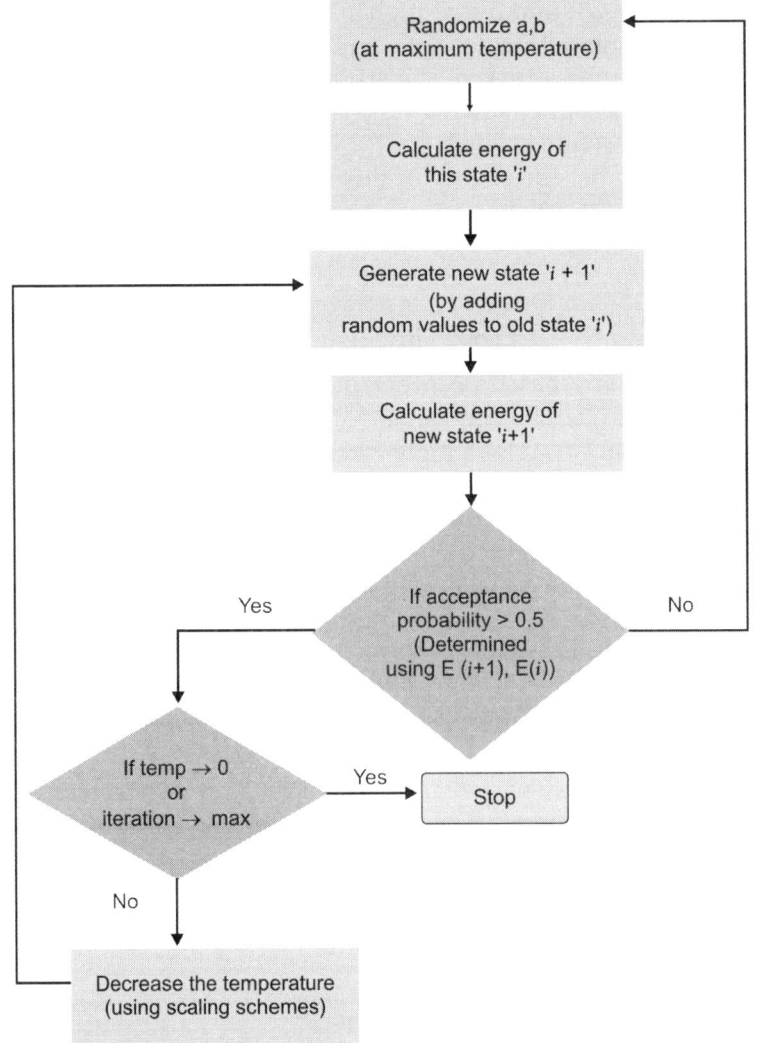

Scheme 2.16: Flow chart showing a simple algorithm for simulated annealing

Beginners can look up http://chemistry.umeche.maine.edu/Modeling/mmminim.html and http://www.wag.caltech.edu/publications/theses/alan/subsection1_4_0_2_2.html to obtain good introduction to the topic.

C3 *The Types*

Energy minimization and energy calculation can be performed with varying levels of detail or accuracy (Hirst, 1990). The choice of the method will be based on:

1. The accuracy of results
2. The size of the system (the number of atoms)
3. The type of interactions/effects that need to be accounted for

For an example of the comparison between C–C bond lengths in ethane, ethylene and acetylene as calculated by methods with varying levels of accuracy, *ref.* Table 2.11. In all, the methods available to calculate the energy of molecules can be broadly classified as in the following paragraphs (also *ref.* Scheme 2.17).

Ab-initio methods: These are methods that calculate energy by accounting for

Molecule	Steric MM	PM3	Ab-Initio	Experimental
Table 2.11: Comparing experimental and calculated C–C bond lengths				
ethane	1.540	1.509	1.541	1.531
ethene	1.540	1.322	1.318	1.339
ethyne	1.540	1.190	1.183	1.203

electronic effects and plunge deep into solving the associated complex integrals. They calculate every quantity from first principles (hence the name). Even if they include approximations for the Schrödinger equation, they yield accurate results (*ref.* Table 2.11). However, they are extremely time-consuming. A single point calculation on a small peptide might take 30 years of computing time! Therefore, these methods are restricted to the calculation of small- to average-sized ligands for which they provide the best energy estimate. A very popular *Ab initio* method is Hartree–Fock (HF) (Leach, 1997). There are several variants to HF method such as the RHF (Restricted Hartree-Fock for closed shell molecules), UHF (Unrestricted Hartree-Fock for open shell molecules of ions and free radicals), etc.

Semi-empirical methods: Calculating orbitals and energy using *Ab initio* integrals leads to identifying, accurately, the conformation corresponding to the energy minimum. However these methods take up a lot of time and consume a large amount of resources. The semi-empirical method does not calculate every quantity from first principles. Instead, certain values are "imported" from experiments and other calculations. This process of substituting values instead of calculating them is referred to as being

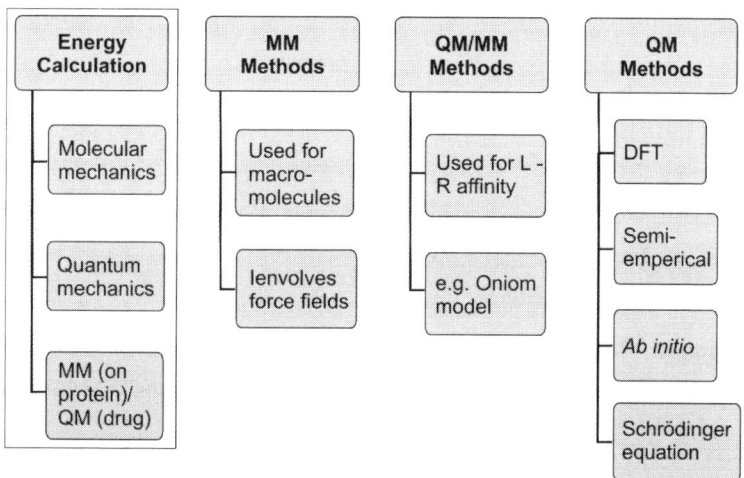

Scheme 2.17: Various methods of calculating energy of molecules

"empirical". The values imported are used for further calculations–and therefore the name semi-empirical calculations. For example, vibrational frequencies of well studied molecules can be imported from IR spectra instead of calculating the frequency of vibrations from quantum effects. Some examples of methods under this category are INDO, MNDO, AM1, PM3, etc. These methods therefore yield moderately accurate results [in Table 2.11, the PM3 (Burkert, et al. 1982) method is known to be perfected to handle organic molecules, hence the accuracy].

DFT methods: The density functional theory is a technique that calculates molecular energies by introducing electron correlation. The calculation is faster, the energy is less accurate, and the frequencies more accurate than *Ab-initio* methods. The method cannot be used for all chemical species. Example: LDA, GGA. Some methods combine DFT and HF in order to gain the advantages of both methods. These are called Hybrids, such as B3LYP, B2PLYP, etc.

Molecular mechanics methods: Molecular mechanics, as discussed, is the only method that can be exploited for calculating the energy of huge macromolecules such as proteins, DNA, RNA, etc. The gain of speed is achieved by ignoring electrons. The Table 2.11 shows the results of a MM calculating with only steric filtering in its force field. Usually force fields include potential energy terms for a large number of molecular parameters (*ref.* section 2.2.10). Examples: Tripos, CHARMM, AMBER, UFF, etc.

QM/MM methods: These use MM on the protein and QM on the ligand. The problem generally arises in defining a boundary between the two. One cannot simply cut through a bond and define half a bond by one method and the other half by the other! So instead, as done in the ONIOM model (Svensson, et al. 1996), there is a region of overlap beyond the ligand atoms that is described by both methods. This technique is being increasingly used to describe protein binding to ligands.

Theoretical calculations on a drug: Several theoretical calculations have been performed on drug molecules to understand their behavior. For example, pindolol, a β-blocker, was analyzed using the HF, DFT and MP2 methods in detail (Nunes, et al.). It was concluded that intramolecular H-bonds were crucial for stabilization of structure (which might have implications in bioavailability as discussed under permeation in section 2.3.2.A1). It must be mentioned that the most significant conformer of pindolol was concluded after analyzing the results of all 3 methods, which is generally the way drug design conclusions are drawn. The examples mentioned under each type of calculation above are not software but methods. An example of software that can handle several of these methods is Gaussian.

Did You Know? 19
About the Gaussian program

*The program **Gaussian** (from Gaussian, inc.) was originally released in 1970 by John Pople. It calculates parameters using all of the above mentioned methods. John Pople shared the Nobel Prize in Chemistry 1998 ("for his development of computational methods in quantum chemistry") with Walter Kohn ("for his development of the density-functional theory")*

C4 *The Structure-Energy Balance*

- *Why we need:* The energy of the specified conformation of the molecule can be calculated, but one does not know how strained this geometry is compared to other possible conformations of the same molecule.

- *Why energy minimization:* So what if the right choice of method is not made from those mentioned under section C3 above? Consider the 3 conformations of hydrogen peroxide (H_2O_2) in Fig. 2.12, labeled cis, trans and gauche. The H_2O_2 molecule is selected here for simplicity. In order to obtain the optimized geometry of this molecule, an energy minimization is carried out on the starting geometry. Say, the cis conformer is inputted into a program such as Gaussian (Gaussian, inc.) by specifying its internal coordinates (*ref.* Discussion 1.6, chapter 2.2). The following comparison will explain the difference between various methods mentioned in this section:

Molecular mechanics minimization: Using a force field with the following expression $V_{tot} = V_{str} + V_{bend} + V_{tors}$, the minimization yields the 'trans' form with H–O–O–H dihedral angle = 180° as the most preferred conformer.

Quantum mechanics minimization: Perhaps a casual reader of this example might also agree with the above result that the transform would have the least conformational strain. However, high level of theoretical calculations using the quantum mechanics approximations-based minimization at B3LYP/6-311++G(d,p) level of theory (mentioned for reference; explanations omitted for clarity) gives the gauche form as the most preferred conformer (actually H_2O_2 has two gauche forms that lie in energy minima having H–O–O–H dihedral angle = 111.5° and 248.5° (Wiberg, et al., 2001)) and places the cis (29.4 kJ/mol) and the trans (4.6 kJ/mol) forms at maxima.

Why the above difference between MM and QM? The MM force field that we have used contains the energy–dihedral angle relationship in its potential energy

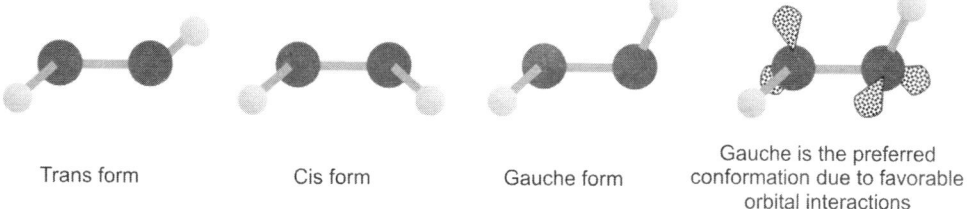

| Trans form | Cis form | Gauche form | Gauche is the preferred conformation due to favorable orbital interactions |

Fig. 2.12: H_2O_2 conformations–will energy minimization arrive at the preferred conformation?

expression and therefore that conformer with maximum H–O–O–H dihedral angle has resulted with least strain. *Ab-initio* (QM) methods on the other hand take no such short-cuts. They derive molecular properties from the behavior of electrons in orbitals and therefore identify the possibility of interaction between $n \rightarrow \sigma^*$ orbitals oxygen lone pairs and empty C–O* orbitals (Coleman, 2008), (Weinhold, et al. 2003).

When such knowledge is available, one can improve molecular mechanics by including a "short-cut expression" in the dihedral angle – energy relationship such that the force field will scan for the presence of H–O–O–H connectivity and reduce the dihedral to 111.5° or 248.5°.

Alternatively, if a more detailed force field is used, such as $V_{tot} = V_{str} + V_{bend} + V_{tors} + V_{h-bo} + V_{e-stat}$, then the hydrogen bonding or electrostatic terms might identify such unique intra-molecular hydrogen bonding relationships (this might not yield the exact angles, but in the least, detailed MM methods might indicate the presence of a favorable gauche of some angle). This is a very simple and well-known example. If a calculation were to miss such important interactions when optimizing the geometry of the ligand, the receptor, or the complex, it is like that

* E_{min} of the ligand is identified erroneously
*   Binding energy is underestimated (erroneous) and the molecule is rejected
*   The wrong ligand-receptor geometry is obtained for lead identification and optimization
*   Entropy penalty of the ligand when bound with the receptor is underestimated and the molecule is erroneously considered a good lead (*ref.* part III, section 3.1.3 for explanations of the components of binding energy).

We know that quantum chemistry based calculations take time even for 15-carbon-alkanes (*ref.* Did You Know? 16 in section 2.2). So it might not be feasible to perform an *Ab-initio* energy minimization (which, as mentioned earlier, includes alternating single point calculations at high detail of theory and conformational change) even on an average-sized ligand molecule (leave alone a protein). So, one has to use molecular mechanics. The least one can do is to select a good force field such as Tripos (Tripos, inc.), CHARMM (Brooks, et al. 2009), AMBER (Cornell, et al. 1995), etc. depending upon the molecules involved.

Just as enantiomerism is one of the life-line principles for designing drugs, so is symmetry, for calculation of molecular properties. The properties of molecules are in a way "constructed" from combinations of points, planes and axes of rotation, reflection, inversion, and other elements of symmetry present in the molecule via orbitals. We know that symmetry is an "all-or-none" parameter. For example, a molecule can either have a plane of symmetry or it cannot. Even if an atom in the molecule is 0.01 Å out of place, the plane of symmetry is abolished (i.e., in other words, atoms in the molecule occur with infinite precision). In this respect, energy minimization plays an important role. When a molecule is built from fragments using molecular modeling software or when its coordinates are obtained from experimental sources, there is very great chance that it is not in its native structure. Calculating orbitals and deriving macroscopic properties from an erroneous conformation can only result in erroneous values (or can end up crashing the program). However, if it has been energy minimized the resulting geometry is more reliable (how much depends on the accuracy of the optimization techniques).

C5 *The Real-life Parallel to the Energy-Minimized State*

The different states in which molecules may occur: We cannot expect that the energy minimized conformation in crystal, in gas-phase, or in solution will coincide with the bioactive conformation in vivo. This is because we cannot expect the energy profile of a molecule to be the same in these different physical states. At this point, we wish to further expand on what was mentioned under approximation #9 (under section 2.2.9)– the medium in which molecules are when their energies are computed and geometry is optimized matters. Consider the following 4 environments in which biomolecules can be found:

  i. Cellular,
 ii. Crystal (solid),
iii. Solution (aqueous),
 iv. Gas-phase

For the sake of simplicity, we do not consider the 'liquid' state and only consider an 'aqueous solution' instead. These 4 states can be characterized as in Table 2.12. From the comparison, one concept is evident–one cannot expect $E_{min(gaseous)}$ to be equal to $E_{min(aq)}$ or $E_{min(cell)}$. If calculations of binding energy, energy minimum, etc. are carried out without including solvent effects, one performs the calculation in gas phase and therefore one cannot compare this result with that obtained from experiments (resulting from aqueous or cellular environments). It cannot be taken for granted that a molecule has identical energy profiles when placed in different environments. Similarly, the resulting geometries are also unique. A conformation optimized in the gas phase must be recalculated in the presence of water molecules in order to obtain the geometry preferred in the aqueous phase. A ligand bound to a protein with an active site not exposed to the surrounding may not vary too much (in conformation or energy) when calculated in the gas phase or in the aqueous phase *(can you tell why?)*. Whereas, if the binding site is situated such that it is accessible to water molecules, then using gas phase values might not be reliable. In this situation, one might have to include solvation *(ref.* chapter 1.3 for this; also *ref.* solvent accessible surface under section 2.3.2E molecular visualization and graphics).

Pros and cons: Some precautions to be followed when obtaining results of an energy minimization process are similar to the precaution needed when using force fields:

• The speed and accuracy of the process depends on the algorithm used and the size of the molecule

• The calculation is performed in the gas phase if solvent effects are not included (as under section 2.2.9)

• The minimum energy conformation, whether it be a protein or ligand, need not be the physiologically/biologically relevant structure

• The accuracy of the result depends on the force field parameters and basis set molecules

Table 2.12: Influence of the environment in energy minimization

	Cellular	Crystalline	Aqueous	Gaseous
Other molecules (of same compound)	+	++	+	-nil-
Environment	+++	++	+ (water)	-nil-
Properties	Dynamic (with constant change due to interaction)	Can be classified as superficial and within the lattice	With dielectric constant	As calculated
Geometry optimization	In balance with water, ions, membrane, 2° messengers, signals, neighboring proteins, substrates, drugs, receptors, chaperones, etc.	In balance with other neighboring molecules packed together into the lattice and their atoms placed close-by	In balance with water as calculated in a solvent box (involving H-bonding, charge, solvation)	Energy minimum arrived at is not influenced by environment and the molecule is isolated
Preferred conformation with respect to energy	Conformations of high energy in the gas phase may be preferred due to drug- receptor interactions, solvation, etc.	That conformation favorably interacting with neighboring molecules in the lattice and accommodating space constraint is preferred.	Conformations that are of higher energy in the gas-phase may be preferred if favorably solvated with water molecules	The global minimum is preferred and conformations of higher energy are not counter-balanced by the environment
The energy profiles are not necessarily equal				
The optimized geometries are not necessarily the same	1) **Silanes:** cyclic in crystal, flexible in gas, open-chain in solution (Hagemann, et al.) 2) **Vitamin B12 – insulin conjugate:** crystal packing can even deform the covalent framework of a molecule (Petrus, et al.) 3) **Ph₃S₈(CH₂)₈S₈Ph₃:** Curved conformation preferred in crystal state; extended, preferred in gas phase (Bettens, et al., 2009)			

- The selection of force field is crucial and is not only dependent on the class of molecules being investigated, but also on the purpose of the research.

C6 *Applications in Research*

So, what role does energy minimization play and where is it used in drug design?

- Energy minimization is used to help to solve experimental structures in NMR and X-ray crystallography techniques (*ref.* part I/ section 1.1.2A and B)
- Energy minimization allows us to directly compare different conformations
  - *Note:* This is mostly the case–energy minimization allows us to compare conformations of the same molecule only and not different configurations or different molecules, even if these latter structures differ only slightly, unless special effects are incorporated in the calculations as mentioned under section 2.2.4 "cautions"
  - Standard algorithms must be used for conformational search: If the conformational space of the molecule is not sampled uniformly, it is likely that a reliable result will not be obtained.

- To build/recognize pharmacophores among molecules in a database, the search needs to be carried out not just on one conformation (that is present in the 3D database) but on several (that need to be generated from that one conformer)
  - This process is extremely time-consuming because of the sheer numbers involved. Spending just 10 CPU seconds to generate conformations for every molecule, a modest database of 250,000 compounds would take 29 days of CPU time to complete conformer generation (Kubinyi, 1995) (CPU time is always either equal to or shorter than clock-time).
- Homology modeling may generate a protein structure that may have steric clashes that need to be eliminated which can be done in the energy minimization step
- When the ligand molecule is built from fragments present in the software, the final molecule needs to be minimized before further processing
- Determining the lowest energy conformation of a molecule, and to compare the preferred conformations of a molecule in a particular environment, e.g. to compare structure in crystal, aqueous phase, gaseous phase, receptor active-site, etc.
- Minimization is performed when calculating the energetics of a reaction. In a sense, the docking of ligands into macromolecules is considered to be a "reaction".

Some examples of force fields, their expressions, relevance and application have been presented in Section 2.2.4. The result always needs to be scrutinized by us:

- Is the structure reasonable? Is the geometry chemically allowed?
- Is there any cause for large strain (large groups very close in space; like charges together, etc.).

Materials:

For basic understanding, look up http://www.shodor.org/chemviz/optimization/teachers/background.html, http://chemistry.umeche.maine.edu/Modeling/mmminim.html.

D. Molecular Visualization and Graphics

The early development of molecular modeling was mainly to visualize molecular structures. Today, however, the term molecular modeling encompasses organizing compounds and their information into databases, simulating the behavior of molecules and their interactions, calculating molecular properties, estimating energies for various interactions, such that visualizing structure in 2D and 3D has become only a small part of the term. As early as the 1970s, visualizing compounds, even if in black and white, was a powerful tool to understand geometry and conformation of a molecule. There was a time when real time rotation (that is, an object rotating with the dragging of a mouse) was not possible and one would have to rotate the molecule by a certain degree using text input, generate a picture, print it out and if not appropriate, change the degree of rotation via the text input. Imagine this process being done to capture the best angle for the docking of a ligand into a protein's binding pocket! For an idea on how a computer deals with visual graphics, *ref.* [(Foye, et al. 2008), (Keil, et al. 2009), (Bohne, et al. 2000)]. Interaction with the computer in real time has increased tremendously since that scenario. It is not uncommon to virtually move a ligand about in the proximity of a protein binding pocket and get a display of the interacting forces simultaneously even in a PC. Effect of depth and three-dimensional shape is called *stereoscopic effect*; this 3D effect, though, is brought out on a 2D screen of a computer's monitor. The appearance is both informative and appealing.

D1 *Visualization in General*

A variety of biological molecules are targeted structures to model. Proteins, nucleotides, ligands, lipids are often modeled for their structure and interaction to get ideas of chemical and physical processes. In protein modeling (or in the modeling of any of the other molecules, for that matter) color is a dimension and not just some decoration. A range of values of a property can be indicated using a smooth gradation of shades from one color to another, where the extremes of colors would correspond to the extremes of values in the range. For example,

- Most electronegative regions of a structure, such as carbonyl oxygen atoms, would be indicated with bright shades of red and most electropositive regions (which would be most electrophilic, such as a quaternized nitrogen), with deep shades of blue.
- Similarly, hydrogens that can be donated for the formation of a hydrogen bond would be colored in blue and the hydrogen acceptor atoms in red. Regions where hydrogen cannot be involved in such bonding interactions (for instance, benzene's hydrogens) would then be colored gray.
- A range of lipophilicity, electron density, charged density, volume indices, conformations (residues with helical/beta-strand/turn conformations),etc can also be indicated using color gradients much like a map of the geography of an area that indicates mountains, valleys, etc.
- Non-physical properties are also mapped. Some examples are regions of the protein that are highly conserved among species, segments of loops that have been subjected to mutations, insertions or deletions, etc.

Instead of coloring the atoms (which are nothing but discrete points in space) and not knowing what color to give the bonds that lie in-between (which are simply lines connecting these atoms), it is easy to imagine mapping a surface around the various atoms of a molecule and coloring the surface with gradients. One cannot just randomly draw a surface: it must be chemically constructed and meaningful. There are a number of rules to construct surfaces that lead to there being surfaces of different types meant to be used for different purposes such as the van der Waal surface, the Lee Richard surface, solvent accessible surface, contour maps, electron density surface, etc as explained in later in this section.

Modeling is carried out to investigate two aspects of biology: The form and the function. It is clear that one is not independent of the other. Arrangement of atoms leads to the formation of a particular structure that can be analyzed in terms of the physicochemical properties as well as the stability of the arrangement. It is the dynamic interrelation between these aspects that results in biological interaction–and hence function. The position of an atom is modeled as a point in space marking the position of its nucleus. However, this is not literally correct because in addition to the presence of protons and neutrons in the nucleus, there is also a cloud of electrons around it. Therefore, atoms are represented as spheres whose radius is the scaled-up value that makes them visible in a simulation and depends on the type of atom. Depending on the study and the presentation, one can chose to represent the atom by its van der Waals radius, atomic radius or a certain percentage of it (say, as a sphere of radius 60% of the atomic radius). A computer shows a "bond" to be a "line" connecting two atoms. It is nothing but a representation of a certain interatomic distance. The more the atomic radius approaches the van der Waals radius, the shorter the "line" connecting the atomic spheres. In the true situation, of course, there is no "line"; there is only overlap between the electron clouds of the two atoms. The distribution of electrons around the nucleus in an atom and in a molecule can be theoretically calculated. Standard software also utilizes this information to generate electron density maps and distribution graphs. Such information helps us to plot and visualize the shape and symmetry of atomic and molecular orbitals that result from advanced theoretical calculations. Similarly vibrations of bonded atoms can be visualized as a "movie" from the calculated frequencies of atoms in a molecule. Some terminology often appears in display software. Some of these are defined in Table 2.13.

Table 2.13: Some terminology in molecular graphics

Term	Definition	Usage - Some Do's & Don'ts
Depth cueing	Changing the hue and colour of an object to reflect its depth in a 3D scene	This is included - atoms look like spheres rather than flat circles
Orthographic view	3D effect without stereoscopic effect	Gives a "real" sense of tilting
Stereoscopic view	The 3D sense of depth obtained when seeing an object with 2 eyes (than with just 1 eye)	Used to highlight protein binding pockets; some images may appear out of scale—this is not preferred when showing small molecule conformation
Contrast	Increases difference between dark and light colors	Useful when colored regions need differentiation from white areas
Brightness	Color appears as if lit-up	Used when colors are dark and become indistinguishable in print

Some types of calculation are performed to trace an entire reaction path (*ref.* section 2.3.2F). Visualizing such calculations can provide us with an excellent means to learn reaction mechanism from the geometries of reactants, the changes that reactants undergo, the geometry of the transition states, any intermediate that is formed, and the details of the final product. All through, information about the vibration modes, shape and orientation of orbitals, changes in electron distribution, shape and volume of the molecules, etc. are very clear when visualized and serve as a means to aid understanding of mechanism of electron transfer and atomic rearrangement in organic chemistry. Molecular visualization also gives us an opportunity to superimpose molecules on top of each other facilitating comparison of shape and properties. This becomes evident from part 1 where structure, chemical functional groups and biological function of proteins were strongly interrelated and used to explain gene composition and functioning. Using visualization software, complicated biomacromolecules can be simplified so that their global shape and structure become evident.

D2 *Visualizing Proteins*

For proteins, there are several representations–ribbons, surfaces, traces, stereo diagrams, ball-and-stick representations, etc. as shown in Fig. 2.13.

D3 *Surfaces*

Construct a ball and stick bench-top model of benzene. Observe that this contains some "free space" in the middle of the ring. Now, using the same kit, construct benzene

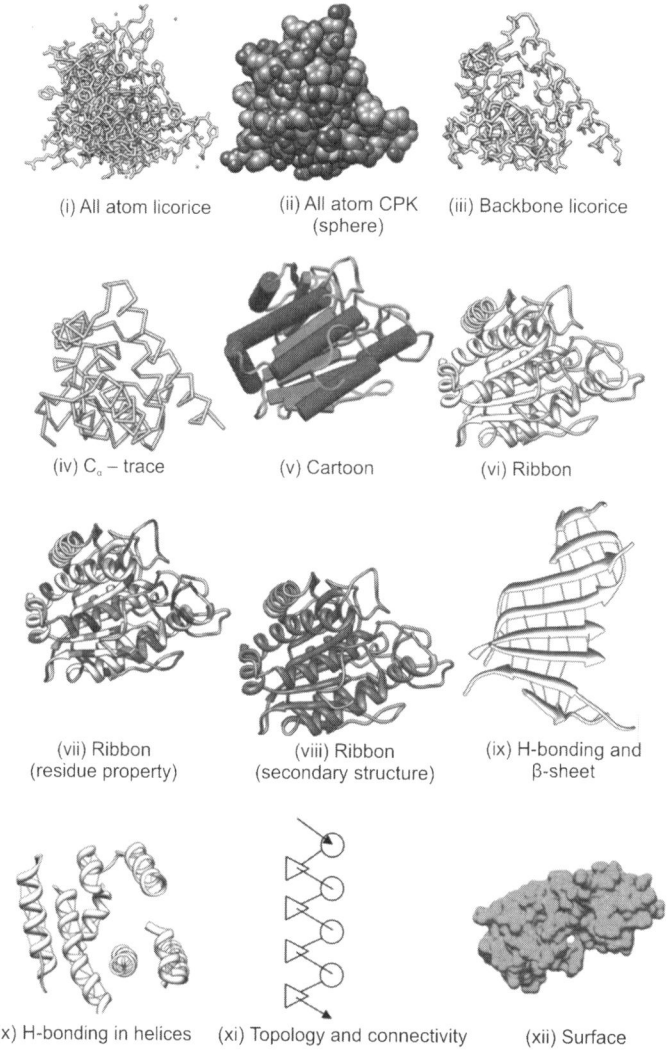

(i) All atom licorice	(ii) All atom CPK (sphere)	(iii) Backbone licorice
(iv) C$_\alpha$ – trace	(v) Cartoon	(vi) Ribbon
(vii) Ribbon (residue property)	(viii) Ribbon (secondary structure)	(ix) H-bonding and β-sheet
(x) H-bonding in helices	(xi) Topology and connectivity	(xii) Surface

Fig. 2.13: Representations of proteins (for color version *see* Plate 3)

using the "space-filling atoms". The free space in the middle of the ring no longer exists. We understand now that the ball and stick model is only a scaled-down version of space-filling model and is used only to increase clarity of the model constructed. The space filling representation (also called the Corey-Pauling-Koltun or the CPK model) indicates the regions in and around a molecule that are accessible (or inaccessible) to other molecules. In case of benzene, the CPK model shows beyond doubt that not even a tiny particle can pass through the benzene ring. Such accessibility and channels are accurately understood by computing surfaces using a computer. This process serves the following purposes:

1. To calculate the volume of drug molecule/protein cavity in order to ascertain drug–receptor steric fit.
2. To exclude, from computations, those atoms of the drug and protein that are not mutually accessible or to the solvent in order to save computer time and resources.
3. Map properties such as charge distribution, electrostatics, lipophilicity, solvent exposure, etc. on the surface of the drug or protein to visualize the respective properties perceived by other molecules (such as solvent or the binding partner) in a semi-quantitative way.

Discussion 2.17: Construction of some basic surfaces

There are 3 fundamental (among several others) surfaces:
- Van der Waal's surface
- Molecular Surface or Solvent Excluded Surface (SES) or Connolly Surface = contact surface + reentrant surface
- Solvent Accessible Surface (SAS) = Lee Richards surface

And several other specialized surfaces:
- Channel surface (that looks for the presence of channels in proteins)
- Separating surface (that constructs ligand-protein (or any intermolecular) interface
- Electron density surface (that contains superficial electron density distributions calculated using the quantum mechanical equations for small molecules and using short cuts for large ones)

Furnished, here, is a description of what is considered as the fundamental surfaces that medicinal chemists must be able to construct and interpret using software.

van der Waals Surface (CPK model)

1. If one fuses the atoms of a molecule as specified with their van der Waals radius, the van der Waals surface is obtained (*ref.* following figure)
2. Calculation of the enclosed volume yields the absolute molecular volume
3. This surface results in very narrow bays (or channels or clefts) that cannot be accessed by even hydrogen molecules. This limits biochemical applicability of this surface

4. *Note:* The van der Waals volume of a molecule is always smaller than the sum of the van der Waals volumes of the constituent atoms: the atoms can be said to "overlap" when they form chemical bonds.

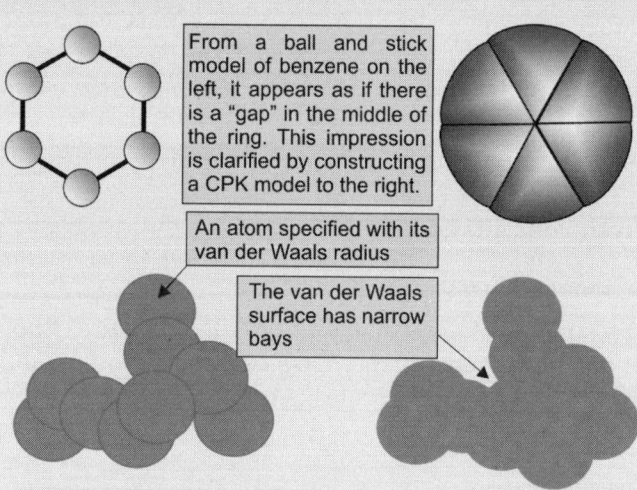

From a ball and stick model of benzene on the left, it appears as if there is a "gap" in the middle of the ring. This impression is clarified by constructing a CPK model to the right.

An atom specified with its van der Waals radius

The van der Waals surface has narrow bays

Fig.: van der Waals surface

Molecular surface or Solvent excluded surface (SES) or Connolly surface

1. The solvent excluded surface is so called because it occupies the defined space by keeping away or excluding water molecules from that area (*ref.* following figure)
   a. Molecular or Solvent Excluded surface is constructed using a spherical probe
   b. The atoms of the molecule are specified by their van der Waals radius
   c. The probe rolls on the molecule–the surface of the molecule is constructed by merging the paths drawn by the surface of the probe as it comes in contact with the atoms of the molecule (*ref.* following figure).
2. After the construction of SES, it is useful to compare this with the van der Waal's surface
   a. There are region on the van der Waals surface that are already well exposed to the surroundings. These remain unchanged in the SES. This surface is common between the van der Waals and the molecular surface and is called contact surface (*ref.* Fig. A1 and A2)
   b. As the probe rolls, it smoothens out the deep clefts of the van der Waals surface that occur when 2 adjacent van der Waals radii (of 2 atoms that occur close by) touch. The newly created surface is the re-entrant surface (Fig. A2, Fig. D).
3. The molecular surface is the most commonly constructed surface for display purposes–when indicating the distribution of properties. More specifically, it is

used to show interaction of hydrophobic ligands with its respective protein as in Fig. C of retinol in the binding pocket of Retinol Binding Protein (PDB ID 1KT6).

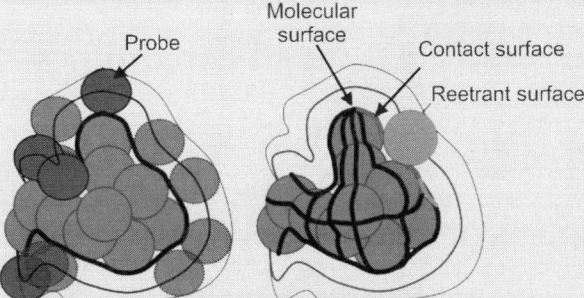

Fig. A1 and A2: (elevation) The rolling ball algorithm to construct solvent excluded surface

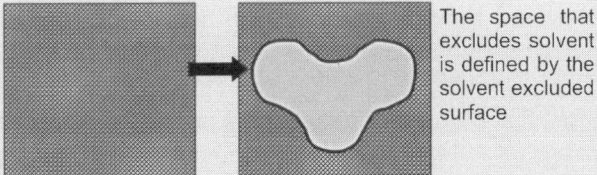

Fig. B: Cross section of an SES in the solvent bulk

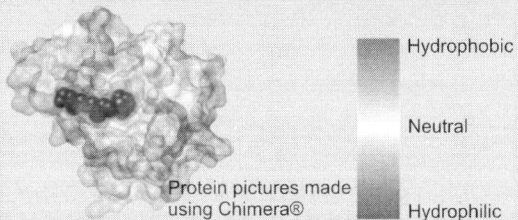

Fig. C: Hydrophobic retinol in the hydrophobic pocket of retinol binding protein is visualized by constructing an SES (for color version *see* Plate 4)

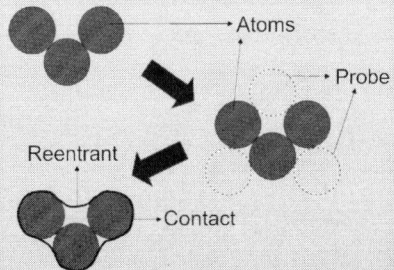

Fig. D: Cross-section of molecule to show solvent excluded surface construction

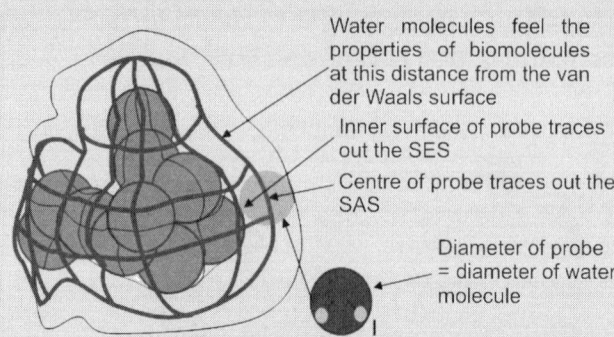

Water molecules feel the properties of biomolecules at this distance from the van der Waals surface

Inner surface of probe traces out the SES

Centre of probe traces out the SAS

Diameter of probe = diameter of water molecule

Fig. E: Solvent accessible surface

Solvent Accessible Surface

1. The SES is created by the circumferance of a probe rolling on the molecule, whereas the SAS is created by the centre. A probe of radius 1.4–1.7 Å is selected (Lee, et al. 1971) (*ref.* Figure).

2. This distance from the van der Waals surface signifies the minimum distance at which long range interactions are initiated. The resulting surface is smooth and indicates only those areas of the molecule that interact with the solvent. The active site of proteins that are usually identified by applying this surface are lined with water molecules.

3. To obtain a more realistic picture, the properties mapped on a solvent accessible surface are incorporated with the influence of the solvent. For example, electrostatic potential is calculated including the effect of dielectric constant of water.

4. Lee-Richard surface is generally considered the Solvent Accessible Surface, but Connolly describes the Solvent-Excluded Surface to contain the contact and re-entrant surfaces traced by the inward facing surface of the probe (Connolly, 1985).

Did You Know? 21
About the Lee-Richard surface

Lee and Richards described the solvent accessible surface in 1971 (Lee, et al. 1971) and the rolling ball algorithm for calculating this surface was developed later (Shrake, et al. 1973).

D4 *Properties on Surfaces*

It has been mentioned that a surface serves as more than just a definition if the outline of a molecule and a shape descriptor–it is used to map molecular properties for semi-quantitative estimate.

1. Calculation of these properties at the van der Waals surface is of chemical relevance. This is because non-bonding interactions are maximal when the van der Waals radii of the non-bonded atoms touch.

2. Calculation of properties on the SAS is of biological importance. This is because
   a. It indicates the level of interaction that the binding site has with surrounding water molecules before the arrival of the ligand
   b. It also shows the approachability of a ligand to the active site, and,
   c. The level of steric hindrance which the ligand faces when binding with the protein (by measuring the volume and describing the shape of the active site)

Some properties generally mapped onto surfaces are:
- Distribution of charges/charged species (Fig. 2.14A)
- Electrostatic potential (Fig. 2.14)
- Lipophilicity/hydrophilicity potential
- Hydrogen donor/acceptor atom distribution (Fig. 2.14B)
- Aromatic/aliphatic groups distribution (Fig. 2.14C)
- Amino acid distribution (Fig. 2.13 (vii) above)
- Secondary structure distribution, etc. (Fig. 2.13 (viii) above)

Advantages of mapping properties on surfaces:
1. Helps graphically view the distribution of values on the molecule grouped into ranges rather than obtain a list of numbers and position
2. Indicates that many properties have a gradient. Consider a point charge; the potential energy obtained when another charge is brought close to it depends on distance. If it is brought really close, the PE increases (whether in the positive or negative direction depends on the nature of the charges). If it is taken farther away, PE drops gradually. So, there is a diffusion of charge (or any other property) in space, the value being maximal on the surface of the atom (at the centre of this is the point charge) and gradually reducing as one moves away from it.

Discussion 2.18: Mapping electrostatics and lipophilicity on surfaces

Mapping electrostatics: $F = q_i q_j / r_{ij}^2$ and potential energy $E = q_i q_j / r_{ij}$ because Energy = Force × Distance. The electrostatic potential EP is slightly different from potential energy PE:
1. For a particular arrangement of atoms, EP is measured at a particular point in space, say, at (x_n, y_n, z_n)

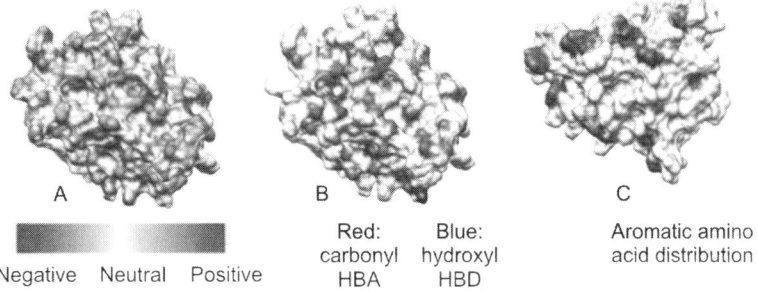

A   B   C

Negative Neutral Positive

Red: Blue:
carbonyl hydroxyl
HBA   HBD

Aromatic amino
acid distribution

Fig. 2.14: Mapping properties on a surface (for color version *see* Plate 4)

2. EP is measured by an ion of charge +1. In other words, it is the change in potential energy that occurs when a probe of +1 charge is introduced
3. The probe (the previous statement) is placed at the point where the electrostatic potential needs to be obtained, i.e., at (x_n, y_n, z_n) (mentioned in point 1 of this bullet list)
4. The, EP at the point (x_n, y_n, z_n) depends on the presence and placement of charged atoms near that point.

Thus, the molecular electrostatic potential (MEP) is a calculation of the electrostatic potential of the atoms of the molecule. This property is mapped on the surface by projecting atomic charges onto it. The surface is first constructed with several points or dots. Each point on the surface is considered i and each atom on the molecule is considered j in the above expression. The EP is mapped by calculating the EP at each ith point on the surface (V_i).

The EP at each ith point is calculated using:

$$V_i = \sum_{j=1}^{N} Q_j / r_{ji}$$

where V_i = projected value on the ith surface dot; Q_j = partial charge of the j atom and r_{ij} = distance between the point i and atom j.

The following inferences are evident from the above relation:

1. The potential Vi at i is inversely proportional to the distance between i and the atom j (as in the above equation)
2. Charges q1 and q2 in the earlier expression is replaced by partial charge Qj of atom j
3. The Vi at i is the sum of the influence of the EP of all atoms (Vi = sum over the Q/r values of $j = 1, j = 2, \ldots j = N$).

Mapping lipophilicity:

Solvent affinity of ligands and macromolecules can be represented by local semi-empirical potentials called the Molecular Lipophilicity Potential (MLP) visualized on molecular surfaces. Similar to the mapping of EP of all j atoms on every ith point on the molecular surface, lipophilicity atomic constants are projected onto the i points. Often, the Broto-Moreau atomic constants are used (Gaillard, et al. 1994). MLP is different from Log P. The latter values are 1D and describe the entire molecule as a single unit. MLPs on the other hand are three-dimensional and 'divide' the molecule into regions of high or low lipophilicity. Therefore, these are used to study ligands, proteins and their interaction. They also aid in topological and stereochemical investigations performed in 3D-QSAR (*ref.* 2.4.2) analyses. The average MLP is used to estimate the Log $P_{[octanol/water]}$. In physical terms, the MLP can be considered to be the attractive or repulsive force exerted by a molecule M (ligand or macromolecule) on surrounding (imaginary) non-polar organic solvent molecules O. If M has lipophilic groups in it, the forces between that fragment and solvent O are attractive (f_i >0 in the expression below); if it contains hydrophilic groups, the respective forces are repulsive (f_i <0). The f_i values are the Recker fragment lipophilicity values (as discussed under 2.4.1) or can be computed by the software itself by considering the atom type, interactions between hydrophilic groups and inter-halogen interactions.

Calculation of Molecular Lipophilic Potential:

$$MLP_M = Ó f_i . g(d_i)$$

where f_i = lipophilicity contribution of the atom i; d_i = distance between the point M and the atom i; $g(d_i) = 1/1+d_i$

MLPs take Log P calculations to the next level. Not only is a 3-dimensional calculation available, but also one is able to calculate Log P changes for various conformers of the molecule. This dynamic aspect is applied to estimate strain energy and binding energy in docking studies (*ref.* part III).

Another technique used to calculate and map lipophilicity is the global hydropathy index (ILM). This property distributes hydrophilic solvent (water) molecules according to the properties of the atoms or groups in the concerned molecule (ligand or macromolecule). The equilibrium distribution of solvent is mimicked and so, more water molecules are placed in the environment of hydrophilic groups and vice versa. The ILM can be mapped on the molecular surface, giving rise to a very detailed local hydropathicity mapping. The solvation is done using a water cluster (see solvation under section 1.3). Molecular dynamics simulation is carried out to calculate ILM (Pedretti, et al. 2000).

Materials:
- Cambridge crystallographic data centre: http://www.ccdc.cam.ac.uk/
- General organic chemistry tutorial http://academic.reed.edu/chemistry/roco/index.html.
- SURFACE: Surface residues and functions annotated, compared and evaluated at http://cbm.bio.uniroma2.it/surface/
- http://www.netsci.org/Science/Compchem/feature14b.html

E. Calculation of thermochemical parameters and relevance

"As far as the laws of mathematics ref. to reality, they are not certain;
as far as they are certain, they do not ref. to reality."

Albert Einstein

Energy is the connection between structure and function. The use of an energetic description of an interacting system has several advantages:
- Connection with experimental work is possible. That is, the methods and formulae may be derived from experimental results; results obtained from theory and

experiment can be compared; and, theoretical calculation can be used to perform experiments. From this, one can predict outcomes of reactions.

• The level of detail of calculating energy may be increased systematically to improve accuracy or may be approximated to shorten calculation time depending on the demands of the research work under focus.

• Established theories and principals that govern interaction of molecules such as reaction rates theory and statistical mechanics can be tested while modeling and perfecting virtual molecular interactions. Thus a thorough verification of our understanding of molecular level interactions that give rise to macroscopic effects is possible. It other words, one tries to imitate laboratory conditions.

Computational tools have theoretical and practical limits. The Heisenberg uncertainty principle (under chapter 2.2) places a theoretical limit on our knowledge of the initial position and momentum of all particles. The various other approximations add to error generated during calculations. Even though it is possible to compute many properties and the many changes in a system from its free energy and its initial conditions, such calculations can be performed only amidst numerous uncertainties. These errors add up, and only with careful planning, their collective effects maybe minimized and made comparable to experimentally derived data. We know that *internal energy* of a molecule is the sum of its vibrational, rotational and translational energy. It results from the atoms in the molecule, i.e. their nuclei and electrons. The energy of molecules that are obtained experimentally includes several types such as those arising from the effects of temperature, solvent, constituting atoms, etc. Invariably, the energy that is determined experimentally is a relative one. In any standard textbook of chemistry, one comes across the expression "enthalpy of formation" and how it is obtained relative to elements in their native form (for example, the enthalpy of hydrogen in the gaseous state, carbon occurring as graphite, etc. are arbitrarily assigned

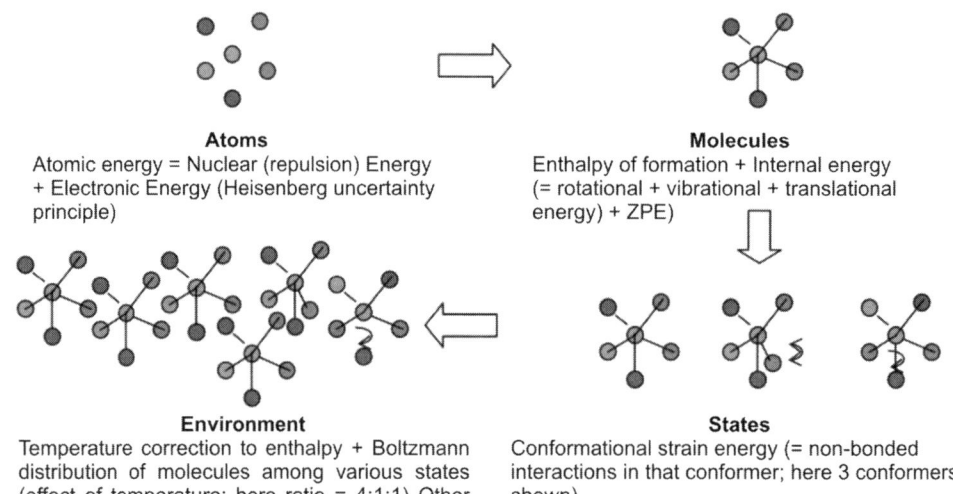

Atoms
Atomic energy = Nuclear (repulsion) Energy + Electronic Energy (Heisenberg uncertainty principle)

Molecules
Enthalpy of formation + Internal energy (= rotational + vibrational + translational energy) + ZPE)

Environment
Temperature correction to enthalpy + Boltzmann distribution of molecules among various states (effect of temperature; here ratio = 4:1:1) Other effects such as solvent can also be included.

States
Conformational strain energy (= non-bonded interactions in that conformer; here 3 conformers shown)

Scheme 2.18: A pictorial representation of some energy terms of molecules

"zero" value. Then, one experimentally measures the difference between the enthalpy of the molecule as a whole and the sum of the individual enthalpies of the constituting elements. This measured quantity is called the *heat of formation* and is calculated in relation to elements that are already formed and existing in nature. It is an enthalpy, and hence is influenced by pressure and temperature).

It is not possible to measure each component of internal energy experimentally (such as rotational energy, translational energy, etc). However, theoretically, internal energy of a molecule can be calculated component-wise and added up. One calculates the *nuclear energy* as the repulsion between nuclei of various atoms in the molecule and *electronic energy* using quantum mechanical methods (orbitals and the Schrödinger's equation). One can also calculate the *zero point energy* (the energy of a molecule at 0 K) and add to it the corrections resulting from exposure to temperatures greater than zero Kelvin. The temperature correction term includes *translational* and *rotational corrections* ($3\frac{1}{2}$ RT each) and the *vibrational correction* ($\Delta E_{vib}{}^T$) at temperature T (*Ref.* Think Box 4).

All these quantities–the electronic energy, ZPE and temperature corrections–are summed up to give the energy E^T of the molecule at the specified temperature. Enthalpy H^T is this energy (E^T) plus RT ($H^T = E^T + RT$). The enthalpy expresses the energy costs necessary to bring atoms together into a particular arrangement (of atoms in the molecule). The *Gibbs* free energy is the difference between the enthalpy HT and TS ($G = H^T - TS$), where S is the entropy. We know that for the same connectivity, several arrangements of atoms are possible (i.e. several conformations). Thus, *entropy* measures the amount of disorder in a system; the idea of entropy is to place individual conformers into the perspective of all possible conformers. It accounts for how many conformers are possible totally and what are their individual energies. Free energy is a thermodynamic quantity. It is a means to quantitatively compare the different possible configurations of a system. Experimentally, one can measure changes that enthalpy or Gibbs free energy undergoes (ΔH^T or ΔG^T, respectively) when one molecule reacts or transforms. Thus, theoretical chemistry deals with calculating all values from first principles – i.e. almost equivalent to assembling the entire molecule electron-by-electron, atom-by-atom, and at every step calculate the energy changes that results from each addition and its effects on the formation of the molecule as a whole including conformations that compete to be formed.

Think Box 4: Energy in chemistry is a relative quantity

Let's say our aim is to "synthesize" the TS complex A–B. The obvious way is to start with A and B. If one tries to put into a box all the atoms of the A–B complex, say 15 carbon atoms, 30 hydrogen atoms, two oxygen atoms, etc. and supplies heat, will the A–B complex form? No. Again, is it possible to isolate a carbon or oxygen atom, store it and put it onto a box for the reaction to take place the way we store colored balls in a molecular model kit? No. We have access to carbon atoms only in the form of chemically combined molecules. It takes some energy to break this combined form of carbon, say CO_2, and recombine into the way we want it... ultimately to achieve the A–B complex. So, one is able to arrive at the A–B complex only through an indirect route. Similarly, it would make perfect sense to calculate relative energies only, rather than the absolute energy of the A–B complex (one can synthesize one compound only from another), yielding an estimate for the investments (in the form of activation energy-reaction enthalpy) and payoffs (the free energy gain). Theoretical methods are approximated to yield this estimate as accurately as possible.

As introduced earlier, molecular mechanics does not consider a molecule to contain electrons and therefore does not calculate the electronic energy. Therefore one starts empirically from the heats of formation and atomization enthalpy of molecules arriving at bond energies. This bond energy is simply averaged over the various conformations and configurations that are encountered among molecules of the basis set and incorporated as a universal term (after statistical treatment) into force fields. Some of the fundamental points that students should understand and remember are enlisted as follows with the help of Fig. 2.15.

Molecules want to have the lowest possible energy. The thermodynamically most stable state that it can possess. This is the driving force for bond breaking and formation: the rearrangement of atoms and electrons.

Molecules are always moving about and therefore possess some kinetic energy. They also possess potential energy–the internal energy–as a sum of their atomic vibrations, rotations and translations. (Remember that even at 0 K wherein one could arrest rotations and translations of atoms, the vibration still exists. The potential energy is due to the electrons and nuclei that are in constant interaction, as worked out at the start of chapter 2.2). This is the *enthalpy factor*.

By the law of conservation of energy, one form of energy can be converted to another. One could imagine things this way:

- The moving about of molecules (kinetic energy) increases the probability of molecules to interact with each other.
- If two types of molecules that we call the reactants of a reaction are mixed together and if we heat up the system (which increases the probability of the molecules "finding each other" to overcome activation barrier), the reaction occurs. One moving molecule of the reactant A has greater chances of approaching another molecule of reactant B.
- Due to various electron and nuclear interactions, A and B feel the presence of each other and form a van der Waals complex. With the formation of A–B complex, the freedom of movement of A and B molecules is substantially reduced. The "freedom" of molecules is calculated in terms of what's called the "degree of freedom". *Ref.* Discussion 2.15 for the famous '3N-6 degrees

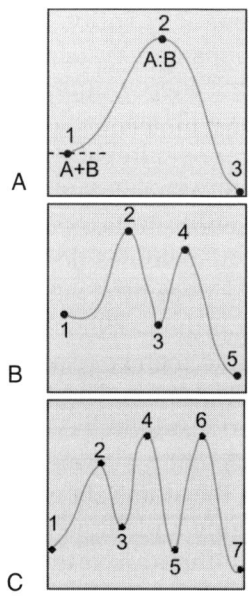

Fig. 2.15: Some reaction curves

of freedom' expression. This "arrest" signifies substantial reduction of kinetic energy of both A and B. This is then converted to potential energy of the complex.

Imagine how high the potential energy of the A–B complex should be (because the kinetic energy has been invested in the formation of weak bonding) and how much stability the system can gain by rearranging into products at point 3 in Fig. 2.15 (say, C and D) that have much lower energy? So the van der Waals complex rearranges, becomes the products and comes rapidly rolling downhill along the slope from transition state (complex) to products. A detailed study of all probabilities of reactions and their corresponding enthalpies for the combination of A and B (and how geometry is affected as a result) is undertaken in a reaction path analysis outlined in Section 2.3.2F.

One important consideration to have in mind in chemistry is that one does not bother with absolute energies. Starting from the calculations of enthalpies of reactions in the early pages of our organic chemistry textbook (you see that one cannot afford to forget the fundamentals) wherein calculations use the heats of formation enthalpies of the constituting elements in their native state (carbon as graphite, etc), and even the definition for atomic mass unit was a relative quantity (the mass of 1 hydrogen atom) and chemistry has always been simplified by making comparisons. In the same spirit, one determines the activation energy alone (difference between energy at points 1 and 2) and not the absolute energy of point 2 as one would have to start with A and B to get to the TS. *Ref.* Think Box 4.

With the breaking up of the A–B complex into products, say C and D, the enormously high potential energy built up in one molecule (the complex) has been expelled. With the restoration of freedom of movement to C and D with respect to the complexed "arrested" state, similar to how A and B were before complex formation, the potential energy is converted to kinetic energy and the products move away.

It must be noted that enthalpy is the cost of bringing molecules together into a particular configuration when many are possible. It is a snapshot of the energy that is present in a system. It is therefore the sum of the kinetic, potential energies of participating molecules and the work done to the system. This however does not completely define enthalpy. To do so, answer the questions: Is enthalpy a constant? What factors influence enthalpy? The high and low energies in Figs 2.15A and B indicate our interest only in the potential energy component of enthalpy as that directly relates to geometry of molecules. At any time during the entire process, enthalpy freely partitions between the kinetic and potential forms as the situation demands.

So what if the reaction's potential energy diagram is as in Fig. 2.15B? Products at point 3 would then be relatively higher in energy content (and of lower stability) than products at point 5. The rule that all systems aim to reach equilibrium having the lowest energy still holds. The energy minimum at point 3 is termed a local minimum and that at point 5 is termed the global minimum. For a system as large as a protein, if one moves the atoms about and calculates energy for each arrangement of atoms, one could imagine a plethora of local minima at various energies. But there will be only one global minimum corresponding to that arrangement of all atoms that yields lowest energy. The search for the global minimum is detailed with methodologies used under section 2.3.2C with applications.

Discussion 2.19: A molecule's states

What we have been discussing about so far is what happens when A and B combine to give C and D. There are, however, many states that each of the product molecules being formed can occupy. Every point along the potential curve in Figs 2.15A to C represents a particular arrangement of atoms of A and B with respect to some parameter, such as the distance between a reacting atom or group on A and its counterpart atom or group on B. For example, the distance between the attacking group and the control atom in an SN2 (nucleophilic substitution) reaction can be varied, and the corresponding changes in energy, studied. Constructing and analyzing such PE curves (2D) and surfaces (3D) by following parameters that changes during the reaction is called reaction path analysis (*ref.* 2.3.2 F for an overview). The parameter is called *reaction coordinate*. At every point along the curve, the arrangement of the atoms of A and those of B are slightly different and indicate the progress of the reaction when read from left to right. States are certain locally stable arrangements such as those occurring on the minima or significant points in the reaction such as the transition state (TS). In the Fig. 2.15,

- When modeling the entire reaction, the energies of both reactants A and B are added up and indicated by one single 'line'. Similarly, the energies of C and D are added up and represented as "products". However, in reality, one must realize that molecules are not ball-and-stick, hard, rigid structures that we make out of molecular model kits.

- The reactant A itself for example can have infinite conformations (depending on its flexibility). If we assume A to be ethane, we know that rotating about the C–C single bond will produce infinite conformations. Some of these conformations are more 'popular' among ethane molecules. For a mono-substituted ethane, if one exaggerates the situation, the perfectly staggered or the anti form would be most populated, and the perfectly eclipsed, least populated. For a di-substituted ethane, the statement would not be an exaggeration.

- At any instant of time and under fixed conditions, referring to 'A' means one refers to the whole bunch of conformations its molecules populate. For example "ethane" is an umbrella term including the eclipsed, staggered and all in-between conformations. 'A' is however generally denoted by its most populated conformer as an effort to save time and space. Each such conformation is referred to as a state. A species of molecules can assume several conformers.

- All the conformers that it can assume, collectively called an *ensemble,* are populated to various extents. Some conformers have very low energy and others have relatively higher energies. The low energy conformers are preferred, but not the only ones present. The probability that an individual state will be adopted is thus related to the energy of the state (Foye, et al. 2008). The Boltzmann expression relates these terms. *Ref.* standard textbooks suggested at the end of this chapter for an understanding.

- It is important to note the wordings in the above statement and its significance. Even though the probability that an individual state will be occupied is proportional to its energy, one must realize that this is only a generalization. Just as many weak interactions can become stronger in terms of total energy than one covalent bond, the presence of many low energy states (local minima) close to the lowest (global minimum) in energy will reduce the preference of molecules for the global minimum, i.e. all the molecules present in the numerous local minima might even outnumber all those in the global minimum. It thus becomes clear that for determining the true probability, one must estimate the probabilities in all the accessible states combined. This is called normalization of the proportionality equation. Thus, the expression is:

$$P(X) \, \alpha \, e^{\frac{\Delta E}{kT}}$$

given that $P(X)$ is the probability of a specific state, ΔE is the difference in energy of that state from the reference, k is the Boltzmann constant and T is the temperature. The probability for a particular state expressed out of the probabilities of all other accessible states becomes the exact probability $P(x)$:

$$P(x) \alpha \frac{e^{-\frac{\Delta E}{kT}}}{\int e^{-\frac{\Delta E}{kT}.dx}}$$

wherein the denominator, the integral over the probability of all other states, is called the partition function.

From the relations in Discussion 2.19, the following inferences must be summarized about the probability function:

- Even if there is only one global minimum for a system, not all molecules would occupy it–there is always a distribution of molecules over other states as well.
- Small increases in energy (relative to kT) dramatically reduce the probability of a state, i.e. the more low energy states there are, the larger the partition function.
- Calculating the probability of a state must include the effects of all possible states.
- Entropy (denoted S) is the property of a system that quantifies its tendency to occupy all possible states. It is well known that as temperature increases, the probability that any one state is preferred decreases due to the increase in disorder and rapid interchanging of the states occupied by molecules. But even when E is low, if there are more local minima, the entropy in the system is high because the global minimum is less likely to be occupied (i.e. compare the distribution of a fixed number of molecules in situation depicted by Figs 2.15B and C: the availability of more states to occupy decreases the probability that most molecules will be going to one state even if it is the global minimum). Thus the entropy 'S' in the system is proportional to number of accessible states (called density of states of the system) denoted by $\omega(E)$ for a given energy and volume:

$$S = k \ln \omega(E)$$

Two aspects become prominent when comparing the methods of theoretical calculations with experimental results:

• Properties measured are actually those that have been averaged over a large number or ensemble (10^5–10^{23}) of molecules and these occupy many different states.

• The quantity that can be compared between the *in-silico* process and the *in vitro/ in vivo* process (whether the process is a chemical reaction, a physical change, etc): *the standard free energy change*. It was mentioned earlier that the sum of enthalpy and entropy terms is termed free energy. Theoretically, the following steps are taken to arrive at this quantity:

  – Calculation of internal energy E (the sum of rotation, vibration and translation energy of a molecule) and zero point correction

  – Calculation of E at 298 K and 1 atm; E + RT gives enthalpy H (including the temperature correction)

  – H – TS = A, the Helmholtz free energy

  – A + PV = G, the Gibb's free energy

  – It is generally the Helmholtz free energy 'A' that is approximated for comparison with experimental results, though 'G' would be the more accurate term. Experimentally, the free energy measured is almost always the *change* in free energy. Theoretically, this is obtained when modeling reactions wherein the difference in G of products and reactants is calculated.

> *"There is a distinct value in being able to anticipate where a thing maybe in the future and what it will look like when it gets there."*.........*(Bergethon, 1998)*

Theoretically one can calculate the energy corresponding to the lowest point in a potential energy diagram E_0 of, say, a homogenous diatomic molecule (the potential energy diagram is as explained under chapter 2.2). This lowest point corresponding to the equilibrium bond length on the abscissa (Fig. 2.16) assumes the entire molecule at 0 K to be "frozen". According to the Heisenberg uncertainty principle, if one estimates the momentum of an electron close to accuracy, the error in its position becomes very large. Thus, an electron can never be still and even at 0 K and it moves about the

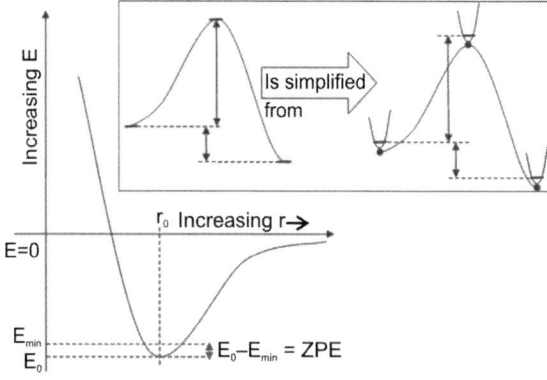

Fig. 2.16: Zero point energy

orbital). This inherent vibration in every atom of a molecule gives rise to zero point energy (ZPE) for the entire molecule.

Did You Know? 22
About the mysteries of the ZPE

Quantum theory predicts, and experiments verify, that the so-called empty space (the vacuum) of the universe contains an enormous residual background energy known as zero-point energy (ZPE). This is the energy that is responsible for elementary particles to continue to exhibit energetic behavior at temperatures of the absolute, i.e. 0 K (−273° Celsius).

We saw that a diatomic molecule has 6 degrees of freedom: 3 for translation, 2 for rotation around 2-axes, and 1 for vibration along the bonding axis. So why isn't its energy (6 × ½ =) 3 kT? Why is it 5/2 kT? This remained a great mystery until the turn of the 19th century when the theories of quantum mechanics were being developed.

According to quantum mechanics, at the sub-atomic level, waves behave as particles and particles as waves. Electrons have wave properties (Heisenberg uncertainty) and light is propagated as packets of energy (called photons) with magnitude hf, where h is Planck's constant and f is the frequency, here with which the atoms in the bond vibrate. The energy can never be 0; the ground state of a molecule occupies a minimum energy of hf/2 and the bonded atoms vibrate with energy that is a higher multiple of hf/2 (i.e., 3hf/2, 5hf/2, etc. or higher). Further explanations on this subject are considered irrelevant to the current topic.

The E_0 in Fig. 2.16 is physically meaningless owing to this phenomenon. The "energy at rest" of the molecule at 0 K is therefore represented by 'E_{min}' a little higher along the PE curve than E_0. Now it is easy to imagine that with increase in temperature, the molecules in the bond vibrate more strongly and its internal energy rises. The bond eventually breaks because the enthalpy of the system prefers to increase its investment in kinetic energy. As mentioned earlier, this occurs at the expense of potential energy

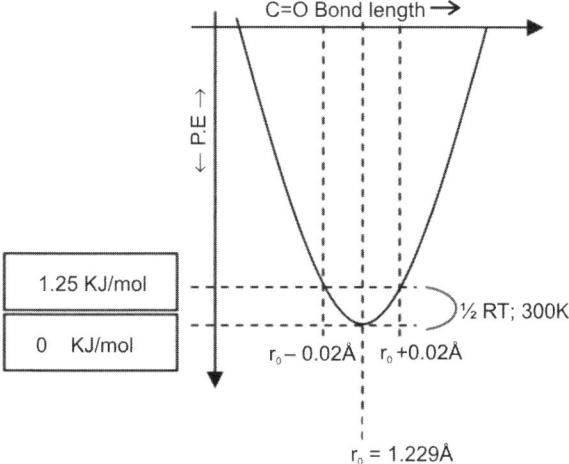

Fig. 2.17: The variations in C = O bond length in a molecule at room temperature

and the molecule need no longer be bonded aiming for low energy (remember that chemical bonding occurs because bound state has lower potential energy than the sum of the energies of the unbound atoms). The following are encountered when calculating these parameters on computers:

- Just as a *single point calculation* is performed to obtain the energy for the specified geometry of a molecule
- A *geometry optimization* is done to determine the geometry that has minimum energy
- A *frequency calculation* is performed to obtain thermochemical data. This calculates the vibrations that atoms undergo and adds this vibrational energy to the calculated electronic energy in a single point calculation. Thus the effect of temperature can be modeled and calculated; the enthalpies and energies become comparable to reactions occurring at room temperature or cellular temperature.

References: (Foye, et al. 2008), (Hirst, 1990), (Höltje, et al. 2008), (Leach, 1997), (Bergethon, 1998)

F. Analyzing the Reaction Path (overview: concept and terminology)

In experimental work, one mixes reagent A, reagent B, some guess that the procedure in the manual is correct, and some hope that it will give good yields. Let's say that the reaction completion is indicated by a color change. If after considerable waiting nothing seems to happen, manipulation of reaction conditions follow wherein factors such as temperature, stirring rates, apparatus set-up, ratio of reactants etc. are tweaked. No success in those steps drives the experimentalist in search of a suitable catalyst C. Failure of even this makes the experimentalist sad that nobody is willing to accept a paper on how A and B do not react even in the presence of catalyst C (this opinion is presented in the light that if 100 molecules can be generated in a series, probably only 1 molecule will become a successful lead. Discovering one unsuccessful molecule out when there are 99 others after intense lab-work might not be called 'success', but is useful information nevertheless). The sadness is not surprising especially if this experimentalist is a PhD student who spent a year or so in trying to get results! The scenario above is an exaggeration, but the point is that without a strong theory (such as a reaction mechanism) any experimental work is like to end up this way. One can imagine that the experiment is left under the sole care of the probability devil that, by Murphy's Law, plays mischief with all those desperate souls who most need something to happen. A theoretical study of the system should yield a list of conditions that are optimal for the reaction to occur.

An investigation of combinations of possible reactions, of what the odds are against obtaining the desired product, the various probabilities of all possible configurations and conformations participating in the reaction, of how the molecules "find each other", of how reactants recognize each other through arrangement of orbitals, and of how the electron density moves about the arranged atoms in turn influencing geometry are the few details modeled in a reaction path analysis. Here, as with other areas above, the computer mathematically mimics the forces that drive chemical reactions. The results obtained are compared to experimental ones in a bilateral way–if computer simulates experimental results correctly, then the microscopic progress of the reaction have been modeled correctly. This will give insights into alternative reactions pathways that are experimentally cheaper to follow and also give higher and/or purer yields of desired product.

A partial list of the various features encountered in reaction curves and surfaces along with their significance are as follows:

The Reaction Path (or curve or surface)

A 2D reaction curve is a plot between a reaction coordinate (explained below) and energy (potential energy or enthalpy changes during the reaction). A 3D surface is obtained when enthalpy is plotted against 2 reaction coordinates. As the human eye cannot perceive greater than 3 dimensions, one cannot include more than 2 reaction coordinates in the analysis plotted versus energy. So, even if many important changes occur during the reaction such as formation of new bonds, breaking of old bonds, rotation of groups, etc., only two of those can be selected to represent the reaction coordinates at a time.

The Reaction Coordinate

This is a specific interatomic distance, angle or dihedral that changes during the reaction–such as that indicated in the SN2 back side attack in Scheme 2.19:

In the above scheme, four suggestions RC1–RC4 (3 distances and 1 angle) for reaction coordinates correspond to the four major changes in geometry that occur during the SN2 substitution reaction. RC1 represents the plane containing the central atom which

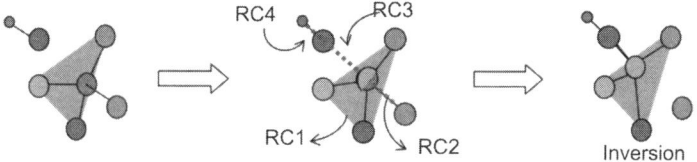

Three atoms lie in the same plane (note how the plane 'cuts through' the central atom of the transition state structure in the middle)

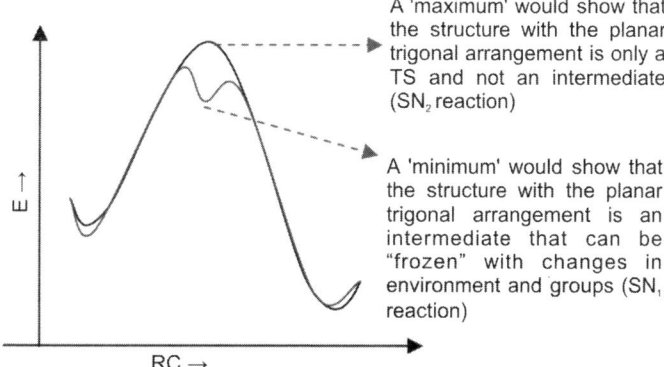

A 'maximum' would show that the structure with the planar trigonal arrangement is only a TS and not an intermediate (SN_2 reaction)

A 'minimum' would show that the structure with the planar trigonal arrangement is an intermediate that can be "frozen" with changes in environment and groups (SN_1 reaction)

Scheme 2.19: The right choice for a reaction coordinate

can be described by a suitable dihedral angle; RC2 indicates the interatomic distance between the leaving atom and the central atom; RC3 represents the interatomic distance between the central atom and the attacking atom; RC4 shows the bonded state of the attacking atom in its reagent molecule and is indicated by interatomic distance again. Plotting 1 or 2 RCs Vs Enthalpy Changes during the progress of the reaction would give the reaction path. The most informative plot is selected for analysis and this would typically inform us of several points including the overall kinetics, rate limiting step, thermodynamics, molecule shape, arrangement of groups, properties of groups that would enhance reactivity, etc.

The Minimum

Indicates an arrangement that is energetically favorable and can be chemically isolated for study (the lower the energy in which the minimum is located, the more stable the arrangement, the easier it is to isolate it from the reaction). Species of interest are located on minima: reactants, products and reaction intermediates. Difference between the various minima (especially that between the reactant and product minima) indicate overall stabilization of the reaction and altering this alters the thermodynamics, *ref.* Fig. 2.18.

The Maximum

A point located in a maximum as in Fig. 2.19 indicates a structure with high energy (the RC is plotted against energy) and that is very unstable. It is only transient during the course of the reaction. A detailed understanding of the structure and forces operating in the TS give us valuable insights on how to reduce the energy barrier and accelerate (improve the kinetics) of the reaction either by changing reactants, or indicating the choice of catalyst.

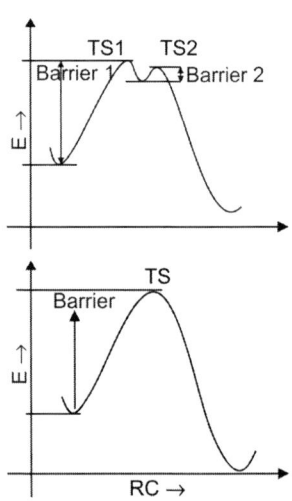

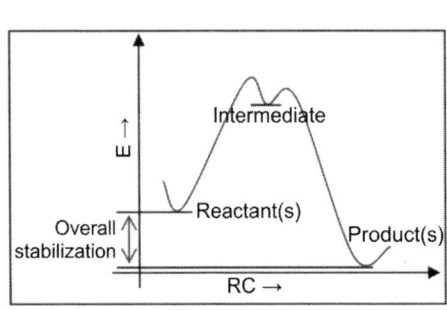

Fig. 2.18: The minima are of chemical interest

Fig. 2.19: Maxima indicate transient structures

Discussion 2.20: To propose one's love with a graphite ring

The activation barrier of carbon converting into diamond is low and so diamond is quickly and easily formed. Carbon requires greater energy to convert into graphite but the product, in this case, is much more stable than the reactant. Thus diamond is the kinetic product of carbon and graphite is the thermodynamic product. Diamond is easily formed (relative to graphite) and easily changed – it is known to rearrange into graphite over a great many years releasing a lot of energy during the process. Thus over time, graphite is more stable and permanent. If this is the kind of relationship you wish to ask of a person you love, would you gift a graphite ring instead of a diamond one?

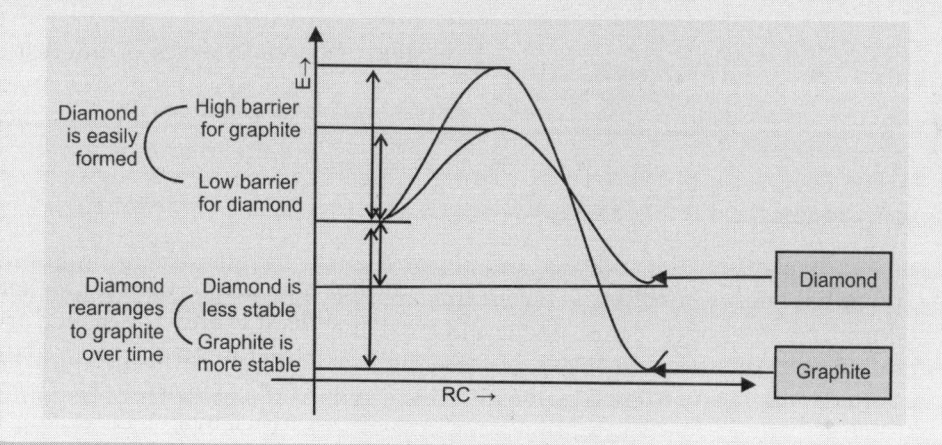

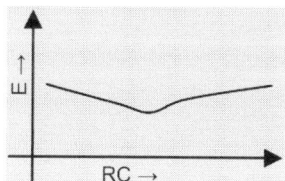

Fig. 2.20: A shallow curve–the minimum is difficult to locate

Some features of reaction surfaces/paths are presented here:

Shallow Minimum

A shallow minimum is one where there is no great stabilization of the minimum over the other conformers/arrangements. Such minima become difficult to locate in calculations.

An "egg-tray" Surface

This kind of a surface is shown in Fig. 2.21 (a cross section is show here in 2D) is very difficult to handle when one searches for the global minimum. Some proteins, when folding, display such extensive "kinetic traps" where the local minima are so deep that the energy minimization algorithm gets trapped in these. It is difficult for these algorithms to scale the energy barriers. This is shown in the boxed part of the surface. *Note:* A surface does not have to be symmetric; the global minimum does not have to be located at the 'centre'.

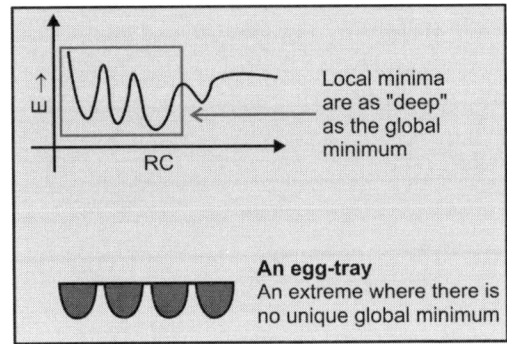

Fig. 2.21: An "egg-tray" like surface

Shoulder or Shelf

These areas are relatively flat and pose another problem when identifying a minimum. As the potential energy function is flat in this area, it appears as if there will be no further lowering of energy. Thus, one could miss the minimum that follows when investigating conformations in Fig. 2.22 from right to left. Special techniques have been reported in literature to capture the minimum even in the presence of a shoulder.

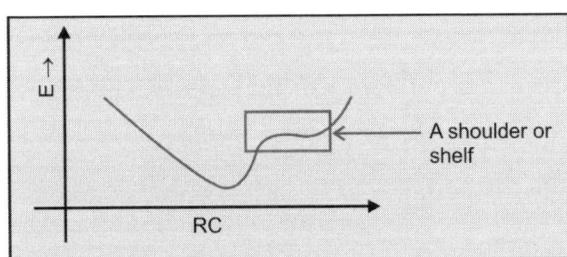

Fig. 2.22: A shelf or a shoulder occurring in a reaction curve

Saddle Point

This is a very important aspect of chemical reactions indicated in Fig. 2.23. A saddle point is point located on a region in the 3D reaction surface that is a minimum in one direction and a maximum along others. The location of the saddle point is important because it corresponds to the TS. On a 2D curve, when one is familiar with the reaction, one can easily locate the maximum and the corresponding TS. But, when one plots the potential energy surface in 3D, location of the TS becomes difficult as several points are located at the maxima in several directions. The TS is therefore the saddle point and it is the maximum in several directions but a minimum in only one.

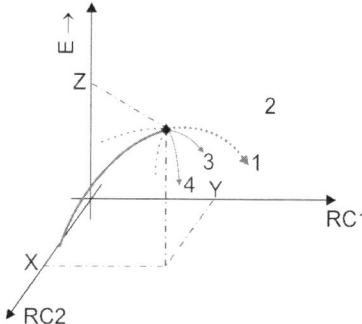

The saddle point (point in black is located at a minimum along the path perpendicular (black line) to the reaction path and at a maximum along every other path (orange, red and purple lines of which the reaction path is in orange) on the reaction surface. Dotted lines indicate that they start from or end on the other side of the black line

Fig. 2.23: A saddle point

The Free Energy Funnel of Protein Folding

The surface that maps the conformational space of a molecule is also a form of a 'reaction surface' involving only one molecule. The free energy funnel is a very important aspect representing the large number of conformations that macromolecules such as proteins can take up. The properties and types of these extensive surfaces are presented in section 1.5.9–11.

A Reaction Surface

With knowledge of these features and their significance, we wish to introduce the readers to a real reaction surface, in the following paragraphs. Consider the surface in Fig. 2.24; actually there are millions of paths that can be traced from the reactant to the product on that surface. However, of chemical interest, are only 3 distinct paths:
1. Reactants → TS1 (not shown) → I–1 → TS2 (not shown) → Products (as in path P1 of the inset)

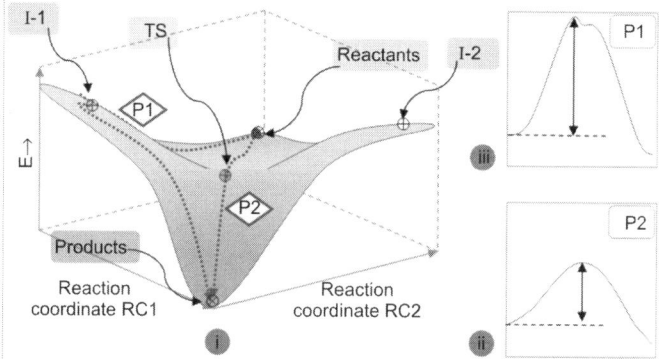

Fig. 2.24: A 3D reaction surface plotting reaction coordinates RC1 and RC2 against energy E showing two possible reaction paths P1 and P2 (with their corresponding 2D versions in the insert). Path P1 includes an intermediate I-1, whereas path P2 includes the transition state TS of the conversion of reactants to products

2. Reactants → TS1 (not shown) → I–2 → TS2 (not shown) → Products (also as in path P1 of the inset)
3. Reactants → TS → Products (as in path P2 of the inset)

We know the location of the minima corresponding to the reactants and products. The intermediate of a reaction is also minima located at higher energy somewhere mid-way between the reactant and product. The TS is located at the saddle point. We say that these points on the potential energy surface listed above are of chemical interest because experimentally, the molecules (and computationally, the structures) on any point of the surface that lies in between the reactants, products, intermediates (including the transition states) are so transient that it is impossible to isolate and study them with the hope to modify them to our gain. The TS, although is also transient as the name suggests, is very important owing to

1. The sudden change in the course of a reaction from uphill to downhill direction
2. The height of the TS (i.e. the energy content of the TS molecule) deciding the kinetics of the reaction.

Figure 2.24 is a schematic representation of the location of reactants, transition state (TS), intermediates (I–1 and I–2) and products on a potential energy surface of a chemical reaction. Two reaction pathways (P1 and P2) are shown on the surface (in *i*) and as 2-D reaction curve representations (*ii* and *iii* of P1 and P2 respectively). An example of Diels-Alder cycloaddition ascribed (Bruice, et al. 2007) to have such a surface and the reaction mechanism when following either of the indicated pathways is shown below.

Applications in Drug Design

1. What is an Enzyme?

We often look for complementary shape and chemical properties between the protein and ligand (whether drug or natural substrate). However, if one took the time to consider the question in Think Box 5, one would be surprised at the blindness of the assumption.

Think Box 5: What is an enzyme?

What is an enzyme? It is a protein that catalyzes a reaction – i.e. it transforms or introduces a change in the structure of the substrate.

Will the structure of the binding site of an enzyme be complementary to the substrate? Consider:

1. What if it was complementary? The ligand would bind with the protein.
2. Then what? The ligand–protein complex would dissociate! There will be an equilibrium between binding and dissociate of the ligand (the mechanism considered here is reversible binding)
3. So where is the catalysis? Even if we consider conformational change in the protein and similar changes in the ligand, the ligand is not undergoing any chemical change!
4. Then, what will the binding site of an enzyme be complementary to? The binding site of an enzyme, either before binding, or after undergoing conformational change on binding, will be complementary to the **transition state of the reaction that the substrate will undergo.**

This complementary shape (or chemical property) that the enzyme possesses to the transition state that the ligand will be going through during the course of the reaction lowers the energy barrier of the reaction and facilitates the formation of product. This is how enzymes serve as catalysts. One such detailed computational analysis was carried out by (Bruice, et al. 2007) comparing the Diels-Alder reaction of a maleimide and an anthracene in water and in the active site of the ribozyme. From the research work, it was concluded that the shape of the enzyme forces the reactants to take up a position that already resembles the TS, even before the reaction began. The anthracene molecule was twisted by 18° toward maleimide in the TS formed at the active site, whereas no such twist was perceived in the TS formed in water. The favorable twist in addition to the two molecules being at van der Waal's distance to each other aids the uphill "climbing" of the reactants to reach the TS. Once at the TS, the reaction proceeds to completion very easily. The ribozyme catalyzed reaction has been estimated to occur 20,000 times faster than the reaction in water (Helm, et al. 2005). Diels-Alder ribozyme is PDB entry 1YKV.

2. Lessons from nature: A warhead on enediyne antibiotics for cancer targeting
Enediyne antibiotics are presented as an example here to show how the knowledge of reaction mechanism can be used in designing drugs. These molecules have multiple unsaturation in their structure and are known to undergo Bergman cyclization (Baroudi, et al. 2010) based on studies in bacteria, etc.

Microorganisms and human beings have one thing in common: Both are attacked by toxic bacteria and viruses. However, microorganisms have been on earth at least 2 billion years longer than human beings, and therefore, they know much better how to protect themselves against bacteria and viruses.

Elfi Kraka & Dieter Cremer
J. Am. Chem. Soc. 2000, 122, 8245

They are used as anticancer drugs but their use was discouraged owing to toxicity due to lack of specificity in biological action (they could not discriminate between normal and cancerous cells). Detailed experimental work reports the synthesis of analogues and the influence of varying groups on biological activity; as a further step, a 'biological warhead was also extensively investigated (Nicolaou, et al. 1992). A "warhead" is a group that targets a certain region in the body. A biological warhead on Dynemicin was aimed to deliver and detach the molecule at the site of the cancerous cell. A lot of research on enediyne antibiotics resulted in a number of strategies in which the warhead could be crafted with a carrier and a trigger. The carrier was coined to physically transport the drug to the site of action upon which the trigger releases the active molecule at the target site. Body temperature, DNA cleaving pharmacodynamic action, kinetic stability, toxicity and other key issues have been critically reviewed (Tuttle, et al. 2005).

2.4 *An Overview of Statistical and Chemometric Methods in Drug Design*

The large number of experiments (whether wet-lab or *in-silico*) performed all round the world, collected and classified in comprehensive databases is a valuable source of information. Extracting correlations between various pairs of variables yield exciting results and have opened up the vast field of the informatics in biology and chemistry. The importance gained by the Quantitative Structure Activity Relationship (QSAR) technique, which lies at the intersection of chemistry, statistics and biology is proof of this concept. Under this chapter, QSAR, 3D-QSAR and chemometric methods are presented. As mentioned under section 2.1.2, Chemometrics involves extracting information from multivariate chemical data (*see* under "Principles of Chemometrics" in this section) by applying statistical and mathematical methods. A data collection task, whether in science, business or any other field, typically involves multivariate data (*ref.* principles of chemometrics: an overview presented later in this section). Using chemometrics as a tool helps to uncover various relationships among all samples and variables by processing the data simultaneously. Chemometrics is primarily used to uncover patterns by which collected data is related, to perform continuous evaluation on the properties of materials (such as in industrial administration), and/or, for setting up classification models (multivariate) for large amounts of data. Literature (Zitko, 1998) mentions that Principal Component Analysis (PCA) and Artificial Neural Networks (ANNs) have been the most widely used methods in chemometrics.

QSAR

There is a dynamic flow of information among the aspects of drug research–the experimental, the theoretical, the PK and the PD perspectives as shown in the Scheme 2.20. Note the reversible arrows; once modifications in structure have been approved by *in silico* predictions of PK and PD, the new structure is synthesized and tested first *in vitro*, and then if promising, *in vivo*. Structure modifications intended for PK improvement may also influence PD properties (and vice versa), predictions and testing are done on both the PK and PD fronts. Experimental results serve as a feedback to further optimization if needed. It is noteworthy that a similar dynamic flow of information cannot be set up for lead discovery as done here during lead optimization.

SAR is not quantitative derivation of correlation; it is only based on similarity: that similar (dissimilar) compounds have similar (dissimilar) activity. This is not always true such as in the case of sulfanilamide and PABA (*ref.* history of drug design strategies under section 2.3.1).

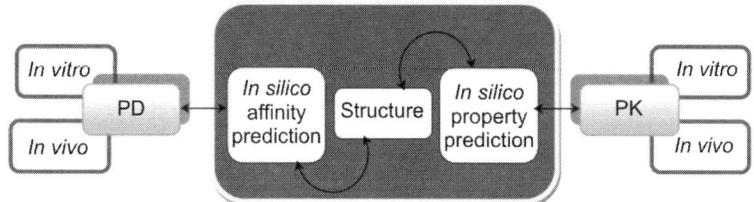

Scheme 2.20: Feedback optimization in drug design

- In SAR studies, chemical structure (or any other descriptor) is converted to some manageable numerical representation
- Similarity in biological activity is predicted from the *numerical distance* between the structures (how different structures are from each other in the numerical representation)
- Condensation to smaller dimension (2D structures to 1D numbers) leads to loss of information, i.e. one cannot exactly capture all that is available in 2D using a 1D description. So it must be ensured that information important to the analysis is not lost
- The robustness of the analysis depends on the authenticity of the type of the relationship between descriptors (numerical description of chemicals as physicochemical properties) and biological activity; this should be known (or derived).

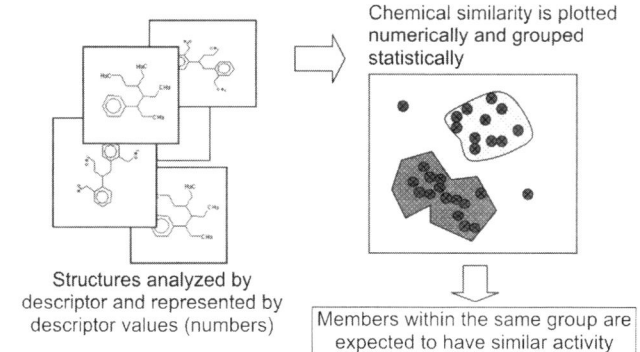

Chemical similarity is plotted numerically and grouped statistically

Structures analyzed by descriptor and represented by descriptor values (numbers)

Members within the same group are expected to have similar activity

Fig. 2.25: Similarity in points on a plot is considered similarity of molecules

What is QSAR? QSAR is a technique that quantitatively tests for the presence of correlation between the structure of a compound and various aspects of its biological activity. It is of 2 types–2D (which is referred to as classical QSAR or simply as QSAR) and 3D (called Comparative Molecular Field Analysis CoMFA; this is detailed under section 2.4.2 in this chapter that deals with chemometric methods).

Methodology Outline
- An equation is set up wherein biological activity is on the left hand side and the list of descriptors (that one thinks is responsible for biological activity) is added on the right hand side. The descriptors are added after multiplying with an unknown

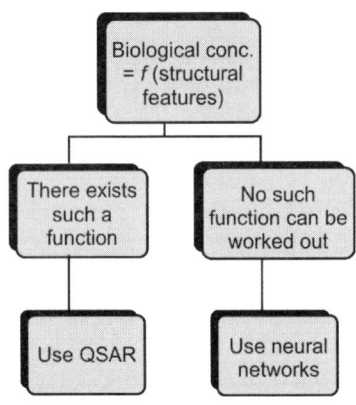

Scheme 2.21: When is QSAR used? biological conc. = biological concentration

coefficient. The goal of QSAR is to find out the coefficients such that the equation becomes valid (such that RHS = LHS)

• In QSAR, an equation is set up wherein every term adds up; the hypothesis is that these terms are linearly related to the biological concentration of the compound (whether this is true or does not need to be tested) and that they can be added up to log 1/C

• *Biological concentration:* This is generally written out as the log of its reciprocal because it is easier to express equipotent molar activities in log scale. In addition, the experimental error has a normal distribution in log scale.

• *Terms:* Every term represents properties of molecules (called molecular descriptors) that can be derived from the structure of the given compound.

• Overlapping descriptions must be avoided when setting up the equation

A fundamental assumption in QSAR is the 'Similarity Principle': Compounds with similar chemical structures usually possess similar physicochemical properties and biological activities. This is used for predicting properties of new compounds. This is an assumption because exceptions do exist to this rule.

Basic requirements in QSAR studies is that the analogs being studied:
• Belong to a congeneric series
• Have the same mechanism of action
• Bind to the target in a comparable manner
• Have predictable effects for isosteric replacement.

Did You Know? 23
The number of molecular descriptors in QSAR

*There are **thousands** of molecular descriptors in QSAR and these can be referred in the books (Karelson, 2000); (Todeschini, et al. 2000).*

The development of a QSAR model requires these three components:
• A list of molecules in their 3D structure: The structure maybe obtained ready-to-use, downloaded from previous research or from experimental sources. If these are not available, the structures maybe constructed; a number of conformations can be generated for each molecule and the best conformation can be selected that closely matches the bioactive one. However, having the right conformation is not as important for 2D QSAR (because this deals with properties of molecules) as it is for 3D QSAR.
• Experimentally determined biological activities for the molecules.
• Software to correlate the data using appropriate statistical methods.
• The molecules may or may not be accompanied by property data; if unavailable from experiments, some data can be calculated.

Discussion 2.21: Molecular descriptors in QSAR

We know that the electronic, steric and hydrophobic properties of molecules determine drug-likeness. So, simple properties like logP, solubility, ionization constant etc. that can be calculated or measured *in vitro* (vide Scheme 2.15: The 3 avenues of investigation in drug design under section 2.3.2.B2) were used as QSAR descriptors. However, there came a need to increase detail of description owing to the vast categories of drugs and targets investigated and discovered. Therefore, this simple list was extended dramatically to include descriptors of molecules such as quantum chemical, minimum energy conformation, etc. that can be inserted into the QSAR equation. This step served to extract various properties related to structure of the molecule to match the increasing heights of experimental techniques and depths of theory. One could also witness the rise in usage of theoretical descriptors such as orbital energies, log P, etc. Once verified in terms of reproducibility, these were found convenient because they can be calculated for many experimentally uninvestigated molecules. In addition, they are unbiased methods and can handle all molecules uniformly.

We wish to expand on three main categories of descriptors:

1. *Lipophilicity (Hydrophobicity):*
   a. log P is expressed as the sum of the π of each substituent present in the compound (Hansch, et al. 1962), (Hansch, et al. 1964). In the absence of intramolecular interactions, the substituent effects stay additive and the relationship between concentration (log 1/C) and $\Sigma\pi$ is linear.
   b. Hydrophobic constants were coined to allow constructing molecular partition from fragments (Rekker, 1977). Rekker's f values are not based on the "substitute H in molecule MH with R" (where H is hydrogen and R is a substituent) principle used by Hansch.

2. *Steric effect:*
   a. Verloop's Sterimol parameters (Verloop, 1987) described the molecular shape by graphical representations which involves measuring the minimal width, length, maximal width, etc. (indicated as L, d1, d2, etc.) of molecules.
   b. Fujita's (Harada, et al. 1997) corrected E_s values for unsymmetrical substituents
   c. The corrected E^c_s values (Hancock, et al. 1961) corrected for the number of α-hydrogens
   d. E_s values (acid-catalyzed hydrolysis of RCOOR′, compared to $CH_3COOR′$) $E_s = \log (k/k_o)_A$
   e. van der Waals radii of symmetric substituents
   f. Corrected atomic radii (or the minimal van der Waals radius of (Charton, 1991), Molar refractivity (Mannhold, et al. 1993)
   g. The Taft's (Taft, 1952) σ^* steric parameters was in prevalent use in many QSAR relations and has been revived recently (Claudia, et al. 2004)

3. *Electronic effect:* The Hammet s (Hammett, 1935) is the most popular descriptor.

Other descriptors are:

4. *Topology:* Molecular connectivity indices of Kier-Hall (electron weighted sub graph counts); spatial disposition as a combination of conformation, geometry, and shape

5. *Chirality:* This is a missing term in 2D QSAR; however, 2.5D QSAR includes configurational information in the form of stereochemical notation of the molecule (R or S)

6. *Quantum chemical descriptors:* HOMO-LUMO energy descriptors (Debnath, et al. 1991), electron density descriptors (Mezey, 2009), etc.

    a. The terms need to contain only linear relationships. If the relationship is non-linear, QSAR cannot be used. It is required that this linear correlation between the descriptor and biological concentration is established *a priori* (meaning beforehand) in order to be included as a term in the QSAR equation. Such 'prior' analysis between descriptor and concentration is done using chemometrics, especially Partial Least Square method, or Neural Networks.

    b. Some software: ADAPT (http://research.chem.psu.edu/pcjgroup/ADAPT.html), OASIS (Mekenyan, et al. 1986), CODESSA (Katritzky, et al.), DRAGON (Todeschini, et al. 2006).

References: (Kubinyi, 1995), (Ramsden, 1990), (Karelson, 2000), (Seydel, 1985), (Wolff, 1994), (Gramatica).

Box 25: CODESSA-PRO

The CODESSA-PRO software (http://www.codessa-pro.com/descriptors/index.htm) categorizes its QSAR descriptors as *Constitutional, Topological, Geometrical, Electrostatic, CPSA* (this includes various charged surface areas), *Quantum-chemical, Molecular Orbital-related* and *Thermodynamic* (Katritzky, et al.).

Did You Know? 24
QSAR is encouraged at a legislative scale

The European Commission (REACH: Registration, Evaluation and Authorization of Chemicals) states the need to use (Q)SAR models to reduce experimental testing (including animal testing). To meet the requirements of the REACH legislation it is essential to use (Q)SAR models that are well validated. It is recommended at the website (http://ec.europa.eu/enterprise/sectors/chemicals/reach/index_en.htm) that reliable QSAR models must be associated with:

1. *A defined endpoint;*
2. *An unambiguous algorithm;*
3. *A defined domain of applicability;*
4. *Appropriate measures of goodness-of-fit, robustness and predictivity;*
5. *A mechanistic interpretation, if possible.*

The ideal QSAR should
- consider an adequate number of molecules for sufficient statistical representation
- must be validated sufficiently to be able to predict new molecule behavior
- have molecules with sufficient distribution of properties in each category (e.g. active and inactive). This increases the robustness of correlation and the range of prediction
- must give an insight on the mechanism of action or the mode of binding

The accuracy of using a QSAR study for correlation or prediction is generally limited by the reliability, precision and accuracy of experimental data available for analysis as given in the European Commission–see Did You Know? 24.

The QSAR Fitness-landscape

The 'fitness-landscape' is the relation between a molecular descriptor called the *landscape* such as log P of molecules with their predictor property called the *fitness* such as the binding affinity. This fitness–landscape correlation is constructed on the projected configurational space of molecules. In simpler words, similar molecules are placed together, in a neighborhood. It follows that when similar molecules have similar properties the fitness-landscape would be smooth. This is an ideal situation; as for real world examples that QSAR deals with, the landscapes are almost always jagged. It is considered that the fitness-landscape is some form of a "potential function" (Stadler, et al. 2002) which indicates that a group of molecules that occur "uphill" have higher correlation between the molecular descriptor and the predictor properties. The parameters that determine landscape are the independent variables on which biological activity, etc. are dependent. The correct choice and usage of the fitness function (the function that is plotted against the landscape) is therefore important. However in QSAR, molecular descriptors can be obtained in an indirect way (by calculation) if experimental values are not available or measurable. Also, the fitness function is not known for all molecules! It is to be remembered that QSAR is conducted to accommodate unknown molecules correctly amidst known ones; the fitness function (such as biological activity) of the unknown is only estimated and not derived. If the function is correct, the estimated biological activity matches with the true value (if available for verification).

A schematic representation of a fitness-landscape: In Fig. 2.26, the X-Y plane contains the landscape, which is, here, the projection of the configurational (and chemical) space of some bi-substituted benzenes. This illustrative example has not been taken from any research work. The fitness function (say, here, binding affinity) estimates which molecules perform the best by placing them "uphill" (for example, here, para-dichlorobenzene).

Examples from publications:
- The expression for mutagenticity of compounds includes terms for lipophilicity (in non-linear relation considering the limits of trans-membrane transport discussed under lipophilicity), energy of LUMO and indicator variables I1 and I2. The QSAR equation takes the form $\log 1/C = a \log P + b \log (\beta P + 1) + c\, \varepsilon_{LUMO} + d\, I_1 + e\, I_2 + f$ wherein a-f represent coefficients that were optimized (Niculescu-Duvâz, et al. 1981)

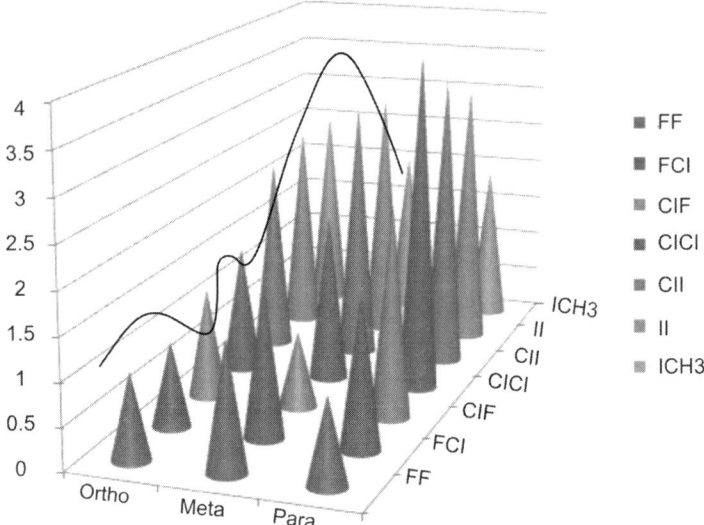

Fig. 2.26: The fitness landscape

- Biological activity is correlated to structural features (Free Wilson analysis), physicochemical properties (Hansch analysis), or fields (CoMFA, CoMSIA). The first two methods handle only comparisons and derivation of relationships from 2D structures and:
  – Obtain information on properties in relation to structure
  – To use this information to improve biological experiments.

Discussion 2.22: Hansch and Free-Wilson analysis

This text does not intend to make itself redundant by entering into a detailed account of the QSAR expressions using Hansch and Free-Wilson analysis. Given here is only an overview.

QSAR-The Hansch equation: $\log(1/C) = ap + bp^2 + cs + dE_s + k$ where a, b, c, d are coefficients, p is a hydrophobic term (e.g. logP), s is an electronic term, E_s is a steric term, k is a constant

- Principle Component Analysis (PCA) can be used to identify the most relevant physical parameters (*ref.* 2.4.3 on PCA)
- At the end of a QSAR analysis, it is assumed that the features identified as an important contributor to property (here, log 1/C) are assumed to occur mainly in drugs and, equally importantly, not in non-drugs
- Plainly, the Hansch equation takes up this structure:

Biological activity = f (transport + binding)
$$= -k1\,(lipo)^2 + k2\,(lipo) + k3(pol) + k4(elec) + k5(ster) + k6$$

where k1 – k6 are unknown constants (weights) that will be assigned appropriate values (optimized) after the QSAR analysis is completed and verified (following the pattern explained in **Discussion 2.14** under section 2.3.2 B2)

QSAR Models: (1) Hansch model (biological property-physicochemical property relationship)

- Parameter π: $\pi_X = \log P_{RX} - \log P_{RH}$
- Linear Hansch model: $\log 1/C = a \log P + b\sigma + c\,MR + ... + k$
- Nonlinear Hansch models
  - $\log 1/C = a\,(\log P)^2 + b \log P + c\,\sigma + ... + k$
  - $\log 1/C = a\,\pi^2 + b\pi + c\,\sigma + ... + k$
  - $\log 1/C = a \log P - b \log (\beta P + 1) + c\,\sigma + ... + k$

(2) Free-Wilson model (structure – property relationship)

- $\log 1/C = \Sigma a_i + \mu$ wherein a_i = substituent group contributions; μ = activity contribution of reference compound

(3) Mixed Hansch/Free-Wilson model

$\log 1/C = a\,(\log P)^2 + b \log P + c\,\sigma + ... + \Sigma a_i + k$

$\log 1/C = a \log P - b \log (\beta P + 1) + c\,\sigma + ... + \Sigma a_i + k$

Caution: Substituents cannot be treated as separate molecules. For example, log P of 1, 2-diphenylethane is not the same as 2 log P of benzene + 2 log P of methane (www.kubinye.de)! For constructing molecular lipophilicity from fragments, the Hydrophobic Fragmental Constants f_i of Rekker must be used (Rekker, 1977)

$$\log P = \Sigma a_i f_i$$

Judging QSAR programs: QSAR is computed on worksheets called Molecular Spread Sheets. Here molecules are accommodated in rows and columns contain the molecular descriptors (*ref.* discussion 2.14 under section 2.3.2.B2). Most QSAR predictions include r^2 and/or q^2 values–generally, q^2 is considered more important than r^2 (van Drie, 2003) and a value of 0.8 or greater is considered a "good" model. QSAR models, during the validation phase need detailed interpretation on how and why certain correlations exist. One cannot simply trust the results of the analysis in deciding whether a molecule is predicted with a good property (such as bioavailability) as in (Drie, 2004). The validity of the QSAR model also depends on the dataset molecules (those used for training as well as those used for validation). An outline of validation is presented in later topics (*ref.* CoMFA for cross validation).

References and Materials

1. The author recommends that readers download the (free access) articles on QSAR and 3D QSAR in drug design Part I and Part II [(Kubinyi, 1997) and (Kubinyi, 1997)] available at www.cmbi.ru.nl/edu/bioinf4/articles/pdf/qsa_kubinyi_1.pdf and www.cmbi.kun.nl/edu/bioinf4/articles/pdf/qsa_kubinyi_2.pdf respectively which are not only authoritative but also easy to read and understand.

2. http://www.qsarworld.com/qsar-datasets.php gives datasets for conducting QSAR evaluations against. The datasets are organized into several categories such as percentage human oral bioavailability, percentage plasma binding, urinary excretion, etc.

3. Perform online calculations (and read descriptions) at http://www.chm. davidson.edu/erstevens/QSAR/QSAR.html

4. http://www.qsari.org/: international QSAR foundation: where use and validation of QSAR is given

5. Free QSAR software download available from the website of the OECD (Organization for Economic Co-operation and Development) http://www. oecd.org/document/23/0,3343,en_2649_34379_33957015_1_1_1_1,00. html#Download_QSAR_AT

6. For tutorials, visit http://www.netsci.org/Science/Compchem/feature19.html

2.4.2 3D-QSAR

> *The ultimate challenge for 3D QSAR is to explain the observed affinities of known drugs.*
> *The ultimate challenge for drug design is to predict the affinities of new drugs...*
>
> *(Andrews, 1993)*

3D QSAR is also an 'SAR determining' method–it assesses similarity of molecules and attempts to relate this to biological activity. However, this is based on the 3D structures of ligands in their protein-bound state. In other words, the supposed bioactive conformation of the ligand is used to describe ligands. 3D-QSAR analysis (CoMFA) has a much broader scope. It starts from 3D structures and correlates biological activities by constructing 3D-property fields.

Advantages

1. Molecules to be analyzed are expected to have the same pharmacophore but not similar structure of scaffolds.

2. The enantiomers and conformations can be distinguished (cannot be done in 2D-QSAR).

It was mentioned earlier that although the pharmacophore is an arrangement of chemical groups in space that a protein recognizes, it is in fact its electron density distribution that draws the protein's attention. Search of the common pharmacophore can be done by selecting a relatively rigid molecule from the set. This reduces the number of conformations that need to be generated for the more flexible molecules of the dataset. One can also consider molecules that have rotatable bonds in different regions of the molecule–the regions that are rigid would be common to all molecules and would suggest a starting point to calculate the pharmacophore. The molecules are aligned and superimposed guided by their pharmacophores. This is the trickiest part in CoMFA (Kubinyi, 1997) especially if the molecules are not from the same 'series'. Superimposed molecules are placed in the centre of a larger box (leaving a clearance of a few Å on all sides) and a 3D grid is constructed (as described under Docking in section 3.2.3C). Each grid point is influenced by attractive and repulsive forces between partners (atom(s) on the molecule and the probe) A probe measures properties at each grid point, the nature of the probe depending on the property being mapped. As mentioned under section 3.2.3C, the most commonly investigated properties to estimate drug-receptor interaction are steric and electrostatic; hydrogen bonding is also considered (Table 2.14).

Table 2.14: Type of interaction, equation used and probes

Type of interaction	Modeled as	Probe used	For the molecule
Steric interaction	van der Waals interaction	carbon atom probe	$^1E_{vdw} = \Sigma$ *over all atoms* $(A.r^{-12} - C.r^{-6})$
Electrostatic interaction	Coulomb interactions	charged atom	$^2E_{estat} = \Sigma$ *over all atoms* $(q_1.q_2/D.r)$
Hydrogen bonds	Geometric or coulombic	Search for atom type: donors and acceptors	

[1]: r = distance between atom on the molecule and the grid point where the probe is located, A and C depend on van der Waals radii of the atom and the probe

[2]: D = dielectric constant, q_1 = partial charge on atom of the molecule, q_2 = charge on the probe

Molecular fields and their calculation: The molecular fields in Table 2.15 are generally calculated (*ref.* Discussion 2.18 on mapping potentials on surfaces under section 2.3.2 D). The molecular fields employ terms that can be calculated by molecular mechanics itself. Therefore, force fields come into play. For example, Tripos force field operates in the programs CoMFA and in VolSurf (see under 2.3.2.B1. Pharmacophore Modeling). The programs Catalyst and Serius use MSI force field. Individual because descriptors of CoMFA and QSAR (2D) are not comparable CoMFA is derived in 3D.

Validation of any QSAR model is most important (for more information, please visit http://ec.europa.eu/enterprise/sectors/chemicals/reach/index_en.htm for the European commission REACH as mentioned in Did You Know? 24 under 2.4.1. QSAR). Results from QSAR study must be considered as a working hypothesis and need to be interpreted in terms of receptor-ligand interactions. It is not true that successful research has implemented all statistical requirements of this method. One of the applications of the *Active Analogue Approach* (Marshall, et al. 1979) is to help in aligning molecules for comparison purposes. Compared to QSAR, 3D-QSAR

- Can handle compounds that are more heterogeneous
- Has better tolerance for alignment of structures as this is done by fields of properties and not atomwise
- The target structure need not be known
- Can allow for variations in binding mechanism of closely related analogues.

Assumptions in 3D QSAR

- The biological effect is produced only by molecules in the dataset (and not by its metabolites)

Table 2.15: The calculation of molecular fields

Molecular Electrostatic Potential	MEP	unit positive charge probe
Molecular Lipophilicity Potential	MLP	(no probe necessary)
Comparitive Molecular Field Analysis	CoMFA	With a probe (sp^3 carbon atom and charge +1.0)
• Steric fields: Lennard-Jones potential used		
• Electrostatic (Coulombic) fields		
• Additional fields: H-bonding and others also calculated		

- The conformation of the molecules in the dataset is the bioactive one (obtained from experiments or computational techniques)
- All molecules being analyzed are known to bind to the same site in the same protein (by the same mechanism)
- Entropic terms are not calculated in 3D-QSAR. Therefore, all molecules have similar entropic changes to free energy during interaction with protein.
- Protein binding directly explains activity; if there is coupling with effector pathway (influence on secondary messengers) it is uniform for all molecules; activity can be mainly explained by enthalpy component of the free energy of binding itself
- Solvent effects are generally not included in 3D-QSAR.

Comparative Molecular Field Analysis (CoMFA)

This is the name of a program (and is available with the Sybyl™ package) (Cramer, et al., 1988). It computes molecular fields on the grid, extract 3D descriptors and computes coefficients of QSAR equation as shown in Scheme 2.22, 2.23 and Fig. 2.27). The molecular fields are calculated using the respective probes (vide Tables 2.14 and 2.15) and the coefficients are optimized using the PLS technique.

Comparative Molecular Similarity Indices Analysis (CoMSIA)

- In CoMSIA, molecules are compared by (i) conformation, and (ii) chemical property distribution, simultaneously
- Similarity is calculated among molecules and expressed as similarity indices
- Similarity fields are mapped on a grid (in contrast to mapping properties directly on grids as done in CoMFA)
- In CoMFA, a small change in distance between atom and probe might drastically change energy. This is owing to the type of functions (equations) used to model properties. Such potentials are referred to as being *hard*. In CoMSIA, the potentials are *softer* and therefore more amenable to calculations of properties with gradual changes in distance within the grid box.

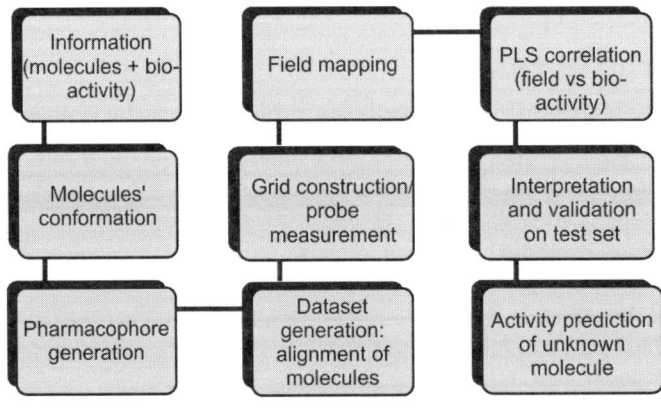

Scheme 2.22: CoMFA workflow

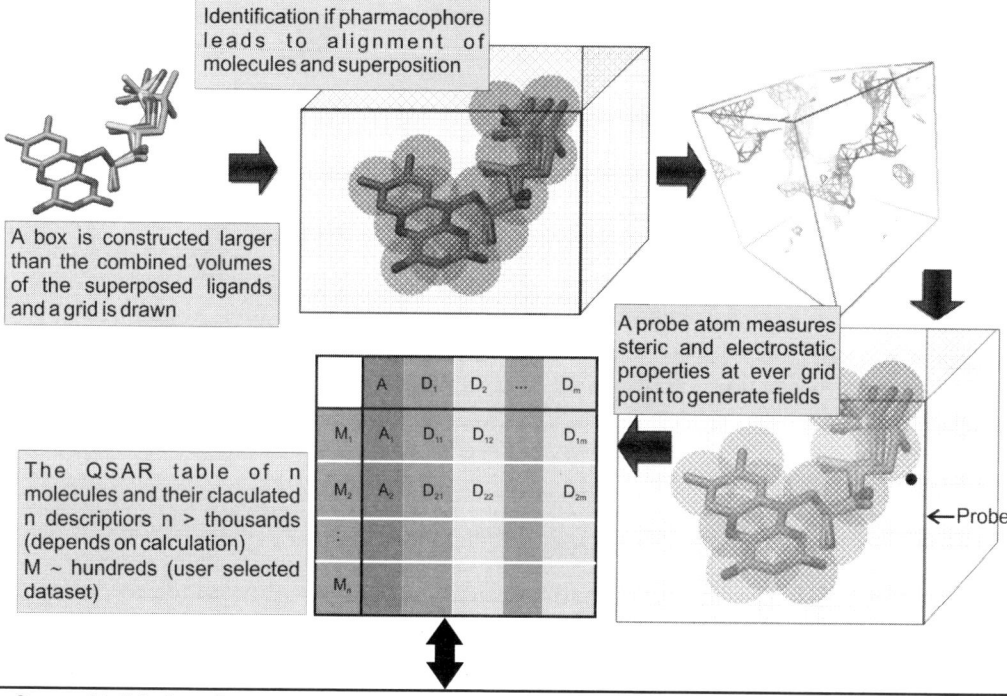

Identification if pharmacophore leads to alignment of molecules and superposition

A box is constructed larger than the combined volumes of the superposed ligands and a grid is drawn

A probe atom measures steric and electrostatic properties at ever grid point to generate fields

	A	D_1	D_2	...	D_m
M_1	A_1	D_{11}	D_{12}		D_{1m}
M_2	A_2	D_{21}	D_{22}		D_{2m}
$\vdots$					
M_n					

The QSAR table of n molecules and their claculated n descriptiors n > thousands (depends on calculation) M ~ hundreds (user selected dataset)

←Probe

Cross–Validation (leave-one-out method)

Molecular descriptors (electrostatic, steric, H-bonding, etc.) are correlated with biological activity as per the QSAR equation:

$A_1 = a_{11}D_{11} + a_{12}D_{12} + ...+ a_{1m}D_{1m}$

$A_2 = a_{21}D_{21} + a_{21}D_{22} + ...+ a_{2m}D_{2m}$

Using a PLS analysis, optimum *a* values are obtained for each equation.

Example: $A_1 = 0.2\ D_{11} + 355\ D_{12} + ...+ 7.9\ D_{1m}$ for M_1 and so on

Each such equation acts as a *model*. Solved equation for molecule M_1 is set as a model and is used to predict the A values of all molecules other than itself (i.e. for molecules $M_2 – M_n$). The number of correct predictions is noted. Similarly, the equation for M_2 attempts to predict the A values of M_1, M_3-M_n.

Calculation of Fit

The comparison of the predicted A values of *m* models (corresponding to *m* molecules and *m* equations) with the respective experimental A values (as in the above QSAR table) is analyzed. Statistical parameters:

• Q^2 : the squared cross-validated correlation coefficient

• r^2 : the squared correlation coefficient

• s : the standard deviation

In general, the Q^2 term is considered an important indicator of validity of the model (with a Q^2 of > 0.8 recommended).

Fig. 2.27: CoMFA steps: Diagrammatic representation

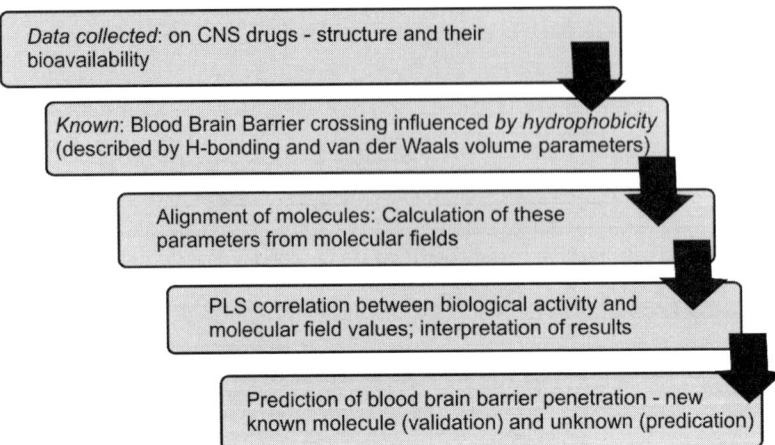

Scheme 2.23: CoMFA example

Principles of Chemometrics: Overview

The chemical discipline that uses mathematical and statistical methods to design or select optimal procedures (and experiments) and to provide maximum chemical information by analyzing chemical data is called *chemometrics* [for standard definitions, *ref.* textbooks (Massart, et al., 1997–1998), (Varmuza, et al. 2009), (Otto, 2007)].

Multivariate Analysis

Upto 3 analytical data for each object can be handled by regular methods (regression and other univariate approaches). But modern computer aided chemistry whether in chemical analysis, in the clinical setting, in design, or other fields handles a lot more than 3 descriptors per object. Therefore multivariate approaches are needed.

The descriptors for one object can be used individually or simultaneously. For example, when one programs the rule "the presence of less than 10 H-bond acceptors makes a good drug" only one data (number of h-bond acceptors) is used. If the user combines this information with other data about the same molecule, the data collected is used simultaneously and successively. For example, "a candidate is a good drug if it satisfies certain conditions with respect to the number H-bond acceptors, donors, molecular weight AND log P".

For example, consider the two methods of plotting data in Figs 2.28 and 2.29

In method 1, the questions "how many molecules have 4 H-bond acceptors?" and "how many molecules have a log P of 2.3" can be answered. These are univariate plots.

By simultaneously considering the number of H-bonds per molecule and the log P of the molecule, one attempts to determine the presence or absence of a relationship between the two variables. This is a bivariate analysis and attempts to answer the question "how many molecules have 4 H-bond acceptors and a log P of 2.3?" as can be done in Fig. 2.29.

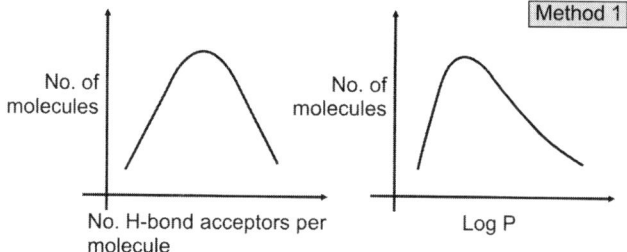

Fig. 2.28: Univariate plots

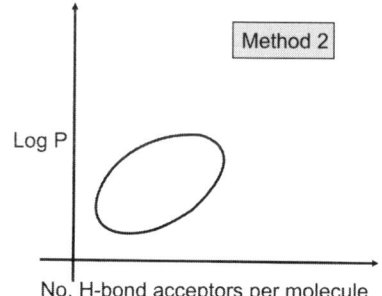

Fig. 2.29: Bivariate plot

Consider a Bivariate Analysis (Fig. 2.30)

- Both parameter X and Y are variables having Gaussian distributions individually
- The dotted lines show the 1σ limit of parameter X and of parameter Y (from respective univariate analyses) and they intersect resulting in a rectangle
- The ellipse describes the 1σ limit of the combination of parameters X and Y
- The axis of the ellipse is oblique (the line) because X and Y are correlated
- The ellipse is also larger than the rectangle (the intersection of 2 independent univariate analyses is not equal to a bivariate analysis).

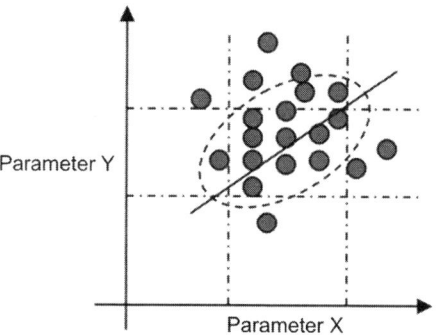

Fig. 2.30: Univariate Gaussian distributions in bivariate plot

Analysis of correlation between 3 (independent) variables would require a 3D plot. The 3D QSAR analysis in the previous section has thousands of variables that need to be correlated with biological activity and a thousands-of-dimensions analysis would follow! Humans are capable of perceiving up to 3 dimensions, therefore the multivariate, multidimensional analysis steps in not only to determine correlations among all those variables, but also to translate data into 2 or 3 dimensions (the PLS method mentioned above is one such statistical method). Points closer (by distance) on the graph represent objects that are similar with respect to the plotted parameter(s) compared to the objects represented by points that are farther apart.

Figure 2.31 plots a bivariate analysis of two independent variables collected from literature or experiments (such as the number of H-bond acceptors and log P). Point P represents an object (here a molecule) that is more similar to Q than it is to R, and is different from S. A clustering of similar points will result in a graph as in Scheme 2.24.

It is noteworthy that such analyses are often considered as a 'pattern recognition' problem and here, one often refers to variables as 'features'. Thus the number of H-bond acceptors and log P are *features*. Each molecule is an *object*. Problems:

- Choice of model–linear, polynomial, etc.
- Visualization
- Interpretation
- Computationally demanding.

2.4.3 PRINCIPAL COMPONENT ANALYSIS (PCA)

A principal component is (Eriksson, et al. 2006)

- A new variable generally denoted by u and represented by the equation $u_i = aX_i + bY_i$ (*components* are also called *latent variables*) wherein, X and Y are two variables on which PCA will be applied
- Constructed from existing data
- Used in condensing information from several dimensions to just one or two
- Set up in such a way as to retain best resolution of groups (to maintain the same differences between various points as present in the representation of high dimensions)

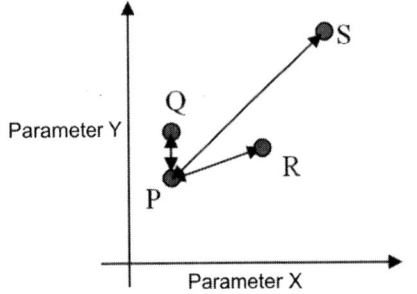

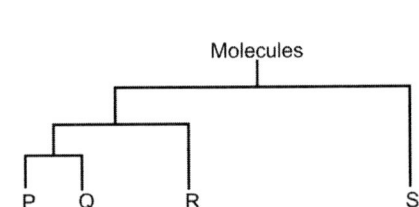

Fig. 2.31: Numerical representation of similarity   **Scheme 2.24:** Hierarchical clustering by similarity

- Plotted on a new line (a line is 1D) which
  - Is different from the m-axes of an m-dimensional plot
  - Is of one dimension and aims to represent points plotted on m-dimensions
  - Is selected to preserve the differences between points evident in the m-dimensional plot (i.e. if 2 groups are evident in a 3D plot, 2 groups must be discernable in the 1D principal component line)

One or two principal component variables can be computed. The first variable (referred to here as PC1) aims to capture as much of the original characteristics of the distribution of points as possible. The second PC variable (here, PC2) is constructed to obtain the rest of the characteristics that could not be described by the first. PC1 and PC2 are not correlated; they are 2 independent observations of the distribution of points obtained in the m-dimensional analysis. PCA involves the calculation of the eigenvalue decomposition of a data covariance matrix or singular value decomposition of a data matrix, usually after mean centering the data for each attribute (Massart, et al. 1997–1998). Details in this direction are not included here as they are beyond the scope of this book.

Extensive data tables such as in QSAR contain a large amount of information not only a lists of numbers but also in the form of relationships between them. These relations remain hidden because the data is too voluminous and complex to be interpreted right away. In such a situation, PCA steps in. PCA helps in the quantitative determination of:

1. The difference between two samples
2. The variables responsible for this difference
3. Whether these variables are correlated
4. The presence of patterns such as the clustering of data points
5. Identify useful information (signal) amidst background information (noise).

Background 1

One should know that variance is calculated for a univariate analysis and that covariance is calculated for a bivariate analysis. When there are more than 2 variables (multivariate analyses include 2 or more variables), the correlation of all possible pair of variables is investigated. Covariance is expressed as a matrix.

Consider 2 variables X and Y collected for every molecule in a dataset; the covariance is calculated as:

$$\begin{pmatrix} cov(X,X) & cov(X,Y) \\ cov(Y,X) & cov(Y,Y) \end{pmatrix}$$

- The diagonal elements of this matrix cov(X, X) and cov(Y, Y) represent univariate variances of X and Y values respectively
- The most important terms are the non-diagonal elements, namely cov(X, Y) and cov(Y, X)
- Again, cov(X, Y) = cov(Y, X) (*ref.* standard text book) and so corresponding elements on either side of the diagonal are equal (there is symmetry across the diagonal)

- Positive non-diagonal element (remember in the above case both non-diagonal elements are equal) indicates positive correlation between X and Y (meaning increase in X leads to an increase in Y) and vice versa.

Background 2

A background of the basics of matrices helps in understanding some simple aspects of PCA analysis. We know that matrices of the same size can be multiplied. When a transforming matrix is multiplied to the left of a vector, the vector is transformed from its original position to a new one. If the transformation is such that the new vector is only longer (by a certain number of times) than the old vector, the vector is called an *eigenvector*. For example, in the equation below the first case is not an eigenvector, but the second is. In the second, the transformation matrix is multiplied to the left of a vector that points to {3, 2} from the origin {0, 0}. The number by which its length is increased (i.e., 4) is the eigenvalue. Qualitatively, pertaining to this section, one can understand the *eigenvalue* as that values which indicates which vector fits the data best.

$$\begin{bmatrix} 2 & 3 \\ 2 & 1 \end{bmatrix} \times \begin{bmatrix} 1 \\ 3 \end{bmatrix} = \begin{bmatrix} 11 \\ 5 \end{bmatrix}$$

$$\begin{bmatrix} 2 & 3 \\ 2 & 1 \end{bmatrix} \times \begin{bmatrix} 3 \\ 2 \end{bmatrix} = \begin{bmatrix} 12 \\ 8 \end{bmatrix} = 4 \times \begin{bmatrix} 3 \\ 2 \end{bmatrix}$$

Eigenvalues can only be found for square matrices (with equal number of rows and columns). However, not all square matrices have eigenvalues or eigenvectors. For square matrices having eigenvectors, there are as many eigenvectors as there are rows (number of rows = no. of columns = no. of dimensions) in the square matrix. The principle that PCA is based on is that each eigenvector is orthogonal (i.e., perpendicular) to the others. If there is a 10 × 10 square matrix with eigenvectors, it will have 10 eigenvectors pointing in 10 perpendicular directions in space. So, instead of using X-Y-Z description, one can simply use the eigenvectors as the axes of data representation.

The Steps in PCA

Data is collected and arranged as rows and columns (say, parameter X and parameter Y form the columns against rows of molecules, as per the example quoted above)

The average of the values of X (= $\overline{X}$) and the average of the values of Y (= $\overline{Y}$) are calculated; the averages are subtracted from the individual values belonging to the respective parameters (X − $\overline{X}$ and Y − $\overline{Y}$ are carried out). After the latter step, the new dataset of values have average = 0. This step shifts the data centre to the origin {0, 0}, as in, from Scheme 2.25 to Scheme 2.26.

The covariance matrix is calculated (*ref.* background 1 and 2) which is a 2 × 2 matrix

$$\text{cov} = \begin{bmatrix} \text{cov}(X,X) & \text{cov}(X,Y) \\ \text{cov}(Y,X) & \text{cov}(Y,Y) \end{bmatrix}$$

The eigenvector and eigenvalues are calculated for the covariance matrix and converted to unit length (by convention) and this is called *scaling*. In this data, there will be two eigenvectors (because it is a 2 × 2 matrix); when plotted, one of them will pass through the data points as a 'line of best fit' and the other vector will be perpendicular to this line.

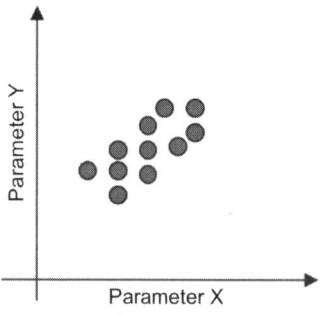

Molecule	Parameter X	Parameter Y
M_1	X_1	Y_1
M_2	X_2	Y_2
:	:	:
	Avg = $\overline{X}$	Avg = $\overline{Y}$

Scheme 2.25: Data arrangement: In rows and columns

Box 26: Arriving at the eigenvector matrix

Feature vector = $\underline{\mathbf{P}}$ = matrix of Eigenvectors = (eig1 eig2...)
Each eigenvector has two elements: eigenvector 1 is represented here by element ∈1,1 (element 1 of vector 1) and ∈2,1 (element 2 of vector 1):

$$eig1 = \begin{pmatrix} \in 1,1 \\ \in 2,1 \end{pmatrix}$$

Similarly, eig2 would contain ∈1, 2 and ∈2, 2
The eigenvector matrix above can be substituted to give:

$$\begin{pmatrix} \in 1,1 & \in 1,2 \\ \in 2,1 & \in 2,2 \end{pmatrix}$$

Each eigenvector indicates the direction in which a vector is pointing to from the origin. For a 2D analysis, such as the one currently considered, the eigenvector has 2 elements.

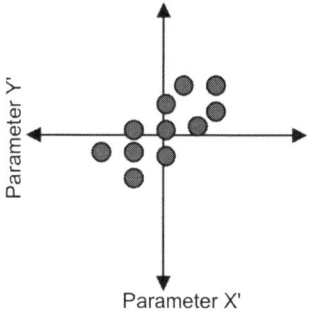

Molecule	Parameter X	Parameter Y
M_1	X_1	Y_1
M_2	X_2	Y_2
:	:	:
	Avg = $\overline{X}$	Avg = $\overline{Y}$

Scheme 2.26: Shifting the data centre to the origin

> **Box 27:** Workflow for data in 3 dimensions
>
> *For a 3D analysis:*
> 3 D → 3 variables → 3 × 3 covaraince matrix → 3 eigenvectors → (each eigenvector having 3 elements to point the direction) → feature vector (also a 3 × 3 matrix because 3 eigenvectors are 3 columns each containing 3 elements distributed in 3 rows)

The eigenvector with the largest eigenvalue is the one that acts as the best fit and will be selected as the principal component (PC1). For a dataset having more parameters, more eigenvectors will result, all of which will be perpendicular to each other. Depending on whether the final result needs mD→1D or mD→2D compression (where m is the number of dimensions of the dataset) the principal component and/ or another representative vector are used.

In this case, let us assume that the aim of executing PCA is to condense 2D data to 1D. In that case, we take only the principal component vector PC1 and simply drop the other vector.

Final feature vector = (eig1) *wherein eig1 is shortened as per Box 26*

The next step would be to project the data onto the selected principal axis:

* Transpose the final feature vector (interchange the rows and columns, as described in any standard textbook) = final feature vector^T

  Transpose the X'–Y' dataset (which is the new dataset obtained after the average was subtracted from the members of each parameter in Scheme 2.26) = X'–Y' dataset^T

* Multiply the transposed feature vector (final feature vector^T above) to the left of the transposed X'–Y' dataset matrix (X'–Y' dataset^T above)

  Final feature vector^T × X'–Y' dataset^T = Result of PCA

$$= \text{new component/latent variable}$$

$$u_i = aX_i + bY_i \ (\textit{ref. under definition of PC})$$

* Thus a set of new variables (called the *components* or the *latent variables*) are generated that are spread over fewer dimensions (1 or 2)

The distance of separation between two points along the 1D axis (PC axis) indicates degree of similarity of the two objects they represent (here, molecules) So, PCA has been successfully used to condense 2D information to just 1D. In Fig. 2.32, we need to focus only on PC1 and the spread of points along this 1D axis. As mentioned earlier, the purpose of performing multivariate analysis is to test for the presence of

* Correlation between variables (in raw data) – presented as a *loading plot*.
* Similarity between objects – obtained from a *score plot*.

Thus one can also determine which of the (many thousand) features (of, say, a QSAR analysis) play a role in determining object (molecule) similarity. The score and loading plots work thus:

* The score and loading plots are 2D and so, here, we consider both PC1 and PC2 (so these plots are used to reduce 3D and higher dimension distribution to 2D).
* The score plot is a plot of row vectors–each point represents objects; it is plotted using the values obtained in the result of the PCA by including PC1 and PC2 in the final feature vector^T expression.

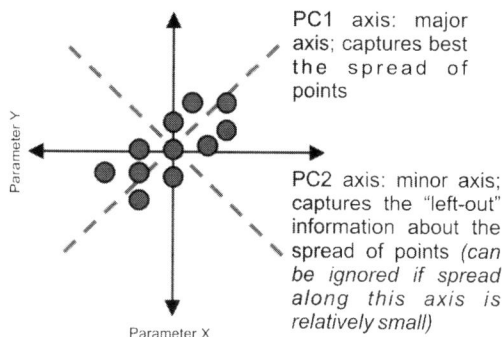

Parameter Y

PC1 axis: major axis; captures best the spread of points

PC2 axis: minor axis; captures the "left-out" information about the spread of points *(can be ignored if spread along this axis is relatively small)*

Parameter X

Fig. 2.32: Two principal component axes

- The loading plot is a plot of column vectors–each point represents features; it is plotted from the **P** feature vector matrix (*ref.* scaling above) in using values of PC1 and PC2.

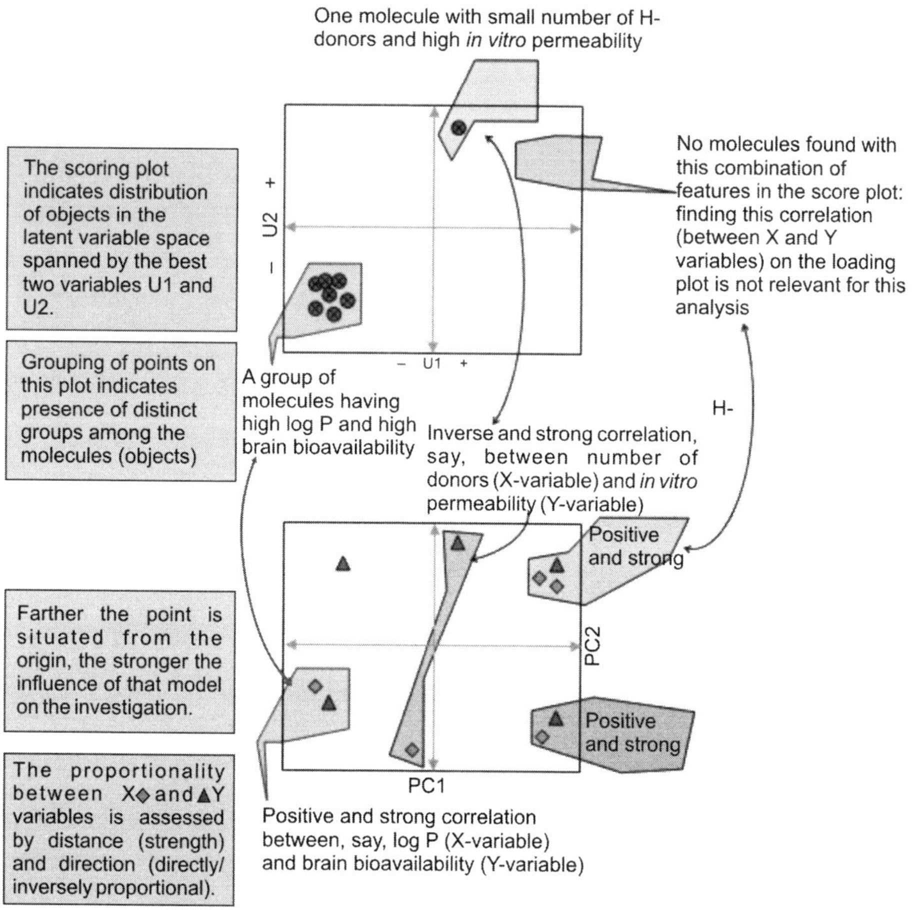

One molecule with small number of H-donors and high *in vitro* permeability

The scoring plot indicates distribution of objects in the latent variable space spanned by the best two variables U1 and U2.

No molecules found with this combination of features in the score plot: finding this correlation (between X and Y variables) on the loading plot is not relevant for this analysis

U2

– U1 +

Grouping of points on this plot indicates presence of distinct groups among the molecules (objects)

A group of molecules having high log P and high brain bioavailability

Inverse and strong correlation, say, between number of donors (X-variable) and *in vitro* permeability (Y-variable)

H-

Positive and strong

Farther the point is situated from the origin, the stronger the influence of that model on the investigation.

PC2

Positive and strong

The proportionality between X◇ and ▲Y variables is assessed by distance (strength) and direction (directly/inversely proportional).

PC1

Positive and strong correlation between, say, log P (X-variable) and brain bioavailability (Y-variable)

Fig. 2.33: Score plot and loadings plots

- It must be noted that in case of datasets having more than 2 parameters, the two eigenvectors with largest eigenvalues are considered (i.e. PC1 and PC2) and are used to construct these plots. The plot can be constructed by including PC3, PC4, etc. as all of the PCs (the latent variables) are independent 'snapshots' of the original dataset, however, these do not give us maximum information (for an analysis with 5 PCs in total PC1 can give, say, 50% information and PC2, say, 25% information. PC3–PC5 together cover only 25% and therefore each PC does not contain as much information as the first two).

The two plots are meant to be read together (they are complementary)–so the same 2 PCs are plotted on both. The loading plot is a means to interpret the scoring plot-the two plots are complementary and equivalent (i.e. a direction in one plot corresponds to the same direction in the other plot).

***Selective reference: (Salkind, 2007)

2.4.4 PARTIAL LEAST SQUARE (PLS) METHODS

Although good correlation can be inferred using PCA from the huge amount of data, in the CoMFA example in Fig. 2.27 under section 2.4.2, PLS is the method of choice. This is because one of the goals of 3D QSAR is to establish a predictive framework based on the data collected (the descriptors of the molecules and the biological activity). In accordance with this goal, PLS is a more a predictive technique than a correlating technique. One cannot expect to obtain an understanding of the relationship of variables as from Principal Component Analysis. The emphasis in PLS is mainly on combining all available information (whether the influence of these information on setting up a model is high or low). This method strikes a balance between

- Variance–which describes how much a feature or variable (such as log P) in the raw data varies among the molecules of study (higher the variance of log P, the greater diversity of log P values one sees among molecules), and
- Correlation–which establishes the strength and direction of relationship between two variables

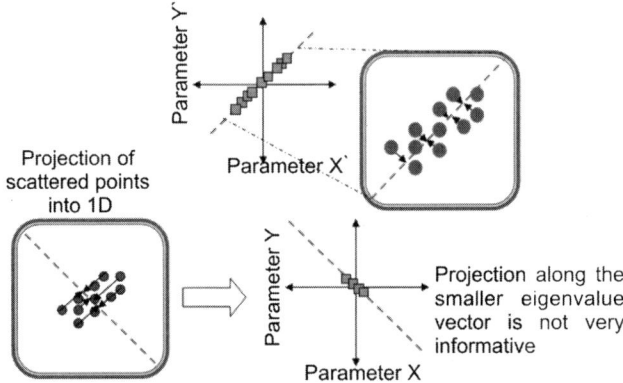

Scheme 2.27: Comparing the efficiency of the two principal components PC1 and PC2

PLS is also a technique deployed to avoid *over fitting of data*. Over fitting is a situation wherein the model fits observed data very well, but is unable to handle predictions! In PLS, the several variables collected in the raw data (the thousands of molecular descriptors) are first condensed to obtain latent variables. Again, as under PCA, latent variables are independent variables that describe the raw data. However, the latent variables under PLS are different from those under PCA. There are fewer latent variables than there are variables. In this way redundancy of information is eliminated. So, the PLS method is also expanded to 'Projection to Latent Structure'

PCA is performed when there are a lot more predictors than there are observations. But in PCA, in contrast to PLS, there is no guarantee that the principal components selected to best describe X, are appropriate for Y also. *Factors* result in *responses*; in this analysis,

- 'X' variables represent *factors* (or *predictor variable*) such as log P, molecular weight, number of hydrogen bonds, etc. of objects (= molecules)
- *Responses* or the Y variables are *dependent variables* which could include bioavailability, blood brain barrier crossing, permeability, excretion rate, etc.
- The X-matrix is constructed with objects and predictors, and the Y matrix with objects and dependent variables

Overall principle: PLS regression concentrates on the components of X that are also relevant for Y. This is carried out in the following steps:

- The components are obtained from the simultaneous decomposition of X and Y such that that the first two eigenvectors best describe the covariance
- Let us consider X decomposition–that it gives T (X-score matrix) and P (X-loading matrix)
- *Two latent variables are calculated:*
  - 'T' is obtained from X (by adding number of constraints; see the next point below) and is also called X-scores
  - 'U', also called Y-scores, is estimated from T (i.e. $U = TBC^T$) wherein B is a diagonal matrix
- (From above) constraints on T: When the first latent variable is obtained, it is subtracted from X and Y (compare with PCA wherein the average of X was subtracted from all values of X and that of Y was subtracted from all Y values). With the calculation of subsequent latent variables, iterative subtraction reduces X to a null matrix.
- Weights obtained from X matrix are stored as C (referred to above) and those obtained from Y matrix, stored as a W-matrix
- Predicted Y weights as U and derived Y weights as C are compared and adjusted
- The final estimation of Y-scores is done from C. Adjustments and estimations at every level involve a process called *normalization*. It involves calculation of the squares of the matrices after transforming those using Z-scores.

Summary: X and Y decomposition yields (after a number of steps, amidst other matrices) X-scores, X-weights, Y-scores, Y-weights and Y-predicted weights. Adjustments ensue based on the comparison between the predicted and derived weights of Y. The prediction of the dependent variables (Y-variables of bioloavailability, etc.) from the independent variables (X-variables of log P, etc.) can be carried out for new molecules. In this way, the aspects of X that most influence Y are favored; thus this decomposition of X with weights adjusted to Y is used to predict Y for unknown molecules. The overall flow is as in Scheme 2.28.

References: (Tobias, 1995; Eriksson, et al. 2006; Salkind, 2007)

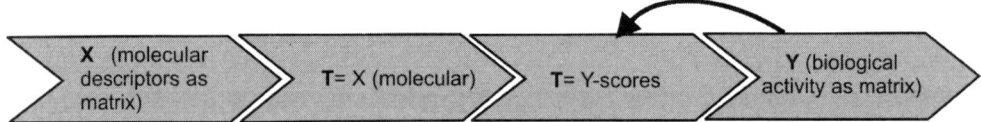

Scheme 2.28: Workflow in Partial Least Squares regression technique

2.4.5 A QUICK INTRODUCTION TO ARTIFICIAL NEURAL NETWORKS

Section contributed by Balaji Raghavan

Artificial Neural Networks (ANNs) have been developed as a generalization of the mathematical model of a biological neural system. In other words, they mimic the performance of a biological neural network. ANNs use a network of "neurons" and uses this network to process information and perform computations. The major advantage is that ANNs are adaptive learning systems that change based on the information flowing through the network in the initial phase, called the *learning/training phase*. ANNs are used extensively for the computational analysis of highly complex models. For example, Fig. 2.34 shows a 3-layered network containing 7-part input, 3-part output and 1 hidden layer in between with 10 nodes. This is called the *architecture* of the network. Other architectures can have several hidden layers.

The Artificial Neural Network is built with a systematic step-by-step procedure to optimize a performance criterion or to follow some implicit constraint, which is commonly referred to as the *learning or training rule*.

The basic processing elements of neural networks are called *artificial neurons*, or simply neurons or nodes. In a simplified mathematical model of the neuron, the effects

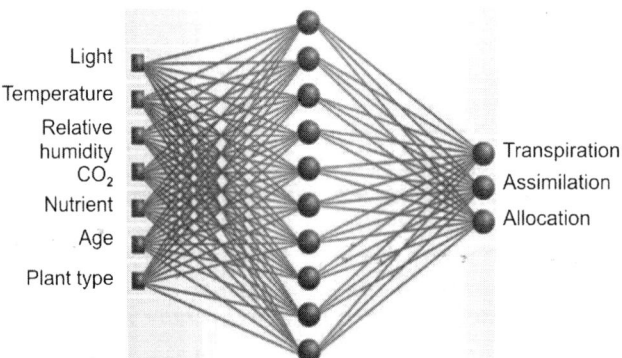

Fig. 2.34: Sample ANN in computational biology[3]—ascertaining the relative contributions of the variables on the left to the processes on the right

of the synapses are represented by *connection weights* that modulate the effect of the associated input signals, and the nonlinear characteristic exhibited by neurons is represented by a *transfer function*. A transfer function is very simply a mathematical operation (multiplication by a constant/variable, integration, differentiation, etc) performed on an input/intermediate variable to obtain an intermediate or final output.

The neuron impulse is then computed as the weighted sum of the input signals, transformed by the transfer function.

Mathematical Model

Figure 2.35 shows the control diagram for a "neural cell" with n synapses in a simple ANN, with corresponding synaptic control weights from 0 to n. The actual activity in this cell is simply adding the p synaptic inputs and applying a transfer function called the "activation function" (example: threshold activation $\varphi(v) = 1$ for non-zero v and 0 otherwise). There are three types of activation functions: threshold, piecewise-linear and sigmoid.

This neural cell may be represented as

$$y(k) = \text{Phi} \left(\Sigma \, \text{weight}_j . \text{input signal}_j \right)$$

Or

$$Y(s) = \text{PHI} \left(\Sigma \, \text{Weight}_j (s). \text{Input signal}_j (s) \right), \text{ in the Laplace form.}$$

The number of hidden neurons affects how well the network is able to separate the data. A large number of hidden neurons will ensure correct learning, and the network is able to correctly predict the data it has been trained on, but its performance on new data (its ability to generalize) is compromised.[5] With too few hidden neurons, the

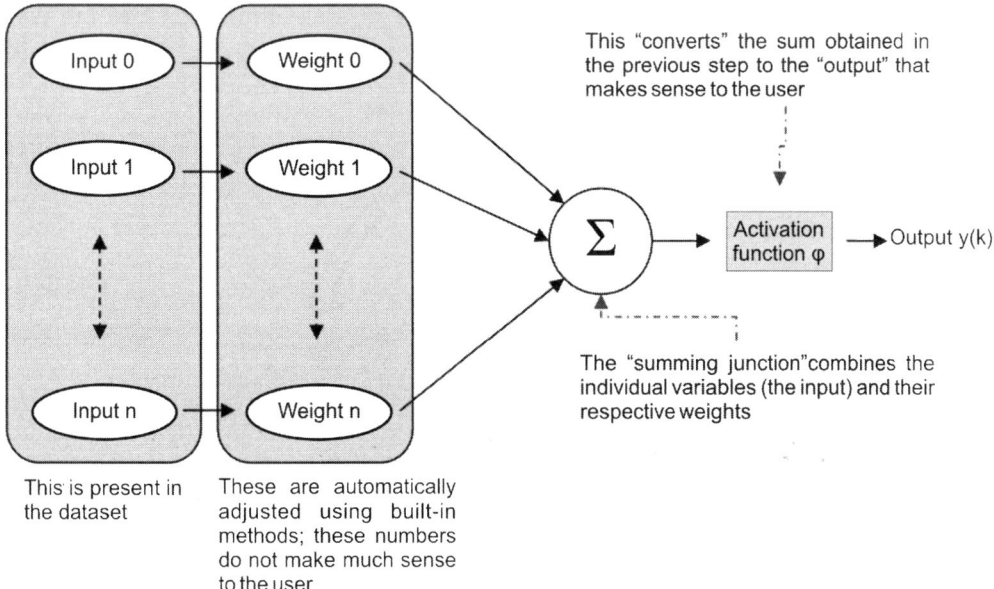

Fig. 2.35: Control diagram for an ANN.[3]

network may be unable to learn the relationships amongst the data and the error will fail to fall below an acceptable level. Thus, selection of the number of hidden neurons is a crucial decision.

Training Phase

In this introduction, we will limit the discussion to a short description of the training phase. The data/information flowing through the ANN are of vital importance in this initial phase. An input is presented to the neural network and a corresponding desired or target response set at the output (when this is the case the training is called supervised). An error is composed from the difference between the desired response and the system output. This error information is fed back to the system, and the system parameters are adjusted in a systematic fashion (the learning rule) as in Fig. 2.36. The "feedback" obtained from the output that is used to adjust the weights corresponding to the signals is referred to as the "Back-propagation algorithm". The learning capability of an artificial neuron in the ANN is achieved by adjusting the connection weights in accordance to the chosen learning algorithm. This process is repeated until the performance of the ANN is acceptable.

It is important to note that if the data does not cover an adequate portion of the operating conditions or if it is too noisy, then ANNs will be unable to solve the problem adequately[5]. On the other hand, if there is sufficient data, then even though the problem may not be properly modeled, ANNs will be capable of obtaining a solution. The performance of the ANN thus hinges heavily on the data available in the learning phase.

Examples of Artificial Neural Networks

There are several ready-made types of neural networks. These have a fixed architecture (referring to the number of hidden layers, the type of algorithm, etc.) and are used depending on the purpose of the problem at hand. Examples:
• Recurrent network

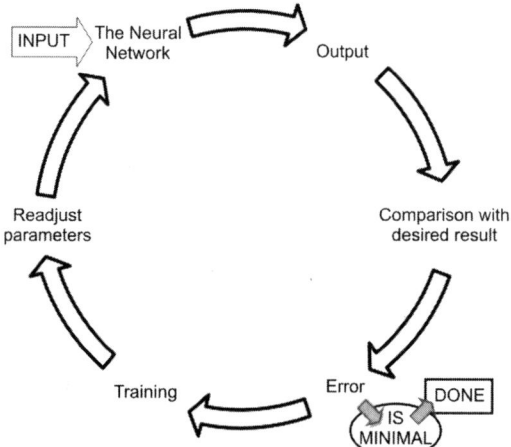

Fig. 2.36: Schematic of training phase[2]; for technical representation

- Stochastic neural network
- Modular neural network
- Physical neural network
- Feedforward neural network
- Radial basis function (RBF) network
- Kohonen self-organizing network.

References

1. M. H. Hassoun. Fundamentals of Artificial Neural Networks MIT Press, 1995.
2. K. Gurney. An Introduction to Neural Networks London: Routledge, 1997.
3. http://en.wikibooks.org/wiki/Artificial_Neural_Networks
4. S. Hayden. Neural Networks: A Comprehensive Foundation, Prentice Hall, 1999.
5. Ajith Abraham. Artificial Neural Networks, Oklahoma State University, Stillwater, OK, USA, 2005.

Applications in Pharmacy

The ANNs were not used much in pharmacy until close to the turn of the millennium. The successful employment of different neural network approaches to distinguish drugs from non-drugs [(Ajay, et al. 1998); (Sadowski, et al. 1998)] is notable. Following this, numerous Neural Network models evolved to ascertain QSAR and 3D-QSAR relationships in various molecules. Some of these works are as mentioned below:

- Barlow, T.W. (1995). Self-organizing maps and molecular similarity. J. Mol. Graphics 13, 24–27.
- Anzali, S., Gasteiger, J., Holzgrabe, U., Polañski, J., Sadowski, J., Tackentrup, A., Wagener, M. (1998). The use of self-organizing neural networks in drug design; in 3D QSAR in Drug Design (Kubinyi, H., Folkers, G. & Martin, Y.C., eds), vol. 2, pp. 273–299, ESCOM/ Kluwer, Dordrecht.
- Polañski, J., Gasteiger, J., Wagener, M. & Sadowski, J. (1998). The comparison of molecular surfaces by neural networks and its application to quantitative structure activity studies. Quant. Struct. Act. Relat. 17, 27–36.
- Jaroslaw Polañski (2000). Self-organizing neural network for modeling 3D QSAR of colchicinoids; Acta Biochimica Polonica 47 (1); 37–45

Recommended read: Gasteiger, J.; Zupan, J. (1993). Neural Networks for Chemists – An Introduction, VCH, Weinheim.

Part III
The Ligand and
the Receptor

"The single most important event in pharmacology is the interaction between a drug molecule and its receptor. The driving force for this spectacular interaction is its chemistry—the steric and electrostatic match between two complementary surfaces which determines their mutual affinity..."

– Andrews, 2005

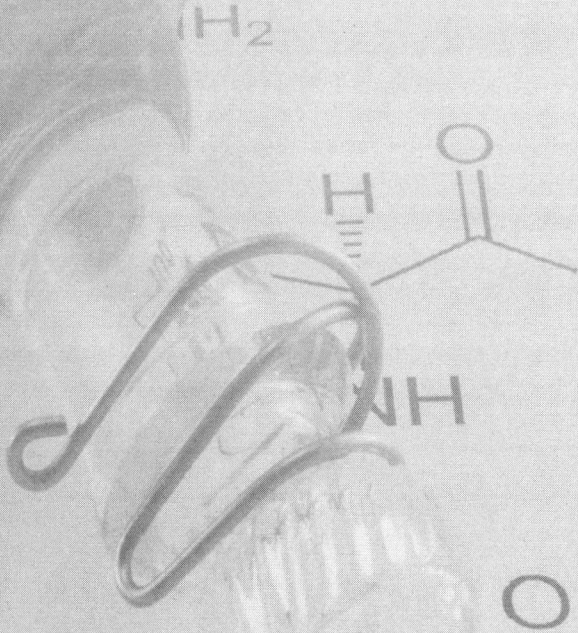

3.1 *Molecular Recognition*

Part III of this book on the modern principles of medicinal chemistry deals with the study of protein–ligand interactions. It is divided into two parts–the first dealing with the biochemical and pharmacological theories of drug receptor binding (under section 3.1 Molecular Recognition) and the second, outlining the use of such theories in predicting binding (under section 3.2 Docking). It is believed that students will be able to appreciate that the knowledge of part I on proteins is as important as the knowledge of part II on ligands. After all, the drugs are the keys and the proteins are the doors that open into a world of reactions cascades, the modulation of which can help us cure diseases and control disorders.

3.1.1 INTRODUCTION

There is an increasing level of complexity in the interaction between various systems from the sub-atomic world to the behavior of compounds. Figure 3.1 demonstrates this concept using water molecule as an example: generally, in order to derive macroscopic properties from sub-atomic level information, one needs greater approximations owing to this increase in complexity. But these approximations inevitably result in less accurate results.

For example, consider the property that water is transparent and is a liquid at room temperature. The calculation of refractive index, the calculation of the wavelength of the emitted light during excited-state→ground-state transition of water molecules (and other quantities that can be calculated from the electronic state of the H_2O molecule) will reveal that water is colorless at room temperature. Similarly, the fact that water is a liquid in the same environmental conditions can also be derived. Such *Ab initio*

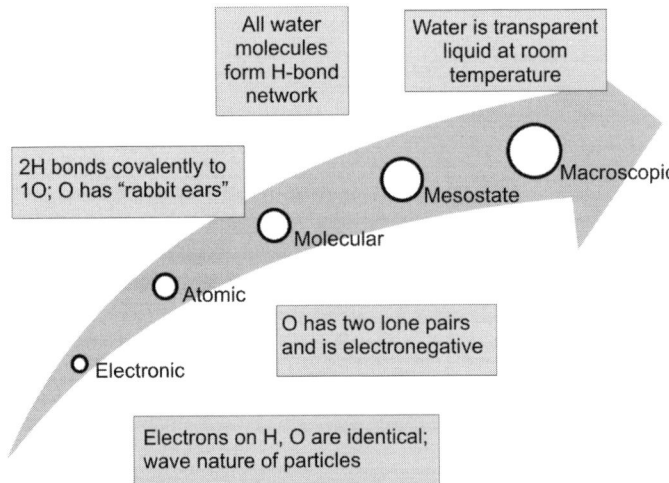

Fig. 3.1: Levels of complexity from sub-atomic state to macroscopic state of water

treatment as mentioned earlier is extremely time-consuming. Introducing approximations in the formulae to save time and computational resources produces corresponding inaccuracies in the derived properties. One can also be semi-empirical in treating this situation–the refractive index of water can be substituted from (experimentally) pre-determined values or the wavelength mentioned above used from values that were (computationally) pre-calculated. From these quantities one could derive the fact that water is transparent. Similarly, given the amino acid sequence of an experimentally un-isolatable receptor (protein), the computer can predict the bioactive structure to that much accuracy as the scientists are clear about the phenomenon (discussed in part I, chapters 1.4 and 1.5). In the same manner, given the structure of a ligand molecule, QSAR studies (as discussed in Part II) can predict binding affinities to that much accuracy as the availability of relevant information from experiments.

It is clear from the above explanation that the scientist specifies the salient points about the calculation to the computer–such as the method used to arrive at macroscopic properties, the geometry of the molecule, atomic composition, electron behavior, etc. in the form of equations that computers can understand–and the computer performs the calculations accordingly to give the result. This concept is summarized in Fig. 3.2.

The so-called 'Docking studies' performed using software is not different in any way. In simple words, the biochemists and pharmacologists convert observations of drug activity into hypotheses on target binding that are written out as equations of intermolecular molecular attractions and tested using docking software. However, it must never be forgotten that any *in-silico* technique even if greatly perfected over generations of research is always limited by computational resources and time when trying to describe the complete biological environment. Molecular pharmacology is extremely complex that no single software can claim to be robust in its predictions of macroscopic effects such as drug binding, inhibitory concentration, etc. Neither can one claim that purely relying on experimental trial-and-error without sound foundation on theory will lead us somewhere worthwhile on the path of discovery and innovation.

3.1.2 THEORIES OF DRUG BINDING

> *"To use an image, I would say that enzyme and glycoside have to fit into each other like a lock and a key, in order to exert a chemical effect on each other."*
>
> *Fischer, 1894*

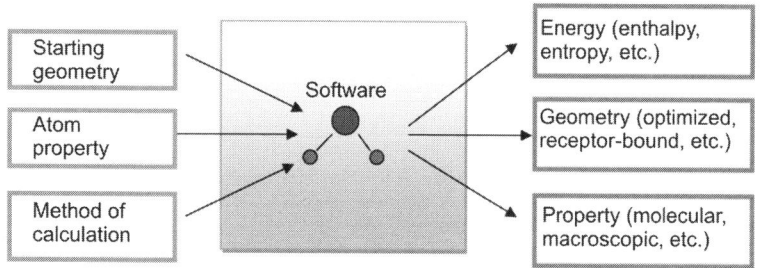

Fig. 3.2: The software and the scientist

Table 3.1: Explanation of some terms relating to drug-protein interaction

Term	Usage
Accessory sites	The site to which competitive antagonists bind[1]
Activated state	The state of the receptor in which it can couple with effector molecules resulting in pharmacological effect
Affinity	Is the ability of a drug to combine with a receptor; it is proportional to the binding equilibrium constant KD. A ligand of low affinity requires a higher concentration to produce the same effect. Both agonists and antagonists have affinity to the receptor
Agonist	Is a substance that interacts with a specific cellular constituent, the receptor, and elicits an observable biological response. It may be endogenous or exogenous substance
Antagonist	Inhibits the effect of an agonist but has no biological activity of its own. It may compete on the same receptor site, that the agonist occupies on an accessory site or it may act on allosteric site
Antimetabolite	A molecular analogue of an intermediate that is formed in the cascade of physiological reactions and replaces the intermediate to halt the formation of a downstream product
Auto receptor	A macromolecule typically found in the nerve ending that regulates the synthesis and/or the release of its own ligand
Heteroreceptor	Is a receptor that regulates the synthesis and/or the release of chemical mediators other than its own ligand
Intrinsic activity	Is a proportionality constant of the ability of the agonist to activate the receptor as compared to the maximally active compound in the series being studied
Inverse agonist or negative antagonist	It acts on the same receptor of the agonist yet produces an inverse effect
Isoreceptors	Different structural and functional forms of a receptor that can be found in different parts of the body. Example—adrenergic isoreceptors react in quantitatively different manner to norepinephrine depending on the organ, the form of the isoreceptor, etc.
Multiplicity of receptors	The property of a receptor to occur as different types - in different parts of the body at pharmacologically distinct points performing different functions. Examples—neurotransmitters and adrenergic receptors
Partial agonists	Acts on the same receptor as agonists, however, regardless of its dose it cannot produce the same maximal biological response as a full agonist
Plasticity of receptor[2]	Ability of the receptor to undergo a conformational change (used in association with approach of complementary ligand)
Receptor down-regulation	Is a phenomenon whereby an agonist actually induces a decrease in the number of those receptors available for binding.
Receptor up-regulation	Is a phenomenon whereby an agonist, actually induces an increase in the number of those receptors available for binding.

[1]In Table 3.1: Originally, the competitive antagonist was expected to bind to the identical active site of the protein as that bound by its agonist. However, in later years, the lack of structural relation between

agonist and competitive antagonists especially evident among neurotransmiters demanded a review (Nogrady, et al. 2005) of the competitive binding hypothesis. Thus, agonist binding sites, competitive antagonist binding sites (*accessory sites*) and non-competitive antagonist binding sites (*allosteric sites*) are recognized. These sites are at discrete loci on the receptor macromolecule and are comprised of specific amino acids held in their respective positions by the scaffold of the rest of the macromolecule. The *accessory sites* theory justifies 3 aspects:

1. The antagonist has an affinity several fold greater than the agonist
2. The antagonist molecule structures are diverse and different from the agonist structures
3. The antagonists have bulky non-polar or even aromatic groups.

   ² In Table 3.1: (Alvarez, et al. 2005), (Waksman, 2005): We are aware of the stereoelectronic complementarity mentioned in the lock and key hypothesis. Is there an equivalent of this in the induced-fit hypothesis? Yes–this is indicated by the plasticity of the receptor. We know that functional proteins are dynamic (part I chapter 1.3) and can occupy several states such as open ↔ closed (for channels) or activated ↔ deactivated (for enzymes and receptors): these different states occupied by the receptor are as a result of its plasticity. Note: Plasticity does not significantly change function.

Did You Know? 25
Stereospecific ligand binding

A ligand should ideally have 3 stereospecific points of interaction (Alvarez, et al. 2005) with the receptor in order to balance

* *The downsides of multiple potential interactions, which is non-specificity binding and*
* *The downsides of very few interaction-specific centres, which is low potency.*

3.1.2A Classical Theories

Ever since it was proposed that there is a receptor in the body to which drugs bind [*ref.* introduction in section 2.3.1 (Langley, 1901); (Ahlquist, 1948)], several theories have been proposed to fit experimental observations. In addition to the famous lock and key theory (Fischer, 1894) and the induced fit theory (Koshland, 1958) which readers would have amply encountered, the following theories were proposed to explain drug-receptor interaction:

Occupation theory (Christopoulos, et al. 1999) : Drugs act on independent binding sites and activate them; the biological response is proportional to the number of drug-receptor complexes formed; on dissociation, the response ceases

$$Drug + Receptor \leftrightarrow Drug - Receptor\ complex$$

Rate theory (Paton, 1961): The biological response to drug administration is proportional to the rate of formation of the drug-receptor complex; the duration of receptor occupation determines whether a molecule is agonist, antagonist or partial agonist.

Macromolecular perturbation theory (Belleau, 1964): The receptor changes its conformation (gets perturbed) on drug binding; the resulting conformation is determined by the type of drug and in turn determines the biological effects that follow binding; agonist → a specific conformation (= type of macromolecular perturbation) → biological response, antagonist → any other perturbation → no biologic response

Activation-aggregation theory (Monod, et al. 1965), (Karlin, 1967): An extension of the macromolecular perturbation theory; the activated (bioactive) state ↔ inactivated (bio-inactive) state are in equilibrium whether the drug is present or not; agonists → bind to the bio-active state, antagonist → bind to bio-inactive state.

3.1.2B Molecular Theories

Two State Receptor Model

Classical theory of activation and aggregation (Monod, et al. 1965) was constantly modified and several variants of the two-state model persist [example, (Samama, et al. 1993), (Leff, et al. 1997)] explaining the dynamic nature of receptors: Some receptors exist in a family of low-energy conformers in equilibrium with each other. In receptors that have multimers, the various subunits influence the state of the entire protein and its state in binding the ligand.

Relaxed/activated ↔ tight/deactivated (in equilibrium)

The agonist → possesses affinity to the relaxed state and shifts equilibrium in its favor

The antagonist → possesses affinity to the tight state and shifts equilibrium in its favor

Partial agonist → possesses partial affinity to both states

Note: In all of the above cases, only shifting of equilibrium occurs and no upregulation.

Receptor Co-operativity Model

This model (Sambrano, et al. 1997) is an extension of the 2-state receptor model in which a group of proteins are involved. This theory is coined from the study of hormones such as the estrogen receptor that bind to a whole variety of proteins (called *promoters*) in order to carry out its function. According to this theory,

1. All proteins (the hormone as well as the promoters) have to reach the active/ relaxed state before eliciting its action (such as opening of a channel).

2. The proteins shift from the T to the R state in a cooperative fashion (*ref.* Part I section 1.5.4.B)

3. As and when the proteins shift to the R state, they
   a. Activate other proteins
   b. Influence (increase) affinity of binding to the substrate

4. Sometimes, the binding of substrate to the receptor may induce the modulators to achieve R state

5. A 1:1 ratio of ligand and receptor need not be present for all proteins to shift to R state.

Did You Know? 26
About effector amplification

The event of a few 1000 molecules of the ligand at 10^{-9}–10^{-10} M concentration is amplified by the effector-chain; this chain
1. Results in the macroscopic effects of modifying the receptor
2. Amplifies the molecular event to a large scale [a single open ion channel in a single impulse allows 10–20 thousand ions to pass through and polarizes (or depolarizes) the membrane].

Did You Know? 27
About the cholera toxin

It was inferred from experiments on rats that the Cholera toxin, a protein called Choleragen, diffuses laterally through the plasma membrane of rat hepatocytes, and enzyme then binds to and stimulates the membrane adenylate cyclase by more than 10-fold. This stimulated enzyme has 3-fold greater sensitivity to glucagon (Bennett, et al. 1975).

3.1.3 ESTIMATION OF BINDING ENERGY

Once more, we wish to clarify the difference between energy and enthalpy. The energy of a molecule is its internal energy (E)–the sum of vibrational, rotational and translational energy. The enthalpy (H) change of a reaction is influenced by changes in either pressure or in volume

$$E = H + PV$$

If either P or V is 0, then E = H. Enthalpy changes are calculated at room temperature and atmospheric pressure. In this sense, one actually calculates the binding enthalpy, but as the term is popularly called binding energy, the same term is used in this text. Presented here are two approaches to the calculation of binding energy–the partitioning approach, which involves breaking up of free energy into contributing pieces, and perturbation approach, which involves calculation of energy in a particular setting and then adding corrections based on the changes in the new setting.

3.1.3A Approach 1: Partitioning the Contributions to Free Energy

The free energy changes (ΔG) that takes place on drug binding (to a receptor) result from intermolecular interactions. However, the net change is lowered at the cost of other energies or entropies taking place in the system or the surroundings during the interaction (*ref.* the *entropic effect* under 2.3.2.E). The interactions can be broadly classified into electrostatic, inductive, non-polar and hydrophobic. These have been discussed in detail elsewhere (chapters 2.2 and 2.4). Changes exist in energies and entropies in addition to the potential energy obtained by summing up the energy of (chemical) interactions between ligand and receptor. Points to remember about the changes that influence free energy changes during drug-receptor binding are summarized in the chart on the previous page (Scheme 3.1).

- Rigid ligands do not loose much entropy after binding—they stay pretty much in the same conformation—so their penalty to free energy change is not high. The entropy penalties to binding free energy are indicated.

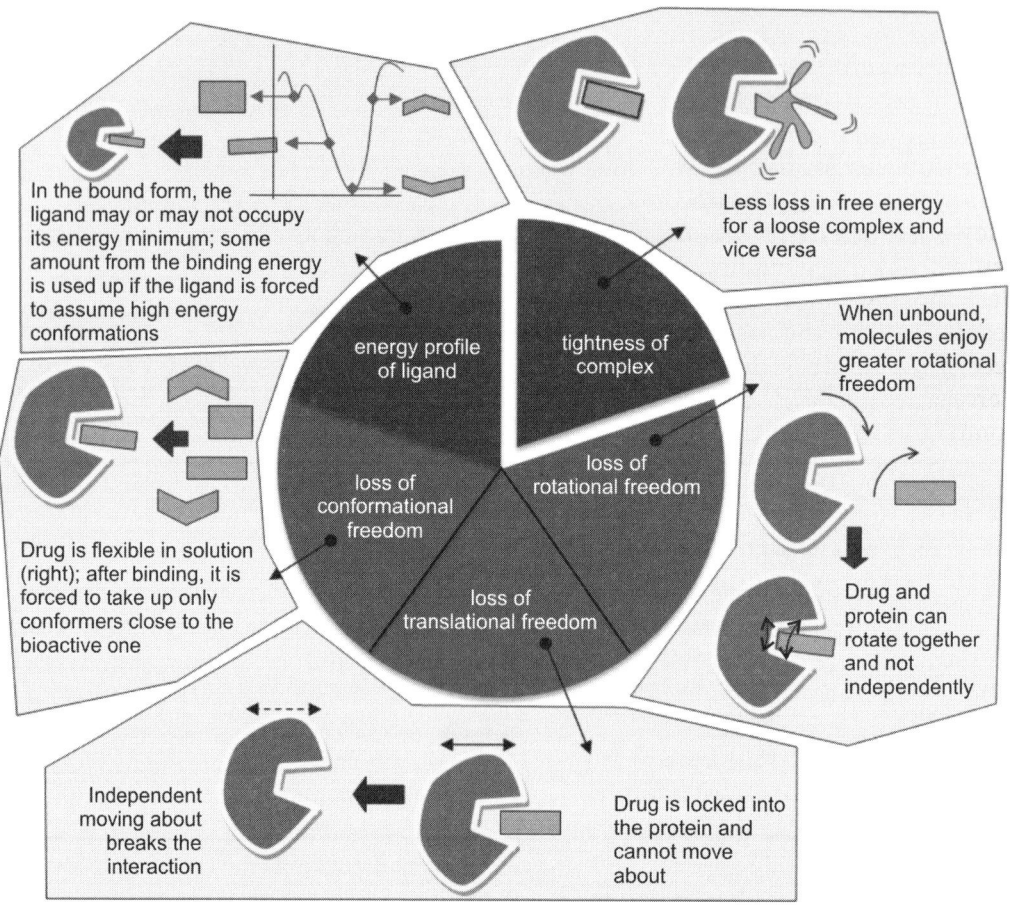

In the bound form, the ligand may or may not occupy its energy minimum; some amount from the binding energy is used up if the ligand is forced to assume high energy conformations

Less loss in free energy for a loose complex and vice versa

When unbound, molecules enjoy greater rotational freedom

Drug is flexible in solution (right); after binding, it is forced to take up only conformers close to the bioactive one

Drug and protein can rotate together and not independently

Independent moving about breaks the interaction

Drug is locked into the protein and cannot move about

energy profile of ligand

tightness of complex

loss of conformational freedom

loss of rotational freedom

loss of translational freedom

Scheme 3.1: General factors that influence free energy of binding of drug to receptor

- Loss of each internal rotation on receptor binding results in an entropy loss that reduces the free energy of binding by an average of 3 KJ/mol. Average binding constant is calculated by summing up the binding energies of the component groups and subtracting the entropy related terms.
- If observed binding energy is greater than this calculated average, drug fits the receptor very well; if it is less than the average, then the fit is not as good as it is in the average case (or the ligand is in a high energy conformation).
- Limitations to such estimates using average values have been discussed in literature (Houk, et al., 2003) and are omitted for clarity. Energy partitioning approach is used by several techniques such as the "Anchor principle", "Site directed mutagenesis approach", "averages approach" etc. descriptions of which are beyond the scope of this book.

The binding energy of each functional group of ligand in its best alignment with respect to its receptor counterpart is summed up to give the *intrinsic binding energy*.

Binding energy of each functional group can be further resolved into several contributing energies and entropies as in Scheme 3.2. In all, 3 rotational and 3 translational degrees of freedom of the ligand are replaced by 6 vibrational degrees of freedom of the complex (i.e. there is relative receptor rigidity and ligand mobility after complex formation. This mobility is called '*residual motion*'. *Ref.* (Krogsgaard-Larsen, et al. 2002)). The freedom enjoyed by the ligand before binding is much greater allowing much larger vibration than the 6 degrees of residual motion that the ligand can perform after binding. When converted to energy, at 310 K this might result in destabilizing binding energy anywhere from 10–50 KJ/mol (=free energy change resulting from the loss of entropy on binding [*ref.* chapter 2: Role of molecular recognition in drug design by Peter Andrews and Michael Dooley in (Krogsgaard-Larsen, et al., 2002)]. The lesser the freedom allowed in the complex (the more rigid complex) the greater the loss binding energy.

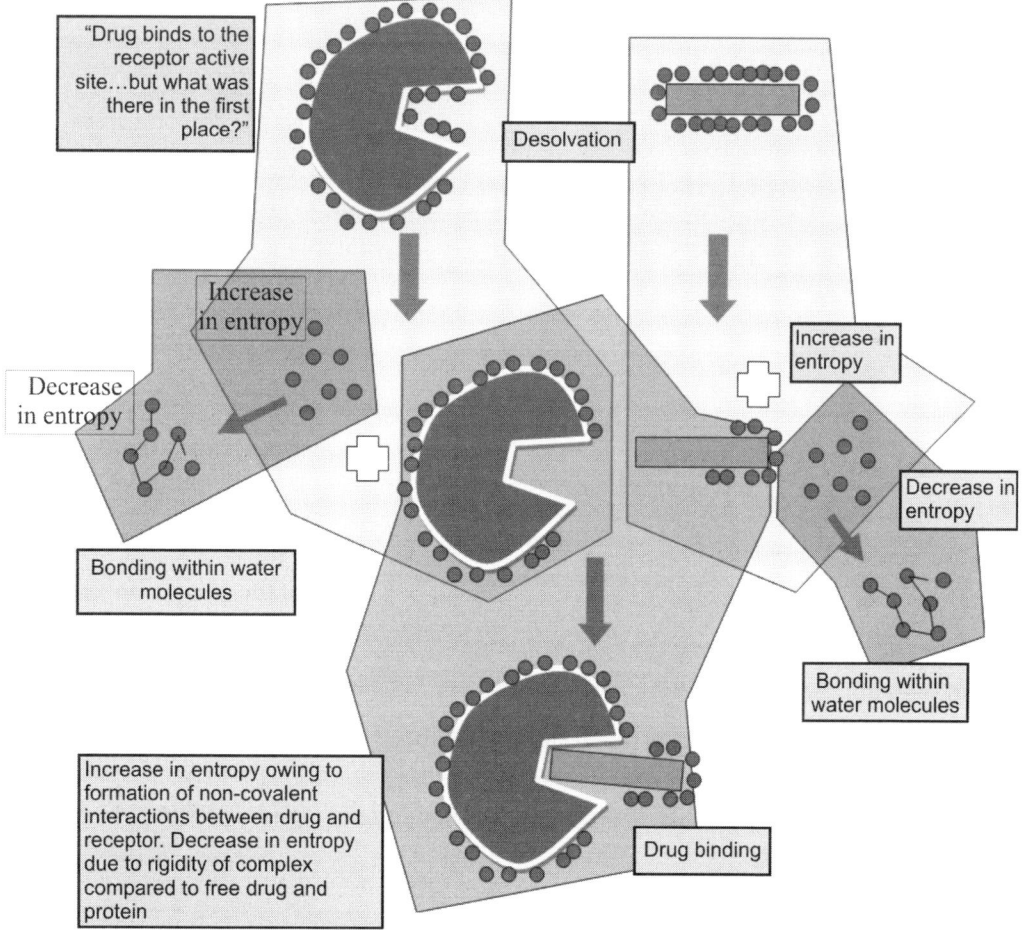

Scheme 3.2: The rise and fall of entropy over the various stages of drug binding with protein indicated qualitatively

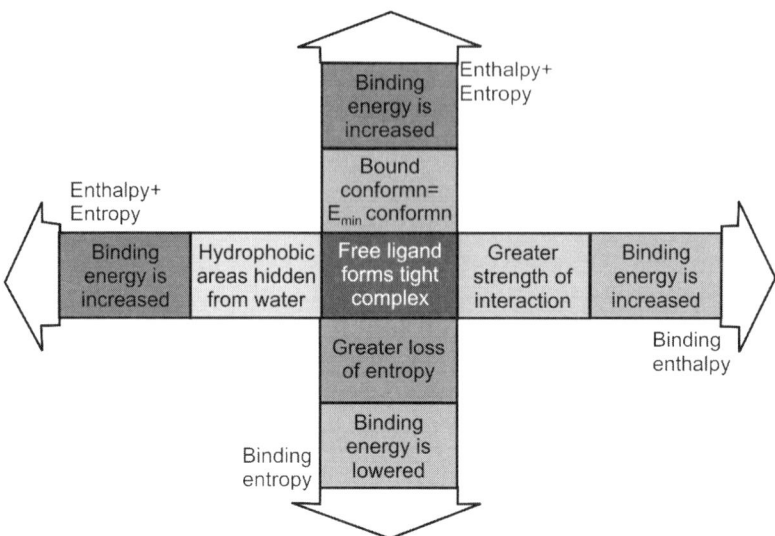

Scheme 3.3: Factors that increase and decrease overall free energy of binding

The translations and rotations above *ref.* to the molecule as a whole. Within the molecule, each rotatable bond also has some degree of freedom taken away from it due to arresting the movement of rotatable bonds (conformational flexibility) after formation of drug-receptor complex. Arresting every rotatable bond results in decrease of binding energy upto 4 kJ/mol (Williams, et al. 1999). Therefore, in general, in drug designing, the binding of a flexible ~300 Da ligand with a ~300 kDa protein might lead to a loss of free energy of binding owing rotational, translational and conformational entropy of ~ 45–60 kJ/mol (several estimates: 45 kJ/mol (Searle, et al. 1992); 58.5 kJ/mol (Böhm, 1998). Increase in binding energy of 0.19 kJ/mol for every square Å of hydrocarbon fragments removed from exposure to water by the binding process has also been calculated (Williams, et al. 1999).

3.1.3.B Approach 2: The Thermodynamic Cycle

The techniques that approach the changes in binding energies as a whole rather than dividing it among the various contributing factors are collectively called *"free energy perturbation"* techniques (Kollman, 1993). If one is still optimizing the structure of molecules based on free energy predictions, the partitioning approaches are the best as they point out what types of changes in structure would improve or destabilize binding energies. When a complete molecule is docked into a protein, the free energy perturbation techniques come handy. One can never be sure that the addition of a group will only affect binding in an additive fashion. In other words, the addition of a group might lead to much greater changes in a molecule, altering its properties globally. In that case, simple additions and subtractions to free energy might not estimate changes correctly. We therefore arrive at a position to distinguish between *intrinsic binding energy* and *apparent binding energy*. The former term refers to the energy (as a sum of enthalpic energy, entropic energy, etc.) obtained when a functional group is conveniently oriented with respect to the protein and the interaction energy calculated. Thus, there is no other factor influencing binding energy values but the presence of that particular functional group in that orientation. The apparent binding energy is that which results from calculations that involve other factors in a global perspective.

The thermodynamic cycle is in principle similar to the Hess's Law (recollect that the latter states that whether a reaction is performed in one or several steps, the overall change in reaction enthalpy is the same) and is applied as follows:

$$\Delta G_{binding\_aq} = \Delta G_{binding\_gas} + \Delta G_{solvation(RL)} - \Delta G_{solvation(R+L)}$$

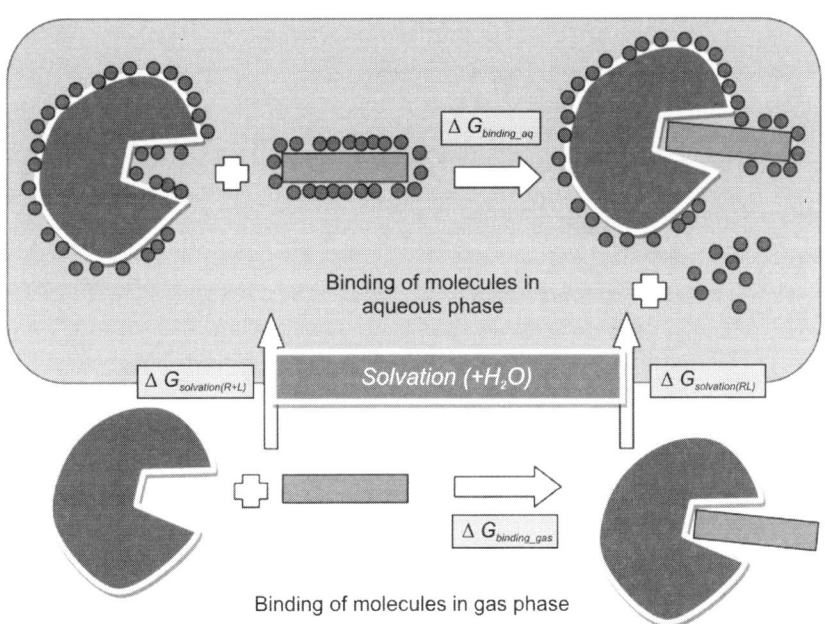

Fig. 3.3: Thermodynamic cycle for calculating aqueous phase binding of ligand

Box 28: What does 'perturbation' mean?

We have come across the word "perturbation" earlier–with reference to perturbation techniques used to calculate molecular orbitals in chapter 2.2, macromolecular perturbation theory earlier in this chapter, as well as the perturbation mean-field approach in fold recognition (chapter 1.4). In this text, the calculation of binding energy is done using a perturbation approach. But, what is the meaning of this term? Perturbation means a change. In methods that follow a perturbational approach, one chooses a similar but simpler situation and compares the current situation with it.

The *difference* is the *change* and is added as a *secondary correction*. Let us consider a simple example: we wish to:

"Predict how a student performs in college"

We know that several factors influence students' performances such as interest of the student, effectiveness of teaching, facilities in the college, etc. One can build up the prediction piece-wise from the mentioned list of parameters and more. This is difficult-how can one account for "interest of student" or "effectiveness of teaching"?

Or one can equate this to a similar situation:

Performance in college = performance in school

Add in second order perturbations:

Performance in college = performance in school + effect of increase in age

Characterize the correction term(s) that has been added

And then check if the correction(s) is sufficient. Some additions greatly improve the description:

Performance in college = Performance in school + effect of increase in age + effect
of change in institution...

For example, in drug design, in the MM3 force field (Allinger, et al. 1989) the $sp^3 - sp^3$ bond stretching potential V_{dist} is not simply the Hooke's law form: $V_{dist} = \frac{1}{2} k\, x^2$. Instead, the Hooke's law ball-and-spring quadratic term is only taken an example situation and cubic and quartic corrections are added to it:

$V_{dist} = \frac{1}{2} k\, x^2 + $ cubic term with $x^3 + $ quartic term with x^4

The simple parabola of Hooke's law was shown to approach the complex Morse potential (ref. section 2.2) by this simple addition that greatly improved the description of bonding by molecular mechanics. Thus one selects a similar and simpler situation and applies *perturbations* to improve it.

3.2 *Docking*

The principles used in docking a ligand into a protein and predicting the affinity are based on the principles of molecular recognition summarized in preceding sections. Even if this event is very restricted in nature, the following aspect explains why a docking study gains considerable importance during the decision making step of whether to promote a drug candidate to the next stage of development or set it aside. The journey of a drug molecule from the port of entry into the body to the site of action is a tedious and uncertain journey often described as a 'random walk'. This is depicted in Fig. 3.4 (from Lecture by Hugo Kubinyi on QSAR parameters at www.kubinyi.de).

When the drug eventually "stumbles upon" the receptor, it must have sufficient *affinity* and *specificity* to bind to it to elicit its action. The specificity of the drug to the receptor lies in the drug being able to complement only those interactions that the receptor seeks. The affinity of the drurg lies in it being able to sufficiently satisfy the demands of the receptor. Some ligands have high affinity but low specificity in which case it becomes a non-specific binder and may never reach the receptor until it saturates all the non-specific sites of binding along its course indicated in the figure.

Such behavior is indicated by the drug's efficacy. In contrast, a ligand with good specificity but low affinity needs to concentrate itself sufficiently around the receptor to be able to elicit the desired action. Thus the effect of the ligand will not manifest unless several of its molecules simultaneously complete their 'walk' and end up accumulating around the receptor. Along the way, a drug candidate will have to encounter millions of molecules. The candidate that is design to cut down on non-specific interactions with other molecules and increase interaction with the protein will be accepted as a good drug candidate. To cut down on the non-specific nature of the drug, one follows rules such as Lipinski's rule of 5 (chapter 2.2) and this improves pharmacokinetics. These concepts are summarized in Scheme 3.4. To increase

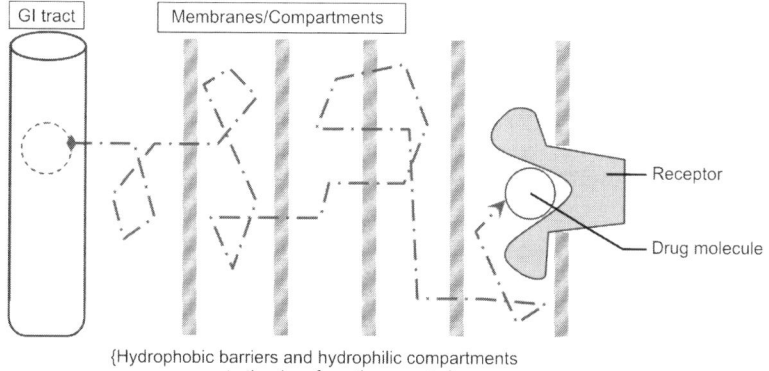

{Hydrophobic barriers and hydrophilic compartments
separate the drug from the receptor}

Fig. 3.4: The drug takes a random walk to reach the receptor

417

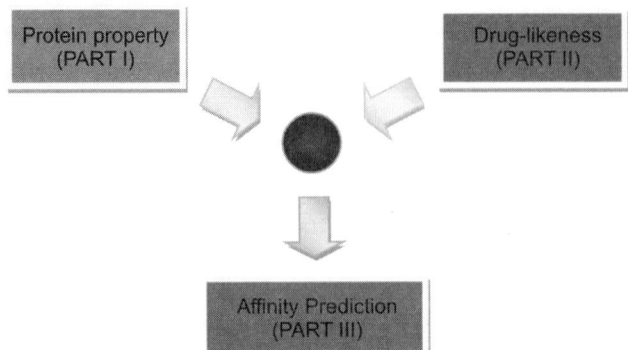

Scheme 3.4: Approaching docking with knowledge about protein and ligand

specificity one needs to complement the drug to the receptor as detailed in this chapter. Here, ligand property meets protein chemistry and the combined knowledge is used to study docking.

3.2.1 INTRODUCTION

"No, this trick won't work...How on earth are you ever going to explain
in terms of chemistry and physics so important a biological phenomenon as first love?"

Albert Einstein

Docking is the process of "molecular recognition" that is computationally simulated. This simply involves placing one molecule in the vicinity of the other and calculating the interacting forces to decide whether they are attractive or repulsive (i.e. whether the receptor will bind the drug or not). When one is trying to complex a small molecule with a larger one, perhaps for formulation or drug delivery purposes, the following needs to be considered:

• Before modeling such interactions, it is important to know whether the force field can describe both the classes of molecules involved.

• It is also important to determine whether the force field can handle the effects that operate in the complex. As mentioned in section 2.2.4, some force fields cannot model special type of interactions such as electron pair interactions, π-conjugations, etc.

• Are the molecules so big to use molecular mechanics to perform this modeling and calculation? Quantum calculations can cover complex formations and molecular mechanical modeling must be used only after investigating whether *Ab-initio*, Semi-empirical and DFT methods (*ref.* section 2.3.E.3 Energy minimization types for an overview) are either inappropriate or end up taxing existing computational resources.

• Is a reasonable 3D structure of the protein and the ligand available? Docking cannot be performed without these files!

• Does literature report at least moderate success in the use of a similar ligand molecule(s)/protein(s) using the default force fields of the docking program? Or are modifications necessary to the force field/scoring function (discussed later in this section)

As described in part 1 and 2, one of the most important aspects of geometry optimization is determination of the global minimum by avoiding or overcoming local minima that act as kinetic traps. Before delving deeper into docking, please read through for a list of terminology and their definitions that will be used throughout Part III.

Table 3.2: Terminology used in docking

Affinity score	A detailed score (including several terms in the force field) is computed after an initial dock score (done including only few terms in the force field)
Degrees of freedom searched	Ligand is searched for translational, rotational, internal degrees of freedom
Dock score	An initial dock score (based on only van der Waal's and electrostatic) is computed
Pose	Each docking mode is called a 'pose' and involves a specific position, conformation or orientation of the ligand in the protein's active site
Score	It is energy, compared and scored; Each pose is scored for affinity based on the degree of match (complementarity) between ligand and receptor

3.2.2 TYPES OF DOCKING

1. *Induced-fit vs Lock-and-key:* The principle of docking can simulate the lock and key theory (Fischer, 1894) or the induced-fit theory (Koshland, 1958) or lie somewhere in between. Based in this, there are three types of docking: the rigid, the flexible and the semi-flexible. A comparison of these methods is given in Table 3.3.

2. *Based on the computational procedure:* A static docking is similar to rigid docking and does not involve movement of atoms. A dynamic docking involves a Molecular Dynamics Simulation (MDS) of the drug-receptor complex where the system is allowed to evolve over time with forces acting on various atoms. Force fields calculate and average the binding energy over several conformations of the drug and the receptor. For details of the technique, *ref.* section 2.3.2E.

3. *Based on user specification:* If the user provides the initial conditions (*ref.* docking theory for details on this term), the process is called manual docking as in SYBYL®-X (Tripos, inc.; Certara™ Company). If the computer investigates various poses in various putative binding site of the protein, the process is called auto-docking. Automated mapping of binding sites in a protein is performed by several software (Schroeder, 2006), (Ewing, 1997), (Laskowski, 1995), two of which are detailed in Discussion 3.1. The term can also *ref.* to the evaluation of various ligand poses in a user-defined active site.

Discussion 3.1: Binding pocket identification techniques

Discussed here are LIGSITE^{csc} and SURFNET which are two methods used to locate and define pockets that can act as tentative binding sites in a protein.

Contd...

Table 3.3: Comparison of rigid, flexible and semi-flexible docking

	Rigid	Semi-Flexible	Flexible
Static and dynamic atoms	Protein + ligand is static	Protein atoms are static; ligand atoms move	Protein + ligand atoms move
Biochemistry	Simulates lock and key hypothesis		Simulates induced fit hypothesis
Entropy arising from conformational flexibility	No entropic factors calculated	Entropy of ligand is considered from the degrees of freedom of the ligand (number of rotatable bonds)	Entropy of the protein can be calculated if the whole protein is allowed to move
Evaluation of steric clash	No van der Waals steric repulsion solved	van der Waals filtering is effective	van der Waals filtering is effective
Algorithms	-	Conformation varied by simulated annealing or GA	Full protein flexibility can be handled using MDS simulation
Time to complete a small calculation	Very quick (one run of few minutes)	Computational time is mainly consumed by conformational search of ligand (~20 minutes for ~10 runs)	Very time consuming (~5 hours when not whole protein but only selective protein atoms are allowed to move)
Generally used variants	–	Ligand conformations are not completely sampled	Only selected protein atoms (around the active site) move; not all ligand conformations are sampled
Applications	Used in virtual screening of a large database (> 200,000 compounds)	Can be used to dock ligands that are members of well-investigated structural series	Used for new molecules; used when binding affinities are needed for

Contd... **Discussion 3.1: Binding pocket identification techniques**

Ligsite (Schroeder, 2006): The protein is snapped onto a 3D grid. It is then scanned in several directions to completely map the free space of a tentative pocket and its boundary with the protein's surface. *Ref.* Fig. (i)

* Ligsite server: http://gopubmed2.biotec.tu-dresden.de/cgi-bin/index.php

Surfnet (Laskowski, 1995): A sphere of 1- 4 Å, which acts as a probe, is placed between two selected superficial atoms of the protein such that it does not penetrate the atoms. Next, it is investigated whether any other neighboring atom overlaps with this probe. The diameter of the probe is progressively reduced until no other atoms overlap (they are only allowed to touch). Several independent spheres are similarly placed until the surface is "saturated". *Ref.* Fig. (ii)

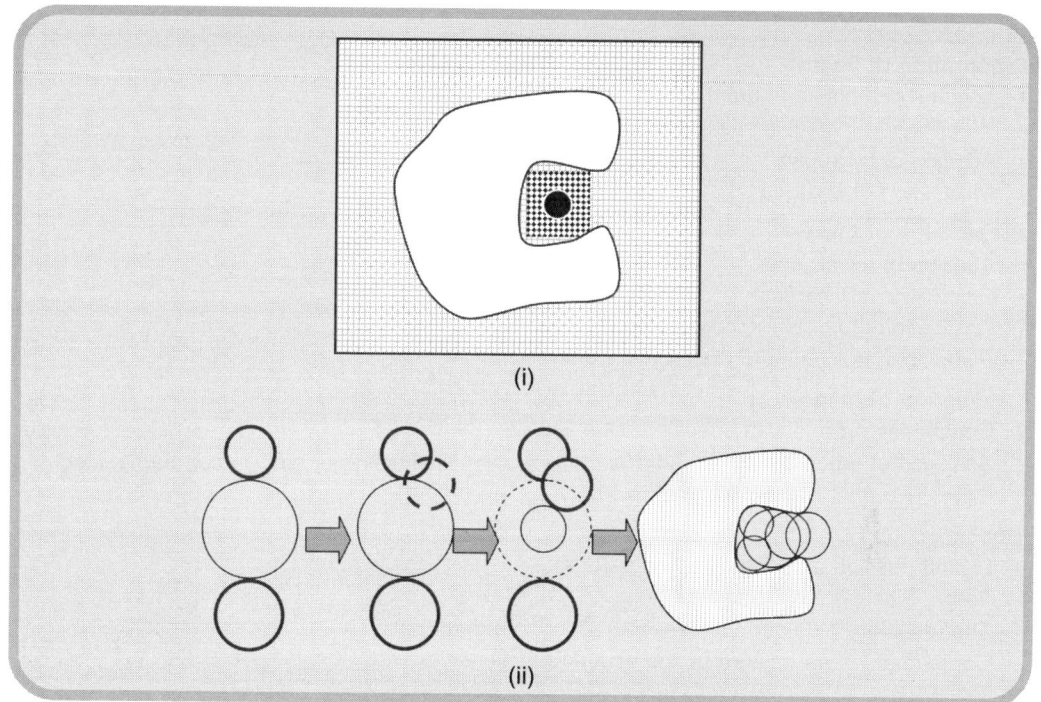

(i)

(ii)

3.2.3 DOCKING THEORY

Independent of the method, the basis of modeling molecular recognition lies in the need for a steric fit as well as complementarity of weak interactions as discussed earlier (section 2.2). Prior to, during, or right after the completion of docking, one can visualize various properties on the surface of the ligand and the protein (more importantly, the binding pocket).

Ref. Scheme 3.5 (and later Fig. 3.5) for an outline of docking principle. The type of properties and its distribution over various atoms being studied are generally "mapped" on the surface of the chemical moiety, whether it is a small part of a protein or the entire ligand itself. Some of the properties that might interest us are lipophilicity, electrostatic charges, hydrogen bond donors and acceptors, aromatic-rings, etc. that are responsible for the weak interactions discussed so far. For details on the visualization process *ref.* section 2.3.2.D.

3.2.3A Docking

The details of docking depend on the software. For example, three salient aspects of AutoGrid in the AutoDock suite (Âsterberg, 2002) are presented in Discussion 3.3. The docking steps can be generalized in the Scheme 3.5 including explanations for each step without reference to any particular software. Notes on the steps of docking with respect to the numbers superscripted in the Scheme 3.5 (p-422).

Preparation of ligand
- Account of atoms and atom types
- Investigating molecular flexibility[1]
- Addition of hydrogen[2]
- Calculation of charges[3]

Preparation of protein
- Addition of hydrogens[2]
- Calculation of charges[3]
- Calculation of flexible residues of protein[11]
- Placement of ligand into the protein's active site[12]

Calculation of maps
- Constructing a grid with specified dimensions[4]
- Selection of probe based on the properties to be calculated[5]
- Mapping properties of the protein as seen by the probe[6]

Docking
- Ligand position and conformation varied[7]
- Steric, Electrostatic, H-bonding, etc. are calculated[8]
- The result are obtained for a number of independent runs[9]
- Conformations are ranked by the scoring functions[10]

Scheme 3.5: Steps in docking (Superscripted numbers are noted below)

[1]: analysis of the number of rotatable bonds and the torsion tree; detection of root

[2]: if hydrogen bonding is calculated, polar hydrogens need to be added; if united atom force fields are used, the hydrogen is 'included' with the carbon–i.e. hydrogen is not considered as a distinct atom

[3]: in general, Gasteiger charges are added onto the ligand and Kollman charges onto the protein (for a word on partial charges *ref.* Box 29)

[4]: the user can specify the grid box enclosing the whole protein, or only enclosing protein atoms around the active site (if known) depending on the purpose of docking

[5]: there are as many probes as there are unique atoms in the ligand

[6]: there are as many maps as there are unique atoms in the ligand

[7]: the manner in which the ligand atoms "view" the protein is calculated using the maps. When the ligand atoms are actually placed in the maps, some atom positions are accepted and some are rejected. The final result is the most advantageous is compromise between best steric and electrostatic fit.

[8]: by default, steric and electrostatic fit are calculated; H-bonding is included in some software

[9]: a "job" submitted to a software contains several "runs". Each run starts from the same initial conditions. "Initial condition" refers to the original placement of the ligand in the protein's active site (that the user submits). This initial position is altered and the energy of the ligand in the newly placed position is calculated. This newly placed ligand is changed for a second time from the current position (and not the original position). Similarly, a series of changes in conformations also take place (by changing the parameters such as bond length, bond angle, etc.). The alteration is mostly done by generating random numbers. Random numbers become values of coordinates when altering the position of the ligand and becomes values for parameters when altering the conformation). A fresh run in the same job starts with the same initial conditions but the result of the second run may or may not be the same as the first run. This is why each run is termed independent and this is the reason random numbers are used to alter the variables of position and parameter. The best conformations are picked and sorted based on scoring rules.

[10]: the scoring function is that function which assigns weights to the various energies of interaction that *result* from *poses* of the docking study. Ultimately, a score is obtained that translates to *ranks* among the various conformations (for simplicity, hereafter, 'positions', is not mentioned). For example, all conformations that have steric clashes with protein atoms are filtered out. Then, the largest (exothermic) binding energy structure is ranked first followed by others. The "best" structure is assessed by the scoring function that ascribes weights to electrostatic, steric, H-bonding, etc. interactions.

[11]: some software such as AutoDock 4 (Âsterberg, 2002) can make selective residues on the protein flexible intending to include an 'induced fit' effect

[12]: this can be done automatically or manually (*ref.* automated and manual docking above under types of docking–section 3.2.2)

Think Box 6: Docking–in a few words

What do you model? The ligand and the macromolecule (receptor, polymer, etc)

What do you calculate? The strain energy of the ligand's bioactive conformation; the electrostatic and steric fit between the ligand and the receptor along with the binding energy and the binding constant

Why is it important? Numbers obtained contribute to the decision-making of accepting to proceed with the development of or discarding an analog

---

Box 29: Addition of partial charges

Kollman partial charges (Kollman, 1993), (Wang, et al. 2006) are added from a look-up table. So it is generally fast and can be used for large macromolecules.

Gasteiger-Marsili empirical atomic partial charges [(Gasteiger, et al. 1978), (Gasteiger, et al. 1980)] are calculated with

$$Q_i = \Sigma_\alpha \, q_i^{<\alpha>}$$

Where $q_i^{<\alpha>}$ is charge determined in several iterations. The calculation is based on electronegativity of orbitals, the ionization potentials and electron affinities of atoms

---

3.2.3B Scoring

The first automated receptor-ligand docking program was DOCK in 1982 (Kuntz, et al., 1982). The "DOCKING" part in Scheme 3.5 consists of steps:

1. Generation of various poses of the ligand (*ref.* conformational search under section 2.3.2.C2.a)
2. Ranking of the energies obtained from various poses (*ref.* Discussion 3.2)

Discussion 3.2: Scoring functions

When a docking is performed, several values are obtained in terms of steric, electrostatic, and if included, hydrogen-bonding energy between various poses of the ligand in the target's binding pocket. A simple addition of all these values can be performed to yield binding energy and the energies of all poses ranked in descending order (most exothermic pose ranked first, followed by the others). However, such an approach is very plain in that one cannot perform an intelligent docking. Instead of sampling 10 poses and ranking them, it would be a lot better if we could obtain 10 low strain-energy poses (remember high strain energy results in low binding energy). It would also be better if the contribution to total binding energy can be weighted—importance also given to van der Waals contacts, desolvation potential, entropic penalties to ligand conformation (and protein conformation) on binding—in order to increase detail. If these terms are included in the force field, a moderate protein and small ligand would take about a week to complete even a small 20-run docking study. Therefore, a reasonable solution would be as in the scheme shown.

Of course, it is assumed that the poses collected in step 2 contains the single truly best docking pose out of all the possible poses that the ligand can take up in the protein's binding pocket (i.e. out of all the sampled and un-sampled poses in step 1). Also, it is assumed that this single best solution will be the solution given by the software in step 3. At this point enter the scoring functions; step 2 is called DOCK-SCORING and step 3 is called AFFINITY-SCORING. The energy of a pose (the fitness in the fitness-landscape–*ref.* section 2.4) consists of:

1. Internal energy of the ligand,
2. Steric interaction energy, and,
3. In some software [GOLD (Jones, 1997)], hydrogen-bonding energy

Scoring functions can be classified similar to the classification of protein structure construction techniques (*ref.* part I, chapters 1.4 and 1.5)—into knowledge-based methods, empirical methods and methods using explicit force fields (Kroemer, 2007) as follows:

Knowledge-based methods: In these methods, known ligand-protein interactions and their binding energies are used to construct knowledge-based potentials (or knowledge-based mean force) that guide the scoring of new ligands in new poses. A large database of crystal structures of protein–ligand complexes is statistically studied for this purpose in terms of variables such as inter-atomic distance, van der Waals contact frequencies, etc. The study also includes successful and unsuccessful binders, to identify what characteristics good binders possess that increases affinity to target that non-binders don't have. Example: DrugScore (Gohlke, et al. 2000)

The other two methods can be collectively called *energy component methods.* They fragment binding energy into several contributions of the various interaction terms (Kroemer, 2007)

$$\Delta G_{binding} = \Delta G_{interaction} + \Delta G_{solvent} + \Delta G_{conformation} + \Delta G_{motion}$$

- Wherein $\Delta G_{interaction}$ = specific ligand – receptor interactions, $\Delta G_{solvent}$ = the interactions of ligand and receptor with solvent, $\Delta G_{conformation}$ = the conformational changes in the ligand and the receptor, and, ΔG_{motion} = the motions in the protein and the ligand during the complex formation.

- The main problem in considering these ΔG values as the true free energy values is that the contributions are calculated for a single structure and not an ensemble (*ref.* section 2.3.2.E and chapter 1.3 for the importance of calculating energy values from an ensemble of molecules)

- *Examples:* Empirical methods use pre-calculated values from experiments and other computational investigations for constructing the scoring function. Examples: the scoring functions of LUDI [(Böhm, 1994)], ChemScore [(Eldridge, et al. 1997)], Autodock3 [(Morris, 1998); (Sotriffer, 2000)], etc.

- *Examples:* Methods using explicit force fields employ a force field such as CHARMM (Brooks, et al. 2009) or assisted model building with energy refinement–AMBER (Cornell, et al. 1995). (The former method is favored for proteins, the latter method for organic molecules, to arrive directly at the binding energy. Example, part of the scoring function in Autodock3 (Morris, 1998).

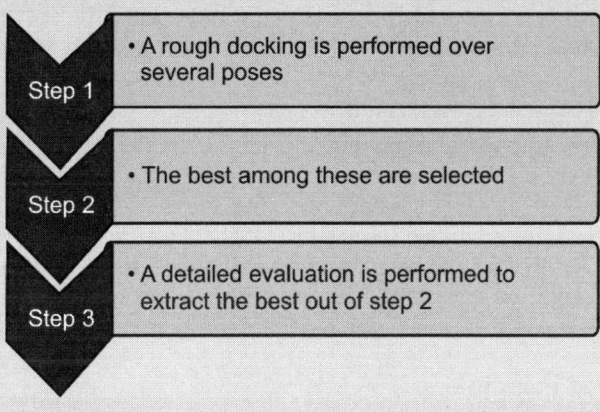

- **Step 1**: A rough docking is performed over several poses
- **Step 2**: The best among these are selected
- **Step 3**: A detailed evaluation is performed to extract the best out of step 2

Box 30: Advanced techniques in docking 1: Target-specific scoring functions

All docking program packages have an *in-house* scoring function that is used by default. These, however, are general functions meant to suite a large variety of proteins. They are developed from a large number of examples found in databases. In addition, these are meant to be used only when relevant predecessors are not available to serve as examples for the ligand or protein in question. Therefore, they are not necessarily the best function for the target in question. One could tweak these functions to suite the target better and this is called target-specific improvement of scoring functions. This can be achieved by training the built-in scoring functions in some software such as FlexX (Rarey, et al. 1996), (Blaney, et al. 1993) using experimental information and by modifying the algorithm (Stahl, 2000). One feeds the software with IC_{50} values or binding affinities for a specific target reported in literature along with the mode of binding for a dataset of ligand molecules. The software adjusts the coefficients with which various components of the scoring function are weighted so as to fit the data (using chemometric methods detailed under section 2.4). This tailored scoring function can be applied in the docking study involving the same target {for details, *ref.* [(Gohlke, 2002), (Kroemer, 2007), (Charifson, 1997)]}.

Although force fields and scoring functions in a docking program are not obvious to the user, many programs provide options through which these can be modified. By fine-tuning the cut-offs, adjusting weighting coefficients, and adding new terms as necessary, one can train the software and greatly improve the results obtained from a docking study, either for a particular receptor (Box 30) or for mimicking solvation effects (Box 31).

Box 31: Advanced techniques in docking 2: Solvation-based scoring

MM-PBSA and MM-GBSA are two techniques known to thoroughly investigate binding energies including solvent effects (Kroemer, 2007).
• MM: Molecular mechanics
• PB : Poisson–Boltzmann
• GB : Generalized Born
• SA : Solvent-accessible surface area
Usually solvent (especially water) mainly exerts electrostatic effects on the ligand and protein. This interaction is generally treated using the Coulomb's law by including the dielectric constant of the solvent. However, in this technique, solvent electrostatics is calculated using PB or GB [(Kollman PA, 2000), (Wang J., 2005)]. Binding energy is calculated by the perturbation approach using the thermodynamic cycle mentioned under section 3.1.3A (Fig. 3.3). The solvation–desolvation process is treated as the sum of polar and apolar contributions depending on the area and properties of the surface of the molecules (Sitkoff, 1998).

3.2.3C Summary of Principle

Docking is the study of the macromolecule–ligand complex and can be summarized using a combination of prepared material and live calculations. The macroscopic implications of docking are presented first, followed by the molecular manipulations involved.

Macroscopic Implications

1. To measure (actually, to calculate) binding energies
2. To establish a likely mechanism of binding, action, and if applicable, toxicity
3. To estimate potency and/or efficacy of the molecule at the receptor level
4. To facilitate decision-making on whether the ligand is worth (in terms of expenditure and effort) promoting to the next stage of development

Microscopic Manipulations

1. *Structure:* The macromolecule is opened in the molecular modeling software and the ligand molecule is placed in it. This is done as per instructions provided in the

software manual. Charges, solvation, or any other parameter is calculated. Remember, every atom on both the molecules are recognized in terms of two aspects:

a. Coordinates (X,Y,Z) indicating the atom location

b. Chemistry (element) indicating the valency, charge, size and other properties of the atom

2. *Flexibility:* Let us assume that a semi-flexible docking is performed. Here, only the ligand molecule's conformation/position/orientation is changed in the macromolecule's pocket. Changes in position and orientation move (translate and rotate, respectively) the entire ligand molecule. Changes in conformation require the application of chemical information (bond length, angles, etc.) to be meaningful.

   a. Step 1: Flexibility in a ligand molecule can take place about bonds that allow free rotation, such as some single bonds. These are collectively termed "rotatable bonds". Step 1 identifies all rotatable bonds in a ligand.

   b. Step 2: A central atom is identified for all these bonds. Systematically, starting from the central atom and moving outward, the bonds are rotated. Let us say that the bond is rotated by 90° steps. We then get four new conformations for every rotation: four conformations for the central atom, another four for each of the next set of atoms adjacent to the central one, yet another four for each of the third round of flexible-bonded atoms, and so on.

   c. Step 3: The above molecules are varied systematically and this resembles a "tree" with four branches at each node. This tree is called the "conformational map", the "conformational tree", or the "torsion tree" of the ligand.

3. *Interactions:* New ligand conformations resulting from the mapping of the torsion tree above is combined with the new ligand positions resulting from translations and new ligand orientations resulting from rotations. Each of these combinations (new locations/orientations/conformations) is called a *pose* as mentioned in the introduction to this chapter on docking. All poses generated are filtered for intra-ligand and protein-ligand steric clashes, calculated based on van der Waals radii. After this elimination, the remaining poses are sorted for the BEST values of electrostatic and steric strain (i.e., the least strain is best) and affinities (i.e. presence favorable interactions in molecules rank them high). Force fields and scoring functions detailed earlier come into play. An easy way to ascertain the strains and affinities is by fixing the macromolecule on a grid and using a probe to measure the required properties. The perspective of the probe—what the probe sees in the macromolecule when standing at that point in the grid—is mapped in the 3D box and is called a *field*.

   Readers are requested to combine the above description with Fig. 3.5, Scheme 2.3 of part II and Scheme 3.6 to follow in this chapter for a comprehensive idea of the major principle applied by software in the docking process.

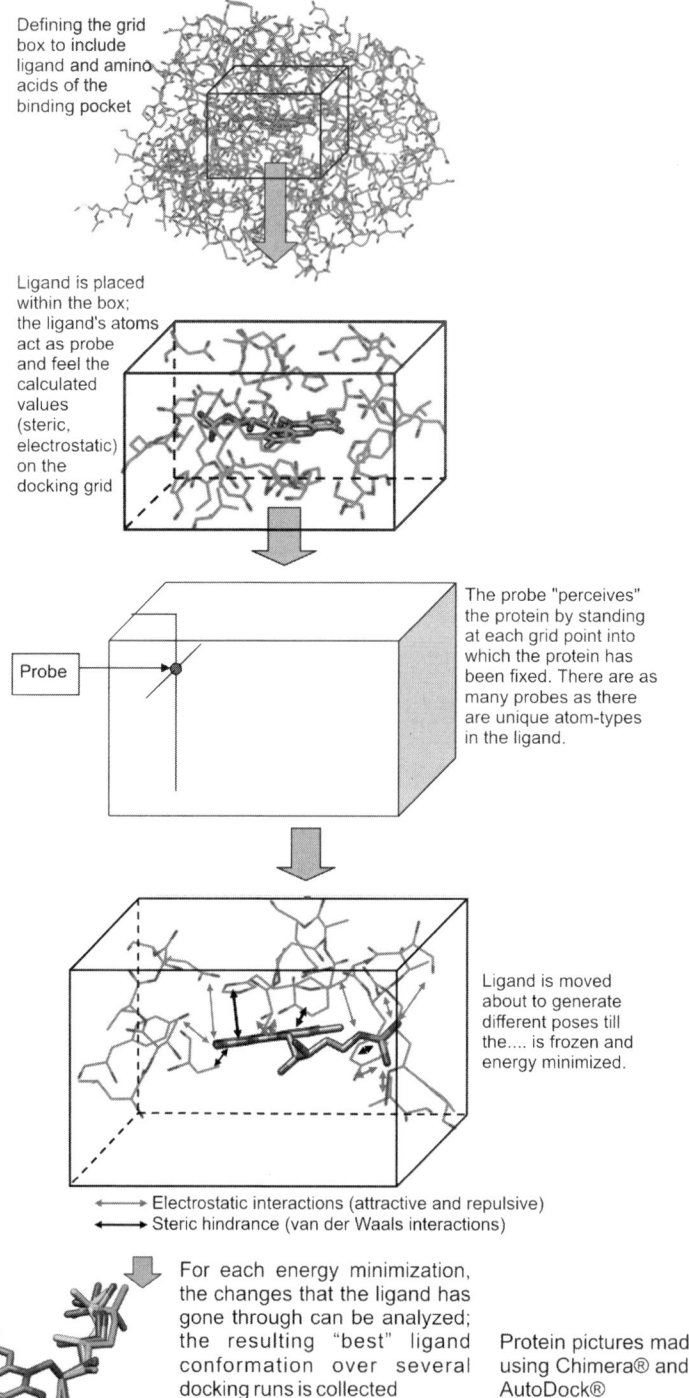

Defining the grid box to include ligand and amino acids of the binding pocket

Ligand is placed within the box; the ligand's atoms act as probe and feel the calculated values (steric, electrostatic) on the docking grid

Probe

The probe "perceives" the protein by standing at each grid point into which the protein has been fixed. There are as many probes as there are unique atom-types in the ligand.

Ligand is moved about to generate different poses till the.... is frozen and energy minimized.

←——→ Electrostatic interactions (attractive and repulsive)
◄——► Steric hindrance (van der Waals interactions)

For each energy minimization, the changes that the ligand has gone through can be analyzed; the resulting "best" ligand conformation over several docking runs is collected

Protein pictures made using Chimera® and AutoDock®

Fig. 3.5: Schematic representation of the principles of docking

Discussion 3.3: AutoDock

The *AutoDock (versions: 3.0, 4.0 (2007)*, latest version: *vina* released in June 2009) is actually a suite of programs developed by the Scripps Research Institute and the University of California at San Diego. Whereas software such as DOCK (Kuntz, et al. 1982), (Ewing, 1997) and Hammerhead (Welch, 1996) dock a fragment of the ligand first and then build up to the whole molecule, AutoDock and other such methods handle the entire ligand as one unit.

Conformational search: AutoDock can use GA, Lamarckian-GA or Simulated annealing to obtain different poses for the ligand in the binding site as per user choice. In accordance with the two GA algorithms, each degree of freedom of the ligand is encoded as a gene (*ref.* section 2.3.2.C2.c)

Scoring: An empirical scoring function is used. The score approximates the free energy of the system. The initial ligand pose is random and lower scores represent lower strain energy or greater stability. The docked conformation gets the lowest score and the highest rank. Ranking of conformations also include structural clustering of the generated poses (similarity is assessed both in terms of ligand conformation and position in the active site).

Docking: AutoDock version 4.0 (Âsterberg, 2002) onwards allows protein flexibility and one can approximate the docking to the induced-fit theory. Residues selected by the user can be made to move within the grid box. In the following expression, N_{tor} refers to the number of rotatable bounds; the ΔG notations are as routinely used in this book:

$$\Delta G = \Delta G_{VDW} + \Delta G_{H-bo} + \Delta G_{elec} + \Delta G_{tor} N_{tor} + \Delta G_{solv}$$

van der Waals interactions: Typically the 12–6 form of the Lennard-Jones potential (*ref.* Discussion 2.4 under section 2.2) are used to model the van der Waals forces experienced between two instantaneous dipoles. The curves in order of increasing well-depth are: HH << CH < NH < OH << CC < CN < CO < NN < NO < OO

Hydrogen bonding: The 12–10 form of the L-J potential (*ref.* Discussion 2.4 under section 2.2) is used to model hydrogen bonds with additional distance constrain (as mentioned in Tables 2.6 and 2.7, section 2.3.2)

Electrostatic potential: AutoGrid calculates Coulombic interactions between the macromolecule and a probe of charge e, $+1.60219 \times 10^{-19}$ C; there is no distance cutoff used for electrostatic interactions.

Solvent effect: A sigmoidal distance-dependent dielectric function is used to model solvent screening, based on the work of Mehler and Solmajer (Mehler, et al. 1991)

$$\in (r) = A + \left[\frac{B}{1 + ke^{-\lambda Br}} \right]$$

where $B = \in_0 - A$; $\in_0$ = the dielectric constant of bulk water at 25°C = 78.4; A = –8.5525, λ = 0.003627 and k = 7.7839 are optimized parameters.

Ligand flexibility: The ΔG value per bond is multiplied by the number of rotatable bonds in the molecule.

Applications:
- Structure refinement in X-ray crystallography (*ref.* Part I section 1.1.2.A)
- Virtual screening, combinatorial library design
- Lead optimization, structure-based drug design
- Chemical mechanism studies
- Protein-protein docking

(i) Focus on the ligand and the protein's residues interacting with it:

(ii) One can almost always find aromatic stacking interactions:

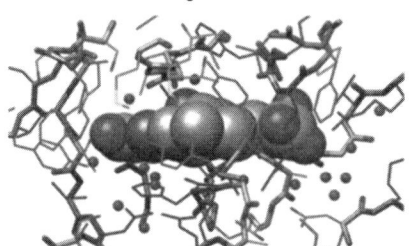

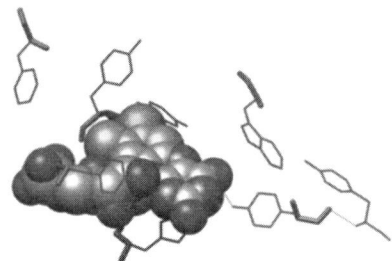

(iii) Water can be found forming a network of H-bonds with the protein active site,....

(iv) ...with each other and also with the ligand.

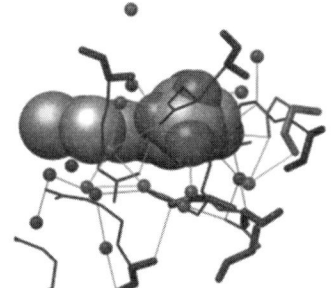

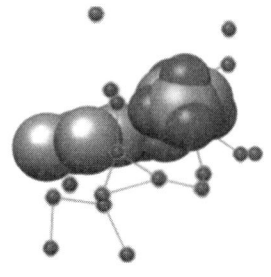

(v) A negative ligand on a bed of positive residues; simultaneously aromatic and non-polar interactions are present to increase the binding

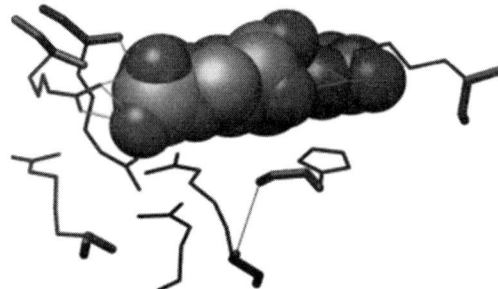

Scheme 3.6: Some snapshots of binding interactions that can be observed from a docking study, pictures of molecules made using Chimera®

Did You Know? 29
About high affinity binding

The binding of natural substrate (endogenous) or drug (exogenous) molecules with a protein can liberate up to 40–50 kJ/mol for binding equilibrium constants of ~10^{-8}–10^{-9}. These molecules are considered to have high affinity to the protein (Nogrady, et al. 2005)

3.2.4 AFTER PERFORMING DOCKING

Did You Know? 30
Time for docking

In a semi-flexible docking study using a ligand of about 30 atoms and a protein of ~ 4000 atoms, 1 docking run calculating ~150 cycles (~ 10^6 energy calculations) on a Pentium4 256MB RAM machine takes ~30min CPU time and much longer in real time (real time = wall clock time).

As with any computational study, the authenticity of the result obtained after calculations depends on the meaningful and valid execution of every step performed by the user. The docking process can be done manually, where you physically move the ligand with the help of a mouse into the receptors binding pocket, or automatically where a cube (called "the box") is defined about the binding pocket and lets the computer determine the best orientation and fit of the ligand with respect to the protein surface. In either case, after the completion of the process, it is of utmost importance to have a look at the results.

• After one gets the docking energy, is the ligand still in the receptor's active site? This might seem to be a very trivial consideration. The process of static docking itself induces small changes in the conformation of the ligand while simultaneously moving the ligand in the tiny space of the receptor's binding pocket. In all probability, when there is a large ligand or when there are several diverse side chains or when the ligand is not correctly placed, automatic docking using simple algorithms might end in a situation where the ligand is gradually pushed out of the defined box. Although giving outstanding values for steric hindrance and electrostatic repulsion, the ligand will actually be standing out of the binding pocket!

> "Well, I never heard it before, but it sounds uncommon nonsense"
> The Mock Turtle in "Through the Looking Glass", by Lewis Carroll

• Concentrate on just the ligand. All the bond distances, angles and dihedrals need to be checked for unusual numbers or chemically impossible arrangement of atoms. For molecules that contain commonly found atoms such as carbon, hydrogen, oxygen, nitrogen, sulfur etc, there should not be fundamental geometry problems. But, if the molecule contains "special atoms" such as transitional metals, or if the molecule has advanced electronic effects such as hyperconjugation or anomeric effects (*ref.* section 2.2.4), one has to clarify beyond doubt whether the force field being used contains a reasonable description for that situation.

- Now superimpose (this means to put one molecule on top of the other so that equivalent atoms are matched) the original conformation of the ligand (that you defined before you started docking) onto the ligand molecule that you get after docking. Is there any difference? Unless the ligand-receptor system is very different from all those that have been investigated so far, studying literature gives useful standard for comparison to determine the amount of conformational change that one can expect in the ligand molecule being studied.

- The starting conformation for the ligand would have been either the energy minimized conformation or the most common conformation as averaged from a large number of data. In the former case, the energy of the ligand can be noted down, whereas in the latter case, a single point calculation (this means calculating the energy of the molecule by freezing it, in other words, without inducing any change in its geometry. Please *ref.* 2.3.2 C energy minimization for details) is needed to determine its energy. The change in energy after docking can then be studied (a single point calculation can be performed on the docked ligand) and correlated with the change in conformation.

- It is meaningful to perform semi-flexible docking. Otherwise, it is useful to energy minimize the protein before docking. Both steps will eliminate the influence of another ligand or the absence of ligand from the binding pocket of the protein when downloaded from the protein data bank or when constructed by homology modeling (*ref.* section 1.4.3.A in part I).

- How much has the receptor structure changed, especially around the binding pocket? There are services available on the web that compare protein structure and point out the differences between two submitted structures as referred to in chapter 1.2.3. Although docking is static (remember: the receptor geometry does not change) it is possible that in some force fields of advanced software the rotamers of side chains of proteins (a detailed discussion of protein structure is given in chapter 1.2) can be made flexible. Sometimes a little flexibility can be allowed in localized regions of the backbone. *Note:* Amino acids chemically combine to form proteins. A continuous chain of N, C_α and $C_{carbonyl}$ from the various amino acids form the backbone and the rest of the amino acid remains dangling from the backbone and is called the "side chain". This side chain can assume a number of conformations and are free to interact with the solvent and other parts of the protein when the protein coils up influencing their rotational conformation called the rotamer sometimes.

Did You Know? 31
Jobs and Runs in docking

A job is the submission of a docking problem to the software. Each job calculates binding energies obtained from several (this is a user specified number) independent docking runs.

- Did you try your best to dock? Did you submit multiple jobs with several runs? Did you get comparable results in all these studies? Did you complement automated docking with a manual trial? It is important to confirm the results of docking as much as possible. What is being modeled is only the steric and electrostatic forces.

One must have in mind that 9 approximations operate as discussed in chapter 2.2 and every effort must be taken to minimize further errors.

- Not only is it necessary to check with our own knowledge and the knowledge that is available to us whether the docking is vaild, not to mention successful, but also mandatory to be able to set up a pharmacological theory (Scheme 3.6) from the results obtained. Before starting docking studies, did you study the structure of your ligand, the class of your protein, and evidence, in literature, of any relation between the two? Based on this understanding, did you predict the ligand to be a successful candidate or did you expect a failure in the docking step? Did the docking study match your ideas and expectations? Study of the protein-pharmacophore complex will give us new ideas for perhaps even better ligands.

- Last, but not the least, did you make good pictures out of your dockings study? The section 2.3.2.D on molecular visualization helps us to understand the importance of conveying ideas through effective pictures, and also what we should know about the atoms, bonds, ribbons and surfaces that appear on the screen.

- Major ongoing work in current docking is conformational sampling of highly flexible ligands, improving force fields, handling solvation, increasing protein flexibility, evaluating various tautomeric forms of the ligand, effect of pH, etc.

Docking in the High throughput Scenario

We wish to add a word on what is expected from docking results when high throughput is required and how the stage of drug design influences the results expected. Table 3.4 outlined this with reference to inhibitors (Kroemer, 2007).

Table 3.4: Affinity of inhibitors as defined by the stage of drug design

Stage	Particulars	Remarks
Lead identification	IC_{50} >100 nM or even > 1μM (weakly active)	Sufficient to identify these molecules
Lead optimization	IC_{50} <100 nM (Potent compounds) IC_{50} >100 nM – 10 μM (moderately/weakly active) IC_{50} >10 μM (inactive)	Should be able to differentiate between these three categories of molecules

"Results! Why, man, I have gotten a lot of results. I know several thousand things that won't work."
Thomas Edison

Other References

1. Ajay, Murcko, M.A. and Stouten, P.F.W. in (Charifson, 1997)
2. Kavraki, L. (2007, March 22). Protein-Ligand Docking, Including Flexible Receptor-Flexible Ligand Docking. Retrieved from the Connexions Web site at http://cnx.org/content/m11456/1.10/

3.3 Protein-Protein Interactions (Overview)

So far, we know that proteins are dynamic, they constantly fold and unfold even under biological folding-favored conditions and their native fully folded state is only slightly lower in energy than the unfolded states. Proteins are the workhorses of the cell and perform their function by a maintaining a dynamic interaction with other molecules. Yet, of the hundreds of molecules in the biological system coming into contact with a protein, only some trigger the protein into its fully functional state. We know that the protein in the form of enzymes, hormones, channels, etc. does not (and is not supposed to) to respond to random molecules. Therefore, more accurate terms that describe protein response is *specificity* and *recognition*. The response may be caused by small molecules as we saw in the previous section 3.2 or to other proteins as outlined in this section.

3.3.1 INTERFACE ANATOMY

The first region of the protein that other molecules feel, and then influence, is its surface. There are specific sites on the surface of a protein that posses the needed physical and chemical properties to perform function [(Vajda, et al., 2006), (Reichmann, et al. 2007)] and these are described in this section. However, some specific points in chapters so far that become relevant to this discussion are presented:

1. Chapter 1.2: proteins possess different structure as they perform different functions; they can be classified by homology into families
2. Chapter 1.3: they breathe and the folded protein structure accommodates this breathing; there is always an ensemble of protein conformations
3. Chapter 1.4: sequence dictates structure; several sequences can form the same structure depending on the presence of 'key' residues
4. Section 2.3.2 A/B: key residues in the receptor active site demand substrates with multiple and specific features in the pharmacophores
5. Chapter 3.2: binding interactions require specificity and strength.

A. Conserved Residues

Proteins related by homology may possess as little as 20% similarities in their sequences. We know that there are some vital residues to the protein whose positions must not be changed. Either the residues themselves or other residues containing their properties are always retained at a particular spot in 3D. These "conserved" residues are attributed to mediate a great number of important functions that a family of proteins perform such as DNA binding, ligand interaction, transmembrane fixation, recognition of other proteins, etc.

B. Hotspots

When two proteins interact, they do not behave like a magnetic sticker that one sticks on the fridge door. The inter-protein surface, also called the protein interface, is not uniform in its binding properties; some amino acids are found to hook into the other surface whereas other residues are not even felt. Correspondingly, some residues contribute more to the binding free energy than others. This heterogeneous distribution of the binding free energy of protein-protein association across the area of the interface [(Clackson, et al. 1995), (Keskin, et al. 2005)] results in localized regions called "hot spots". A hot spot is a group of residues that contribute 0.2 kCal/mol or more to the binding energy. Site-directed mutagenesis and alanine scanning (*ref.* textbooks such as (Waksman, 2005)) experimentally disturb the arrangement of hotspot-residues to determine any change in recognition. Investigations on several families of proteins known to bind to each other [such as (Keeble, et al. 2006)] demonstrate that hotspots were structurally strongly conserved. The 3D similarity of structure (even in the absence of sequence conservation) indicates similarity in the functions performed by proteins and in the stability of the proteins under various conditions (Hemerta, et al. 2008). Extensive computational modeling of interfaces has been performed taking into account H-bonds, solvent and packing interactions (Filizola, et al. 2005). Now, hotspots can be predicted.

C. Anchor

One of the theories explaining protein-protein interactions (Rajamani, et al. 2004) propose that the smaller protein attaches to the larger through specific points called "anchors". These are the side chains of amino acids that dock into narrow, relatively rigid grooves of the larger protein where the conformations of the surrounding residues are conformationally restricted. The *'groove'* is always in a favorable conformation. This induces a conformational change in the anchor. The anchor is however not forced into this new conformation owing to its flexibility. It is known to take up this structure even in the absence of the partner protein. Such studies have been found to explain the action of several hormone receptors that are known to bind to a host of other proteins (called promoters) such as estrogen receptor.

D. Binding Pockets

Regions of the interface are almost always "pitted" and these pits are called binding pockets. The centers of these pits are not solvent exposed, have a rigid conformation that is ready-made, does not seem to change much after binding, and contains energetic hot spots. The residues around the pocket form a ring, and in MD simulations [such as (Brown, et al. 2005)], show that 16 out of the 18 analyzed complexes (Launay, et al. 2008) have very small r.m.s deviations, of less than 1 Å. Thus they undergo very little conformation change after binding and do not loose much entropy. It is evident that proteins do all they can to maximize binding (reduce entropy penalty) and the size of the molecules are not as convenient as in the case of the interaction between ligand and receptor.

3.3.2 INTERFACE CHARACTERISTICS

Figure 3.6 shows diagrammatically the characteristics of interfaces in protein 1N0J (chains labeled A and B). Among proteins that interact, a number of variables can be studied:

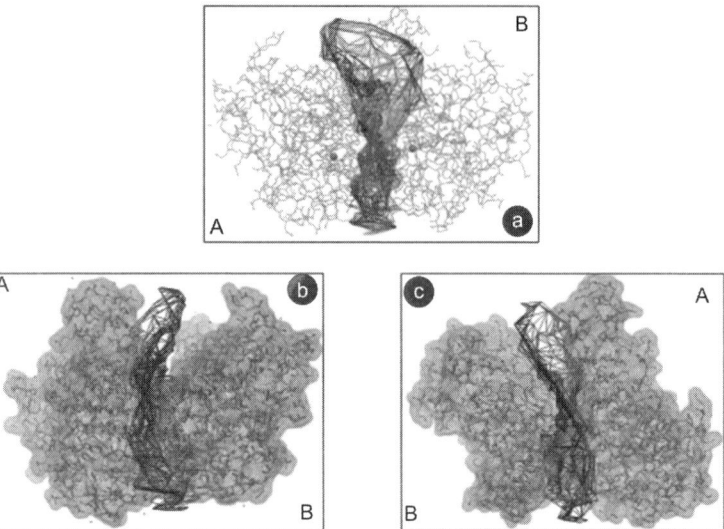

Fig. 3.6: Study of the interface of a dimer protein 1NOJ. Shown here are 3 perspectives (a), (b) and (c) of chains A and B dimerizing to form a protein. The 'lines' representation is depicted in (a) and a transluscent surface around 'sticks' is used in (b) and (c). Interface orea is inapped by dense network of lines. Protein picture, interface and surface construction made using Chimera®

A. Interface Size

Interfacial changes depend on the symmetry of the multimer. Change in terms of area in a homodimer is less than in the other cases. Studies also indicate that area changes among conserved residues are less than in the other residues. Conserved residues are already stabilized by hydrogen bonding in a particular conformation. After dimerization, the type of interaction alone changes to van der Waals attraction. The number of conserved residues is also proportional to the interface contact area (Ma, et al. 2003).

B. Interface Shape

Interfaces have different shapes, depending on the nature of the proteins involved. A homodimer's interface is known to be somewhat "rugged" with several complementary pockets. Other interfaces are known to be relatively planar and more uniformly accessible. Smooth interfaces come in contact transiently and this plays a role in the protein's functioning.

C. Interface Texture

Surfaces that bind other proteins similar to those that bind ligands have binding pockets. These resemble pits and the solvent inaccessible regions of the pits are rich in conserved residues. The pockets lack conformational flexibility—they are always present in the bound conformation. Cutting down entropy loss on binding is important. Some theories (Li, et al. 2009) explain that these conformationally constrained areas are the hot spots. They also propose that the reason they are located in "pits" and shielded from the solvent is to amplify the electrostatic contrast between the amino acid side chains and the space immediately surrounding it. When in contact with the solvent bulk charges are dissipated owing to the high dielectric constant of the aqueous medium. It is noteworthy that conserved residues are not localized to hot spots although the latter are rich in conserved residues.

D. Packing at Subunit Interface

Homodimers are known to be better packed than other interfaces (Zhanhua, et al., 2005). At the pockets, due to rigidity in conformation, dense packing is observed to increase van der Waals interactions.

E. Hydrophobicity at Interface

Proteins with exposed hydrophobic surfaces come together and bond in order to avoid the exposure of these surfaces to the aqueous solvent. This attempt to reduce total exposed surface area is called communal aggregation. Obligate complexes (complexes that are absolutely necessary for biological action) have such "sticky" hydrophobic patches (leading to as in the case of mutant hemoglobin aggregation in sickle cell anemia) whereas the interfaces of transient complexes such as those of enzyme and inhibitors are known to be more hydrophilic with polar residue patches. Hydrophobic interactions as explained under chapter 3.1 increase entropy of water and reduce the area of 'oil'-water interface.

F. Flexibility of Backbone Conformation at Interacting Sites

The following are the opinions found in corresponding literature:

a. The interfacial residues even in unbound state are known to assume the bound conformation during an MD simulation, the justification proposed is that

  i. First, it is easy and quick to find the bound conformation as the need for detailed conformational sampling is avoided, and

  ii. Second, the rigidity before protein-protein binding does not lead to a very great loss of entropy, after binding (Smith, et al. 2005).

b. *Conserved residue behavior:*

  i. Conserved residues were found to visit restricted regions of the Ramachandran map (Yogurtcu, et al. 2008). It has been mentioned earlier under chapter 1.2 on protein structure that this is possible if the residue is counter-balanced by strong favorable interactions such as hydrogen bonding as occurs here.

  ii. The spread and average of the φ, ψ value distributions were also found to be different for conserved and non-conserved residues.

  iii. Conserved residues before and after binding were found not to vary significantly in their φ, ψ conformations.

  iv. Clusters of neighboring conserved residues were found to cause rigidity in certain non-conserved residues as well.

c. It is interesting to portray the above aspect in a different light as done by Steinberg and Scharega. Consider two protein interfaces interacting; the concerned residues are able to take up conformations that are usually disallowed in a self-existing protein. The "new flexibility" in conformation is itself an indication of increased entropy. The accessibility of new structures by the complex that was not accessible by the two independent monomers is a type of configurational entropy (Steinberg, et al. 1963). Therefore the rotational and translational degrees of freedom are reduced, but there is an increase in configurational entropy. In other words, an interaction between two biomacromolecules (protein, DNA, RNA, etc.) increases the local flexibility the complex (Lyubchenko, et al. 1993).

G. Hydrogen Bonding Tendency

a. In an MD simulation, there is constant motion of atoms. The geometry of the arrangement of hydrogen acceptor, hydrogen and the hydrogen donor constantly changes. At specific distances, the H-bond is capable of forming; when this distance increases, it is broken. The mean gemometry needs to be favorable for an H-bond to be consistently present. An average of the number of H-bonds formed by each residue through all frames of an MD simulation (and this means snapshots over time as described in chapter 1.3) is called *H-bond residence time*.

b. Buried residues in binding pockets contribute to less H-bonding with water.

c. These residues are also involved in intra-chain H-bonding within the pits of the binding pockets, as mentioned above. Hotspots were favored to form interfacial H-bonds but no consistent trend has been observed.

d. After complexation, interfacial H-bonding of residues in pockets are negligible. Only van der Waals interactions have been indicated in the anchoring and interaction.

H. Amino acid Propensity at the Interface

Hotspot residues are often found to be large and aromatic in nature (Zhou, et al. 2001) independent of the interacting proteins. Conserved residue backbone conformations were found to differ from others except for Ala, Pro, and Thr.

I. Function

Protein function depends on interactions with other molecules such as ligands that change protein conformation and structure, signaling messengers, substrates in which the protein catalyzes configurational changes, and other proteins that lead to microscopic as well as macroscopic changes influencing biochemical pathways. Thus proteins function as workhorses only through various interactions that they participate in. Proteins that perform similar functions have strongly conserved residues especially among those that mediate interactions. The role of water can never be overemphasized in influencing enthalpy, entropy, surrounding dielectric constant, charge distribution, etc. with regard to stabilizing folded structure, influencing correct folding, mediation of enzyme action, aiding specificity in molecular recognition, etc. (Raschke, 2006). *Other references:* (Joachimiak, et al. 2006; Keskin, et al. 2005; Fuller, et al. 2009)

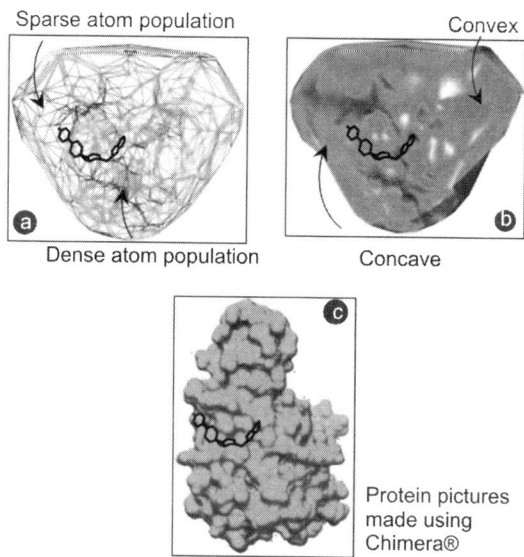

Sparse atom population

Dense atom population

Convex

Concave

Protein pictures made using Chimera®

Fig. 3.7: Protein interface inhibitors which prevent protein-protein interaction. A representation of only the interface is shown to put forth the principle

3.3.3 PROTEOMICS ROADMAP TO MEDICINAL CHEMISTRY–5

All discoveries are worth the trouble only when applied. This is especially so in the health care sector where there still exist unmet medical challenges. Extensive study of protein-protein interfaces are used in the design of interface inhibitors. This group of drugs prevent binding and interaction between two specific proteins by either preventing their physical aggregation (leading to precipitation) or by breaking the pharmacological reaction cascade. The former principle is applied in protein misfolding and aggregation disease such as Alzheimer's and Parkinson's disease (discussed in detail under section 1.5.12. proteomics roadmap to medicinal chemistry–4). The latter of the two strategies mentioned above is used to prevent dimer (or multimer) formation. Possible drug candidates being investigated especially among the G-protein Coupled Receptor class aim to prevent the formation of the fully functional protein multimer form.

Example

Estrogen is a steroidal hormone and it interacts with the cellular Estrogen Receptor (ER) to elicit its physiological effects (Edwards, 2005). These ERs are of two types corresponding to two different and independent (Revankar, et al. 2005) pathways of estrogen action:

1. Nuclear control by binding with nuclear ERs. The ERs act as transcription factors that modify the expression levels of gene products (such as proteins) and these

effects take longer to show. They are well known and belong to steroid hormone receptor family including those for androgens, mineralocorticoids, etc.

2. Cytoplasmic action via ERs on the cell surface that belong to the G protein-coupled receptor family (Simoncini, et al. 2003). Via this route estrogen acts much faster.

The nuclear ERs interact with a large group of modulator proteins (called transcription coregulators) that bind in succession to modify the activity of the receptor protein and in turn the DNA. Tight binding ligands that target the receptor or its modulators prevent this interaction and block estrogen action; an example is the recently discovered binding site of hydroxytamoxifen (Wang, et al. 2006). Such drugs are therefore useful in estrogen-dependent cancers. The advantage of this principle is that these drug can be designed independent of the active site of the protein.

Other references: (Tsai, et al. 1994; Carino, et al. 2008; Nagler, et al. 2007)

3.4 *Successful Drug Designing in Real-world Medicinal Chemistry*

Various approaches of medicinal chemistry have mushroomed because of the success demonstrated in using them on specific cases of molecules. Overall success lies in regularizing these different approaches and using them in harmony to generate a systematic workflow that can be applied to any molecule. This is the core of rational drug design and modern medicinal chemistry. The results obtained from a blend of techniques discussed so far in the three parts of this book are presented here. The authors hope that this will serve as an inspiration to students aspiring to contribute to research in medicinal chemistry. Table 3.5 shows a comprehensive list of some details regarding the drugs and targets involved in some therapeutic classes.

Often, relatively simple systems can serve as an example for drugs with complex structure. Readers are referred to the description of hydrogen peroxide structure discussed in section 2.3.2.E. The peroxide arrangement occurring in several molecules was critically reviewed from experimental structures (data stored in CCCBDB at http://cccbdb.nist.gov/—a crystallographic database referred to in Did You Know? 2 in chapter 1.1; (Mahler, et al. 2008)) and theoretical calculations (Kittredge, et al. 2008; Weinhold, et al. 2003) with respect to geometry, charges, etc. From these observations, the minimal energy conformation of albendazoles and the role of d-orbitals in determining geometry and reactivity have been noted (Coleman, 2008). The same paper also recommends the use of H_2O_2 as a model system for studying albendazoles. In drug discovery, by and large, one does not get to perform such a focused study until the very end of the lead optimization stage. Almost always, one needs to scan through a large number of putative ligands in a library. The process becomes target-oriented with the availability of a target protein. One has to then take account:

1. To identify the various binding modes of the protein
2. To identify a receptor model that would be representative of several isoforms if necessary
3. To minimize the number of false positives
4. To "enrich" the selection process by including actives.

We wish to mention, as an example, a research work (Schuster, et al. 2010) that follows this methodology. Cyclooxygenase (COX) is a precious pharmaceutical target; it is a prostaglandin H2 synthase (enzyme classification code EC 1.14.99.1) having isoforms 1 and 2. The X-ray crystal structure is available with a large number of bound inhibitors. Its active ligands have also been well studied. The mentioned paper constructs several pharmacophore models for COX 1 and COX 2 and uses this to screen databases of molecules (trying to distinguish between known actives and known false positives).

The structures of all pharmaceutical enzymes have not been elucidated as with COX. Readers are reminded of the Protein Structure Initiative mentioned in

Table 3.5: Antimetabolites, substrates, and their corresponding therapeutic targets and some PDB files of interest

Used with permission from the Journal of Chemical Education, Vol. 82, Feb, 2005, page 588, copyright ©2005, Division of Chemical Education, Inc. *Reference:* Medicinal Chemistry and Molecular Modeling: An Integration for the Teaching of Drug Structure–Activity Relationship and the Molecular Basis of Drug Action; Ivone Carvalho, Áurea D. L. Borges and Lílian S. C. Bernardes

Group	Therapeutic class	Enzyme substrate	PDB file	drug/ antimetabolite
I Antineoplastic	Thymidylate synthase	Deoxyuridylate monophosphate	1tls, 1tsn, 1hzw, 1kzi, 1hvy, 1bq1, 1cif,1tsw	5-fluorouracil, trifluorothymidine
II Anti-HIV	Reverse transcriptase	Deoxythymidylate monophosphate	1cot, 1cou, 1dtq, 1fkp, 1hmv, 1hvu	Zidovudine, lamivudine, stavudine, didanosine
III Anti-HIV	HIV Protease	Poliprotein	1hvp,1kzk, 2aid,2bpv, 2bpw, 7upj	Saquinovir, indinavir, ritonavir
IV Antibiotic	Transpeptidase and Carboxypeptidase	Acil-D-Ala-DAla	1cef, 1ceg, 1es2, 1es3	Penicillin G, oxacillin, ampicillin, carbenicillin, cephalexin
V Hipolipemic	HMGO-CoA reductase	HMGO-CoA	1dqa, 1hw8, 1hw9, 1hwj, 1qax, 1qay	Lovastatin, simvastatin, fluvastatin, atorvastidina
VI Antihypertensive	Dopa descarboxilase	L-Dihydroxy-phenylalanine	1js3, 1js6, 5pah, 4pah, 1phh, 1d7l	Methyldopa, methyldopamine, methylnorepine-phrine
VII Antineoplastic	Dihydrofolate reductase	Dihydrofolic acid	1rb3, 1rg7, 1rh3, 1ra3, 7dfr, 3d	Methotrexate, piritrexim, trimetrexate
VIII Antiinflammatory	Cyclooxygenase	Arachidonic acid	1dcx, 1cqe, 1cvu, 1ddx, 1cx2, 1pgf	Ibuprofen, indomethacin, naproxen, acetylsalicylic acid
IX Cholinergic	Acetylcholinesterase	Acetylcholine	2ace, 1gqr, 2ack, 1dx4, 2clj, 1qti	Neostigmine, tacrine, pyrido-stigmine, echothiophate, demecarium, pralidoxime

Discussion 1.3 under section 1.1 that takes major efforts to accelerate the experimental elucidation of pharmaceutically important proteins. Until then, what should one do if a target's structure is not available? Chapter 1.4 discusses how homology modeling can be used to generate 3D structure of proteins of known sequence if the structures of (approximately) similar proteins (by sequence) are available. This enables the screening of more databases of ligands for several unexplored disease conditions and pharmacological pathways. Pertaining to this scenario we wish to present Discussion 3.4 as a background to the remarkable case of the G-Protein Coupled Receptor (GPCR). The G-Protein in the GPCR has an extracellular domain, an intracellular domain and a domain with 7-transmembrane helices. It spans the lipoidal plasma membrane with the 7 helices arranged parallel to each other and spanning the membrane. To remain submerged in the lipoidal phase, the helices possess long strips of hydrophobic residues. Protein–isolating experiments involve homogenizing the cell, separating the protein fraction and then extracting the GPCR from this mixture. Such an isolated and purified GPCR molecule is subjected to X-ray studies or NMR spectroscopy. What do you expect the structures to look like? WILL IT RESEMBLE THE BIOLOGICAL STRUCTURE? No; because the lipid phase is missing! In an aqueous solution hydrophobic residues prefer to be buried into the interior of the protein rather than be exposed to the surroundings as a hydrophobic strip on a helix. So the biological arrangement cannot be expected to remain intact. HOW do we then get a GPCR protein for drug design (given that a majority of the drugs act via the G-proteins)? This is where computations have been used both in the form of homology modeling/receptor mapping with available ligands, and in evaluating the stability of the protein in an 'imaginary' lipid bilayer environment constructed in a simulation. GPCR protein coordinates are available in the PDB for computational use.

Discussion 3.4: Cell signaling and the G-protein coupled receptors

The scope of this discussion is to let the student appreciate the process of cell signaling in the context of drug discovery. Therefore a sketchy outline of the fundamental process is alone presented herein. It is not intended to cover in depth every aspect of cell signaling.

Living organisms are able to see, taste, hear, smell and feel because of sensory signals they receive from the environment. At the cellular level, cells in different organs communicate with one another by means of molecular signals, which are generated extracellularly and received by other cells which have specific receptors on the surface of the cell. This external signal is relayed to the interior of the cell by signal transduction systems. Non polar hydrophobic molecules are conveyed into the cell rather easily, e.g. Steroidal hormones. It is the polar hydrophillic molecules that cannot pass through the lipid bilayer that require signal transduction systems. The signal relayed into the interior of the cell interacts with one or more intracellular proteins, which relay the message to the effector proteins resulting in changes in metabolic activity, gene expression patterns or changes in cell shape or movement. Effective communication between the cells of the various organs is fundamental to the functioning of the organism as a whole. The broad outline of the cell signaling process can be summarized as follows:

- Extracellular signaling molecules interact with proteins that are transmembrane in nature spacing the plasma membrane. Such proteins are referred to as receptors.
- These receptors being transmembrane have an extracellular projection and an intracellular projection.
- Signals from the outside are relayed via the extracellular projection into cell.
- The intracellular projection relays the signal within the cell by interacting with intracellular signaling proteins.
- The intracellular signaling proteins relay the message to the effector proteins, which in turn mediate the appropriate response.

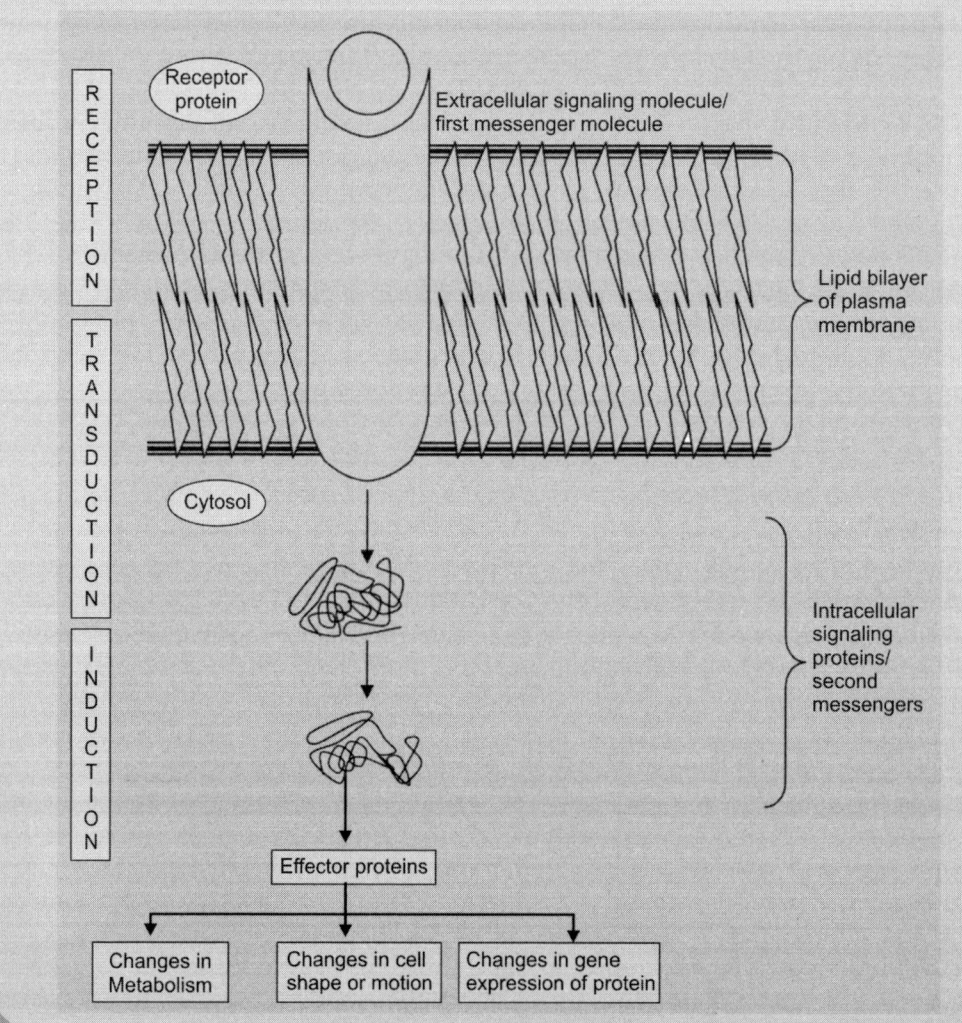

Signal transduction: Extracellular signaling molecules like steroidal hormones are nonpolar in nature, i.e. lipophilic and easily traverse through the lipid bilayer of the plasma membrane and enter into the cytosol of the cell. This is not possible with the polar molecules which are hydrophilic. The relay of the signal by these molecules is facilitated by the process of signal transduction. So, signal transduction is the ability of a cell to convert external stimuli into cellular events, ultimately leading to a cellular response.

The entire signal transduction process can be studied as a cascade of reactions involving different stages and various agents. The interactions for the sake of simplicity and ease of understanding can be divided as follows:

1. The interaction between the extracellular signal molecule–the receptor and the G-protein
2. The interaction between G-protein and adenylyl cyclase (adenylate cyclase)
3. Activation of protein kinase A
4. The interaction between G-protein and phospholipase C
5. Role of small G-proteins.

1. ***The interaction between the extracellular signal molecule, the receptor and the G-protein***

   Let us first have a look at the different players involved in this interaction.

   Extracellular signal molecules: The extracellular fluid may contain different molecules that have been secreted by the endocrine glands, e.g. hormones or they may be drug molecules that have been administered. These molecules are referred to as first messengers or ligands.

   Receptor: When the signal molecules are too polar or are too large to diffuse through the cell membranes, the information that signal molecules are present must be transmitted across the cell membranes without the molecules themselves entering the cell. This is made possible by a plasma membrane associated protein receptor that performs the task of transferring information across the membrane. As these proteins span across the plasma membrane they are called Transmembrane proteins. As they have seven helices, the domains are referred to as 7-transmembrane Helix. When such a receptor is bound at the intracellular portion to a G-protein it is called G-protein coupled receptor or GPCR. Adrenergic receptors, neurotransmitter receptors, opioid receptors, olfactory receptors and rhodopsin belong to the GPCR family of receptors.

   G-proteins: G-proteins are important molecules involved in the signal transducing process. They are bound to the inner surface of the cell membrane. They bear the name G- proteins because they bind the guanine nucleotides GDP and GTP. They are heterotrimeric, i.e. composed of three different sub units referred to as $G\alpha$, $G\beta$ and $G\gamma$ sub units. The $G\alpha$ sub unit contains the binding site for the nucleotides, GDP/GTP. The G-proteins are anchored to the inner cell surface via lipid anchors. There are different types of G-proteins and sub types within them. Some of the types of G-proteins are G_s, G_i and G_q. These G-proteins are referred to as large G-proteins. Apart from these large G-proteins which are heterotrimeric and activated by GPCRs there are also other G-proteins called small G-proteins. Structurally they are homologous to the sub unit of the heterotrimeric large G-proteins. The small G-proteins are also involved in signal transduction. In the inactive or resting state it is bound to GDP which it swaps for GTP when in the active state. When the extra cellular signal molecule or first messenger interacts with the 7-transmembrane protein and brings about a conformational change, which is relayed to the intracellular portion, it facilitates the $G\alpha$ subunit to release GDP and binds itself to GTP. In this process the $G\alpha$ and the $G\beta/G\gamma$ subunits are activated.

The process of transduction:
1. When an extra cellular signal molecule interacts with the receptor (7-transmembrane helix), i.e. GPCR there is a change in the tertiary structure of the receptor affording a new binding site in its intracellular portion.
2. A G-protein now binds to the new binding site. This leads to a change in the shape of the binding site of the guanyl nucleotide.
3. This renders the $G\alpha$ subunit more accessible to the cytosol where the concentration of the GTP is more than the concentration of the GDP. This in turn leads to the release of GDP by the $G\alpha$ subunit and binding to GTP. This is referred to as GDP-GTP exchange.
4. The binding of GTP brings about another conformational change leading to the dissociation of the $G\alpha$ subunit with the attached GTP from the $G\beta/G\gamma$ complex. Both these fragments also leave the receptor. The $G\beta/G\gamma$ dimer is called passive subunits of the G-protein because they are dissociated from the $G\alpha$ subunit when it carries out the important function of relay of the message.

Signal amplification: Before the extra cellular signal molecule detaches from the receptor, the complex is able to activate many G-proteins leading to amplification of the signal.

2. *The interaction between G-protein ($G_{s\alpha}$ sub unit) and adenylyl cyclase (adenylate cyclase)*

   G-protein: As we have seen in the previous stage the G-protein is by now split into two fragments-the $G\beta/G\gamma$ dimer and $G\alpha$ subunit with the attached GTP. Irrespective of the type of G-protein the above splitting remains the same. But further stages of transduction are dependant on the type of G-protein. Let us consider the case of G_s protein which produces the $G_{s\alpha}$ sub unit. This specific sub unit is capable of activating adenylyl cyclase (also known as adenylate cyclase).

   Adenylyl cyclase: It is an enzyme on the inner surface of the plasma membrane. It is a transmembrane protein. It catalyzes the conversion of ATP into Cyclic AMP also written as cAMP. This cAMP is called a second messenger. It relays the signal from the cell membrane into the cell.

$$ATP \rightarrow cAMP + PP_i$$

The phosphodiestrase enzymes, catalyze the hydrolysis of cAMP into AMP

$$cAMP + H_2O \rightarrow AMP$$

Second messengers: Apart from cyclic AMP, several other molecules within the cell act as intracellular messengers. Calcium ions, cGMP, phosphotidylinositol derivatives such as phosphotidylinositol triphosphate (PIP_3), diacylglycerol (DAG), inositol triphosphate (IP_3) and nitric oxide are some of them. The increased concentration of calcium ions in the cell can kick start changes like contraction and motility of cells or even activation of signaling pathways. A change in the levels of nitric oxide is accompanied by altered smooth muscle relaxation.

The process of signal transduction: When the α-subunit of the G_s (with the GTP) protein is bound to adenylyl cyclase it activates the adenylyl cyclase which catalyzes the conversion of ATP into cAMP. But the α subunit of the G_s protein possesses GTPase activity, i.e. the ability to catalyze the hydrolysis of GTP to GDP. This change leads to the restoration of the Gβ/Gγ dimer with the Gα-GDP sub-unit, forming the original G_s protein which is inactive. When the Gα subunit remains bound to the GDP, it is said to be in switch-off mode. When the Gα subunit is bound to GTP, it is said to be in switch-on mode.

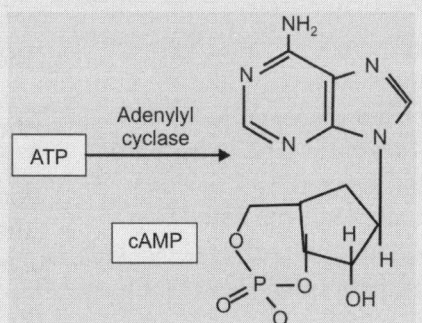

Signal amplification: Before the deactivation occurs, i.e. until the α-subunit is bound to the adenylyl cyclase, several molecules of cAMP are produced leading to signal amplification.

3. *Activation of protein kinase A—Deactivation of cAMP*

Let us have a brief look into what the Protein Kinases are.

Protein kinases: Signals are transmitted by activated receptors through intracellular signaling proteins called kinases. These protein kinases transfer the terminal phosphate of ATP to a hydroxyl group on the protein. This is called phosphorylation. The amino acids serine, tyrosine and threonine contain the hydroxyl group. Depending upon whether the amino acid involved is serine, tyrosine or threonine, the protein kinase is called serine kinase, tyrosine kinase or threonine kinase. The receptor bound to tyrosine kinase is referred to as RTK or Receptor Tyrosine Kinase. The process of phosphorylation alters the activity of enzyme by bringing about conformational changes and so changes in enzyme activity and conformation of proteins ultimately leading to changes in cellular activity. The phosphorylation reaction is shown.

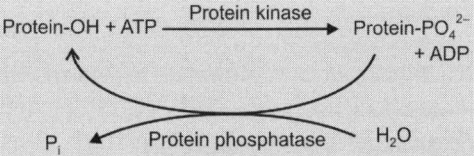

Protein phosphorylation is not irreversible. The reversal of the phosphorylation reaction is brought about by the Hydrolytic reaction catalysed by the enzyme Protein Phosphatase. Protein Phosphatases are a means of terminating a signaling process. If signaling process is not terminated, cells will loose their responsiveness to new signals. If the signaling process is not terminated properly it can lead to uncontrolled cell growth and the possibility of cancer.

The process of signal transduction: Cyclic AMP activates the protein kinase A. The protein kinase A is an inactive tetramer made up of two regulatory units and two catalytic subunits. These sub units are dissociated by cyclic AMP resulting in the formation of active catalytic sub units. The latter catalyze phosphorylation and activation of other enzymes with function very specifically to that cell/organ. Protein Kinase Inhibitors (PKIs) modulate the activity of the catalytic subunits. Phosphorylation that is catalyzed by Protein Kinase A activates the enzyme phosphodiesterase that cleaves cyclic AMP. So cyclic AMP stimulates its own degradation, acting as a switch off mechanism.

Example: Let us consider the series of phosphorylations by the protein kinase enzymes involved in the formation of glucose from glycogen in the liver and the resultant activation/deactivation of the target enzyme .The extracellular signal molecule in this case is the hormone adrenaline and the receptor is the β-adrenoceptor. All the events like the formation of cAMP and activation of Protein Kinase A occur as stated earlier. The enzyme Phosphorylase Kinase is phosphorylated which in turn catalyzes the phosphorylation of the inactive enzyme phosphorylase into the active form which ultimately catalyzes the breakdown of glycogen. Other phosphorylations that favour the production of glucose include the phosphorylation of the molecule Phosphorylase Inhibitor. Upon phosphorylation, this molecule inhibits the phosphatase enzyme which converts the active phosphorylase into inactive form. The enzyme Glycogen Synthase when phosphorylated is converted into an inactive form which cannot synthesize glycogen. So there is a three pronged effort to produce glucose in the liver cells.

Signal amplification: The catalytic subunits of Protein Kinase A catalyze the phosphorylation of several proteins before the cAMP self destructs. This leads to significant signal amplification.

4. *The interaction between G-protein and Phospholipase C*
   Phospholipase C: We have already seen that there are different types and subtypes of G-proteins like the G_s, G_i, and G_q. The enzyme phospholipase is activated/deactivated when certain receptors bind to a G_q protein. Phospholipases are involved in transmitting signals arising from the interaction of an extra cellular signal molecule and the receptor in the plasma membrane to the cell.

The process of signal transduction:
When the G_q protein interacts with an extracellular signal molecule all events until the the split of the a subunit remains the same excepting the fact that now the active fragment is a subunit of a G_q protein. From now on the signaling path takes a

different course. The nature of the released subunit decides whether the phospholipase would be activated or deactivated. Activation of phospholipase C catalyzes the hydrolysis of phosphatidylinositol diphosphate (PIP_2) which produces the second messengers inositol phosphate (IP_3) and Diacylglycerol (DAG).

- The DAG has a role in the activation of the enzyme Protein Kinase C (PKC)
- Activation of phospholipases affects Protein Kinase C. PKC is active in the presence of the second messengers calcium ions and diacylglycerol (DAG). The activated PKC catalyzes the phosphorylation of proteins with serine and threonine residues. These activated enzymes in turn catalyze other reactions resulting in various responses.
- The second messenger IP3 opens up the calcium ion channel and activates calcium dependant protein kinases which results in a cascade of reactions leading to activation of cell specific enzymes. The calcium ions bind to the protein calmodulin
- The second messengers IP3 and DAG reunite to form phosphatidylinositol diphosphate (PIP2) after their task is completed.

5. *Role of small G-proteins*

   Small G-proteins: Small G-proteins are also proteins involved in the signaling process and bind to GDP/GTP. They are referred to as small G-proteins because they are only about two thirds in size as compared to the large G-proteins. Just like the large G-proteins they bind to GDP in the resting state and exchange with GTP in the activated state. Guanine Nucleotide Exchange Factors (GEFs) promote the GDP/GTP exchange. The hydrolysis of GTP to GDP is autocatalysed or

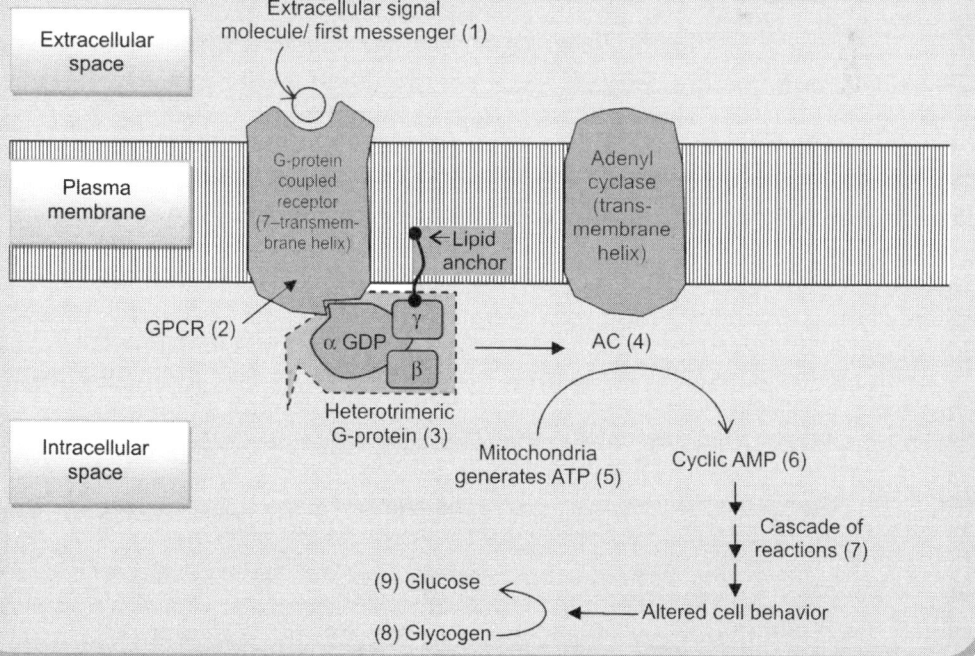

facilitated by GTPase Activating Proteins (GAPs). So the small G-proteins are controlled either way by the GEF and GAP. Mutations that prevent the proteins to hydrolyse the bound GTP keep them permanently activated leading to unrestricted cell growth.

Some of the small G-proteins are:
- Ras-involved in growth factor signal cascades
- Rab-involved in vesicle targeting and fusion
- Ran-involved in transport of proteins into and out of the nucleus
- Rho-involved in regulation of actin cytoskeleton

All these proteins differ in conformation depending upon whether they are bound to GDP or GTP at their nucleotide binding site.

The process of signal transduction: Small G-proteins play a major role in transmission of signal from the activated Receptor Tyrosine Kinase (RTK) into the cell. These small G-proteins act as molecular switches which upon activation are responsible for proteins that participate in the signaling process.

Signal amplification: Activated RTKs activate small G-proteins which in turn activate GEF. These activated exchange factors can now activate several small G-proteins which leads to amplification of the receptors initial signal.

Conclusion

An important function of cell signaling is to control and maintain normal physiological balance within the body. Continued proliferation and death of cells, alterations in metabolism and activation of genes are some of the cellular responses to extra cellular stimuli that needs signal transduction. An initial stimulus can set off a cascade of reactions like expression of genes which in turn can lead to the activation of a number of physiological events like increased uptake of glucose from the blood stream stimulated by insulin or migration of neutrophils to sites of infection stimulated by bacterial products. Mammalian cells need stimulation as well as control, not only for cell division but also for cell survival. However, in the absence of growth factor stimulation, cell death occurs. From all these we understand that signal transduction pathways are critical for biological processes and diseases can result in the event of their derangement. So GPCRs are attractive targets in the sphere of drug discovery. Although several hundred GPCRs have been established, the functions for most of them have not been unraveled. The number of drugs that target the GPCRs is bound to increase as the functions of the GPCRs are discovered.

References and Literature for Further Reading (for this discussion)

1. Graham L, Patrick; An introduction to Medicinal Chemistry; fourth edition.
2. Wesley K. Kvoeze, Douglas J. Sheffer and Bryan L. Roth (2003) G-protein coupled receptors at a glance. *Journal of Cell Science* 116, 4867–69.
3. Nevin A. Lambert, et al; Regulation of G-proteins accelerate GPCR signaling kinetics and govern stability solely by accelerating GTPase activity. *PNAS*.

4. "Peptide Hormone Signal Transduction", Animation by Larry Keedey, Professor Emeritus of Entomology, Texas A&M university.
5. Uerik Gether; Uncovering molecular mechanisms involved in activation of G-protein Coupled Receptors. *Endocrine reviews.*

Using experimentally determined or homology modeled target structures, rational drug design is the "intelligent" design of drugs—the medicinal chemistry approach that has come to stay. As mentioned earlier in this section, the current challenge is to use several strategies simultaneously towards achieving our goals. For example, the paper mentioned above that constructed and validated COX pharmacophore models (Schuster, et al., 2010) was not only able to validate the COX model but also apply it in ethnopharmacology. It was used to screen for new leads in the Thai traditional medicine used for the treatment of dysmenorrhea called "Prasaplai". This traditional medicine is known to be composed of 10 crude drugs:

- Sodium chloride
- Camphor
- The roots of *Acorus calamus* L. [sweet flag]
- The bulbs of *Allium sativum* L. [garlic]
- The pericarps of *Citrus hystrix* DC. [kaffir lime]
- The rhizomes of *Curcuma zedoaria* Roscoe [white turmeric]
- The bulbs of *Eleutherine americana* (L.) Merr. [type of croton]
- The seeds of *Nigella sativa* L. [Fennel Flower]
- The fruits of *Piper chaba* Hunt [type of chilly pepper]
- The fruits of *Piper nigrum* L. [black pepper]
- The rhizomes of *Zingiber cassumunar* Roxb [type of ginger]
- The rhizomes of *Zingiber oficinale* (Roscoe) [ginger]

The prasaplai database was earlier established (Tangyuenyongwatana, et al. 2008) and has 683 compounds. The screening of these compounds against the COX pharmacophore models lead to the identification of fatty acid derivatives and phenolic compounds. We know that one structure-based pharmacophore model represents a particular binding mode and so, to investigate several binding modes, one has to use several models. Some models are constructed using only the receptor as template whereas other models incorporate known ligands as well. In addition to modeling just the active site (using the pharmacophore), one can also dock the ligand(s) into a complete receptor for studying pharmacodynamics. In this light, we wish to connect two points mentioned separately earlier:

1. *Section 2.3.2.A (lead identification):* Aims to (amidst other things) successfully characterize "drug-likeness"–i.e. distinguish the drug from the non-drug (remember: independent of the target/applicable to any target/not target specific).
2. *Section 3.2 (docking):* Aims to (amidst other things) determine if a particular drug will bind to a particular receptor with enough specificity and strength (remember: independent of other factors/assuming that the drug would reach the target site)

We can therefore view the former as a *pharmacokinetic* aspect and the latter as the *pharmacodynamic* aspect. Let us now consider experimental high throughput screening (HTS) and virtual screening—are we doing the same thing twice? Recent studies clarify this point. Soichet and coworkers (Doman, et al. 2002) performed

- *HTS:* By creating 400,000 compound in-house library and experimentally screening it.

- *Virtual screening:* On molecules present in libraries containing commercially available compounds.

These were performed for the type 2 diabetes target protein tyrosine phosphatase 1B. The compounds obtained by HTS and by virtual screening were later compared experimentally. It was found that the group identified by virtual screening was more drug-like and had 1700-fold better performance than that identified by HTS. In yet another analysis (Paiva, et al. 2001), the exact same library of compounds was investigated theoretically and experimentally. They reported that

- Each method found a different group of molecules without overlap

- Virtual screening resulted in more potent molecules

- The two methods are complementary.

Several inhibitors have been identified for thrombin, Factor Xa, DNA gyrase, peroxisome-proliferator activated receptor (PPAR) ligands, etc. (Schuster, et al. 2010; Makino, et al. 2001; Liebeschuetz, et al. 2002; Markt, et al. 2008) using a combination of computational and experimental techniques such as those described above.

Docking investigates the mechanism of action of the drug in influencing the receptor. An example of how certain macroscopic responses of organisms to drugs can be justified by looking at the molecular behavior is discussed using piperine as an example. It is known that piperine is a natural agonist of the vanilloid receptor (TRPV1 channel). The receptor is important in the perception of thermal and nociceptive stimuli. It is known that the molecule (and also analogue methylpiperate) has antidepressant properties in addition. How? Does it influence any enzyme involved in the brain? The binding of piperine to Mono Amine Oxidase (MAO; EC 1.4.3.4; there are A and B forms) was therefore investigated by docking. In addition to establishing that it does indeed bind, the following inferences also resulted when performing flexible docking (*ref.* section 3.2):

1. The MAO enzyme has an "aromatic cage" that determines ligand positioning

2. The methylenedioxyphenyl (MDP) ring of piperine fails to dock comfortably between the phenolic side chains of Tyr407 and Tyr444 in human MAO-A in a flexible docking simulation (NOTE: no such behavior was observed in rigid docking; *in-silico* methods need to be as close to real situation in order to observed complete molecular behavior)

3. The MDP ring docked well in the MAO-B receptor form in both rigid as well as flexible docking!

4. Not only does piperine bind to MAO to produce its result, it is actually a selective modulator of the enzyme binding to MAO-B but not to MAO-A

Binding affinity can be measured experimentally by NMR, Surface Plasmon Resonance spectroscopy (SPR), Isothermal Titration Calorimetry (ITC), etc. The latter method can also indicate the mechanism of binding. Experiments and computations need to go hand in hand and it is possible to synchronize both with careful planning. The results obtained by docking can be confirmed by these techniques before launching molecules to the next phase of drug development. An example is the development of inhibitors of Pin 1 (peptidyl prolyl cis/trans isomerase–an anticancer target) (Potter, et al. 2010). NMR-based screening resulted in a fragment hit. This was followed by computational development into analogues that possessed nM potency against Pin1 and further into molecules that behaved as reversible inhibitors of the enzyme. Another example of the coordinated efforts of theory and experiment (Boehm, et al., 2000) is the search for an inhibitor for DNA gyrase. Virtual screening hits were confirmed by SAR, re-evaluated by NMR and biophysical experiments, and ultimately the DNA-gyrase–analogue complex was elucidated by X-ray study! Authors hope that these snapshots of examples will inspire readers with new ideas on how theory and experiment can be combined in the path to discovery using these modern principles of medicinal chemistry.

Important references: (Potter, et al.), (Schuster, et al. 2010), (Rahman, et al. 2010), (Shoichet, et al. 2002).

Bibliography

Abkevich, V.I., Gutin, A.M. and Shakhnovich, E.I. 1994. Specific nucleus as the transition-state for protein-folding - Evidence from the lattice model. Biochemistry. 1994, Vol. 33, pp. 10026–10036.

Agre, P., Johnson, P. F. and McKnight, S. L. (1989) Cognate DNA binding speci®city retained after leucine zipper exchange between GCN4 and C/EBP. Science. Vol. 246, pp. 922–926.

Agrestia, Jeremy J., et al. 2010. Ultrahigh-throughput screening in drop-based microfluidics for directed evolution. PNAS. 2010, Vol. 107, 9, pp. 4004–4009.

Ahlquist, R.P. 1948. A study of the adrenotrophic receptors. Am J Physiol. 1948, Vol. 155, pp. 586–600.

Ajay, WP, Walters and MA, Murcko. 1998. Can we learn to distinguish between 'drug-like' and 'nondrug-like' molecules? J Med Chem. 1998, Vol. 41, pp. 3314–3324.

Albert, A. 1951. Selective Toxicity. London: Methuen, 1951.

Allen, M. P. and Tildesley, D. J. 1989. Computer Simulation of Liquids. s.l. : oxford university press, 1989.

Allen, Michael P. 2004. Introduction to Molecular Dynamics Simulation. [book auth.] Norbert Attig, et al. Computational Soft Matter: From Synthetic Polymers to Proteins, Lecture Notes . s.l. : NIC Series, 2004, Vol. 23, pp. 1–28.

Allinger, N. L., Yuh, Y. H. and Lii, J. H. 1989. J. Amer. Chem. Soc. 1989, Vol. 111, p. 8551.

Allinger, Norman L. 1977. J. Amer. Chem. Soc. 1977, Vol. 99, p. 8127.

Altschul, SF, et al. 1990. Basic local alignment search tool. J Mol Biol. 1990, Vol. 215, 3, pp. 403–410.

Alvarez, uan and Shoichet, Brian. 2005. Virtual screening in drug discovery. Boca Raton, Florida : CRC Press, 2005.

An and Friesner. 2002.

Anderson Claus AF, Rost B. 2003. Secondary structure assignment. Structural Bioinformatics, pp. 341–363.

Andrews, Peter. 2005. 3D QSAR in Drug Design: theory methods and applications. [book auth.] Hugo Kubinyi. 2005, p. 13.

Anfinsen, C, et al. 1961. Proc. Natl. Acad. Sci. USA. 1961, Vol. 47, p. 1309.

Anfinsen, C.B. 1973. Science. 1973, Vol. 181, pp. 223–30.

Anson, ML. 1945. Protein Denaturation and the Properties of Protein Groups. Advances in Protein Chemistry. 1945, Vol. 2, pp. 361–386.

Arab, Shahriar, et al. 2007. Helix segment assignment in proteins using fuzzy logic. Iranian Journal of Biotechnology. 2007, Vol. 5, 2, pp. 93–99.

Armstrong, Jason W. 1999. A review of high-throughput screening approaches for drug discovery. Combinatorial Chemistry Review. 1999, Vol. April, p. 26. free download available at http://www.combichemistry.com/review.html.

Arnautova, Yelena A., Scheraga, Harold A. and Jagielska, Anna. 2006. A new force field (ECEPP-05) for peptides, proteins, and organic molecules. Journal of Physical Chemistry B. 2006, Vol. 110, 10, pp. 5025–5044.

Artymiuk, P.J., et al. 1979. Nature. 1979, Vol. 280, pp. 563–568.

Asaf A Salamov, Victor V Solovyev. 1995. Prediction of protein secondary structure by combining nearest-neighbor algorithms and multiple sequence alignments. J. Mol. Biol., Vol. 247, pp. 11–15.

Âsterberg, F., Morris, G.M., Sanner, M.F. and Olson, A.J. 2002. Proteins. 2002, Vol. 46, pp. 34–40.

Aung, Zeyar and Tan, Kian-Lee. 2006. MatAlign: Precise Protein Structure Comparison by Matrix Alignment. Journal of Bioinformatics and Computational Biology. 2006, Vol. 4, 6, pp. 1197–1216.

Balaram, P. and Ramaseshan, S. G N Ramachandran Festschrift. Bangalore : Indian Academy of Sciences.

Barlow, DJ and Thornton, JM. 1988. Helix geometry in proteins. J. Mol. Biol. 1988, Vol. 201, pp. 601–619.

Barone, S.R., et al. 1993. Newtonian Chaos + Heisenberg Uncertainty = macroscopic indeterminacy. American Journal of Physics. 1993, Vol. 61, 5.

Baroudi, Abdulkader, Mauldin, Justin and Alabugin, Igor V. 2010. Conformationally Gated Fragmentations and Rearrangements Promoted by Interception of the Bergman Cyclization through Intramolecular H-Abstraction: A Possible Mechanism of Auto-Resistance to Natural Enediyne Antibiotics? J. Am. Chem. Soc. 2010, Vol. 132, pp. 967–979.

Barton. 2005. Creation and analysis of protein multiple sequence alignments. [book auth.] Andreas D. Baxevanis and B. F. Francis Ouellette. Bioinformatics: A Practical Guide to the Analysis of Genes and Proteins. s.l. : John Wiley & Sons, Inc., 2005, pp. 333–336.

Bateman, A., et al. 2002. The Pfam protein families database. Nucleic Acids Res. 2002, Vol. 30, pp. 276–280.

Baxevanis, Andreas D. and Ouellette, B. F. Francis. 2005. Bioinformatics: A Practical Guide to the Analysis of Genes and Proteins. s.l. : John Wiley & Sons, Inc., 2005. p. 224.

Becktel, W. J. and Schellman, J. A. 1987. Biopolymers. 1987, Vol. 26, pp. 1859–1877.

Belleau, B. 1964. A molecular theory of drug action based on induced conformational perturbations of receptors. J. Med. Chem. 1964, Vol. 7, p. 776.

Benedetti E, Blasio B D, Pavone V, Pedone C, Santini A, Crisma M, Toniolo C. 1991. The 3–10 and alpha-helical conformation in peptides. [book auth.] Balaram... Molecular conformations and biological interactions. Bangalore : Indian Institute of Science, 1991, pp. 497–502.

Benkovic, Stephen J. and Hammes-Schiffer, Sharon. 2006. Enzyme Motions Inside and Out. Science. 2006, Vol. 312, 5771, pp. 208–209.

Bennett, Vann, O'keefe, Edward and Cuatrecasas, Pedro. 1975. Mechanism of Action of Cholera Toxin and the Mobile Receptor Theory of Hormone Receptor-Adenylate Cyclase Interactions. Proc. Nat. Acad. Sci. USA. 1975, Vol. 72, 1, pp. 33–37.

Bergethon, Peter R. 1998. The Physical Basis of Biochemistry: The Foundations of Molecular Biophysics. New York : Academic Press, 1998.

Berman H M, Westbrook J, Feng Z, Gilliland G, Bhat T N, Weissig H, Shyndalyov I N, Bourne P E. 2000. The Protein Data Bank. Nuclei acid research, Vol. 28, pp. 235–242.

Bettens, Ryan P. A., et al. 2009. The influence of crystal packing effects upon the molecular structures of Ph3Sn(CH2)nSnPh3, n = 1 to 8, as determined by X-ray crystallography and DFT molecular orbital calculations. Supramolecular aggregation patterns sustained by C–H interactions. Cryst Eng Comm. 2009, Vol. 11, pp. 1362–1372.

Blaney, JM and Dixon, JS. 1993. A good ligand is hard to nd: automated docking methods. Perspect Drug Discovery Design. 1993, Vol. 1, pp. 301– 319.

Blouin C, Butt D, Roger A J. 2004. Rapid evolution in conformational space: a study of loop regions in a ubiquitous GTP binding domain. Protein Sci., Vol. 13, pp. 608–616.

Blum, L.C. and Reymond, J.-L. 2009. J. Am. Chem. Soc. 2009, Vol. 131, 25, pp. 8732–8733.

Boehm, HJ, et al. 2000. Novel inhibitors of DNA gyrase: 3D structure based biased needle screening, hit validation by biophysical methods, and 3D guided optimization. A promising alternative to random screening. J Med Chem. 2000, Vol. 43, pp. 2664–2674 .

Böhm, H.-J. 1994. J. Comput.-Aided Mol. Des. 1994, Vol. 8, pp. 243–256.

Böhm, Hans-Joachim. 1998. Prediction of binding constants of protein ligands: A fast method for the prioritization of hits obtained from de novo design or 3D database search programs. Journal of Computer-Aided Molecular Design. 1998, Vol. 12, 4.

Bohne, A., Lang, E. and Von der Lieth, C.-W. 2000. Molecular visualization programs on the web. Drugs of the Future. 2000, Vol. 25, 5, p. 489.

Bower, Michael J., Cohen, Fred E. and Jr, Roland L. Dunbrack. 1997. Prediction of Protein Side-chain Rotamers from a Backbone-dependent Rotamer Library: A New Homology Modeling Tool. J. Mol. Biol. 1997, Vol. 267, pp. 1268–1282.

Boyer, Joshua A. and Lee, Andrew L. 2008. monitoring aromatic picosecond to nanosecond dynamics in proteins via 13C Relaxation: Expanding Perturbation Mapping of the Rigidifying Core Mutation, V54A, in Eglin c. Biochemistry, 2008, Vol. 47, 17, pp. 4876–4886.

Branden, C. and Tooze, J. 1999. Introduction to Protein Structure. second edition. s.l. : Garland Publishing, 1999.

Brannigan, James A. and Wilkinson, Anthony J. 2002. Protein engineering 20 years on. Nature Reviews Molecular Cell Biology. 2002, Vol. 3, pp. 964–970.

Brevern, AG de and Hazout, S. 2001. compacting local protien folds with the "hybrid protein" models. Theor Chem. Acc. 2001, Vol. 106, pp. 36–47.

Brinda et al. 2005.

Brooks BR, Bruccoleri RE, et al. 1983. CHARMM—A program for macromolecular energy, minimization, anddynamics calculations. J. Comput. Chem. 1983, Vol. 4, pp. 187–217.

Brooks, BR., et al. 2009. CHARMM: The Biomolecular simulation Program. J. Comp. Chem. 2009, Vol. 30, pp. 1545–1615.

Brown, RJ, et al. 2005. Model for growth hormone receptor activation. Nat Struct Mol Biol. 2005, Vol. 12, pp. 814–821.

Bruccoleri, R. E. and Karplus, M. 1987. Prediction of the folding of short polypeptide segments by uniform conformational sampling. Biopolymers. 1987, Vol. 26, p. 137.

Bruice, Xiaohua Zhang and C., Thomas. 2007. Diels-Alder Ribozyme Catalysis: A Computational Approach. J. Am. Chem. Soc. 2007, Vol. 129, pp. 1001–1007.

Bryngelson, J.D. and Wolynes, P.G. 1989. Intermediates and barrier crossing in a random energy model (with applications to protein folding). J. Phys. Chem. 1989, Vol. 93, pp. 6902–6915.

Buck, Patrick M. and Bystroff, Christopher. Simulating protein folding initiation sites using an alpha-carbon-only knowledge-based force field. Proteins: Structure, Function, and Bioinformatics. Vol. 76, 2, pp. 331–342.

Burke D F, Deane C M, Blundell T L. 2000. Browsing the SLoop database fo structurally classified loops connecting elements of protien secondary structure. 6, 2000, Bioinformatics, Vol. 16, pp. 513–519.

Burkert, U. and Allinger, N.L. 1982. Molecular Mechanics. ACS Monograph 177. Washington, D.C.: American Chemical Society, 1982, pp. 64–72.

Busch, SJ and et al. 1990. Trends Genet. 1990, Vol. 6, pp. 36–40.

Bychkova, VE and Ptitsyn, OB. 1993. Stostoianie rasplavlenno- globuly belkovykh molekul stanovitsia skoreepravilom. chem iskliucheniem. Biofizika. 1993, Vol. 38, 1, pp. 58–66.

Carignano, M.A. 2002. Monte Carlo simulations of small water clusters: microcanonical vs canonical ensemble. Chemical Physics Letters. 2002, Vol. 361, pp. 291–297.

Carino, Andrea, et al. 2008. Endocrine Disrupter adsorbed on plastic debris and its environmental implications on fish. 2008.

Cartailler JP, Luecke H. 2004. Structural and functional characterization of pi bulges and other short intrahelical deformations. Structure (Camb), Vol. 12, pp. 133–144.

Carugo, Oliviero. 2006. Rapid Methods for Comparing Protein Structures and Scanning Structure Databases. Current Bioinformatics. 2006, Vol. 1, pp. 75–83.

Cecconi, C, et al. 2005. Direct observation of the three-state folding of a single protein molecule. Science. 2005, Vol. 309, pp. 2057–60.

Chakraborty, Atanu, Paul, Bindu Diana and Nagaraja, Valakunja. 2007. Bacteriophage Mu C protein is a new member of unusual leucine zipper-HTH class of proteins. Protein Engineering, Design & Selection. 2007, pp. 1–5.

Chakravarthy, S, et al. 2008. Systematic analysis of the effect of multiple templates on the accuracy of comparative models of protein structure. BMC Struct Biol. 2008, Vol. 8, p. 31.

Chan AW, Hutchinson EG, Harris D, Thornton JM. 1993. Identification, classification and analysis of beta bulges in protiens. Protein Sci, Vol. 2, pp. 1574–1590.

Chance M R, Fiser A, Sali A, Pieper U, Eswar N, Xu G, Fajardo J E, Radhakannan T, Marinkovic N. 2004. High-throughput computational and experimental techniques in structural genomics. Genome Res., Vol. 14, p. 2145.

Charifson, P.S. 1997. Practical Application of Computer-Aided Drug Design. New York : Marcel Dekker, 1997.

Charton, 1991.

Chelvanayagam, Gareth, Heringa, Jaap and Argos, Patrick. 1992. Anatomy and evolution of proteins displaying the viral capsid jellyroll topology. J. Mol. Biol. 1992, Vol. 228, pp. 220–242.

Chothia, et al. 1983.

Chothia, C. and Lesk, A.M. 1987. Canonical structures for the hypervariable regions of immunoglobulins. J Mol. Biol. 1987, Vol. 196, 4, pp. 901–917.

Chothia, C., et al. 1983. Nature. 1983, Vol. 302, pp. 500–505.

Chothia, Cyrus and Lesk, Arthur M. Conformation of strand entry into parallel β-sheets. Bangalore: s.n.

Chou, P. Y. and Fasman, G. D. 1974. Biochemistry. 1974, Vol. 13, 2, p. 211.

Chou, Peter Y and Fasman, Gerald D. 1977. Beta-turns in proteins. J Mol. Biol. 1977, Vol. 115, pp. 135–175.

Christopoulos, A and El-Fakahany, EE. 1999. Qualitative and quantitative assessment of relative agonist efficacy. Biochem. Pharmacol. 1999, Vol. 58, 5, pp. 735–48.

Clackson, T and Wells, JA. 1995. A hot spot of binding energy in a hormone–receptor interface. Science. 1995, Vol. 267, pp. 383–386.

Clark, DE. 2002. Computational methods for prediction of ADME and toxicity. Advanced drug delivery reviews. 2002, Vol. 54, pp. 253–254.

Clark, M., Cramer, R.D. and Van Opdenbosch, N. 1989. Validation of the General Purpose Tripos 5.2 Force Field. J. Comp.Chem. 1989, Vol. 10, pp. 982–1012.

Claudia, BABIJ and J., POë Anthony. 2004. Deconstruction of Taft's σ^* parameter: QSAR meets QALE. Journal of physical organic chemistry. 2004, Vol. 17, 2, pp. 162–167 .

Clementi, C, Nymeyer, H and Onuchic, JN. 2000. Topological and energetic factors: What determines the structural details of the transition state ensemble and "en-route" intermediates for protein folding? An investigation for small globular proteins. J. Mol. Biol. 2000, Vol. 298, pp. 937–53.

Coleman, William F. 2008. Molecular Models of Peroxides and Albendazoles. Journal of Chemical Education. 2008, Vol. 85, 12, p. 1710.

Collins, Francis S., Morgan, Michael and Patrinos, Aristides. 2003. The Human Genome Project: Lessons from Large-Scale Biology. Science. 2003, Vol. 300, pp. 286–290.

Colloc'h N, Etchebest C, Thoreau E, Henrissat B, Mornon J-P. Comparison of three algorithms for the assignment of secondary structure in proteins: the advantages of a consensus assignment. Vol. 6, pp. 377–382.

Connolly, Michael L. 1985. J. Am. Chem. Soc. 1985, Vol. 107, 5, pp. 1118–1124.

Cornell, WD, et al. 1995. A Second Generation Force Field for the Simulation of Proteins, Nucleic Acids, and Organic Molecules. J. Am. Chem. Soc. 1995, Vol. 117, pp. 5179–5197.

Cramer, Christopher J. 2005. Essentials of computational chemistry: theories and models. London : John Wiley, 2005.

Cramer, R. D., Petterson, D. E. and Bunce, J. D. 1988. Comparitive Molecular Field Analysis -? J. Am. Chem. Soc. 1988, Vol. 110, pp. 5959–5967.

Cramer, R.D., III, Patterson, D.E. and Bunce, J.D. 1988. Comparative Molecular Field Analysis (CoMFA). 1. Effect of shape on Binding of steroids to Carrier proteins. J. Am. Chem. Soc. 1988, Vol. 110, pp. 5959–5967.

Crawford JL, Lipscomb WN, Schellman CG. 1973. Proc. Natl. Acad. Sci. USA, Vol. 70, pp. 538–542.

Creamer, TP and Rose, GD. 1994. A-helix-forming propensities in peptides and proteins. Proteins. 1994, Vol. 19, pp. 85–97.

Creighton, Thomas E. 1990. Protein folding. Biochem. J. 1990, Vol. 270, pp. 1–16.

—. 1993. Proteins: Structures and molecular properties. S.I.: WH Freeman, 1993.

Crippen, Gordon M. 1978. The tree structural organization of proteins. J. Mol. Biol. 1978, Vol. 126, 3, pp. 315–32.

Cruciani and et al. 2000. Molecular fields in quantitative structure-permeation relationships: the VolSurf approach. J. Mol. Struct. (Theochem). 2000, 503, pp. 17–30.

Crum-Brown, A. and Fraser, T.R. 1869. Trans. R. Soc. Edinburgh. 1869, Vol. 25, 151, pp. 1868–1869.

Cuff, J., et al. 1998. JPRED: a consensus secondary structure prediction server. Bioinformatics. 1998, Vol. 14, pp. 892–893.

Cummings, JL, et al. 2002. Guidelines for managing Alzheimer's disease: Part II. Treatment. Am Fam Physician. 2002, Vol. 65, 12, pp. 2525–34.

Dahl, David B, et al. 2008. Assessing side-chain perturbations of the protein backbone: a knowledge-based classification of residue Ramachandran space. Journal of molecular biology. 2008, Vol. 378, 3, pp. 749–58.

Dalal, S, Balasubramanian, S. and Regan, L. 1997. Protein alchemy: changing beta-sheet into alpha-helix. Nat structure biology. 1997, Vol. 4, 7, pp. 548–52.

Dasgupta, B, et al. 2004. Expanded turn conformations: characterization and sequence structure correspondencein alpha-turns with implications in helix folding. Protiens. 2004, Vol. 55, pp. 305–315.

Dauber-Osguthorpe, P, et al. 1988. Structure and energetics of ligand binding to proteins: Escherichia coli dihydrofolate reductase-trimethoprim, a drug-receptor system. Proteins. 1988, Vol. 4, 1, pp. 31–47.

Day R, Beck D A, Armen R S, Daggett V. 2003. A consensus view of fold space: combining SCOP, CATH and the Dali domain dictionary. Protein Science, Vol. 12 (10), pp. 2150–2160.

Dayhoff, M.O., Schwartz, R. and Orcutt, B.C. 1978. A model of Evolutionary Change in Proteins. Atlas of protein sequence and structure. s.l. : Nat. Biomed. Res. Found., 1978, Vol. 5, pp. 345–358.

Deane, C. M. and Blundell, T. L. CODA: a combined algorithm for predicting the structurally variable regions of protein models. Protein Sci. Vol. 10, p. 599.

Debnath, AK, et al. 1991. J Med Chem. 1991, Vol. 34, pp. 786–797.

Di, Li and Kernsy, Edward H. 2003. Profiling drug-like properties in discovery research. Current Opinion in Chemical Biology. 2003, Vol. 7, pp. 402–408.

Dill, K. A. 1985. Theory for the folding and stability of globular proteins. Biochemistry. 1985, Vol. 24, 6, pp. 1501—1509 .

Dill, KA and Chan, HS. 1997. From Levinthal to pathways to funnels. Nat. Struct. Biol. 1997, Vol. 4, pp. 10–19.

Dill, Ken A. 1990. Dominant forces in protein folding. Biochemistry. 1990, Vol. 29, pp. 7133–55.

—. 1999. Polymer principles and protein folding. Protein Sci. 1999, Vol. 8, pp. 1166–80.

Dill, Ken A., et al. 2008. The Protein Folding Problem. Annu. Rev. Biophys. 2008, Vol. 37, pp. 289–316.

Dixon, Steven L. and Merz. Jr., Kenneth M. 1997. Fast, accurate semiempirical molecular orbital calculations for macromolecules. J. Chem. Phys. July 15, 1997, Vol. 3, p. 107.

Dobzhansky, Theodosius. Anything in biology makes sense only in the light of evolution. American Biology Teacher. Vol. 35, pp. 125–129.

Doig, A J, et al. 1997. Structure of N-termini of helices in protiens. Protein Science. 1997, Vol. 6, pp. 147–155.

Doig, AJ. 2008. The alpha-Helix as the Simplest Protein Model: Helix–Coil Theory, Stability, and Design. [book auth.] V. Muñoz. Protein Folding, Misfolding and Aggregation: Classical Themes and Novel Approaches. London : Royal Society of Chemistry, 2008.

Dokholyan, N. V. and Shakhnovich, E. I. 2001. J. Mol. Biol. 2001, Vol. 312, pp. 289–307.

Dokholyan, Nikolay V., Shakhnovich, Boris and Shakhnovich, Eugene I. 2002 . Expanding protein universe and its origin from the biological Big Bang. PNAS. 2002 , Vol. 99, 22, pp. 14132–14136.

Doman, TN, et al. 2002. Molecular docking and high-throughput screening for novel inhibitors of protein tyrosine phosphatase-1B. J Med Chem. 2002, Vol. 45, pp. 2213–2221.

Drie, J. H. van. 2004. The importance of being Earnest. [book auth.] P. Bultinck, et al. Computational Medicinal Chemistry for Drug Discovery. s.l. : Marcel Dekker, 2004.

Duan, Y. and Kollman, P. A. 1998. Pathways to a protein folding intermediate observed in a 1-microsecond simulation in aqueous solution. Science. 1998, Vol. 282, pp. 740–744.

Dupuis, Franck, Sadoc, Jean-Francois and Mornon, Jean-Paul. 2004. Protein secondary structure assignment through Voronoi Tessellation. Protiens. 2004, Vol. 55, 3, pp. 519–528.

Dyson HJ, Wright PE. 2006. According to current texbooks, a well defined three-dimensional structure is a prerequisite for the function of a protein. is this correct? : s.n., IUBMB Life, Vol. 58(2), pp. 107–109.

Dyson, H. Jane and Wright, Peter E. 2005. Intrinsically Unstructured Proteins and their Functions. Nature reviews. 2005, Vol. 6, p. 197.

Dyson, H.Jane and Wright, Peter E. 1993. Peptide conformation and protein folding. Current Opinion in Structural Biology. 1993, Vol. 3, 1, pp. 60–65.

Eaton, W.A., et al. 2000. Annu. Rev. Biophys. Biomol. Struct. 2000, Vol. 29, pp. 327–359.

Edwards, D.P. 2005. Regulation of signal transduction pathways by estrogen and progesterone. Annu. Rev. Physiol. 2005, Vol. 67, pp. 23.1–23.42.

Efimov, A V. 1984. A novel supersecondary structure of protiens and the relation between structure and amino acid sequence. FEBS, Vol. 166(1), pp. 33–38.

Efimov, A V. 1986. [Standard structures in protein molecules I: a-b-Hairpins]. Molekulyarnaya Biologiya, Vol. 20(2), pp. 329–339.

Efimov, A V. 1986. [Standard structures in protein molecules II: α-β-Hairpins]. Molekulyarnaya Biologiya, Vol. 20(2), pp. 340–345.

Efimov, A V. 1987. Pseudo-homology of protein standard structures formed by two consecutive β-strands. FEBS letters, Vol. 224(2), pp. 372–376.

Efimov, A V. 1991. Structure of coiled β-β-hairpins and β-β-corners. FEBS, Vol. 284(2), pp. 288–292.

Efimov, A V. 1991. Structure of α-α-hairpins with short connections. Protein engineering, Vol. 4, pp. 245–250.

Efimov, A V. 1993. Patterns of loop regions in proteins. Curr. Opinion Struct. Biol., Vol. 3, pp. 379–384.

Efimov, A V. 1993. Standard structures in proteins. Prog. Biophys. molec. Biol. 1993, Vol. 60, pp. 201–239.

Efimov, A V. 1997. A structural tree for proteins containing 3β-corners. FEBS letters, Vol. 407, pp. 37–41.

Eldridge, M.D., et al. 1997. Empirical Scoring Functions. I. The Development of a Fast, Fully Empirical Scoring Function to Estimate the Binding Affinity of Ligands in Receptor Complexes. J. Comput.-Aided Mol. Design. 1997, Vol. 11, pp. 425–445.

Elliott, William H. 2009. Biochemistry and Molecular Biology. s.l. : Oxford University Press , 2009.

Ellis, RJ. 2001. Macromolecular crowding: an important but neglected aspect of the intracellular environment. Curr Opin Struct Biol . 2001, Vol. 11.

Eriksson, Lennart, et al. 2006. Megavariate analysis of environmental QSAR data. Part I – A basic framework founded on principal component analysis (PCA), partial least squares (PLS), and statistical molecular design (SMD). [book] Molecular Diversity. 2006, Vol. 10, pp. 169–186.

Espadaler, J., et al. 2004. ArchDB: automated protein loop classification as a tool for structural genomics. Nucleic Acids Res. 2004, Vol. 32, p. D185.

Eswar N, Ramakrishnan C, Srinivasan N. 2003. Stranded in isolation: structural role of isolated extended strands in protiens. Prot Eng , Vol. 16, pp. 331–339.

Ewing, T.J.A. and Kuntz, I.D. 1997. Critical evaluation of search algorithms for automated molecular docking and database screening. J. Comput. Chem. 1997, Vol. 18, pp. 1176–1189.

Ferguson, D. M. and Raber, D. J. 1989. J. Am. Chem. Soc. 1989, Vol. 111, p. 4371.

Fernandez-Fuentes, N., et al. 2005. Prediction of the conformation and geometry of loops in globular proteins: testing ArchDB, a structural classification of loops. Proteins. 2005, Vol. 60, pp. 746–757.

Fernandez-Fuentes, Narcis, Oliva, Baldomero and Fiser, Andras. 2006. A supersecondary structure library and search algorithm for modeling loops in protein structures. Nucleic Acids Research. 2006, Vol. 34, 7, pp. 2085–2097.

Fersht, A R. 1995. Optimization of rates of protein folding: the nucleation-condensation mechanism and its implications. Proc Natl Acad Sci U S A. 1995, Vol. 92, 24, pp. 10869–10873.

Fersht, A. 1985. Enzyme Structure and Mechanism. San Francisco : Freeman, 1985.

Fersht, AR, et al. 1985. Hydrogen bonding and biological specificity analysed by protein engineering. Nature. 1985, Vol. 314, pp. 235–38.

Fetrow, JS. 1995. Omega Loops: non-regular secondary structures significant in protein structres and stability. FASEB J. 1995, Vol. 9, pp. 708–717.

Fidelis K, Stern P S, Bacon D, Moult J. Comparison of systematic search and database methods for constructing segments of protein structure. 1994, Protein Eng., Vol. 7, p. 953.

Filizola, M and Weinstein, H. 2005. The study of G-protein coupled receptor oligomerization with computational modeling and bioinformatics. FEBS J. 2005, Vol. 272, 12, pp. 2926–38.

Fink, AL. 1995. Compact intermediate states in protein folding. Annu Rev Biophys Biomol Struct. 1995, Vol. 24, pp. 495–522.

Finkelstein, A.V. and Badretdinov, A.Ya. 1997. Fold. Des. 1997, Vol. 2, pp. 115–121.

Fischer, D. 2006. Servers for protein structure prediction. Curr Opin Struct Biol. 2006, Vol. 16, 2, pp. 178–182.

Fischer, E. 1894. Einfluss der Configuration auf die Wirkung der Enzyme. Ber. Dtsch. Chem. Ges. 1894, Vol. 27, p. 2985.

Fiser, A., Do, R.K. and Sali, A. 2000. Modeling of loops in protein structures. Protein Sci. 2000, Vol. 9, p. 1753.

Flaherty, K M, et al. 1991. Similarity of the three-dimensional structures of actin and the ATPase fragment of a 70-kDa heat shock cognate protein. PNAS. 1991, Vol. 88, 11, pp. 5041–5045 .

Fodje, M.N. and Al-Karadaghi, S. 2002. Occurance, conformational features and amino acid propensities for the pi-helix. Protien Engg. 2002, Vol. 15, pp. 533–558.

Fourier, L, Benros, C and Brevern, A G de. 2004. Use of a structural alphabet for the analysis of short loops connecting rpititive structures. BMC Bioinformatics. 2004, Vol. 5, p. 58.

Foye, William O., Lemke, Thomas L. and Williams, David A. 2008. Foye's principles of medicinal chemistry. 6. s.l. : Lippincott Williams & Wilkins, 2008.

Francesco V Di , Garnier J, Munson P J. 1997. Protein topology recognition from secondary structure sequences: applications of the Hidden Markov Models to the alpha class protiens. J Mol Biol, Vol. 267, pp. 446–463.

Freddolino, Peter L., et al. 2008. Ten-Microsecond Molecular Dynamics Simulation of a Fast-Folding WW Domain. Biophysical Journal: Biophysical Letters. 2008, Vol. 94, 10, pp. L75–L77.

Freire, Ernesto, Haynie, Donald T. and Xie, Dong. 2004. Molecular basis of cooperativity in protein folding IV. Core: A general cooperative folding model. Proteins. 2004, Vol. 17, 2, pp. 111–123.

Frenkel, Daan and Smit, B. 2001. Understanding Molecular Simulation, 2001.

Frishman, Dmitrij and Argos, Patrick. 1985. Knowledge-based protein secondary structure assignment. PROTEINS: structure, fuction and genetics. 1985, Vol. 23, pp. 566–579.

—. 1994. The FSSP database of structurally aligned protein fold Families. Nucleic Acids Research. 1994, Vol. 22, 17, pp. 3600–3609.

Fuller, Jonathan C., Burgoyne, Nicholas J. and Jackson, Richard M. 2009. Predicting druggable binding sites at the protein–protein interface. Drug Discovery Today. 2009, Vol. 14, 3/4.

Gaillard, P., et al. 1994. J. C.A.M.D. 1994, Vol. 8, p. 83.

Galzitskaya, Oxana V., Ivankov, Dmitry N. and Finkelstein, Alexei V. 2001. Folding nuclei in proteins. FEBS Letters. 2001, Vol. 489 , pp. 113–118.

Garnier, J and Robson, B. 1990. [book auth.] G. D. Fasman. Prediction of Protein Structure and the Principles of Protein Conformation. New York & London : Plenum Press, 1990, pp. 417–465.

Gasteiger, J. and Marsili, M. 1978. Tetrahedron Lett. 1978, p. 3181.

—. 1980. Itera partial equalization of orbital electronegativity–a rapid access to atomic charges. Tetrahedron 1980, pp. 3219–3228.

Gerstein, M., Lesk, A. and Chothia, C. 1991. Biochemistry. 1991, Vol. 22, pp. 6739–6749.

Ghose, Arup K., et al. 2006. Knowledge-based chemoinformatic approaches to drug discovery. Drug Discovery Today. December 2006, Vol. 11, 23/24.

Gö, N and Taketomi, H. 1978. Respective roles of short- and long-range interactions in protein folding. Proc. Natl. Acad. Sci. USA. 1978, Vol. 75, pp. 559–63.

Godzik, Adam and Jaroszewski, Lukasz. 2000. Search for a new description of protein topology and local structure. Proc Int Conf Intell Syst Mol Biol. 2000, Vol. 8, pp. 211–217.

Gohlke, H. and Klebe, G. 2002. Angew. Chem. Int. Ed. 2002, Vol. 41, pp. 2644–2676.

Gohlke, H., Hendlich, M. and Klebe., and G. 2000. Knowledge Based Scoring Function to Predict Protein-Ligand Interactions. Journal of Molecular Biology. 2000, Vol. 295, pp. 337–356.

Goldman, B.B. and Wipke, W.T. 2000. QSD quadratic shape descriptors. 2. Molecular docking using quadratic shape descriptors (QSDock). Proteins. 2000, Vol. 38, pp. 79–94.

Gottlieb, Scott and fellow, Clegg. 1998. Is the FDA approving drugs too fast? BMJ. 1998, Vol. 317, 7163, pp. 899–900.

Gough, J, et al. 2001. Assignment of Homology to Genome Sequences using a Library of Hidden Markov Models that Represent all Proteins of Known Structure. J Mol Biol. 2001, Vol. 313, 4, pp. 903–919.

Gramatica, Paola. A short history of QSAR evolution. QSAR Research Unit in Environmental Chemistry and Ecotoxicology. Vol. http://www.qsar.it.

Grant, Guy H. and Richards, W. Graham. 2003. Computational Chemistry. [book auth.] Alan Hinchliffe. Molecular Modelling for Beginners. 2003.

Gribbon, Philip and Sewing, Andreas. 2005. High-throughput drug discovery:what can we expect from HTS? Drug Discovery Today. 2005, Vol. 10, 1.

Gromiha, MM. 2005. A statistical model for predicting protein folding rates from amino acid sequence with structural class information. J Chem Inf Model. 2005, Vol. 45, 2, pp. 494–501.

Gutin, A.M., Abkevich, V.I. and Shakhnovich, E.I. 1995. Biochemistry. 1995, Vol. 34, pp. 3066–3076.

Hadley, Caroline and Jones, David T. 1999. A systematic comparison of protein structure classifications: SCOP, CATH and FSSP. Structure. 1999, Vol. 7, pp. 1099–1112.

Hagemann, Michael, et al. N,N-Dimethylaminopropylsilane: A Case Study on the Nature of Weak Intramolecular Si...N Interactions. Chemistry - A European Journal. Vol. 14, 35, pp. 11027–1038.

Halgren, Thomas A. 1996. Merck molecular force field. I. Basis, form, scope, parameterization, and performance of MMFF94. J. Comp. Chem. 1996, pp. 490–519.

Hall, J. G. and Frieden, C. 1989. Proc. Natl. Acad. Sci. U.S.A. 1989, Vol. 86, pp. 3060–3064.

Hamada, D, Segawa, S and Goto, Y. 1996. Nat. Struct. Biol. 1996, Vol. 3, pp. 868–73.

Hammett, Louis P. 1935. Some Relations between Reaction Rates and Equilibrium Constants. Chem. Rev. 1935, Vol. 17, 1, pp. 125–136.

Hancock, CK, Meyers, EA and Yager, BJ. 1961. J Am Chem Soc. 1961, Vol. 83, pp. 4211–4213.

Hansch, C. and et al. 1990. Comprehensive Medicinal Chemistry. s.l. : Pergamon Press, 1990.

Hansch, C. and Fujita, T. 1964. J. Am. Chem. Soc. 1964, Vol. 86, p. 1616.

Hansch, C., et al. 1962. Nature. 1962, 194, p. 178.

Harada, N., Fujita, K. and Watanabe, M. 1997. Enantiomer. 1997, Vol. 2, p. 359"366.

Hardman, J.G., Limbird, L.E. and Gilman, A.G. 2001. Goodman & Gilman's The Pharmacological Basis of Therapeutics. 10th ed. New York : McGraw-Hill, 2001.

Harrison, Andrew, et al. 2003. Recognizing the fold of a protein structure. 2003, Vol. 19, 14, pp. 1748–1759.

Harrison, S. C. and Durbin, R. 1985. Proc. Natl. Acad. Sci. U.S.A. 1985, Vol. 82, pp. 4028–4030.

Harvel, Edward and Di, Li. 2008. Drug-like properties : concepts, structure design and methods : from ADME to toxicity optimization. [ed.] Kerns. Amsterdam; Boston : Academic Press, 2008.

Hashem, Yaser and Auffinger, Pascal. 2009. A short guide for molecular dynamics simulations of RNA systems. Methods. 2009, Vol. 47, pp. 187–197.

Hecht, M.H., et al. 2004. De novo proteins from designed combinatorial libraries. Protein Sci. 2004, Vol. 13, pp. 1711–23.

Hecht, Stefan and Huc, Ivan. 2007. Foldamers: structure, properties, and applications. Weinheim : Wiley-VCH, 2007.

Helm, M., et al. 2005. J. Am. Chem. Soc. 2005, Vol. 127, 30, pp. 10492–10493.

Hemerta, Formijn J. van, et al. 2008. Mosaic amino acid conservation in 3D-structures of surface protein and polymerase of hepatitis B virus. Virology. 2008, Vol. 370, 2, pp. 362–372.

Henikoff, S. and Henikoff, J.G. 1992. Amino Acid Substitution Matrices from Protein Blocks. PNAS. 1992, Vol. 89, pp. 10915–10919.

Hill, D. J., et al. 2001. A Field Guide to Foldamers. Chem. Rev. 2001, Vol. 101, pp. 3893–4011.

Hirst, D.M. 1990. A Computational Approach to Chemistry. [book auth.] ?? Oxford : Blackwell Scientific Publications, 1990, pp. 108–111; 400–403.

Hockenmaier, J, Joshi, AK and Dill, KA. 2006. Routes are trees: the parsing perspective on protein folding. Proteins. 2006, Vol. 66, pp. 1–15.

Hogue, Christopher W.V., Ohkawa, Hitomi and Bryant, Stephen H. A dynamic look at structures: WWW-Entrez and the Molecular Modeling Database. Trends in Biochemical Sciences. Vol. 21, pp. 226–229.

Holm, Liisa, et al. 1992. A database of protein structure families with common folding motifs. Protein Science. 1992, Vol. I, pp. 1691–1698.

Holm, Liisa and Sander, Chris. 1991. Database algorithm for generating protein backbone and side-chain co-ordinates from a Cα trace: Application to model building and detection of co-ordinate errors. Journal of Molecular Biology. 1991, Vol. 218, 1, pp. 183–194 .

—. 1993. Parser for protein folding units. Proteins. 1993, Vol. 19, pp. 256–268.

—. 1993. Protein structure comparison by alignment of distance matrices. J. Mol. Biol. 1993, Vol. 233, pp. 123–138.

—. 1993. Proteins: Structures and molecular properties. s.l. : W.H. Freeman, 1993.

—. 1994. The FSSP database ofstructurally aligned protein fold Families. Nucleic Acids Research. 1994, Vol. 22, 17, pp. 3600–3609.

—. 1996. Mapping the protein universe. Science. 1996, Vol. 273, 5275, pp. 256–268.

—. 1997. Proteins. 1997, vol. 28, pp. 72–82.

Höltje, Hans-Dieter, et al. 2008. Molecular Modeling – basic principles and applications. s.l. : Wiley-Vch, 3rd edn, 2008.

Honig and Yang. 1995. 1995.

Hooft, R.W., et al. 1996. WHATCHECK: Errors in protein structures. Nature. 1996, Vol. 381, 6580, p. 272.

Houk, K. N., et al. 2003. Binding Affinities of Host-Guest, Protein-Ligand, and Protein-Transition-State Complexes. Angewandte Chemie International Edition. 2003, Vol. 42, 40, pp. 4872–4897.

HovmoÈller, Sven, Zhou, Tuping and Ohlson, Tomas. 2002. Conformations of amino acids in proteins. Acta Cryst. 2002, Vol. D58, pp. 768–776.

Humphrey W, Dalke A, Schulten K. 1996. VMD-Visual Molecular Dynamics. J Molec. Graphics, Vol. 14(1), pp. 33–38.

Hutchinson, E.G. and Thornton, J.M. 1994. A Revised Set of Potentials for Beta-Turn Formation in Proteins. Protein Sci. 1994, Vol. 3, pp. 2207–2216.

Ing, H. R., Kordik, P. and Tudor-Williams, D. P. H. 1952. The structure-action relationship of the choline group. Brit. J. Pharmacol. Chemother. 1952, Vol. 7, pp. 103–116.

Ioannis Michalopoulos, Gilleain M Torrance,David R Gilbert, David R Westhead. 2004. An enhanced database of protein structural topology. Nucleic Acid research. 2004, Vol. 32, pp. D251–D254.

Islam, S.A., Luo, J. and Sternberg, M.J.E. 1995. Identification and analysis of domains in proteins. Protein Eng. 1995, Vol. 8, pp. 513–525.

—. 1952. J. Am. Chem. Soc. 1952, Vol. 74, p. 3120.

—. 1987. J. Am. Chem. Soc. 1987, Vol. 109, p. 3150.

—. 1993. J Med Chem. 1993, Vol. 36, pp. 1450 – 1460.

Jackson, S.E. 1998. Fold. Des. 1998, Vol. 3, pp. R81–R91.

Jacobsa, Steven and Cuatrecasas, Pedro. 1976. The mobile receptor hypothesis and "cooperativity" of hormone binding. Application to insulin. Biochimica et Biophysica Acta (BBA) – Biomembranes. 1976, Vol. 433, 3, pp. 482–495.

Joachimiak, LA, et al. 2006. Computational design of a new hydrogen bond network and at least a 300-fold specificity switch at a protein–protein interface. J Mol Biol. 2006, Vol. 361, pp. 195–208.

Johnson(III), Russell D. 2010. NIST Computational Chemistry Comparison and Benchmark Database. NIST Standard Reference Database Number 101. [Online] February 15, 2010. http://cccbdb.nist.gov.

Jones, D. 1999. Protein secondary structure prediction based on position specific scoring matrices. J. Mol. Biol. 1999, Vol. 292, pp. 195–202.

Jones, David T and McGuffin, Liam J. 2003. Assembling novel proteins from super-secondary structural fragments. PROTEIN: structure, function, and genetics. 2003, Vol. 53, pp. 480–485.

Jones, David T. 2001. Predicting novel protein folds by using FRAGFOLD. Proteins: Structure, Function, and Bioinformatics. 2001, Vol. 45, suppl 5, pp. 127–132.

Jones, G., Willett, P., Glen, R.C., Leach, A.R. and Taylor, R. 1997. J. Mol. Biol. 1997, 267, pp. 727–748.

Jónsdóttir, Svava Ósk and Rasmussen, Kjeld. 2000. The Consistent Force Field. Part 6: An optimized set of potential energy functions for primary amines. New J. Chem. 2000, Vol. 24, pp. 243–247.

Jorgensen, W. L., Maxwell, D. S. and Rives, J. Tirado. 1996. Development and testing of the OPLS all-atom force field on conformational energetics and properties of organic liquids. J. Am. Chem. Soc. 1996, Vol. 118, pp. 11225–11236.

Kabsch, Wolfgang and Sander, Christian. 1983. Dictionary of secondary structure of proteins: pattern recognition of hydrogen-bonded and geometrical features. Biopolymers. 1983, Vol. 22, 12, pp. 2577–2637.

Karelson, M. 2000. Molecular Descriptors in QSAR/QSPR. New York : Wiley-InterScience, 2000.

Karlin, A. 1967. The acetylcholine receptor channel in the absence of exogenously applied cholinergic agent. J Theor Biol. 1967, Vol. 16, p. 306.

Karlsson, A. J., et al. 2006. J. Am. Chem. Soc. 2006, Vol. 128, pp. 12630–12631.

Karpen M E, De-aseth P L, Neet K E. 1992. Differences in amino acid distribution of 3(10)-helices and alpha-helices. Protein Science, Vol. 1, pp. 1333–1342.

Karpen, Mary E., Pieterl, De Haseth and Neet, Kenneth E. 1992. Differences in the amino acid distributions of 310-helices and a-helices. Protein Science. 1992, Vol. 1, pp. 1333–1342.

Karplus, M. and Weaver, D.L. 1994. Protein folding dynamics: the diffusion-collision model and experimental data. Protein Sci. 1994, Vol. 3, pp. 650–68.

Katritzky, Alan R., Karelson, Mati and Petrukhin, Ruslan. The CODESSA PRO project (COmprehensive DEscriptors for Structural and Statistical Analysis).

Kaur, Harpreet and Raghava, G.P.S. 2004. Prediction of -Turns in Proteins Using PSI-BLAST Profiles and Secondary Structure Information. PROTEINS: Structure, Function, and Bioinformatics. 2004, Vol. 55, pp. 83–90.

Kauzmann, W. 1959. Adv. Protein Chem. 1959, Vol. 14, pp. 1–63.

Kawasaki, H. and Kretsinger, R.H. 1995. Calcium-binding proteins 1: EF-hands. Protein Profile. 1995, Vol. 2, pp. 297–490.

Keeble, AH, et al. 2006. Calorimetric dissection of colicin DNase–immunity protein complex specificity. Biochemistry. 2006, Vol. 45, pp. 3243–3254.

Keil, M, et al. 2009. Molecular visualization in the rational drug design process. Front Biosci. Jan 1 2009, Vol. 14, pp. 2559–83.

Kendrew, J C, et al. 1958. A Three-Dimensional Structure of the Myoglobin Molecule Obtained by X-ray Analysis. Nature. 1958, Vol. 181, pp. 662–666.

Keskin, O, et al. 2005. Protein–protein interactions: organization, cooperativity and mapping in a bottom-up systems biology approach. Phys Biol. 2005, Vol. 2, pp. S24–S35.

Khanna, Richie, et al. 2010. The pharmacological chaperone isofagomine increases the activity of the Gaucher disease L444P mutant form of -glucosidase. FEBS Journal. 2010, Vol. 277, 7, pp. 1618–1638.

Kim, David E., et al. 2005. Automated Prediction of Domain Boundaries in CASP6 Targets Using Ginzu and RosettaDOM. PROTEINS: Structure, Function, and Bioinformatics Suppl. 2005, Vol. 7, pp. 193–200.

Kim, S.T., et al. 1999. Enhanced conformational diversity search of CDR-H3 in antibodies: role of the first CDR-H3 residue. Proteins. 1999, Vol. 37, pp. 683–696.

Kim, You Jung and Patel, Jignesh M. 2006. A framework for protein structure classification and identification of novel protein structures. BMC Bioinformatics. 2006, Vol. 7, p. 456.

Kister, Alexander E. and Phillips, James C. (2008) 1–17. 2008. The most severe test for hydrophobicity scales: Two proteins with 88% sequence identity but different structure and function. arXiv.org, e-Print Archive, Condensed matter, pp. 1–17.

Kittredge, M. C., et al. 2008. J. Chem. Educ. 2008, Vol. 85, pp. 1655–1657.

Klebe, G. and Abraham, U. 1999. Comparitive Molecular Similarity Indices Analysis. J. Comput.-Aided Mol. Design. 1999, Vol. 13, pp. 1–10.

Klepeis, J. L. and Floudas, C. A. 2003. ASTRO-FOLD: A Combinatorial and Global Optimization Framework for Ab Initio Prediction of Three-Dimensional Structures of Proteins from the Amino Acid Sequence. Biophysical Journal. 2003, Vol. 85, pp. 2119–2146.

Kolinski, A. 2004. Protein modeling and structure prediction with a reduced representation. Acta Biochim Polon. 2004, Vol. 51, pp. 349–371.

Kollman PA, Massova I, Reyes C, Kuhn B, Huo S, Chong L, Lee M, Lee T, Duan Y, Wang W, Donini O, Cieplak P, Srinivasan J, Case DA and Cheatham TE III. 2000. 2000, Acc. Chem. Res., Vol. 33, pp. 889–897. Kollman PBSA solvent scoring function.

Kollman. 1993.

Konkoli Z, Kraka E, Cremer D. 1997. Unified reaction valley approach mechanism of the reaction CH3+ H2 —> CH4 + H. J. Phys. Chem. A, Vol. 101, pp. 1742–1757.

Kopp, Jürgen and Schwede, Torsten. 2004. The SWISS-MODEL repository of annotated three-dimensional protein structure homology models. Nucleic acids research. 2004, Vol. 3, database issue, pp. D230 – D234.

Koretke and et al. 1999.

Koshland, D.E. 1958. Application of a theory of enzyme specificity to protein synthesis. Proceedings of the National Academy of Sciences USA. 1958, Vol. 44, 2, pp. 98–104.

Koyack, M. J. and Cheng, R. P. 2006. Methods Mol. Biol. 2006, Vol. 340, pp. 95–109.

Kraka, E. 1998. Reaction Path Hamiltonian and its Use for Investigating Reaction Mechanisms. [book auth.] Allinger NL, Clark T, Gasteiger J, Kollman PA, Schaefer III HF, Schreiner PR Schleyer PvR. Encyclopedia of computational chemistry. Chichester, UK : John Wiley, 1998, Vol. 4, p. 2437.

Kreyszig, Erwin. 1991. Differential geometry. s.l. : Dover publications, 1991.

Krishna, MMG, et al. 2006. Order of steps in the cytochrome c folding pathway: evidence for a sequential stabilization mechanism. J.Mol. Biol. 2006, Vol. 359, pp. 1411–20.

Kroemer, Romano T. 2007. Structure-Based Drug Design: Docking and scoring. Current Protein and Peptide Science. 2007, Vol. 8, pp. 312–328.

Krogsgaard-Larsen, Povl, Liljefors, Tommy and Madsen, Ulf. 2002. Textbook of drug design and discovery. London : Taylor and Francis, 2002.

Kryshtafovych, Andriy, et al. 2009. Protein structure prediction center in CASP8. Proteins: Structure, Function, Bioinformatics. 2009, Vol. 77, (Suppl 9), pp. 5–9 .

Kubelka, J, et al. 2006. Sub-microsecond protein folding. J. Mol. Biol. 2006, Vol. 359, pp. 546–53.

Kubinyi, Hugo. 1997. QSAR and 3D-QSAR in drug design Part 1: methodology. Drug Discovery Today. 1997, Vol. 2, 11, p. 457.

—. 1997. QSAR and 3D-QSAR in drug design. Part 2: applications and problems. Drug Discovery Today. 1997, Vol. 2, 12, p. 538.

—. 1995. The quantitative analyisis of structure-activity relationships. [book auth.] Manfred E Wolff. Burger's Medicinal Chemistry and Drug Discovery. s.l. : Wiley-Interscience, 1995, pp. 497–571.

Kubinyi. 3D QSAR in drug design: theory methods and applications.

Kumar, S, Bansal, M and Velavan, R. 2000. HELANAL: a program to characterize helix geometry in proteins. J Biomol. Struct. Dyn. 2000, Vol. 17, pp. 811–819.

Kuntz, I D. 1972. J Am Chem Soc. Vol. 94, pp. 4009–4012.

Kuntz, I.D., et al. 1982. A Geometric Approach to Macromolecule-Ligand Interactions. J. Mol. Biol. 1982, Vol. 161, pp. 269–288.

Kuntz, I.D., et al. 1999. The maximal affinity of ligands. Proc. Natl. Acad. Sci. U.S.A. 1999, Vol. 96, pp. 9997–10002.

Kuwajima, K. and Sugai, S. 1978. Biophys. Chem. 1978, Vol. 8, pp. 247–254.

Kwasigroch J-M, Chomilier J, Mornon J-P. 1996. A global taxonomy of loops in globular protiens. J Mol Biol, Vol. 259(4), pp. 855–872.

Kyle, DJ and et al. 1991. Med Chem. 1991, Vol. 34, p. 2649.

Laity, J. H., Dyson, H. J. and Wright, P. E. 2000. DNA-induced α-helix capping in conserved linker sequences is a determinant of binding affinity in Cys2-His2 zinc fingers. J. Mol. Biol. 2000, Vol. 295, pp. 719–727.

Lander, Eric S. and et al. 2001. Initial sequencing and analysis of the human genome. Nature. 2001, Vol. 409, pp. 860–921.

Langley, J. 1901. On the stimulation and paralysis of nerve cells and of nerve-endings. Part 1. J Physiol. 1901, Vol. 27, 3, pp. 224–236.

Laskowski, R A, et al. 1993. PROCHECK: a program to check the stereochemical quality of protein structures. J. App. Cryst. 1993, Vol. 26, pp. 283–291.

Laskowski, R. 1995. SURFNET: a program for visualizing molecular surfaces, cavities and intermolecular interactions. J Mol Graph. 1995, Vol. 13, pp. 323–330.

Laskowski, R.A., et al. 1996. AQUA and PROCHECK-NMR: programs for checking the quality of protein structures solved by NMR. J Biomol. NMR. 1996, Vol. 8, 4, pp. 477–486.

Lau, K.F. and Dill, K.A. 1989. A lattice statistical mechanics model of the conformational and sequence spaces of proteins. Macromolecules. 1989, Vol. 22, pp. 638–642.

Launay, Guillaume and Simonson, Thomas. 2008. Homology modelling of protein-protein complexes: a simple method and its possibilities and limitations. BMC Bioinformatics. 2008, Vol. 9, 427.

Lazaridis, T. and Karplus, M. 2000. Effective energy functions for protein structure prediction. Curr Opin Struct Biol. 2000, Vol. 10, 2, pp. 139–145.

Leach, Andrew. 1997. Molecular Modelling: Principles and Applications. 2. s.l. : Prentice Hall, 1997.

Lee KH, Benson DR, Kuczera K. 2000. Transitions from alpha to pi helix observed in molecular dynamics simulations of synthetic peptides. Biochemistry, Vol. 39, pp. 13737–13747.

Lee, B. and Richard, F.M. 1971. The interpretation of protein structures: estimation of static accessibility. J Mol Biol. 1971, Vol. 55, pp. 379–400.

Lee KH, Benson DR, Kuczera K. 2000. Transitions from alpha to pi helix observed in molecular dynamics simulations of synthetic peptides. 2000, biochemistry, Vol. 39, pp. 13737–13747.

Leff, P, et al. 1997. Trends Pharmacol. Sci. 1997, Vol. 18, p. 355.

Leo, A. 1993. Estimating LogPoct from structures. Chem. Rev. 1993, Vol. 5, pp. 1281–1306.

Leopold, PE, Montal, M and Onuchic, JN. 1992. Protein folding funnels: a kinetic approach to the sequence-structure relationship. Proc. Natl. Acad. Sci. USA. 1992, Vol. 89, pp. 8721–25.

Leszczynski, J.F. and Rose, G.D. 1986. Loops in globular proteins: A novel category of protein secondary structure. Science. 1986, Vol. 234, pp. 849–855.

Levinthal, Cyrus. 1968. J. Chim. Phys. Chim. Biol. 1968, Vol. 65, pp. 44–45.

Levitt, Michael and Greer, Jonathan. 1977. Automatic identification of secondary structure in globular proteins. J. Mol. Biol. 1977, Vol. 114, pp. 181–293.

Lewis, P.N., Momany, F.A. and Scheraga, H.A. 1973. Chain Reversals in Proteins. Biochem. Biophys. Acta. 1973, Vol. 303, pp. 211–229.

Li, Jinyan and Liu, Qian. 2009. 'Double water exclusion': a hypothesis refining the O-ring theory for the hot spots at protein interfaces. Bioinformatics. 2009, Vol. 25, 6, pp. 743–750.

Li, W, Liu, W and Lai, L. 1999. Protien loops on structurally similar scaffolds: database and conformationally similar analysis. Biopolymers. 1999, Vol. 49, pp. 481–95.

Liebeschuetz, JW, et al. 2002. PRO_SELECT: combining structure-based drug design and arraybased chemistry for rapid lead discovery. 2. The development of a series of a series of highly potent and selective factor Xa inhibitors. J Med Chem. 2002, Vol. 45, pp. 1221–1232.

Limbird, L.E. 2005. Cell Surface Receptors: A Short Course on Theory and Methods. s.l. : Springer, 3rd Edn, 2005.

Limbird, LE. 2004. The receptor concept: A continuing evolution. Mol. Interv. 2004, Vol. 4, 6, pp. 326–36.

Linderstrøm-Lang, Kaj Ulrik. 1952. Proteins and Enzymes. Lane Medical Lectures. s.l. : Stanford University Press, 1952, Vol. VI.

Linusson, A., et al. 2000. Statistical molecular design of building blocks for combinatorial chemistry. J. Med. Chem. 2000, Vol. 43, 1320–1328.

Lipinski, Christopher A. 2003. Chris Lipinski discusses life and chemistry after the Rule of Five. Drug Discovery Today. 2003, Vol. 8, 1, pp. 12–16.

Lipton, M. and Still, W. C. 1988. J. Comput. Chem. 1988, Vol. 9, p. 343.

Liszewski, Kathy. 2006. drug discovery: successful lead optimization strategies. Genetic Engg & biotech news. august 1, 2006, Vol. 26, p. 14.

Liwo, A., et al. 1993. Calculation of protein backbone geometry from a-carbon coordinates based on peptide-group dipole alignment. Protein science. 1993, Vol. 2, pp. 1697–1714.

Longhi, S. and et al. 2003. The C-terminal domain of the measles virus nucleoprotein is intrinsically disordered and folds upon binding to the C-terminal moiety of the phosphoprotein. J. Biol. Chem. 2003, Vol. 278, pp. 18638–18648.

Loo, TW and Clarke, DM. 2007. Chemical and pharmacological chaperones as new therapeutic agents. Expert Rev Mol Med. 2007, Vol. 9, pp. 1–18.

Lovell, Word, Richardson, J.S. and D.C., Richardson. 2000. The penultimate rotamer library. Proteins. 2000, Vol. 40, pp. 389–408.

Lu, Guoguang. 2000. TOP: A new method for protein structure comparisons and similarity searches. J Appl Cryst. 2000, Vol. 33, pp. 176–83.

Lyubchenko, Yuri L., et al. 1993. CA runs increase DNA flexibility in the complex of lambda. Cro protein with the OR3 site. Biochemistry. 1993, Vol. 32, 15, pp. 4121–4127.

Ma, Buyong, et al. 2003. Protein-protein interactions: Structurally conserved residues distinguish between binding sites and exposed protein surfaces. PNAS. 2003, Vol. 100, 10, pp. 5772–5777.

Mahler, G., et al. 2008. J. Chem. Educ. 2008, Vol. 85, pp. 1652–1654.

Maity, H., et al. 2005. Protein folding: The stepwise assembly of foldon units. Proc. Natl. Acad. Sci. 2005, Vol. 102, pp. 4741–4746.

Majumdar I, Krishna SS, Grishin NV. 2005. PALSSE: A program to delineate linear secondary structural elements from protein structures. BMC Bioinformatics, Vol. 6, p. 202.

Makino, S, et al. 2001. Discovery of a novel serine protease inhibitor utilizing a structure-based and experimental selection of fragments technique. J Comput Aided Mol Des. 2001, Vol. 15, pp. 553–559.

Makino, S., Ewing, T.J. and Kuntz, I.D. 1999. DREAM++: flexible docking program for virtual combinatorial libraries. J. Comput. Aided Mol. Des. 1999, Vol. 13, pp. 513–32.

Mannhold, R., Krogsgaard-Larsen, P. and Timmerman, H. 1993. QSAR: Hansch Analysis and Related Approaches. [book auth.] H. Kubinyi. Methods and Principles in Medicinal Chemistry. s.l. : VCH, 1993.

—. 1996. Mapping the protein universe. Science. 1996, Vol. 273, 5275, pp. 595–603.

Markt, P., et al. 2008. J. Med. Chem. 2008, Vol. 51, pp. 6303–6317.

Marrone, Tami J., Briggs, James M. and McCammon, J. Andrew. 1997. Structure-Based Drug Design: Computational advances. Annu. Rev. Pharmacol. Toxicol. 1997, Vol. 37, pp. 71–90.

Marshall, Garland R., et al. 1979. The Conformational Parameter in Drug Design: The active analogue approach. [book auth.] Edward C. Olson and Ralph E. Christoffersen. Computer-Assisted Drug Design. s.l. : American Chemical Society, 1979, Vol. 112, pp. 205–226.

Martin J, Lettelier G, Marin A, Taly J-F, Brevern A-G-de, Gibrat J-F. 2005. Protein secondary structure asignment revisited: a detailed analysis of different asiignment methods. BMC Structural Biology, Vol. 5, p. 17.

Martin, A.C., Cheetham, J.C. and Rees, A.L. 1989. Modeling antibody hypervariable loops: a combined algorithm. PNAS. 1989, Vol. 86, pp. 9268–9272.

Massart, D.L., et al. 1997–1998. Handbook of Chemometrics and Qualimetrics. s.l. : Elsevier, 1997–1998.

Matouscheck, A., et al. 1995. Biochemistry. 1995, Vol. 34, pp. 13656–13662.

Matsuda, H, Taniguchi, F and Hashimoto, A. 1997. An approach to the detection of protien structural motifs using an encoding scheme of backbone conformations. Pacific Symposium on Biocomputing. 1997, Vol. 2, pp. 280–291.

Mattos C, Petsco GA, Karplus M. 1994. Analysis of two-residue turns in proteins. J Mol Biol, Vol. 238, pp. 733–747.

Mayo, Stephen L., Olafson, Barry D. and III, William A. Goddard. 1990. DREIDING: A Generic Force Field for Molecular Simulations. J . Phys. Chem. 1990, Vol. 94, pp. 8897–8909.

McGovern, SL, et al. 2002. A common mechanism underlying promiscuous inhibitors from virtual and high-throughput screening. J Med Chem. 2002, Vol. 45, pp. 1712–1722.

McGuffin, Liam J. 2007. Benchmarking consensus model quality assessment for protein fold recognition. BMC Bioinformatics. 2007, Vol. 8, p. 345.

McPherson, J. D. and et al. 2001. Nature. 2001, Vol. 409, p. 934.

Mehler, E.L. and Solmajer, T. 1991. Electrostatic effects in proteins: comparison of dielectric and charge models. Protein Engineering. 1991, Vol. 4, pp. 903–910.

Mekenyan, O. and Bonchev, D. 1986. Acta Pharm Jugosl. 1986, Vol. 36, p. 225.

Mendieta-Wejebe, Jessica E., et al. 2008. Comparing the electronic properties and docking calculations of heme derivatives on CYP2B4. J Mol Model. 2008, Vol. 14:, pp. 537–545.

Meyer, H. 1899. Arch. Exp. Pathol. Pharmakol. 1899, Vol. 42, p. 109.

Mezei, M. 1998. Chameleon sequences in the PDB. Protein Eng. 1998, Vol. 11, pp. 411–14.

Mezei, Mihaly. 2003. A novel fingerprint for the characterization of protein folds. Protein Engineering. 2003, Vol. 16, 10, pp. 713–715.

Mezey, Paul G. 2009. QSAR and the ultimate molecular descriptor: the shape of electron density clouds. Journal of Mathematical Chemistry. 2009, Vol. 45, 2.

Michalopoulos, Ioannis, et al. 2004. TOPS: An enhanced database of protein structural topology. Nucleic Acid research. 2004, Vol. 32, pp. D251–D254.

Michalsky, E, Goede, A and Preissner, R. 2003. Loops In Proteins (LIP) - a comprehensive loop database for homology modelling. Protein Engg. 2003, Vol. 16, 12, pp. 979–85 .

Miles, Andrew J., Sansom, Clare E. and Wallace, Bonnie A. 2005. Protein Structure and its Classification. [book auth.] Moss, Jelaska and Pongor. Essays in Bioinformatics. s.l. : IOS Press, 2005.

Miller, Clark A., Abbott, Nicholas L. and Pablo, Juan J. de. 2009. Surface Activity of Amphiphilic Helical {beta}-Peptides from Molecular Dynamics Simulation. Langmuir. 2009, Vol. 25, pp. 2811–2823.

Mills, J.E. and Dean, P.M. 1996. Three-dimensional hydrogen-bond geometry and probability information from a crystal survey. J Comput Aided Mol Des. 1996, Vol. 10, 6, pp. 607–622.

Milner-White, J E. 1988. Recurring loop motif in proteins that occurs in right-handed and left-handed forms Its relationship with alpha-helices and beta-bulge loops. J Mol Biol, Vol. 199(3), pp. 503–511.

Milner-White, J E. 1990. Situation of Gamma turns in proteins. Their relatio to alpha-helices, beta-sheets and lignad-binding sites. J Mol. Biol. 1990, Vol. 216, 2, pp. 386–397.

Miyazawa, Sanzo and Jernigan, Robert L. 1996. Residue-residue potentials with a favorable contact pair term and an unfavorable high packing density term, for simulation and threading. Journal of Molecular Biology. 1996, pp. 623–644.

—. 2000. Molecular basis for modulation of biological function by alternate splicing of the Wilms' tumor suppressor protein. Proc. Natl Acad. Sci. USA. 2000, Vol. 97, pp. 11932–11935.

Monod, J, Wyman, J and Changeaux, J.-P. 1965. J Mol Biol. 1965, Vol. 12, p. 88.

Montgomery, John A, et al.

Morris, G.M., Goodsell, D.S., Halliday, R.S., Huey, R., Hart, W.E., Belew, R.K. and Olson, A.J. 1998. Automated docking using a Lamarckian genetic algorithm and an empirical binding free energy function. J. Comput. Chem. 1998, Vol. 19, pp. 1639–1662.

Moult, J and James, M. N. 1986. An algorithm for determining the conformation of polypeptide segments in proteins by systematic search. Proteins. 1986, Vol. 1, p. 146.

Zhang J, Quin M, Wang W. 2005. Multiple folding mechanisms of protien ubiquitin. 2005, Proteins: structure, function and bioinformatics, Vol. 59 (3), pp. 565–579.

Murzin AG, Finkelstein AV. 1988. General archtecture of the alpha-helical globule. J. Mol. Biol., Vol. 204, pp. 749–769.

Murzin, A.G., et al. 1995. SCOP: a structural classification of proteins database for the investigation of sequences and structures. J. Mol. Biol. 1995, Vol. 247, pp. 536–540.

Myers, J.K. and Oas, T.G. 2001. Preorganized secondary structure as an important determinant of fast protein folding. Nat. Struct. Biol. 2001, Vol. 8, pp. 552–58.

Nagler, James J., et al. 2007. The complete nuclear estrogen receptor family in the rainbow trout: Discovery of the novel ER2 and both ER isoforms. Gene. 2007, Vol. 392, pp. 164–173.

National Research Council, USA: Committee on challenges. 2003. Beyond the Molecular Frontier: Challenges for Chemistry and Chemical Engineering. Washington DC : National Academic Press, 2003.

Navizet, Isabelle, Cailliez, Fabien and Lavery, Richard. 2004. Probing Protein Mechanics: Residue-Level Properties and Their Use in Defining Domains. Biophysical Journal. 2004, Vol. 87, pp. 1426–1435.

Needleman, Saul B. and Wunsch, Christian D. 1970. A general method applicable to the search for similarities in the amino acid sequence of two proteins. Journal of Molecular Biology. 1970, Vol. 48, 3, pp. 443–53.

Nelson, David and Cox, Michael. 2008. Lehninger Priniciples of Biochemistry. s.l. : W. H. Freeman, 2008.

Nicolaou, K. C. and Dai, W. M. 1992. Molecular design and chemical synthesis of potent enediynes. 2. Dynemicin model systems equipped with C-3 triggering devices and evidence for quinone methide formation in the mechanism of action of dynemicin A. J. Am. Chem. Soc. 1992, Vol. 114, 23, pp. 8908–8921.

Niculescu-Duvâz, et al. 1981. A quantitative structure-activity analysis of the mutagenic and carcinogenic action of 43 structurally related heterocyclic compounds. Carcinogenesis. 1981, Vol. 2, 4, pp. 269–275.

Nogrady, Thomas and Weaver, Donald F. 2005. Medicinal chemistry: a molecular and biochemical approach. 3rd edn. Oxford : Oxford University Press, 2005.

Noguchi T, Onizuka K, Akiyama Y, Saito M. PDB-REPRDB: A Database of Representative Protein Chains in PDB (Protein Data Bank) 1997. Menlo Park, CA. : AAAI press, 1997. Proceedings of the Fifth International Conference on Intelligent Systems for Molecular Biology.

Notredame, C., Higgins, D. and Heringa, J. 2000. T-COFFEE: a novel method for fast and accurate multiple sequence alignment. J. Mol. Biol. 2000, Vol. 302, pp. 205–217.

Nunes, Sandra C.C., et al. Conformational study of isolated pindolol by HF, DFT and MP2 calculations.

O'Brien, Robert A. 1986. Receptor binding in drug research. s.l. : Marcel Dekker Inc, 1986.

O'Shea, EK and et al. 1989. Science. 1989, Vol. 243, pp. 538–542.

Offmann, Bernard, Tyagi, Manoj and Breverne, Alexandre G de. 2007. Local protein structures. Current Bioinformatics. 2007, Vol. 2, 3, pp. 165–202.

Ofran and Rost. 2005. Predictive methods using protein sequences. [book auth.] Andreas D. Baxevanis and B. F. Francis Ouellette. Bioinformatics: A Practical Guide to the Analysis of Genes and Proteins. s.l. : John Wiley & Sons, Inc., 2005, pp. 198–219.

—. 2002. On the sequencing of the human genome. Proc Natl Acad Sci U S A. 2002, Vol. 99, 6, pp. 3712–3716.

Onuchic, J. N., et al. 1995. Toward an outline of the topography of a realistic protein-folding funnel. PNAS USA. 1995, Vol. 92, 8, pp. 3626–3630.

Onuchic, José Nelson, et al. 1996. Protein folding funnels: the nature of the transition state ensemble. Folding & Design. 1996, Vol. 1, pp. 441–450.

Onuchic, Jose Nelson, Luthey-Schulten, Zaida and Wolynes, Peter G. 1997. Theory of Protein Folding: The Energy Landscape Perspective. Annu. Rev. Phys. Chem. 1997, Vol. 48, pp. 545–600.

Oprea, T. I. 2001. Rapid estimation of hydrophobicity for virtual combinatorial library analysis. SAR QSAR Environ. Res. 2001, Vol. 12, pp. 129–141.

Oprea, T.I., Zamora, I. and Svensson, P. 2001. Qvo vadis, scoring functions? Toward an integrated pharmacokinetic and binding Affinity Prediction Framework. [book auth.] A. K. Ghose and V. N. Viswanadhan. Combinatorial Library Design and Evaluation for Drug Design. New York : Marcel Dekker Inc., 2001, pp. 233–266.

Oprea, Tudor Ionel. 2002. ADME Filters for Virtual Screening. Molecules. 2002, Vol. 7, pp. 51–62.

Orengo, C.A., et al. 1997. CATH- A Hierarchic Classification of Protein Domain Structures. Structure. 1997, Vol. 5, 8, pp. 1093–1108.

Orth, P., et al. 1998. Conformational Changes of The Tet Repressor Induced by Tetracycline Trapping,. J.Mol.Biol. 1998, Vol. 279, p. 439.

Osapay, Klara and Case, David A. 1991. A new analysis of proton chemical shifts in proteins. J. Am. Chem. Soc. 1991, Vol. 113, 25, pp. 9436–44.

Otto, Matthias. 2007. Chemometrics: statistics and computer application in analytical chemistry. Weinheim : Wiley-Vch, 2007.

Overton, C.E. 1901. Studien Uber die Narkose. Fischer, Jena, Germany : s.n., 1901.

Ozkan, S. Banu, et al. 2007. Protein folding by zipping and assembly. PNAS. 2007, Vol. 104, 29, pp. 11987–11992.

Pace, CN. 1975. The Stability of Globular Proteins. CRC Critical Reviews in Biochemistry. 1975, Vol. 1, p. 43.

Paiva, AM, et al. 2001. Inhibitors of dihydrodipicolinate reductase, a key enzyme of the diaminopimelate pathway of *Mycobacterium tuberculosis*. Biochim Biophys Acta. 2001, Vol. 1545, pp. 67–77.

Pal L, Basu G, Chakrabarthi P. 2002. Variants of 3(10) helices in protiens. Protiens, Vol. 48, pp. 571–579.

Pal L, Basu G. 1999. Novel protein structural motifs containing two-turn and longer 3(10) helices. Protien Eng, Vol. 12, pp. 811–814.

Panchenko, Anna R., Luthey-Schulten, Zaida and Wolynes, Peter G. 1996. Foldons, protein structural modules and exons. Proc. Natl. Acad. Sci. 1996, Vol. 93, pp. 2008–2013.

Pang, Xiaodong, et al. 2008. Nature Precedings 2008.

Papandreou N, Berezovsky IN, Lopes A, Eliopoulos E, Chomilier J. 2004. Universal positions in Globular proteins. Eur J Biochem, Vol. 271, pp. 4762–4768.

—. 1993. Parser for protein folding units. Proteins. 1993, Vol. 19, pp. 256–268.

Parthasarathy, S. and Murthy, M.R.N. 2000. Protein Eng. 2000, Vol. 13, pp. 9–13.

Paton, W. D. M. 1961. A Theory of Drug Action Based on the Rate of Drug-Receptor Combination. Proceedings of the Royal Society of London. Series B, Biological Sciences. 1961, Vol. 154, 954, pp. 21–69.

Pauling L, Corey R B, Branson H R. 1951. The structure of protiens: two hydrogen bonded helical configurations of the polypeptide chain. Proc Natl Acad Sci, USA, Vol. 37, pp. 205–211.

Pavone, V., et al. 1996. Discovering Protein Secondary Structure: Classification and Description of Isolated alpha- Turns. Biopolymers. 1996, Vol. 38, pp. 705–721.

Payne, Philip W. 1993. Reconstruction of protein conformations from estimated positions of the C, coordinates. Protein Science. 1993, Vol. 2, pp. 315–324.

Pearson, WR and Lipman, DJ. 1988. Improved tools for biological sequence comparison. Proceedings of the National Academy of Sciences USA. 1988, Vol. 85, 8, pp. 2444–8.

Pedretti, A., et al. 2000. Internet Journal of Chemistry. 2000, Vols. 45 (7), Art. 13.

Penzotti, Julie E., et al. 2002. A Computational Ensemble Pharmacophore Model for Identifying Substrates of P-Glycoprotein. 2002, Vol. 45(9).

Perutz, M. F., Kendrew, J. C. and Watson, H. C. 1965. J. Mol. Biol. 1965, Vol. 13, pp. 669–678.

Petrus, Amanda K., et al. Exploring the Implications of Vitamin B12 Conjugation to Insulin on Insulin Receptor Binding. Chem Med Chem. Vol. 4, 3, pp. 421–426.

Pettitt, Chris S., McGuffin, Liam J. and Jones, David T. 2005. Improving sequence-based fold recognition by using 3D model quality assessment. Bioinformatics. 2005, Vol. 21, 17, pp. 3509–3515.

Phillips, CM, Mizutani, Y and Hochstrasser, RM. 1995. Proc. Natl. Acad. Sci. USA. 1995, Vol. 92, pp. 7292–96.

—. 1970. Physical Organic Chemistry. 2nd ed. New York : McGraw-Hill, 1970.

Pichierri, Fabio. 2002. Molecular orbital study of the E-selectin/sialyl Lewis interaction. RIKEN. 2002, Vol. Review No. 46. RIKEN: review no. 46; Focused on Intermolecular Interactions in Molecular Assemblies and Biological Systems.

Pillardy, J., et al. 2001. Development of physics-based energy functions that predict medium resolution structure for proteins of α, β, and α/β structural classes. J. Phys. Chem. B. 2001, Vol. 105, pp. 7299–7311.

—. 1994. PROMOTIF - A Program to Identify and Analyse Structural Motifs in Proteins. Protein Sci. 1994, Vol. 5, pp. 212–220.

Potter, Andrew, et al. 2010. Structure-guided design of a-amino acid-derived Pin1 inhibitors. Bioorg. Med. Chem. Lett. 2010, Vol. 20, pp. 586–590.

Prabhu, Ninad V. and Sharp, Kim A. 2005. Heat capacity in proteins. Annu. Rev. Phys. Chem. 2005, Vol. 56, pp. 521–48.

Prentis, R. A., Lis, Yvonne and Walker, S. R. 1988. Pharmaceutical innovation by the seven UK-owned pharmaceutical companies (1964–1985). Br. J. clin. Pharmac. 1988, Vol. 25, pp. 387–396.

Protein Data Bank. www.rcsb.org/pdb. [Online]

Przytycka, T, Aurora, R and Rose, GD. 1999. A protein taxonomy based on secondary structure. Nat Struct Biol. 1999, Vol. 6, 7, pp. 672–82.

Ptitsyn, O. B. 1973. Sequential mechanism of protein folding. Doklady Akademii Nauk SSSR. 1973, Vol. 210, pp. 1213–1215.

Radford, Sheena E. and Dobson, Christopher M. 1995. Insights into Protein Folding Using Physical Techniques: Studies of Lysozyme and α-lactalbumin. Philosophical Transactions: Biological Sciences (Protein Folding). 1995, Vol. 348, 1323, pp. 17–25.

Rahman, Taufiq and Rahmatullah, Mohammed. 2010. Proposed structural basis of interaction of piperine and related compounds with monoamine oxidases. Bioorganic & Medicinal Chemistry Letters. 2010, Vol. 20, pp. 537–540.

Rajamani, Deepa, et al. 2004. Anchor residues in protein-protein interactions. Proc Natl Acad Sci U S A. 2004, Vol. 101, 31, pp. 11287–11292.

Rajashankar, K.R. and Ramakumar, S. 1996. Pi-Turns in Proteins and Peptides: Classification, Conformation, Occurrence, Hydration and Sequence. Protein Sci. 1996, Vol. 5, pp. 932–946.

Ramachandran, G. N. and Sasisekharan, V. 1968. Adv. Protein Chem. 1968, Vol. 23, pp. 283–437.

Ramachandran, GN, Ramakrishnan, C and Sasisekharan, V. 1963. Stereochemistry of Polypeptide Chain Configuration. J.Mol.Biol. 1963, Vol. 7, pp. 95–99.

Ramadevi, N., Rodriguez, Javier and Roy, Polly. 1998. A Leucine Zipper–Like Domain Is Essential for Dimerization and Encapsidation of Bluetongue Virus Nucleocapsid Protein VP4. Journal of virology. 1998, pp. 2983–2990.

Ramji, Dipak P. and Foka, Pelagia. 2002. CCAAT/enhancer-binding proteins: structure, function and regulation. Biochem. J. 2002, Vol. 365, pp. 561–575.

Ramsden, CA. 1990. Quantitative drug design, Vol. 4. [book auth.] PG Sammes, JB Taylors C Hansch. Comprehensive Medicinal Chemistry. Rational drug Design, Mechanistic Study, and Therapeutic Application of Chemical Compounds. Oxford : Pergammon Press, 1990.

Ranganathan S; Izotov D; Kraka E; Cremer D. 2008(2). Automated and accurate protein structure description: distribution of ideal secondary structural units in natural proteins. (unpublished) submitted to: Journal of Physical Chemistry B. 2008–2.

Ranganathan S; Izotov D; Kraka E; Cremer D. 2008–3. Projecting Three-dimensional Protein Structure into a One-dimensional Character Code Utilizing the Automated Protein Structure Analysis Method. (unpublished) submitted to: Proteins: structure, function, and bioinformatics. 2008–3.

Ranganathan S; Izotov D; Kraka E; Cremer D. 2008–4. Classification of supersecondary structures in proteins using the Automated Protein Structure Analysis method. (unpublished). 2008–4.

Ranganathan S; Izotov D; Kraka E; Cremer D. 2009. Description and recognition of regular and distorted secondary structures in proteins using the automated protein structure analysis method. Proteins: Structure, Function, and Bioinformatics. 2009, Vol. 76, 2, pp. 418–438.

Rao, S T and Rossman, M G. 1973. Comparison of supersecondary structures in proteins. J. Mol. Biol. 1973, Vol. 76, pp. 211–256.

Rapaport, D. C. 2004. The Art of Molecular Dynamics Simulation. 2004.

Rappé, Anthony K. and Casewit, Carla J. 1997. Molecular mechanics across chemistry. Sausalito, California : University Science Books, 1997.

Rarey, M, et al. 1996. A fast flexible docking method using an incremental construction algorithm. J Mol Biol. 1996, Vol. 261, 3, pp. 470–489.

Raschke, TM. 2006. Water structure and interactions with protein surfaces. Curr Opin Struct Biol. 2006, Vol. 16, pp. 152–159.

Raveh, Barak, et al. 2007. Rediscovering secondary structures as network motifs- an unsupeervised learning approach. Bioinformatics. 2007, Vol. 23, 2, pp. e163–e169.

Regan, L. and DeGrado, W. F. 1988. Science. 1988, Vol. 241, pp. 976–978.

Reichmann, Dana, et al. 2007. The molecular architecture of protein–protein binding sites. Current Opinion in Structural Biology. 2007, Vol. 17, pp. 67–76.

Rekker, R. 1977. The Hydrophobic Fragmental Constant. Amsterdam : Elsevier, 1977. p. 479. Vol. 14.

Revankar, C.M., et al. 2005. A transmembrane intracellular estrogen receptor mediates rapid cell signaling. Science. 2005, Vol. 307, pp. 1625–1630.

Rice PA, Goldman A, Steitz TA. 1990. A Helix-turn-strand structural motif common in α-β proteins. PROTEINS: Structure, function, and genetics, Vol. 8, pp. 334–340.

Richards, Frederic M and Kundrot, Craig E. 1988. Identification of structural motifs from protien coordinate data: secondary and first level supersecondary structure. Protiens. 1988, Vol. 3, pp. 71–84.

Richardson, J S. 1977. Nature (London), Vol. 268, pp. 495–500.

Richardson, J.S. 1981. The anatomy and taxonomy of protein structure. Advan. Prot. Chem. 1981, Vol. 34, pp. 167–339.

Richardson, J.S. and Richardson, D.C. 1989. Principles and patterns of protein conformation. [book auth.] G.D. Fasman. Prediction of Protein Structure and Principles of Protein Conformation. New York : Plenum Press, 1989, pp. 1–98.

Ring, C.S., et al. 1992. Taxonomy and conformational analysis of loops in proteins. Journal of Molecular Biology. 1992, Vol. 224, pp. 685–699.

Ringe, Dagmar and Petsko, Gregory A. 2009. Q&A: What are pharmacological chaperones and why are they interesting? Journal of Biology. 2009, Vol. 8, p. 80.

Robson, B. and Pain, R. H. 1971. Analysis of the code relating sequence to conformation in proteins: possible implications for the mechanism of formation of helical regions. J. molec. Biol. 1971, Vol. 58, pp. 237–259 .

Roche, O, et al. 2002. Development of a virtual screening method for identification of 'frequent hitters' in compound libraries. J Med Chem. 2002, Vol. 45, pp. 137–142.

Rose, G.D. 1997. Protein folding and the Paracelsus challenge. nature structural biology. 1997, Vol. 4, pp. 512 – 514.

Rose, G.D., Gierasch, L.M. and Smith, J.A. 1985. Turns in peptides and proteins. Adv Prot Chem. 1985, Vol. 37, pp. 1–109.

Rose, George D. 1979. Hierarchic organization of domains in globular proteins. J. Mol. Biol. 1979, Vol. 134, pp. 447–470.

Rost, B. 1997. Folding Des. 1997, Vol. 2, pp. S19–S24.

Rost, B. and Sander, C. 1994. Combining evolutionary information and neural networks to predict secondary structure. Proteins. 1994, Vol. 19, pp. 55–71.

Rost, B., Schneider, R. and Sander, C. 1997. Protein fold recognition by prediction-based threading. J Mol Biol. 1997, Vol. 270, pp. 471–480.

Rost, Burkhard, et al. 2003. Prediction of protein structure through evolution. [ed.] J Gasteiger and T Engel. Handbook of Chemoinformatics - From Data to Knowledge. New York : Wiley, 2003, pp. 1789–1811.

Sadowski, J and Kubinyi, H. 1998. A scoring scheme for discriminating between drugs and nondrugs. J Med Chem. 1998, Vol. 41, pp. 3325–3329.

Saini, H K and Fischer, D. 2005. domain prediction meta-server. Bioinformatics. 2005, Vol. 21, 12, pp. 2917–2920.

Sakharov, DV and Lim, C. 2009. Force fields including charge transfer and local polarization effects: Application to proteins containing multi/heavy metal ions. J Comput Chem. 2009, Vol. 30, 2, pp. 191–202.

Salamov Asaf A, Solovyev Victor V. 1995. Prediction of protein secondary structure by ombining nearest-neighbor algorithms and multiple sequence alignments. 1995, J. Mol. Biol., Vol. 247, pp. 11–15.

Salkind, Hervé Abdi Neil. 2007. Partial Least Square Regression. Thousand Oaks (CA) : Sage, 2007.

Samama, P, et al. 1993. J Biol Chem. 1993, Vol. 268, p. 4625.

Sambrano, Gilberto R., Terpstra, Valeska and Steinberg, Daniel. 1997. Independent Mechanisms for Macrophage Binding and Macrophage Phagocytosis of Damaged Erythrocytes: Evidence of Receptor Cooperativity. Arteriosclerosis, Thrombosis, and Vascular Biology. 1997, Vol. 17, pp. 3442–3448.

Saraste, M., Sibbald, P.R. and Wittinghofer, A. 1990. The P-loop—a common motif in ATP- and GTP-binding proteins. Trends Biochem. Sci. 1990, Vol. 15, pp. 430–434.

Saunders, M. 1989. J. Comput. Chem. 1989, Vol. 10, p. 203.

Saunders, M., et al. 1990. J. Am. Chem. Soc. 1990, Vol. 112, p. 1419.

Schaftenaar G, J H Noordik. 2000. 2000, J. Comp.-Aided.Mol.Des., Vol. 14, p. 123.

Scheerlinck, Jean-Pierre Y., et al. 1992. Recurrent αβ-loop structures in TIM barrel motifs show a distinct pattern of conserved structural features. PROTEINS: Structure, Function, and Genetics. 1992, Vol. 12, pp. 299–313.

Schellman, JA. Denaturant m values and heat capacity changes: relation to changes in accessible surface areas of protein unfolding. Protein Sci. 4. Vol. 4, pp. 2138–2148.

—. 1994. The thermodynamics of solvent exchange. Biopolymers. 1994, Vol. 34, pp. 1015–1026.

Schlick, Tamar. 2002. Molecular Modeling and Simulation : An Interdisciplinary Guide. Secaucus, NJ, USA : Springer-Verlag New York, Inc., 2002.

Schmid, F. X., et al. 1986. Proc. Natl. Acad. Sci. U.S.A. 1986, Vol. 83, pp. 872–876.

Schrauber, Eisenhaber and Argos. 1993. Rotamers: to be or not to be? An analysis of amino acid Side-chain confirmations in globular proteins. Journal molecular biology. 1993, Vol. 230, pp. 592–612 .

Schroeder, Bingding Huang and Michael. 2006. LIGSITE csc: predicting protein binding sites using the Connolly surface and degree of conservation. BMC structural Biology. 2006, Vol. 6, p. 19.

Schuster, Daniela, et al. 2010. Predicting Cyclooxygenase Inhibition by Three-Dimensional Pharmacophoric Profiling. Part IModel Generation, Validation and Applicability in Ethnopharmacology. Mol. Inf. 2010, Vol. 29, pp. 75 – 86.

Searle, M.S. and Williams, D.H. 1992. J Am Chem Soc. 1992, Vol. 114, p. 10690.

Segawa, S.-I. and Sugihara, M. 1984. Biopolymers. 1984, Vol. 23, pp. 2473–2488.

Seydel, JK, [ed.]. 1985. QSAR and the strategies in the design of bioactive compounds: Proceedings of the 5th symposium on QSAR, Bad Segenburg, 1984. Weinham : VCH, 1985.

Shang, Li, et al. 2007. pH-dependent protein conformational Changes in Albumin: Gold Nanoparticle Bioconjugates: A Spectroscopic Study. Langmuir. 2007, Vol. 23, 5, pp. 2714–2721.

Shen, Tongye, et al. 2002. Molecular Dynamics of Acetylcholinesterase. Acc. Chem. Research. 2002, Vol. 35, pp. 332–340 .

Shoichet, Brian K, et al. 2002. Lead discovery using molecular docking. Current Opinion in Chemical Biology. 2002, Vol. 6, pp. 439–446.

Shrake, A. and Rupley, J.A. 1973. Environment and exposure to solvent of protein atoms. Lysozyme and insulin. J Mol Biol. 1973, Vol. 79, 2, pp. 351–71.

Siddiqui, AS and Barton, GJ. 1995. Continuous and discontinuous domains: an algorithm for the automatic generation of reliable protein domain definitions. Protein Sci. 1995, Vol. 4, 5, pp. 872–884.

Silverman, Richard B. 2004. The Organic Chemistry of Drug Design and Drug Action. second. s.l. : Elsevier Academic Press, 2004.

Simoncini, T. and Genazzani, A.R. 2003. Non-genomic actions of sex hormones. Eur. J. Endocrinol. 2003, Vol. 148, pp. 281–292.

Simons, K.T., et al. 1997. Assembly of protein tertiary structures from fragments with similar local sequences using simulated annealing and Bayesian scoring functions. J Mol. Biol. 1997, Vol. 268, pp. 209–225.

Sippl, M.J. and Wiederstein, M. 2008. A note on difficult structure alignment problems. Bioinformatics. 2008, Vol. 24, pp. 426–427.

Sippl, Manfred J, Weitckus, Sabine and Flockner, Hannes. 1994. In search of protein folds. [book auth.] M Merz Jr. and S Le Grand. The protein folding problem and tertiary structure prediction. Boston : s.n., 1994.

Sippl, MJ. 1995. Knowledge-based potentials for proteins. Curr Opin Struct Biol. 1995, Vol. 5, pp. 229–235.

Sitkoff, D., Sharp, K.A. and Honig, B. 1998. J. Phys. Chem. 1998, Vol. 98.

Skolnick, Jeffrey, Kolinski, Andrzej and Mohanty, Debasisa. 1999. De Novo Predictions of the Quaternary Structure of Leucine Zippers and Other Coiled Coils. International Journal of Quantum Chemistry. 1999, Vol. 75, pp. 165–176.

Smit, Berend and Frenkel, Daan. 2001. Understanding Molecular Simulation. 2nd edition. s.l. : Academic Press, 2001.

Smith, GR, Sternberg, MJE and Bates, PA. 2005. The Relationship between the Flexibility of Proteins and their Conformational States on Forming Protein–Protein Complexes with an Application to Protein–Protein Docking. Journal of molecular biology. 2005.

Smith, T.F. and Waterman, M.S. 1981. Identification of common molecular subsequences. J. Mol. Biol. 1981, Vol. 147, pp. 195–197.

So much more to know... Science. 2005, Vol. 309, pp. 78–102.

Sotriffer, C.A., Ni, H. and McCammon, J.A. 2000. J. Med. Chem. 2000, Vol. 43, pp. 4109–4117.

Sridevi, K, et al. 2004. Increasing stability reduces conformational heterogeneity in a protein folding intermediate ensemble. J. Mol. Biol. 2004, Vol. 337, pp. 699–711.

Sridhar, B. and Ravikumar, K. 2009. Lamotrigine, an antiepileptic drug, and its chloride and nitrate salts. Acta Crystallographica. 2009, Vol. C65, 9, pp. 0460–0464.

Srinivasan N, Sowdhamini R, Ramakrishnan C, Balaram P. 1991. Analysis of short loops connecting secondary structural elements in proteins. [book auth.] S Ramaseshan P Balaram. Molecular conformation and biological interactions. Bangalore : Indian Academy of Sciences, 1991.

Stadler, Christian M., Reidys and F., Peter. 2002. Combinatorial Landscapes. SIAM Review. 2002, Vol. 44, 1, pp. 3–54.

Stahl, Martin. 2000. Modifications of the scoring function in FlexX for virtual screening applications. Perspectives in Drug Discovery and Design. 2000, Vol. 20, 1.

Steinberg, I.Z. and Scheraga, H.A. 1963. Entropy changes accompanying association reactions of proteins. J. Biol. Chem. 1963, Vol. 238, 172–181.

Stone, John E., et al. 2009. High Performance Computation and Interactive Display of Molecular Orbitals on GPUs and Multi-core CPU. GPGPU. 2009, Vol. March 8.

Stote, R.H. and et al. 2004. Biochemistry. 2004, Vol. 43, pp. 7687-7697.

Stouch, T. R., Gudmundson, O. and Ge, S. E. 2001. Prediction of PGP transporter activity using calculated molecular properties. 221st National Meeting of the American Chemical Society, 2001. Abstr. Pap. - Am. Chem. Soc. pp. BTEC-037.

Sugita, Y and Okamoto, Y. 1999. Replica-exchange molecular dynamics method for protein folding. Chem. Phys. Lett. 1999, Vol. 314, pp. 141–51.

Sun, S. 1993. Reduced representation model of protein structure prediction: statistical potential and genetic algorithms. Protein Sci. 1993, Vol. 2, pp. 762–785.

Sun, Zhirong and Blundell, Tom. 1995. The patter of common supersecondary structure (motifs) in protien database. Proceedings of the 28th Annual Hawaii International Conference on System Sciences. 1995, p. 312.

Sun, Zhi-Rong, et al. 1996. A vector projection method for predicting supersecondary motifs. J Protien Chem. 1996, Vol. 15, 8, p. 721.

Svensson, Mats, et al. 1996. ONIOM: A Multilayered Integrated MO + MM Method for Geometry Optimizations and Single Point Energy Predictions. A Test for Diels"Alder Reactions and Pt(P(t-Bu)3)2 + H2 Oxidative Addition. J. Phys. Chem. 1996, Vol. 100, 50, pp. 19357–19363.

Swillens, S and Dumont, JE. 1977. The mobile receptor hypothesis in hormone action: a general model accounting for desensitization. J Cyclic Nucleotide Res. 1977, Vol. 3, 1, pp. 1–10.

Swindells, M.B. 1995. A procedure for detecting structural domains in proteins. Protein Sci. 1995, Vol. 4, pp. 103–112.

Swindells, Mark B. and Overington, John P. 2002. Prioritizing the proteome: identifying pharmaceutically relevant targets. Drug Discovery Today. 2002, Vol. 7, 9, pp. 516–520.

Taft, R. W. 1952. J. Am. Chem. Soc. 1952, Vol. 74, p. 2729.

Tai, Kaihsu, et al. 2001. Analysis of a 10-ns Molecular Dynamics Simulation of Mouse Acetylcholinesterase. Biophysical Journal Volume. 2001, Vol. 81, 2, pp. 715–724.

Tainer, J.A., Thayer, M.M. and Cunningham, R.P. 1995. DNA repair proteins. Curr. Opin. Struct. Biol. 1995, Vol. 5, pp. 20–26.

Tangyuenyongwatana, P and Gritsanapan, W. 2008. A study on artifacts formation in the Thai traditional medicine Prasaplai. Planta Med. 2008, Vol. 74, pp. 1403–1405.

Taylor H S. 1941. 1941, Proc Am Phyl Soc, Vol. 85, p. 1.

Taylor, J.S. and Burnett, R.M. 2000. DARWIN: A program for docking flexible molecules. Proteins. 2000, Vols. 41,, pp. 173–191.

Taylor, W. R., Flores, T. P. and Orengo, C. A. 1994. Multiple protein structure alignment. Protein Sci. 1994, Vol. 3, pp. 1858–1870.

Taylor, William R. 2002. A 'periodic table' for protein structures. Nature. 2002, Vol. 416, pp. 657–660.

Taylor, WR. 1999. Protein structural domain identification. Protein Engineering. 1999, Vol. 12, 3, pp. 203–216.

Teichmann, S. A., Chothia, C. and Gerstein, M. 1999. Curr. Opin. Struct. Biol. 1999, Vol. 9, pp. 390–399.

Thompson, J., Higgins, D. and Gibson, T. 1994. CLUSTAL-W: improving the sensitivity of progressive multiple sequence alignment through sequence weighting, position specific gap penalties and weight matrix choice. Nucleic Acids Res. 1994, Vol. 22, pp. 4673–4680.

Tobias, D.J., Martyna, G. J. and Klein, M. L. 1993. Molecular dynamics simulations of a protein in the canonical ensemble. J. Phys. Chem. 1993, Vol. 97, pp. 12959–12966.

Tobias, Randall D. 1995. An Introduction to Partial Least Squares Regression. s.l. : SUGI Proceedings, 1995.

Todd, A., Orengo, C. and Thornton, J. 2001. Domain assignment for protein structures using a consensus approach: characterization and analysis. J. Mol. Biol. 2001, Vol. 307, pp. 1113–1143.

Todeschini, R. and Consonni, V. 2000. Handbook of Molecular Descriptors. Weinheim (Germany) : Wiley-VCH, 2000.

Todeschini, R., et al. 2006. DRAGON—Software for the calculation of molecular descriptors. Ver. 5.4 for Windows, Talete srl, Milan, Italy, 2006.

Toniolo C, Crisma M, Formaggio F, Peggion C, Broxterman Q, Kaptein B. 2005. Peptide Beta bend and 310 helix: from 3D structural studies to applications as templates. J Inclusion phenomena and macrocyclic chemistry, Vol. 51, pp. 121–136.

Topham, C M, et al. 1993. Fragment ranking in modeling of protein structure. J Mol. Biol. 1993, Vol. 229, pp. 194–220.

Tosatto, S., et al. 2002. A divide-and conquer approach to fast loop modeling. Protein Eng. 2002, Vol. 15, pp. 279–286.

Tress, Michael, et al. 2005. Assessment of Predictions Submitted for the CASP6 Comparative Modeling Category. PROTEINS: Structure, Function, and Bioinformatics Suppl. 2005, Vol. 7, pp. 27–45 .

Tripos, inc.; a Certara Company. SYBYL(TM) -X.

Tsai, J., et al. 1999. The packing density in proteins: standard radii and volumes. J. Mol. Biol. 1999, Vol. 290, p. 253.

Tsai, M.-J. and O'Malley, B.W. 1994. Molecular mechanisms of action of steroid/ thyroid receptor superfamily members. Annu. Rev. Biochem. 1994, Vol. 63, pp. 451–486.

Tsaioun, Katya, et al. 2009. ADDME – Avoiding Drug Development Mistakes Early: central nervous system drug discovery perspective; . BMC Neurol. 2009, Vol. 9(Suppl 1).

Tuffery, Etchebest and Hazout. 1997. Prediction of protein side-chain confirmations: a study on the influence of backbone accuracy on conformation stability in the rotamer space. Protein engineering. 1997, Vol. 10, pp. 361–372.

Tuttle, Tell, Kraka, Elfi and Cremer, Dieter. 2005. Docking, Triggering, and Biological Activity of Dynemicin A in DNA: A Computational Study. J. Am. Chem. Soc. 2005, Vol. 127, 26, pp. 9469–9484.

Tyagi, M., et al. 2006. Protein Block Expert (PBE): a web-based protein structure analysis server using a structural alphabet . Nucleic Acids Research. 2006, Vol. 34, Web Server Issue W119–W123.

Uversky, V. N. 2002. Natively unfolded proteins: a point where biology waits for physics. Protein Sci. 2002, Vol. 11, pp. 739–756.

Vajda, S and Guarnieri, F. 2006. Characterization of protein–ligand interaction sites using experimental and computational methods. Curr Opin Drug Discov Devel. 2006, Vol. 9, pp. 354–362.

van Drie, J. H. 2003. Beware of Q2. Curr. Pharm.Des. 2003, Vol. 9, p. 1649.

van Gunsteren, W.F. and Karplus, M. 1982. Biochemistry. 1982, Vol. 21, pp. 2259–2274.

Varley, P. G. and Pain, R. H. 1991. Relation between stability, dynamics and enzyme activity in 3-phosphoglycerate kinases from yeast and Thermus thermophilus. J. Mol. Biol. 1991, Vol. 220, pp. 531–538.

Varmuza, Kurt and Filzmoser, Peter. 2009. Introduction to Multivariate Statistical Analysis in Chemometrics. s.l. : CRC press, 2009.

Veber, D.F and et al. 2002. Molecular Properties That Influence the Oral Bioavailability of Drug Candidates. J. Med. Chem. 2002, Vol. 45, pp. 2615–2623.

Vedani, Angelo. 1988. YETI: An interactive molecular mechanics program for small-molecule protein complexes. Journal of Computational Chemistry. 1988, Vol. 9, 3, pp. 269–280.

Venkatachalam CM. 1968. Stereochemical criteria for polypeptides and proteins: conformaitonof a system of three linked peptide units. 1968, Biopolymers, Vol. 6(10), pp. 1425–1436.

Veerapandian, Pandi. 1997. Structure-based drug design. s.l. : Marcel Dekker, 1997.

Venter, J. C. and et al. 2001. Science. 2001, Vol. 291, p. 1304.

Veretnik, S, et al. 2004. Toward consistent assignment of structural domains in proteins. J. Mol. Biol. 2004, Vol. 339, 3, pp. 647–678.

Verloop, A. 1987. The STERIMOL approach to drug design. New York : Marcel Dekker, 1987.

Vijayakumar S, Bugg C E, Cook W J. 1987. Structure of ubiquitin refined at 1.8 A resolution. 531–544, 1987, J Mol Biol, Vol. 194.

—. 2002. Virtual Screening in Lead Discovery: A Viewpoint. Molecules. 2002, Vol. 7 , pp. 51–62.

Vitkup, Dennis, et al. 2000. Solvent mobility and the protein 'glass' transition. Nature structural biology. 2000, Vol. 7, 1.

Waksman, Gabriel. 2005. Proteomics and protein-protein interactions: biology, chemistry, bioinformatics and drug design. [book auth.] M. Zouhair Atassi. Protein Reviews. 2005, Vol. 3.

Wallner, B, Fang, H and Elofsson, A. 2003. Automatic consensus-based fold recognition using Pcons, ProQ, and Pmodeller. Proteins. 2003, Vol. 53, 6, pp. 534–541.

Wallner, B. and Elofsson, A. 2003. Can correct protein models be identified? Protein Sci . 2003, Vol. 12, 5, pp. 1073–1086.

Wand, Josh. 2006. Introduction: Protein Dynamics and Folding. Chem. Rev. 2006, Vol. 106, 5, pp. 1543–1544.

Wang J., Kang X., Kuntz I.D. and Kollman P.A. 2005. J. Med. Chem. 2005, Vol. 48, pp. 2432–2444.

Wang, J., et al. 2006. automatic atom type and bond type perception in molecules mechanical calculations. Journal of Molecular Graphics and Modelling. 2006, Vol. 25, pp. 247–260.

Wang, Yong, et al. 2006. A second binding site for hydroxytamoxifen within the coactivator-binding groove of estrogen receptor . PNAS. 2006, Vol. 103, 26, pp. 9908–9911.

Waterston, Robert H., Lander, Eric S. and Sulston, John E. 2003. More on the sequencing of the human genome. Proc Natl Acad Sci U S A. 2003, Vol. 100, 6, pp. 3022–3024.

Weber, L., et al. 1995. Optimization of the biological activity of combinatorial compound libraries by a genetic algorithm. Angew. Chem., Int. Ed. 1995, Vol. 34, 2280–2282.

Weiner SJ, et al. 1984. A new force-field for molecular mechanical simulation of nucleic acidsand proteins. J. Am. Chem. Soc. 1984, Vol. 106, pp. 765–784.

Weinhold, F. and Landis, C. R. 2003. Valency and Bonding: A Natural Bond Orbital Donor–Acceptor Perspective. Cambridge, UK : Cambridge University Press, 2003.

Welch, W., Ruppert, J. and Jain, A.N. 1996. Chem. Biol. 1996, Vol. 3, pp. 449–462.

Wermuth, Camille George. 2008. The Practice of Medicinal Chemistry. Third edition. s.l. : Academic press, 2008.

Wetlaufer, D. B. 1973. Proc. Natl. Acad. Sci. U.S.A. 1973, Vol. 70, pp. 697–701.

White, GWN, et al. 2005. Simulation and experiment conspire to reveal cryptic intermediates and a slide from the nucleation - condensation to framework mechanism of folding. J. Mol. Biol. 2005, Vol. 350, pp. 757–75.

Wiberg, Egon, Wiberg, Nils and Holleman, Arnold Frederick. 2001. Inorganic chemistry. s.l. : Academic press, 2001.

Wierenga, R.K., Terpstra, P. and Hol, W.G. 1986. Prediction of the occurrence of the ADP-binding beta alpha beta-fold in proteins, using an amino acid sequence fingerprint. J. Mol. Biol. 1986, Vol. 187, pp. 101–107.

Williams, David A, Lemke, Thomas L and Foye, William O. 2002. Foye's Principles of Medicinal Chemistry. s.l. : Lippincott Williams & Wilkins, 2002.

Williams, Dudley H. and Bardsley, Ben. 1999. Estimating binding constants – The hydrophobic effect and cooperativity. Perspectives in Drug Discovery and Design. 1999, Vol. 17, 1, pp. 43–59.

Williams, J. O., Alsenoy, C. van and Schäfer, Lothar. 1981. Ab initio studies of structural features not easily amenable to experiment : Part 6. Quantitative estimate of the effect of bond delocalization on structure and hyperconjugative interaction of the amide group. Journal of Molecular Structure: THEOCHEM. 1981, Vol. 76, 2, pp. 171–177.

Wilmot, C.M. and Thornton, J.M. 1988. Analysis and the prediction of different types of beta turns in proteins. J. Mol. Biol. 1988, Vol. 203, pp. 221–232.

Wishart. 2005. Protein structure prediction and analysis. [book auth.] Andreas D. Baxevanis and B. F. Francis Ouellette. Bioinformatics: A Practical Guide to the Analysis of Genes and Proteins. Third Edition. s.l. : John Wiley & Sons, Inc., 2005, pp. 224–247.

Wojcik, J, Mornon, J P and J, Chomilier. 1999. New efficient statistical sequence dependent strucvture prediction of short to medium sized protein loops based on an exhaustive loop classification. J Mol Biol. 1999, Vol. 289, pp. 1469–90.

Wolfenden, R. 2007. Experimental measures of amino acid hydrophobicity and the topology of transmembrane and globular proteins. J. Gen. Physiol. 2007, Vol. 129, pp. 357–62.

Wolff, Manfred E., [ed.]. 1994. Burger's Medicinal Chemistry and Drug Discovery. 5. s.l. : John Wiley & Sons Canada, Ltd., 1994.

Xiang, Z., Sotot, C. and Honig, B. 2002. Evaluating conformational free energies: the colony energy and its application to the problem of loop prediction. Proc. Natl. Acad. Sci. USA. 2002, Vol. 99, pp. 7432–7437.

Xu and et al. 2001. 2001.

Yamaguchi, Atsuko, et al. December 19–21, 2005. A New Method of Computing Ligand-Based. Pharmacophore Models for Flexible Chemical Compounds. 16th International Conference on Genome Informatics. Yokohama Pacifico, Japan : s.n., December 19–21, 2005.

Yogurtcu, O., et al. 2008. Restricted Mobility of Conserved Residues in Protein-Protein Interfaces in Molecular Simulations;. Biophysical Journal. 2008, Vol. 94, 9, pp. 3475–3485.

Yuan, Zheng, Zhao, Ju and Wang, Zhi-Xin. 2003. Flexibility analysis of enzyme active sites by crystallographic temperature factors. Protein Engineering. 2003, Vol. 16, 2, pp. 109–114.

Zagrovic, B, et al. 2002. Simulation of folding of a small -helical protein in atomistic detail using worldwide-distributed computing. J. Mol. Biol. 2002, Vol. 323, pp. 927–37.

Zhang, H.L., Song, S.Y. and Lin, Z.J. 1999. Sci. China. 1999, Vol. 42, pp. 225–232.

Zhang Jian, Quin Meng, Wang Wei. 2005. Multiple folding mechanisms of protein ubiquitin. 3, 2005, Proteins: structure, function and bioinformatics, Vol. 59(3), pp. 565–579.

Zhang, M. Chen, C. He, Y. Xiao, Y. 2005. Improvement on a simplified model for protein folding simulation. Physical Review, Series E, Vols. 72 (5), Part 1, p. 051919 .

Zhanhua, Cui, et al. 2005. ; Protein subunit interfaces: heterodimers versus homodimers. Bioinformation. 2005, Vol. 1, 2, pp. 28–39.

Zhi, Degui, et al. 2006. Representing and comparing protins structure as paths in three-dimensional space. BMC Bioinformatics. 2006, Vol. 7, pp. 460–475.

Zhou, HX and Shan, Y. 2001. Prediction of protein interaction sites from sequence profile and residue neighbor list. Proteins. 2001, Vol. 44, pp. 336–343.

Zimm and Bragg. 1959. 1959.

Zitko, V. 1998. Chemometrics in environmental analysis. Chemomet Intel Lab Sys. 1998, Vol. 40, pp. 119–120.

Zu-Kang, Feng and Sippl, Manfred J. 1996. Optimum superimposition of protein structures: ambiguities and implications. Folding & Design. 1996, Vol. 1, pp. 123–132.

Index

485